LABORATORY TESTS AND DIAGNOSTIC PROCEDURES

with NURSING DIAGNOSES

8th Edition

Jane Vincent Corbett, RN, EdD
Professor Emerita
School of Nursing and
Health Professions
University of San Francisco
San Francisco, California

Angela Denise Banks, RN, PhD
Associate Professor
School of Nursing and
Health Professions
University of San Francisco
San Francisco, California

PEARSON

Boston   Columbus   Indianapolis   New York   San Francisco   Upper Saddle River
Amsterdam   Cape Town   Dubai   London   Madrid   Milan   Munich   Paris   Montreal   Toronto
Delhi   Mexico City   São Paulo   Sydney   Hong Kong   Seoul   Singapore   Taipei   Tokyo

Library of Congress Cataloging-in-Publication Data

Corbett, Jane Vincent.
  Laboratory tests and diagnostic procedures : with nursing diagnoses / Jane Vincent Corbett, Angela
Denise Banks. —8th ed.
     p. cm.
  Includes bibliographical references and index.
  ISBN-13: 978-0-13-237332-6
  ISBN-10: 0-13-237332-7
  1. Diagnosis, Laboratory. 2. Diagnosis. 3. Nursing diagnosis. I. Banks, Angela Denise. II. Title.
  RT48.5.C67 2012
  616.07'5—dc23

                                                                                    2012000722

Notice: Care has been taken to confirm the accuracy of information presented in this book. The
authors, editors, and the publisher, however, cannot accept any responsibility for errors or omissions
or for consequences from application of the information in this book and make no warranty, express or
implied, with respect to its contents.

The authors and publisher have exerted every effort to ensure that drug selections and dosages set
forth in this text are in accord with current recommendations and practice at the time of publication.
However, in view of ongoing research, changes in government regulations, and the constant flow of
information relating to drug therapy and reactions, the reader is urged to check the package inserts of
all drugs for any change in indications or dosage and for added warning and precautions. This is particularly important when the recommended agent is a new and/or infrequently employed drug.

Publisher: Julie Levin Alexander
Publisher's Assistant: Regina Bruno
Senior Acquisitions Editor: Kelly Trakalo
Assistant Editor: Lauren Sweeney
Director of Marketing: David Gesell
Marketing Manager: Phoenix Harvey
Marketing Specialist: Michael Sirinides
Marketing Assistant: Crystal Gonzalez
Production Project Manager: Debbie Ryan
Production Editor: Sandeep Rawat/Aptara®, Inc.

Media Project Managers: Rachel Collett/
  Leslie Brado
Senior Design Director: Maria Guglielmo
Art Director: Jayne Conte
Cover Photo: Rob Bouwman/Fotolia
Cover Designer: Bruce Kenselaar
Art Director: Jayne Conte
Printer/Bindery: RRD/Crawfordsville
Cover: Lehigh-Phoenix Color/Hagerstown
Composition: Aptara®, Inc.

10 9 8 7 6 5 4 3 2 1

PEARSON

ISBN-10:   0-13-237332-7
ISBN-13: 978-0-13-237332-6

Dedication

To Rod Corbett, who gave me the space
and time to make this book a reality
and whose contributions were invaluable.
And to our daughter Rhonda Jane
and her husband, Jorge Luis Eyzaguirre,
and my two grandchildren,
Mateo Rodney Eyzaguirre
Raquel Grace Eyzaguirre.
Each of you is such a joy for me! (JVC)

To my husband, Rev. Beryl Banks,
and my son, Caleb Joshua Banks.
Thank you both for your unwavering love
and support during the preparation
and completion of this book. (ADB)

Contents

Preface   vi
Acknowledgments   viii
Reviewers   x

PART I   Laboratory Tests   1

Chapter 1   Using Laboratory Data   2

Chapter 2   Hematology Tests   22

Chapter 3   Routine Urinalysis and Other Urine Tests   59

Chapter 4   Renal Function Tests   82

Chapter 5   Four Commonly Measured Electrolytes   102

Chapter 6   Arterial Blood Gases and Related Tests   127

Chapter 7   Three Less Commonly Measured Electrolytes and Vitamin D   157

Chapter 8   Tests to Measure the Metabolism of Glucose and Other Sugars   180

Chapter 9   Tests to Measure Lipid Metabolism and Other Cardiac Risk Factors   209

Chapter 10   Tests Related to Serum Protein Levels, Tumor Markers, and Cancer Genomics   228

Chapter 11   Tests to Measure the Metabolism of Bilirubin   257

Chapter 12   Tests to Measure Enzymes and Cardiac Markers   273

Chapter 13   Coagulation Tests and Tests to Detect Occult Blood   297

Chapter 14   Serologic Tests: Immunohematology Microbiology and Immunology   332

Chapter 15   Endocrine Tests   373

Chapter 16   Culture and Sensitivity Tests and Rapid Tests for Infections   414

Chapter 17   Therapeutic Drug Monitoring and Toxicology Screens   447

Chapter 18   Tests Performed in Pregnancy, the Newborn Period, and for Genetic Screening   473

PART II   Case Studies   495

Chapter 19   Practice Interpretation of Laboratory Data   496

PART III   Diagnostic Procedures   505

Chapter 20   Diagnostic Radiologic Tests   506
Chapter 21   Body Scans: CT, DXA, MRI, PET, and SPECT   537
Chapter 22   Nuclear Scans: Diagnostic Tests with Radionuclides or Radioisotopes   558
Chapter 23   Diagnostic Ultrasonography   580
Chapter 24   Common Noninvasive Diagnostic Tests   599
Chapter 25   Common Invasive Tests   622
Chapter 26   Stress Tests, Cardiac Catheterizations, Electrophysiologic Studies, and Syncope Tests   648
Chapter 27   Endoscopic Procedures   665
Chapter 28   Diagnostic Procedures Related to Childbearing Years   681
Appendix A   Reference Values for Newborns and Children Compared with Adult Values   700
Appendix B   Possible Alterations in Reference Values for the Aged   702
Appendix C   Altered Reference Values for Common Laboratory Tests in Normal Pregnancies   704
Appendix D   Units of Measure   706
Appendix E   SI Conversion Factors   708
Appendix F   Diagrams of Laboratory Results   714

Index   715

This eighth edition continues to focus on how nurses can use data from laboratory tests and diagnostic procedures to plan nursing care. The extensive reference list for each chapter supports the best-practice approach based on current literature in the field. To further strengthen this evidence-based approach, over 100 websites for many practice guidelines are included. Although much has changed in health care since the first edition of this book in 1982, many tests remain the same and many now have expanded use. These new uses are discussed and compared with the past to provide the reader with a historical perspective. Additionally, for this edition, a few tests were deleted and several new tests added with even more emphasis on genetic testing. Of particular interest are the many rapid tests now available for point-of-care testing by the nurse and wide range of tests available to the consumer for home use. The use of picture archiving and communication system (PACS) and of electronic health records (EHR) is another technological advance discussed in this edition. As before, examples abound with clinical significance and reference values over the entire life span from newborns to aged. Two chapters (Chapters 18 and 28) are devoted to the pregnant client.

Related tests or procedures are grouped so that common nursing diagnoses can be highlighted. The nursing diagnoses presented in this book are not meant to be used in cookbook form. The nurse can read about the test and possible nursing diagnoses, but then must evaluate the actual clinical situation and apply what seems appropriate. The purpose of this book is to make nurses think more, not less. The case studies in Part II give the reader an opportunity to practice interpreting lab data to formulate nurse's diagnoses.

As health care becomes more and more technical, the multitude of diagnostic procedures and laboratory tests continue to grow. Nurses can become dazzled by the technical details and discouraged about keeping pace with these advances. This book is based on the belief that the nurse's role in relation to diagnostic testing should continue to focus on the human element. Professional nurses are involved on health teaching, client preparation, and assessment for adverse reactions to diagnostic procedures. The pathophysiologic conditions that cause altered laboratory values are explained in an easy-to-understand format. A discussion of usual medical intervention for a particular set of circumstances is included to show how nursing use is related to and yet different from medical use of laboratory data. The independent role of the nurse is emphasized throughout.

Each chapter of this book is organized as an independent study unit complete with objectives, an organizing theme with background information (called an expository organizer), and test questions. The organization and content of the chapters are based on research conducted by the primary author (Corbett, 1985, 1997; Corbett & LaBorde, 1994). This book, meant to be both scholarly and practical, is intended for use in both the academic and the clinical setting. Following are some examples:

1. Undergraduate and graduate nursing students can use the book as a textbook in theory classes that integrate laboratory data as one aspect of nursing care.

2. Practicing nurses can use the book to update themselves in specific areas. The content in this book has been used extensively in continuing education courses for RNs.

3. Nurses in clinical settings can use the book as a quick reference. By consulting the index or the listing for each chapter, the nurse can retrieve information about one specific test.

It is intellectually challenging to broaden one's knowledge in a field, and in nursing we often have the added benefit of seeing that our increased knowledge is of direct benefit to the client. Our enthusiasm and sense of purpose in writing this book stem from our belief that students and practicing nurses will be able to use the information in this book to improve the care of many clients. We hope the reader finds the book informative and useful in the practice of nursing. We welcome written comments, which can be sent to me or my co-author at the following addresses:

Dr. Jane Vincent Corbett, RN, EdD
Professor Emerita, School of Nursing and Health Professions
University of San Francisco
2130 Fulton Street
San Francisco, CA 94117

Email: corbett@usfca.edu

Dr. Angela Denise Banks, RN, PhD
Associate Professor, School of Nursing and Health Professions
University of San Francisco
2130 Fulton Street
San Francisco, CA 94117
Email: adbanks@usfca.edu

Corbett, J. V. (1985). *The effects of two types of preinstructional strategies on two levels of cognitive learning from a written study unit.* Dissertation for School of Education, University of San Francisco. Reprints available from University Microfilms International, Ann Arbor, MI.

Corbett, J. V. (1997). An exploration of the independent use of laboratory data to make nursing diagnoses [Abstract]. In: M. J. Rantz and P. Lemone (Eds.), *Classifications of nursing diagnoses: Proceedings of the twelfth conference* (p. 380). Glendale, CA: Cinahl Information Systems.

Corbett, J. V., & LaBorde, A. (1994). Nurses' perceptions of usefulness of laboratory data for nursing practice. *Journal of Continuing Education in Nursing, 25*(4), 175–180.

Acknowledgments

For the eighth edition, I am pleased to have Dr. Angela Denise Banks, a co-author for the first time. It has been wonderful to find a colleague who brings new ideas and enthusiasm to this project. I am grateful to the University of San Francisco (USF) for granting me my first sabbatical in 1978 to do the research that culminated in the first edition of this book. During my 35-year tenure at USF, I had three more sabbaticals that gave me time to do the research needed for updating each edition. One sabbatical gave me the opportunity to interview nurses in Israel, and my fourth sabbatical was spent interacting with students and faculty at St. Bartholomew's School of Nursing in London. Now as Professor Emerita at USF, I continue to learn from my colleagues and students.

A large number of nurses from various clinical settings continue to participate in my continuing education courses. Their questions and discussions about cases in their own practice have helped me update content for this edition. I am particularly grateful to the Hospital Consortium Education Network of Northern California, who sponsored my classes for nearly 20 years. Other providers of continuing education such as Stanford University Hospital and the University of California at San Francisco Medical Center have also sponsored me for many years. A newer provider, American Health Education, has given me another avenue for teaching and learning about laboratory tests from practicing nurses.

The format for this book was based on work completed for my doctoral dissertation. I am grateful to S. Alan Cohen, EdD; Joan Hyman, EdD; and William Schwartz, EdD, who helped me gain an in-depth knowledge about how written strategies such as behavioral objectives and expository organizers can influence cognitive learning from study units. Eleanor Hein, RN, EdD; Jean Nicholson, RN, MS; Mae Timmons, RN, EdD; and Ginny Jones, RN, BS, also helped a great deal with their careful critiques of Chapter 13, which was used as the prototype chapter.

Carol Bailey, RN, MS (formerly of Kaiser Hospital, San Francisco), has been most helpful in obtaining information for each edition. Other people at Kaiser, such as Sunny Holland, RN, Cardiac Catheterization Lab, and Elaine Vaughn, Director of Diagnostic Imaging Services, have also been helpful in answering many of my questions and allowing me to observe numerous types of diagnostic procedures. The University of California at San Francisco (UCSF) provided me with excellent library resources and the opportunity to observe clinical tests and consult with various experts. (JVC)

First and foremost, I am grateful to Dr. Jane Vincent Corbett for giving me the opportunity to co-author this wonderful book. However, this privilege would not have been possible without the love and support of my wonderful husband, Rev. Beryl Banks. Beryl, there are no words to describe my gratitude and appreciation for your understanding during the writing and revising of this book. I thank you for believing in me and allowing me to pursue my dream of becoming an author.

Caleb Banks, my wonderful son. Thank you for supporting me and believing that your Mom could do just about anything. You are a tremendous inspiration and blessing to me.

Dr. Anna Kwong, my dear friend. You have always been there for me throughout my journey during the revisions of this book, and I sincerely thank you for your kindness, consideration, and encouragement. You have been a gift to my family and me from the moment we met, and you have changed the way I view life because it is so much more meaningful since you have become a part of it. (ADB)

Reviewers

Our heartfelt thanks go out to colleagues from schools of nursing across the country who have given their time generously to help us create this exciting new edition of the book. We have reaped the benefit of your collective experience as nurses, teachers, and students, and we have made many improvements due to your efforts. Among those who gave us their encouragement and comments are the following:

Angelique Allemand, DNP, RN, ACNP-C, CNS
Nicholls State University
Thibodaux, LA

Lisa Aymong, ANP, MPA, BS, RN
Suffolk County Community College
Selden, NY

Mary C. Bielski, EdD, MSN, CNE, RN
Triton College
River Grove, IL

Sevilla Bronson, MSN, ARNP
Florida Agricultural and Mechanical University
Tallahassee, FL

Steve Campbell, RN, BSN, MSN, CCRN
Polk State College
Winter Haven, FL

Michelle Dufrene, RN
Nicholls State University
Thibodaux, LA

Christine Eisenhauer, PhD(c), CNE, APRN-CNS
University of Nebraska Medical Center Northern Division
Norfolk, NE

Jacqueline Guhde, MSN, RN, CNS
University of Akron
Akron, OH

Kris Hale, RN, MSN
San Diego Community College District
San Diego, CA

Saul Jones, EdD, RN
Contra Costa College
San Pablo, CA

Jo Ann King, RN, MSN, NCS
Elizabethtown Community and Technical College
Elizabethtown, KY

Magda Sandra McCarthy, MSN, RN, CNE
Houston Community College
Houston, TX

Barbara McGraw, MSN, RN, CNE
Central Community College
Grand Island, NE

Linda Piacentine, PhD, RN, ACNP-BC
Marquette University College of Nursing
Milwaukee, WI

Deborah A. Raines, PhD, EdS, RN, ANEF
Walden University
Minneapolis, MN

Jean Storey, RN, MNSc
Texarkana College
Texarkana, TX

Darlene J. Street, PhD, RN
North Carolina Central University
Durham, NC

Jill K. Thornton, RN, MSN, ANP, APRN-BC
Suffolk County Community College
Selden, NY

Susan L. Woods, PhD, RN
University of Washington School of Nursing
Seattle, WA

LABORATORY
TESTS

Using Laboratory Data

- Laboratory Reports, Evidence-Based Practice, and the Nursing Process 3
- Nursing Functions in Laboratory Testing 6
- "Normal" Reference Values and the Variability of Test Results 12
- False-Positive and False-Negative Tests 14

- New Technology for Diagnostic Testing 14
- Measurements in Laboratory Reports 16
- Metabolic Panels and Other Screening Tests 17
- Laboratory Personnel 18
- Changes Related to Healthcare Reform 19

OBJECTIVES

1. Describe how laboratory data can be used in the framework of the nursing process and how the use of data differs in nursing and medicine.
2. Describe the functions of nurses in relation to laboratory tests, including genetic testing.
3. Explain the meaning of CLIA waived tests for point-of-care testing.
4. Identify the two nondisease factors that cause the greatest variations in normal reference values for laboratory tests.
5. Compare the meanings of the terms *specificity* and *sensitivity* in relation to diagnostic tests.
6. Explain the meaning of the measurement symbols in the conventional laboratory system and in the SI system.
7. Describe the purpose of each of the basic diagnostic screening tests recommended for asymptomatic adult populations.
8. Define how nurses can foster smooth working relationships with personnel in the laboratory department.

In discussing several issues that are pertinent to the nurse's utilization of laboratory data, this chapter touches briefly on the nursing process, on the differences between nursing care and medical care, and on the traditional roles of the nurse in relation to diagnostic tests. Technological advances have now made it possible for nurses to perform many tests at the point of care. Emphasis is given to the many factors that influence test results, such as physiology, drug interference, and the statistical methods used to determine "normal" ranges. A comparison of conventional measurements and SI units is included, and the purpose of screening tests is explored. The last section in the chapter discusses ways that the nurse can effectively work with personnel in other departments.

LABORATORY REPORTS, EVIDENCE-BASED PRACTICE, AND THE NURSING PROCESS

Up to the early 1970s, problem solving was emphasized as a way of thinking about the needs of clients. About that time, most nursing educators started turning to the nursing process, which is an elaboration of the problem-solving technique used by all disciplines. In essence, the *nursing process* is a way of systematically identifying the needs of patients or clients and then logically planning the appropriate nursing actions to meet those needs. (The term *client* is used in this book, but *patient* may be substituted if one wishes.) Most practicing nurses use the nursing process even though they may be unsure about how to describe it step-by-step in writing. However, nursing students learn to develop care plans based on the nursing process in a very systematic manner. Yet, whether written or not, the nursing process, as a way of thinking, helps the nurse provide nursing care that is based on more than guesswork or generalizations about clients. This process is a deliberate way of using data to make the assessments and to identify the problems that are under the jurisdiction of the nurse. The evaluation and modification of care are also essential components of the nursing process. The format for a written nursing care plan is shown in Table 1–1.

Table 1–1 Use of Laboratory Data in Nursing Process

Collection of Data (Assessment)	Nursing Diagnosis or Statement of Problems (Analysis)	Client/ Nurse Goals (Planning)	Interventions (Nurse-to-Nurse Orders Implementation)	Evaluation and Modification Needed (Evaluation)
Cannot use left arm to hold glass; mouth is dry; skin turgor poor; I&O for last 24 h I = 800 O = 600 s.g. = 1.036 Hct 50% BUN 35 mg	Deficient fluid volume related to inability to feed self	Client remains hydrated with an s.g. 1.020 or less *Short term:* Client drinks at least 1,000 mL on the day shift and 600 mL on the evening shift	Give mouth care at least once a shift Ask client what type of fluids are wanted—does not like *water* Assist client to drink out of glass—likes straw In addition to meals, offer 250 mL of fluids at: 10 AM, 2 PM, 4 PM, and 8 PM	Intake for 2–10: 7–3 PM 1,000 mL 3–11 PM 650 mL Client's s.g. now 1.015 on 2–11 2–11: Continue with plan

Note: Although a nursing diagnosis may arise from the use of one or two laboratory tests, more often, many tests and much clinical data are needed to fashion an individualized care plan. This text helps the reader by suggesting nursing diagnoses related to specific abnormal test results. The nurse must then gather relevant clinical data to validate the use of those diagnoses in a given situation.

I, intake; O, output; s.g., specific gravity; Hct, hematocrit; BUN, blood urea nitrogen.

Collection of Data (Assessment)

Nurses use a variety of ways to collect data, including physical assessment and interviewing; laboratory data constitute only one small part of the entire clinical situation. Consequently, one can never use the laboratory data apart from other clinical data. For example, although an increased specific gravity is one objective sign of dehydration, or a fluid volume deficit, the nurse must collect other data that may be relevant to this client's situation. If the client has just undergone diagnostic tests with radiopaque dye (Chapter 20), the specific gravity is not a meaningful contribution to data collection.

Nursing Diagnosis

Taking all the collected data, nurses then formulate a *nursing diagnosis*, which is a problem within the scope of nursing practice. In a national conference held in 1973, nurses identified a list of nursing diagnoses that were generally agreed to be under the control of the nurse. Since then the list has been periodically updated by national meetings of nurses, the official organization, the North American Nursing Diagnosis Association (NANDA), was founded in 1982 and was advanced to an international status in 2002. NANDA International periodically publishes a book that contains all the approved diagnoses including definitions, defining characteristics, risk factors, and other related information (Herdman, 2009). Information on the next publication is available at www.nanda.org. Although many nurses use this official and quite specific list of nursing diagnoses, others may prefer to use their own words to describe client problems. Various nurse practice acts define the nursing process in different ways. In a recent study, out of the 50 states in the United States, more than 80% used diagnosis as a subtheme and over 60% used nursing diagnosis language (Jarrin, 2010). The important point is that nurses must make sure the diagnosis or problem is truly within the scope of nursing and that other healthcare workers understand the terminology.

A nursing diagnosis is not the same as a medical diagnosis. Although medicine is focused on the diagnosis and treatment of disease, nursing focuses on the care, comfort, and support of people whose patterns of daily life are in some way threatened. Nursing focuses on restorative support, nurturance, comfort measures, and health teaching. Over the years, nursing diagnosis has moved from a basic concept about the nature of nursing toward theory-based diagnostic categories that can be tested in clinical practice.

Many client problems can be identified by means of the nursing process. For example, through assessment, the nurse may discover that Mr. Smith's urine has become concentrated because he cannot feed himself and no one has been offering him any fluids between meals. Thus, the nursing diagnosis would be a deficient fluid volume caused by an inability to obtain fluids. However, dehydration, or a deficient fluid volume, may be caused by a serious medical problem such as ketoacidosis. The second case warrants medical interventions such as insulin administration and intravenous fluids (Chapter 8). Other examples are as follows:

1. An elevated direct bilirubin often causes itching in clients. What measures by the nurse may be effective? (Readiness for enhanced comfort)
2. A client has a low serum potassium level. What *health teaching* does the client need about foods rich in potassium? (Deficient knowledge)

3. A woman is to undergo a hysterosalpingogram as part of an infertility workup. The nurse observes that the client is very anxious. What can the nurse do to prepare the woman and to give her *nurturance*? (Moderate anxiety)

4. A young child has a low hemoglobin reading. What can the nurse teach the parents that would be *restorative support*? (Imbalanced nutrition)

The nursing process is effective if one knows the answers to go with the questions raised in the preceding list. Hence, the subsequent chapters provide the information necessary for planning individualized client care. Only potential nursing diagnoses are listed for each test. The nurse must decide if the diagnosis is really appropriate for a particular client. Students, clinicians, and researchers must continue to be flexible and creative in the use and validation of nursing diagnoses.

Writing Goals for Client Outcomes

With the nursing diagnosis, the nurse can write client/nurse goals in behavioral terms. The goal should be acceptable to the client and compatible with medical goals. For example, in Mr. Smith's case, an immediate short-term goal is to have him drink so many milliliters of fluid during each shift. The long-term goal is that he not show any signs of dehydration (i.e., his specific gravity remains in a normal range).

Nursing Interventions (Implementation)

The nurse then plans the nursing actions or interventions needed to reach the goals. She or he may consult with the client about how to best achieve a mutually acceptable goal. Maybe Mr. Smith needs to be fed completely. Maybe he could feed himself and drink fluids if he were properly positioned. Maybe the client would drink juice better than water. Collaboration with the physician and with other health team members (such as the dietitian) is often necessary.

Nurses write goals and interventions in various ways. These interventions, called *nurse-to-nurse orders*, need to be written in the client's record. The important point is to differentiate between actions that depend on physicians' orders and independent nursing actions. Too often, nurses communicate their own orders only by word of mouth. While nursing as a profession becomes more assured of its uniqueness, one hopes that nurse-to-nurse orders will become a more common practice. Another way to define the collective expertise of nurses has been the *Nursing Interventions Classification* (NIC) system, which lists and defines 336 nursing interventions. The NIC, first published in 1992, is designed to make the contributions of nurses visible in health information systems. Research continues on the use of NIC and other nomenclatures in various settings. Muller-Staub (2009) and Carpenito-Moyet (2010) discuss strategies that help the student learn to use nursing diagnoses at each level of the curriculum. Ongoing research conducted by the investigative teams at the University of Iowa is focused on supporting critical thinking by the use of NOC (Nursing Outcomes Classification) and NIC with NANDA-I (Johnson et al., 2012). The NOC, another group working closely with NANDA, is trying to unify nursing languages as electronic health records (EHR) and require the use of standardized nursing languages.

Evaluation of Goals or Expected Outcomes

Evaluation is necessary to see if the goals or expected outcomes are met. If goals are not achieved, what needs to be modified? For example, a specific gravity measurement can be considered evidence that the client has regained a normal fluid balance. *Responsibility* and *accountability* in nursing mean that nurses take responsibility for the quality of client care and that they are accountable if the care does not meet certain standards. Hence, evaluation is an integral part of accountability.

NURSING FUNCTIONS IN LABORATORY TESTING

Integrating Laboratory Data into Nursing Practice

As health care has become more complex and technological, nurses have been increasingly expected to integrate laboratory data into their practice. Although nurses are expected to use laboratory data in their nursing practice, not all nurses may feel comfortable with this role. Nearly 20 years ago, a nursing research study identified a lack of knowledge about clinical importance and time constraints as the two most common barriers to the use of laboratory data (Corbett & LaBorde, 1994). These two barriers may still exist. In addition to using laboratory data to formulate nursing diagnoses, nurses must determine if the results of a test need to be reported immediately to a physician or if the report is not urgent. Nurses may also need to alert other healthcare workers or the client and family about symptoms to watch for or precautions to take. Although abnormal results may require immediate attention, normal results may also have great diagnostic importance in ruling out certain diseases. The importance of both normal and abnormal results is emphasized for each of the tests in the following chapters. Reviewing outpatient laboratory results in a timely manner is also a challenge. The use of electronic systems similar to an e-mail inbox that highlights abnormal results helps clinicians review these results first. Another challenge is reviewing a client's laboratory test results from various locations. Laboratories have devised programs to store laboratory data from multiple sources into a single electronic medical record (EMR) or an EHR (Staes et al., 2006). Clients may also access their laboratory results by using the electronic records. Even though laboratory reports are all computerized, there are some clinicians who may use a shorthand way to summarize results, as shown in Appendix F.

Using Critical Thinking in Judging the Value of Laboratory Data

Strategies such as judging the value of laboratory data and learning to recognize patterns are useful in interpreting laboratory data. Judging the value does not mean just comparing a number to a reference value. How low is "low"? The critical thinker must assess the credibility of the test and the contextual relevance. For example, when is a sudden drop in hematocrit of the greatest concern? Why may a client have more symptoms with an abrupt low hematocrit compared to a client who has a chronically low hematocrit? What factors, such as fluid balance, must be considered in judging the value? Do clients with low hematocrits exhibit a pattern of symptoms? What other assessment data suggest a low hematocrit? What factors may change those patterns? Interpreting laboratory data does require this kind of critical thinking in order for the nurse to become expert in using laboratory data.

Striving for an Evidence-Based Practice

Over the past few years, the use of current, relevant, and defensible research to help with clinical judgment has become known as evidence-based practice. Although evidence-based practice is ideal, a recent study by Pravikoff, Tanner, and Pierce (2005) found that registered nurses (RNs) in the United States were not well prepared for evidence-based practice. Two main barriers were their attitude toward research and a lack of understanding of how to use electronic databases. These researchers identified several sources to help nurses improve their practice. Thus, the reader of this text, whether a novice nurse or an expert, is encouraged to supplement the information here with the many current resources available on the Web. This new edition has many websites listed for each chapter so that the reader can verify guidelines from various professional organizations. An outstanding website (www.labtestsonline.org) is sponsored by the laboratory professionals who do the testing. This peer-reviewed site is constantly being updated.

Reimbursement for Laboratory Tests

Insurance companies will reimburse only tests warranted as "medical necessity." For Medicare, physicians or nurse practitioners must provide the laboratory with the ICD-9 (International Classification of Diseases) diagnostic code to justify the laboratory test. Many private insurance carriers also require that an appropriate diagnostic code be provided when the test is requested, and some may have other guidelines to determine eligibility coverage. Patients without third-party insurance may be asked to pay before the test is done or referred to Social Services for assistance with obtaining financial help.

Protecting Client Confidentiality

The federal Health Insurance Portability and Accountability Act (HIPAA) legislates for confidentiality regarding all aspects of health care, including data related to laboratory tests and diagnostic procedures. Nurses must follow HIPAA guidelines as well as any additional state laws related to sharing or reporting laboratory test results, such as those for sexually transmitted diseases (STD). The use of DNA testing, discussed later, has created new concerns about privacy. Roche and Annas (2006) discussed the dangers of unregulated market on the Internet and stressed that clients need to know that the privacy protection they may take for granted in health care may not apply to DNA tests available on the Web.

Preparation of the Client for a Laboratory Test

The nurse's role includes preparing the client physically and psychologically. As a client advocate, the nurse can make sure that the client has adequate knowledge of what is to be performed. As information giver or health teacher, the nurse can also seek additional input from other members of the health team so that the client gives informed consent. The responsibilities of nurses in implementing a doctrine of informed consent are related to their role within the health team, the facility at which health care is given, and current law. In the past few years, there has been more emphasis on clients' rights, which may now be called informed decision making.

See www.informedmedicaldecisions.org for current research in this area.

Standard Precautions: Blood and Other Specimen Collection

The premise for Standard Precautions, formerly called Universal Precautions, is that all patients should be considered as potentially infectious. Standard precautions are now routine in all institutions. Healthcare workers handling blood or other body fluids must follow the Occupational Safety and Health Administration (OSHA) guidelines to reduce the risk of exposure to infections. Current OSHA guidelines must be part of the orientation for every worker in a healthcare setting. In November 2000, Congress enacted the Needlestick Safety and Prevention Act, and enforcement began July 2001. Nurses need to be familiar with the protective devices used in a particular setting and request additional training in response to new technology. At the present time the primary concerns for bloodborne pathogens are human immunodeficiency virus (HIV), hepatitis B virus (HBV), hepatitis C virus (HCV), and West Nile virus (WNV) (see Chapter 14).

Collection and Transportation of Specimens

Venous Samples

Nurses often draw venous blood for blood work. When they do, they must avoid the following possible causes of hemolysis, which invalidates tests such as potassium or lactic dehydrogenase (LDH) determination:

1. Skin too wet with antiseptic
2. Moisture in the syringe or collection tube
3. Prolonged use of a tourniquet or clenching of fist
4. Use of a small-gauge needle to withdraw a large volume of blood
5. Use of suction on the syringe
6. Vigorous shaking of the blood specimen
7. Not removing the needle from the syringe before expelling the blood into the collection tube
8. Vigorous expulsion of blood from the syringe into the collection tube

Other precautions are not drawing blood from an arm in which there is an intravenous catheter because the values are changed by the solution being infused. Blood samples may be obtained by vascular access devices or central venous catheters when peripheral draws are not possible.

The meanings of the various colors for tubes are explained in Table 1–2. For example, a red top on a tube means *no additives*. Most venous blood samples for chemistry are collected without additives or in the red-and-black tube that separates the serum; the tubes are noted as serum separator tubes (SSTs). These tubes are

Table 1–2 Meaning of Conventional Color Code for Blood Specimens

Color of Tube Top	Contents	Use
Red	No additives No separator	Most chemistry, serology, and blood banking
Red and black	Silicone gel to separate serum from cells[a]	Most chemistry and serology
Green	Heparin	Special tests such as ammonia levels, blood gases
Lavender	EDTA	Hematology, some chemistry, and blood banking
Blue	Sodium citrate	PT, PTT, and other coagulation tests
Gray	Glycolytic inhibitor such as oxalate and fluoride	Glucose

[a]The use of silicone gel, which separates the cells from the plasma, makes it easier for the laboratory worker to obtain the serum. But the gel is rather expensive. Tubes should be rotated if additive is present so it will mix with the specimen.

EDTA, ethylenediaminetetraacetate; PT, prothrombin time; PTT, partial thromboplastin time.

often referred to as "tiger tops" or "speckled reds." Chapter 13 describes techniques for arterial blood samples. Except for tubes that are intended to allow blood to clot, all tubes should be inverted several times to mix the additive with the blood. The nurse should note that complete filling of the tube is important for some tests.

Order of Collection Tubes of Blood

Although some institutions may have a different sequence for collection of multiple tubes of blood, the usual order is as follows:

1. Blood cultures (yellow top)
2. Nonadditive tubes (red top)
3. Coagulation tubes (light blue top)
4. Serum separator tubes (tiger top)
5. Heparin tubes (green top)
6. EDTA tubes (lavender top)
7. Oxalate fluoride (gray top)

If venous access is poor the nurse should consult with the physician and/or the laboratory and consider drawing the most necessary test first.

Finger, Earlobe, and Heel Sticks

For many tests performed with a portable analyzer, capillary blood obtained with a finger stick is used, rather than blood obtained by means of venipuncture. The earlobe may occasionally be used for tests such as hematocrits. The usual procedure is to cleanse with 70% alcohol, dry with a gauze sponge, and puncture with a sterile blade deep enough to get a free flow of blood. Enough blood is collected to fill a capillary tube supplied by the laboratory or a drop of blood may be put onto special filter paper. It is important not to squeeze to obtain capillary blood because the squeezing causes tissue fluids to dilute the sample. Warming the site a few minutes before the puncture greatly increases blood flow, as does selecting a lancet with the needed puncture depth. In infants, heel sticks are used to obtain capillary blood. The lateral aspects of the heel are used to avoid the plantar artery. Instant disposable chemical heat packs are used routinely for neonates. Although these packs are usually safe and effective, adverse events have occurred when nurses failed to follow the suggested guidelines by the manufacturer and the institution's policy and procedures (Dwyer, 2009). Research has suggested that the use of swaddling and bringing a preterm infant to an alert state before the heel stick may help the infant tolerate the procedure without expending as much energy (Evans et al., 2005; Morrow, Hidinger, & Wilkinson-Faulk, 2010).

Urine and Other Specimens

The procedure for urine collection, including 24-hour testing, is detailed in Chapter 3. Chapter 16 gives explicit details on all the types of specimens collected for cultures.

After a specimen is collected, the way it is stored and transported to the laboratory can affect the test values. For example, blood gases or anaerobic cultures must not be exposed to the air. The nurse must check with the laboratory to determine if there are any special requirements about the transportation of specimens.

Seeing That Stat Tests are Stat

The word *stat* means "at once." Because a stat request interrupts the normal laboratory routine, a test should be marked "*stat* only" when the results really do need to be known as soon as possible. The nurse should be familiar with the preparation needed and with the expected results of stat tests because these tests are done in emergency situations when there is little time to review. Table 1–3 lists 22 tests done stat by almost all hospitals.

Point-of-Care Testing and Clinical Laboratory Improvement Act

The availability of sophisticated wet and dry chemistry systems (automatic analyzers) that can be used outside the traditional centralized laboratory has made it possible to perform many tests in the physician's office or in small clinics. Handheld portable analyzers that require only a few drops of blood can simultaneously perform many measurements such as electrolyte, glucose, blood urea nitrogen (BUN), and hematocrit values within 2 minutes. These portable analyzers have proved useful in many settings. Not having to send specimens to a laboratory usually means faster results at a lower cost. Proficiency testing for quality control in laboratories had been voluntary for many years. However, with the passage of the Clinical Laboratory Improvement Act of 1988 (CLIA), effective in 1992, proficiency testing became mandatory. All tests are categorized as "waived," moderately complex, or highly complex. The level of test is determined by assessing the relative difficulty of doing the test and the relative risk to the client if the test is performed incorrectly. (See www.fda.gov/cdrh/clia for current information on all waived tests.)

Table 1–3 Tests Most Commonly Done As Stat Procedures

Name of Test	Discussed In
Complete blood count (CBC)	Chap. 2
Urinalysis (UA)	Chap. 3
Blood urea nitrogen (BUN)	Chap. 4
Electrolytes (Na, K, Cl, CO_2 as bicarb)	Chap. 5
Blood gases	Chap. 6
Calcium	Chap. 7
Glucose	Chap. 8
Acetone (serum)	Chap. 8
Bilirubin	Chap. 11
Amylase	Chap. 12
Prothrombin time (PT) with international normalized ratio (INR)	Chap. 13
Partial thromboplastin time (PTT)	Chap. 13
Platelet count	Chap. 13
Fibrinogen	Chap. 13
Type and crossmatch	Chap. 14
Direct Coombs'	Chap. 14
Transfusion reaction investigation	Chap. 14
Inoculate media for cultures	Chap. 16
Gram stains	Chap. 16
Alcohol	Chap. 17
Salicylates	Chap. 17
Cerebrospinal fluid (CSF)	Chap. 16

See McPhee, Papadakis, and Rabow (2011) for more information on stat procedures.

Laboratories that perform moderately complex or highly complex tests are subject to biennial inspections and must meet more stringent protocols than laboratories that perform waived tests. Waived testing laboratories must be registered and must perform the tests according to the manufacturer's instructions. (Some states may set standards that are higher than the minimum requirements of CLIA.) A "CLIA waived" test means that nurses can do the test as point of care with supervision by a laboratory that has CLIA certification.

Common point-of-care testing (POCT), sometimes called patient testing in hospitals, includes those for glucose, coagulation, blood gases, hematocrit, and electrolytes. Many new point-of-care tests, also called rapid tests, are available for infections, such as those for influenza, respiratory syncytial virus (RSV), and vaginitis (Chapter 16). Issues revolve around the need to document staff competence, quality assurance, and the cost versus benefits of POCT. Some nurses have complained that simple tests, such as those for specific gravity or fecal occult blood, are no longer on the nursing units because ensuring competency makes them cost prohibitive (Pellico, 2005). Authorities recommend that institutions have a standing committee to address these issues and provide resources for nurses.

Table 1–4 Examples of FDA-Approved Home Testing by Consumers and CLIA Waived for Nurses

Name of Test	Discussed In
Alcohol scans	Chap. 17
Allergies (send-in sample)	Chap. 10
Cholesterol	Chap. 9
Drug screening	Chap. 17
Fecal occult blood tests (FOBT)	Chap. 13
FSH for menopause and fertility	Chaps. 15–28
Glucose	Chap. 8
Hemoglobin for anemia	Chap. 2
Hgb A1C	Chap. 8
Hepatitis C (send-in sample)	Chap. 14
HIV (send-in sample)	Chap. 14
Ketones	Chap. 8
LH for ovulation	Chap. 15
Microalbumin in urine	Chap. 10
Pregnancy HCG	Chap. 18
Prothrombin time/INR	Chap. 13
Semen analysis	Chap. 28
Thyroid (TSH)	Chap. 15
Urine dipsticks for UTI	Chap. 3

Note: All these tests may also be done by nurses as point-of-care testing. See the text on other examples of rapid testing.

Educating Consumers About the Use of Home Test Kits

Advanced technology has made it possible for many tests to be approved by the U.S. Food and Drug Administration (FDA) for use by consumers. The first such home tests, in 1977, were for pregnancy (Chapter 18). Now a variety of home test kits are available for screening, such as the ones for serum cholesterol, HIV, and prothrombin time (PT). Consumers need to understand that they are self-testing not self-diagnosing. Nurses need to be knowledgeable about the home test kits available and how clients may use them for self-monitoring. Many are available online. See Table 1–4 for examples of FDA-approved home tests.

"NORMAL" REFERENCE VALUES AND THE VARIABILITY OF TEST RESULTS

Laboratory values in the medical literature are referred to as *normal reference values* or *reference values* and not as *normal values* because each laboratory must determine what is "normal" for a test performed in a specific laboratory. *The use of any of the reference values in this book may be hazardous to the well-being of clients unless values are verified by the local laboratory. No book can be the authority on what is normal for a specific laboratory.* Because reference ranges are specific to the laboratory that performs the test, the nurse must use the ones provided by the laboratory for a specific client.

For a few tests such as cholesterol (Chapter 9), glucose (Chapter 8), prostate-specific antigen (Chapter 10), and INR (Chapter 13), there have been major efforts to standardize test methods and determine a cut-off number instead of a reference range that is used for clinical decision making. In addition, other tests such as electrolytes rarely vary much from one laboratory to the next.

For the most part, the reference values used throughout this book are those periodically published in the *New England Journal of Medicine.* These values, based on the ones used at Massachusetts General Hospital, have been published periodically since 1946. Reference values for some tests were gained from various hospitals in San Francisco, California. Other sources for reference values are listed in each chapter and with the tables in the appendices.

Variables That Affect Test Results

Besides the obvious differences in technique and method, many other variables can influence laboratory reference values. Age and sex are the chief physiologic factors that change the "norms." Pregnancy alters the normal reference values. (See the tables in Appendices A, B, C, and D for examples of changes in values in different populations.) Computer printouts of values are usually adjusted for age and sex.

Other physiologic factors, such as diet, time of day, activity level, and stress, may alter what is "normal" for a test. For example, hormones (Chapter 15) have a diurnal variation, so the time of day must be recorded when the specimen is drawn. Geographic location, altitude, temperature, and humidity may also affect results. Racial or ethnic variation can also cause different reference values for different groups, but usually ethnic or racial differences are not of much importance for most tests. How much a drug alters a laboratory value may depend on the dosage, timing, physiology of the client, and other variables such as the mixture of drugs. The reader must consult pharmacology references or other more specialized texts than this book for details on drug interactions, from both the physiologic effects and the chemical effects on laboratory results. Only the more common drug interferences are included in this text.

Critical Test Results (Panic Values)

Extreme test results, such as a potassium less than 3 or over 6 mEq/L (mmol/L for SI), that could be life threatening are called to the healthcare provider who ordered the test and the hospital unit of inpatients. The date and time of this notification later appear on the computer printout. The use of personal phones for nurses means the laboratory can give results directly to the nurse caring for the client. Phone-reported laboratory values must be read back to the caller. Each laboratory maintains a list of the panic values that require immediate notification. Some prefer the term *critical values* as "panic values" has a negative connotation. Nurses should be aware of these values for a given setting. The time interval from sending a specimen to the laboratory to the first intervention to correct a critical or panic value has been used as one of the ongoing measurements of nursing care (Curley & Hickey, 2006). (See the website of the Joint Commission [www.jointcommission.org] for standards of laboratory testing.)

FALSE-POSITIVE AND FALSE-NEGATIVE TESTS

Specificity

If a test is 100% *specific*, it reacts positively only when the client actually has the condition being tested. No laboratory test is 100% specific because there is always a factor, such as drugs, that can effect a false-positive reaction. For example, the radioimmunoassay (RIA) test for pregnancy is very specific because almost all women who have a positive test are indeed pregnant. However, the VDRL (Venereal Disease Research Laboratory) test for syphilis is not highly specific (i.e., a large number of people can have a positive VDRL even though they do not have syphilis). The danger of false positives is that the client may receive additional tests and treatments that are unnecessary.

Sensitivity

The *sensitivity* of a test is the degree to which a test detects disease without yielding a false-negative diagnosis. No test is 100% sensitive because there is always some possibility that the test will not reveal the abnormality even though it is present.

In disease states, false-negative tests mean that clients are misclassified as not needing treatment or care when actually they *do* need treatment. For example, the electrocardiogram (ECG) is not a sensitive test for coronary artery disease before a myocardial infarction. In other words, coronary artery disease is not detected by this particular test. Thus, a person may have a "normal" ECG one day and a myocardial infarction the next.

NEW TECHNOLOGY FOR DIAGNOSTIC TESTING

Specificity and sensitivity are important criteria when a new test is introduced into practice. Some questions to ask may be as follows:

1. Does the new procedure provide a greater specificity and sensitivity than current methods?
2. Is the new information valuable in client management?
3. Is the new approach as effective in routine clinical practice as it is in selected populations of a university center?
4. Does the test provide answers not provided by clinical findings and established diagnostic procedures?
5. In light of the other four factors, is the test cost-effective?

The past few years have seen an amazing array of new technology for diagnostic testing. Many of these techniques have improved the sensitivity and specificity of testing by labeling specific antigens and antibodies so that very small amounts of a hormone, a drug, or other substance can be identified. The technique for labeling first used radioisotopes and was thus called radioimmunoassay (RIA). Rosalyn Yalow received a share of the 1977 Nobel Prize for the development of this technique. Alternative labels to radioisotopes, which are less expensive and do not have the problems associated with radioactive materials, have been developed. These newer techniques include enzyme immunoassay (EIA), fluorescence immunoassay (FIA), enzyme-linked immunosorbent assay (ELISA), and others. These initials may be used with the test to let the clinician know the type of testing used.

The polymerase chain reaction (PCR) is a technique used to make copies of a sequence of DNA. Amplification makes it possible to study very small amounts of biologic material, even dried blood spots. RNA can also be used, provided it is first converted to DNA with a reverse transcriptase step. For example, PCR is very useful to assay the RNA in the hepatitis C virus. PCR, introduced in 1985 and first used in a court case in 1986, is also used in the clinical setting to identify sample mix-ups of blood and even urine. To make a match of DNA, a nucleic acid probe is needed. A nucleic acid probe is a replica or construct of the DNA or RNA of the cell or organism to be detected. The probe is labeled with a radioisotope or other tag. Commercial kits that rely on nucleic acid probes with PCR (NA-PCR) have been available since 1990. For commercial kits, the amplified sample of DNA fragments is probed by a complementary fragment of DNA bound to membrane strips. Testing for organisms (Chapter 16) and for genetic diseases (Chapter 18) are examples of the use of techniques that may be called DNA probes, PCR tests, or just DNA testing.

Chapter 21 describes the many types of scans now available. In many other chapters, the impact of technology on the development of new tests or on improvement of the sensitivity and specificity of older tests is evident.

Genetics/Genomics

Although DNA testing, as discussed earlier in chapter, has been available for several years, the completion of maps of the human genome in 2003 has added another dimension to understanding the genetic makeup of an individual. Genetics refers to the study of the role of genes in the inheritance of certain traits (blue eyes) or conditions (sickle cell anemia). Genomics is a broader term meaning the study of a person's genes including interaction of those genes with each other and with the individual's environment.

Genetics tests used during pregnancy include those such as phenylketonuria (PKU), Down syndrome, and several others (Chapter 18). Genetic testing may also be used to predict future disease such as breast cancer, colon cancer, alpha-1-antitrypsin emphysema (Chapter 10), or coagulation problems. (Chapter 13). A newer field of pharmacogenomics studies how genetic testing helps determine an individual's ability to metabolize certain medications (Chapter 13 on warfarin and Chapter 17 for others).

Many ethical and legal issues arise when these tests are used for decision making. The first federal law to address the misuse of genetic testing was the 2008 Genetic Information Nondiscrimination Act (GINA). This law prohibits the use of genetic information by employers and health insurance providers. States also have other laws that help protect consumers. In addition to legal and ethical questions, the proliferation of over 1,600 genetic tests raises questions on cost and the benefit to the individual and the society (Calzone et al., 2010). DNA can be stored from terminally ill patients for use later when tests are developed. DNA banking, a tool that allows genetic material to be saved for later testing, is offered through commercial and university-based laboratories at a cost to clients who may be interested. In addition to banking DNA for future testing, clients may also purchase home test kits that claim to identify health risks based on an individualized genome. However, these kits may vary in accuracy and reliability in relation to predicting diseases. Information about genetic tests and points to consider are available at www. genetests.org and www.genome.gov.

Nurses should be incorporating genetic and genomic information in many settings, as discussed in the following chapters. One of the important roles of the nurse is to obtain a thorough family history to screen for possible referrals for genetic counseling. The International Society of Nurses in Genetics (www.isong. org) has excellent resources including position statements and standards of practice for nurses involved in genetics/genomics.

MEASUREMENTS IN LABORATORY REPORTS

Conventional Measurements

Probably most of the measurements used in laboratory reports, such as mL (milliliter) or mg (milligram), are already very familiar. A list of the common abbreviations used for metric measurements is included in Table 1–5, and a more complete list is included as Appendix D. Note that mg/dL means so many milligrams in a deciliter, which is 1/10 of a liter, or 100 mL. In other words, a serum glucose report of 90 mg/dL is the same as 90 mg/100 mL.

The terms *picogram* (pg) and *nanogram* (ng) are also commonly used, now that it is possible to detect trace amounts of substances such as hormones and drugs.

The measurement used for electrolytes is *milliequivalent* (mEq). The exact meaning of this term, as well as how milligram can be converted to milliequivalent, is

Table 1–5 Metric Measurements Used in Laboratory Reports[a]

Nonmetric Equivalent

Length	
Meter (m)	39.37 in
Centimeter (cm) = 1/100 m	2.5 cm = 1 in
Millimeter (mm) = 1/1,000 m	
Weight	
Kilogram (kg)	2.2 lb
Gram (g)	453 g = 1 lb
Milligram (mg) = 1/1,000 of a g	
Microgram (μg) = 1/1,000 of a mg	
Nanogram (ng) = 1/1,000 of a mg	
Picogram (pg) = 1/1,000 of a ng	
Femtogram (fg) = 1/1,000 of a pg	
Volume	
Liter (L) = 1,000 mL (or 1,000 cc[b])	1.05 qt
Deciliter (dL) = 100 mL or 1/10 of a L	
Milliliter (mL) = 1/1,000 of a L	
Microliter (μL) = 1/million of a L	
Nanoliter (nL) = 1/billion of a L	

[a]See Appendix D for an expanded list of measurement terms used in laboratory reports.

[b]Note that "mL" and "cc" are interchangeable.

explained in Chapter 5. *Milliosmoles* (mOsm) is used to express the concentration of body fluids. (See Chapter 4 for a definition of milliosmoles in relation to urinary osmolality.) Note that *mOsm* is different from *mmol*, which is discussed next.

SI Measurement System

SI units are based on a comprehensive form of the metric system called *Le Système Internationale d'Unités* (hence SI). The rationale for the adoption of this international system is to provide a common language for all the various disciplines all over the world. Used not only for the biologic sciences but also for all sciences, SI uses *moles* as the basic unit for the amount of a substance and *kilograms* for its mass. (A mole is the amount of substance that contains as many elementary particles [e.g., atoms, electrons, ions, etc.] as there are atoms in 0.012 kg of carbon-12.) Length is still by *meter*.

The most profound change in laboratory reports effected by SI is that concentration is expressed as an amount per volume (moles or millimoles per liter) rather than as a mass per volume (grams or milligrams per 100 mL or dL). For some laboratory tests, the numbers stay the same even though the unit is new. For example, the normal range for potassium (K) in the conventional system is 3.5–5.0 mEq/L and in SI it is 3.5–5.0 mmol/L. Some of the other tests involve a radical change in numbers, so health workers must totally relearn the reference values. For example, the conventional reference value for glucose of *70–100 mg/dL* becomes *3.9–5.6 mmol/L* in SI.

Because of the drastic change in many laboratory reports, the conversion is taking place slowly in the United States. Many laboratories report results in both conventional and SI units (Wu, 2006). Appendix E gives the reference values in both conventional and SI units.

METABOLIC PANELS AND OTHER SCREENING TESTS

Metabolic panels consist of a battery of tests, usually 7 or 14, in which the client's individual results are compared against the normal reference values. A basic metabolic panel includes the four electrolytes (Chapter 5), BUN and serum creatinine (Chapter 4), and glucose (Chapter 8). (See Appendix F KEEP THIS as a way to diagram the results.)

Laboratory tests and other diagnostic procedures should be determined by the nature of the client's problem, which must be detected by means of careful history-taking and physical examination. See the earlier discussion on reimbursement issues.

In the past few years, several expert panels have identified screening tests that are recommended for all asymptomatic adults. One of the newest tests is routine HIV screening for clients ages 19–64 (Chapter 14). The most agreement is for routine blood pressure measurements, serum cholesterol levels every 5 years (Chapter 9), mammograms for women every year or two (Chapter 20), and Pap smears every 1–3 years for women (Chapter 25). Other tests are colonoscopy (Chapter 27) or occult blood testing (Chapter 13) and sigmoidoscopy (Chapter 27) as routine screens for colorectal cancer. Some authorities question the prostate-specific antigen (PSA) (Chapter 14) to screen men for prostatic cancer. Screening tests for older women may include thyroid-stimulating hormone (TSH) for detecting hypothyroidism (Chapter 15) and bone density scans (Chapter 21) to assess for osteoporosis. Ultrasound screening for abdominal aneurysm is recommended for men between 65 and 75 years who have been smokers (Chapter 23). For both sexes, glucose screening (fasting plasma glucose or hemoglobin A1C) may be offered every 3 years beginning at age 45 (Chapter 8). Although these are the basic screening tests, panels do not always agree on what screening tests are essential for all people. Many professional organizations make recommendations for screening as does the U.S. Preventive Services Task Force (www.uspreventiveservicestaskforce.org). These panels are made up of experts appointed by the federal government to evaluate evidence and then make recommendations for the use or nonuse of screening tests. These recommendations are not legislative mandates, but some insurers do base coverage on these guidelines. Benefits versus cost is constantly being evaluated. Nurses need to be aware of the recommended screening tests so they can educate clients about practical and cost-effective primary care.

LABORATORY PERSONNEL

Who Works in a Clinical Laboratory?

The Pathologist

The laboratory is directed by a physician with a specialty in pathology, which focuses on the use and interpretation of laboratory tests in the diagnosis and treatment of disease. Because they often interpret the results of laboratory tests to the attending physician, pathologists are often called the "doctor's doctors." In addition to helping with clinical decision making, the pathologist plays an important role in the accreditation and inspection of the laboratory.

Medical Technologist

The actual management of the laboratory is carried out by a medical technologist who has had additional training in management and administration. Usually the director of the laboratory establishes the policies and procedures that affect nursing. In most states, medical technologists have a bachelor's degree in a biologic science, which includes a year or more of study in a school of medical technology. States have their own medical technology examination, but a national examination is also available for certification.

Medical technologists typically become specialists in different areas, such as serology, hematology, or bacteriology. Nurses should understand how the laboratory is organized well enough that they do not call the chemistry section, for example, for the results of a culture and sensitivity test.

Cooperating with Laboratory Personnel

Laboratory personnel complain that specimens are not marked correctly—that they are lost or otherwise ineptly handled by the nursing staff. Clients are not always correctly assessed by point-of-care testing, or the laboratory personnel are not informed about quality control issues. On the other hand, nurses complain that the laboratory personnel are insensitive to the individual needs of the client, are late with stat requests, do not notify nurses of changes in procedures, and so forth. Unfortunately, both departments often have legitimate reasons for complaining, but poor communications between the departments often allow small problems to become large frustrations.

The information in the rest of this book should enable nurses to function better in preparing the client for laboratory testing, as well as make them sensitive to what the laboratory personnel need to know about any special problems with clients. For example, if the nurse knows a client is disoriented and potentially combative, the laboratory personnel should be warned about this attitude before they draw blood or perform other procedures.

CHANGES RELATED TO HEALTHCARE REFORM

It is too early to determine the impact of the new health reform on laboratories. But in 2006, when the state of Massachusetts passed a law requiring all adults to purchase health insurance, clinics and outpatient settings observed more clients seeking medical assistance and preventive care earlier than compared to the past where clients waited longer or for symptoms to appear prior to seeking medical assistance (Malone, 2010). The net effect in Massachusetts was receiving clients sooner who were not as ill. We are unable to determine if this trend will continue, but if clients across the country who are now insured become proactive in their medical care, then the trend may very well spread.

Questions

1. A client has a urine specific gravity of 1.030 and other clinical signs of a deficient fluid volume. In using the nursing process, the nurse should use this information about specific gravity not only to make an assessment of the problem but also to
   a. Diagnose the pathophysiology or underlying disease
   b. Initiate treatment of the disease
   c. Evaluate the effectiveness of nursing interventions
   d. Determine the rate of intravenous infusion of fluids

2. The traditional functions of the nurse in relation to laboratory tests have never included
   a. Transcribing physicians' orders and writing requisitions for the laboratory
   b. Collecting and transporting specimens to the laboratory
   c. Conducting simple testing on the unit
   d. Scheduling the times when tests are performed by laboratory personnel on the unit

3. Which of these two factors are generally the most common reasons for variations in normal reference values for laboratory tests?
   a. Genetic factors and drugs
   b. Sex and drugs
   c. Activity levels and stress
   d. Geographic location and diet

4. If a test yields too many false positives, the test is described as
   a. Not very sensitive
   b. Too sensitive
   c. Not specific
   d. Highly specific

5. In conventional laboratory reports, the smallest amount of a substance would be measured by weight as a
   a. ng
   b. pg
   c. μg
   d. mg

6. Laboratory results measured in SI units are reported as amount per volume as expressed by
   a. Milliequivalents (mEq)
   b. Milliosmoles (mOsm)
   c. Millimoles (mmol)
   d. Milligrams (mg)

7. Which of the following tests is of questionable value as a basic screening test for asymptomatic adult populations 50–65 years of age?
   a. Annual blood pressure checks
   b. Complete blood count (CBC) and urinalysis every 2 years
   c. Mammograms for women every 1–2 years
   d. Serum cholesterol levels every 5 years

8. The new nurse manager wants to help her staff develop a good relationship with the laboratory personnel. Which of the following actions by the nursing staff would be counterproductive to achieving this goal?
   a. Calling the laboratory to seek information about client preparation for an unfamiliar test
   b. Seeing that stat specimens are hand-delivered to the laboratory and that only real emergencies are marked stat
   c. Making sure that special needs of the client are conveyed to personnel from other departments who must interact with the client
   d. Complaining to other nurses about the lack of communication with laboratory personnel

References

Calzone, K. A., Cashion, A., Feetham, S., Jenkins, J., Prows, C. A., Williams, J. K., et al. (2010). Nurses transforming health care using genetics and genomics. *Nursing Outlook, 56*(1), 26–34.

Carpenito-Moyet, L. J. (2010). Invited paper: Teaching nursing diagnosis to increase utilization after graduation. *International Journal of Nursing Terminologies and Classifications, 21*(3), 124–133.

Corbett, J. V., & LaBorde, A. (1994). Nurses' perceptions of usefulness of laboratory data for nursing practice. *Journal of Continuing Education, 25*(4), 175–180.

Curley, M. A., & Hickey, P. (2006). The nightingale metrics. *American Journal of Nursing, 106*(10), 66–70.

Dwyer, D. (2009). Use heel warmers with care. *Nursing 2009, 30*(4), 59.

Evans, J. C., McCartney, E., Lawhon, G., & Galloway, J. (2005). Longitudinal comparison of preterm pain responses to repeated heelsticks. *Pediatric Nursing, 31*(5), 216–221.

Herdman, T. H. (2009). *NANDA International nursing diagnoses: Definitions and classifications 2009–2011* (2nd ed.). Hoboken, NJ: Wiley-Blackwell.

Jarrin, O. G. (2010). Core elements of U. S. nurse practice acts incorporation of nursing diagnosis language. *International Journal of Nursing Terminologies and Classification, 21*(4), 166–176.

Johnson, M., Moorhead, S., Bulechek, G. M., Butcher, H. K., Maas, M. L., & Swanson, E. (2012). *NOC and NIC linkages to NANDA and clinical conditions: Supporting critical reasoning and quality care* (3rd ed.). St. Louis, MO: Mosby.

Lunney, M. (2006). Helping nurses use NANDA, NOC and NIC: Novice to expert. *Nurse Educator, 31*(1), 40–46.

Malone, B. (2010). Healthcare reform arrives: How will labs fare in the new era? *Clinical Laboratory News, 26*(6), 1–6.

McPhee, S. J., Papadakis, M. A., & Rabow, M. W. (Eds.). (2011). *Current medical diagnosis and treatment* (50th ed.). New York: McGraw-Hill.

Morrow, C., Hidinger, A., & Wilkinson-Faulk, D. (2010). Reducing neonatal pain during routine heel lance procedures. *MCN: The American Journal of Maternity and Child Nursing, 35*(6), 347–354.

Muller-Staub, M. (2009). Evaluation of the implementation of nursing, diagnosis, interventions and outcomes. *International Journal of Technologies and Classifications, 20*(1), 9–15.

Pellico, L. H. (2005). Where's my stuff? *American Journal of Nursing, 105*(7), 13.

Pravikoff, D. S., Tanner, A., & Pierce, S. (2005). Readiness of U.S. nurses for evidence-based practice. *American Journal of Nursing, 105*(9), 40–51.

Roche, P. A., & Annas, G. (2006). DNA testing, banking, and genetic privacy. *New England Journal of Medicine, 355*(6), 545–546.

Staes, C. J., Bennett, S., Evans, S., Narus, S., Huff, S., & Sorensen, J. (2006). A case for manual entry of structured, coded laboratory data from multiple sources into an ambulatory electronic health record. *Journal of American Medical Informatics Association, 13*, 12–15.

Wu, A. H. (Ed.). (2006). *Tietz clinical guide to laboratory tests* (4th ed.). St. Louis, MO: Saunders Elsevier.

Websites

www.fda.gov/cdrh/clia (Information on the Clinical Laboratory Improvement Act.)
www.genome.gov (Information on the Genome project and current research.)
www.informedmedicaldecisions.org. (Research and guidelines on informed decision making.)
www.isong.org (Standards of practice for the International Society of Nurses in Genetics.)
www.jointcommission.org (Standard for laboratory testing.)
www.labtestsonline.org (Peer-reviewed site for information on laboratory tests.)
www.nanda.org (Updates on nursing diagnoses.)
www.ncbi.nlm.nih.gov/sites/GeneTests (Information on available gene tests and DNA banking.)
www.uspreventiveservicestaskforce.org (Evidence-based recommendations for screening tests.)

Answers

1. c, 2. d, 3. b, 4. c, 5. b, 6. c, 7. b, 8. d

- Red Blood Cell Count 25
- Hematocrit 27
- Hemoglobin 31
- Home Test for Hemoglobin 33
- Methemoglobin 33
- Erythrocyte Indices 33
- Red Blood Cell Distribution Width 35
- Serum Folic Acid and Vitamin B_{12} 37
- Methylmalonic Acid (MMA) and Homocysteine Levels 37
- Serum Iron Levels, Total Iron-Binding Capacity, Transferrin Saturation, and Serum Ferritin Levels 39
- Glucose-6-Phosphate-Dehydrogenase 41
- Reticulocyte Count 42
- Erythropoietin Assay 43
- EPO Urine Test as Drug Screen 44
- Peripheral Blood Smear 44
- Erythrocyte Sedimentation Rate or Sed Rate 45
- Total White Blood Cell Count and Differential 46
- Lymphocyte Immunophenotyping by Cluster of Differentiation (CD) 54

OBJECTIVES

1. Describe the purpose of each of the different tests done by hematology analyzers.
2. Identify appropriate nursing diagnoses for clients with increased and decreased hemoglobin (Hgb) and red blood cell (RBC) levels.
3. Anticipate how a change in the hydration status of a client affects hematocrit (Hct) results.
4. Describe how acute and chronic blood loss, iron deficiency anemia, and pernicious anemia change the erythrocyte indices.
5. Prepare teaching plans, which include specific information on drugs and diet, for clients with abnormal serum folic acid, B_{12}, iron, or glucose-6-phosphate-dehydrogenase (G-6-PD) levels.
6. Give examples of clinical situations in which an elevated reticulocyte count is an expected physiologic response.
7. Plan appropriate nursing interventions for a client who has an increasing erythrocyte sedimentation rate (sed rate, or ESR).
8. Compare and contrast reference values for the differential (diff) white blood cell (WBC) count in children, in adults, and in pregnant women.

9. Define the meaning of the phrase "shift to the left" with regard to the WBC differential count.

10. Identify appropriate nursing diagnoses for clients with increased and decreased levels of the different types of leukocytes.

Routine hematology tests can be performed by automatic counters, so the results are more reliable than the older method of counting under a microscope. Table 2–1 lists the tests routinely completed with a hematology analyzer, a standard instrument in all laboratories. If the WBC count is abnormal, it is necessary to know which of the five types of WBCs is increased or decreased. The test of the five WBC types is called a *differential*. Some laboratories call the tests listed in Table 2–1 a *hemogram* to distinguish this battery of tests from a complete blood count (CBC), which includes a WBC differential and a platelet count.

Sometimes only one component of CBC is needed. For example, if the primary concern is assessing blood loss, an Hct performed a few hours after the bleeding gives an index of the severity of the blood loss. With undiagnosed anemia, it would be important to have RBC, Hgb, and Hct values. The following three different measurements of the erythrocytes (red blood cells [RBCs]) are the figures used to compute the erythrocyte indices: (1) mean corpuscular volume (MCV), (2) mean corpuscular hemoglobin (MCH), and (3) mean corpuscular hemoglobin concentration (MCHC).

A reticulocyte count gives an indication of the rate of production of RBCs. One test that involves erythrocytes and that is discussed in this chapter is the sed rate, or ESR, but it really has nothing to do with erythrocyte production or function. The sed rate, or ESR, is a test for inflammatory reactions. A peripheral smear of blood is prepared to look for abnormal blood cells. This chapter mentions some of the common terms used on laboratory reports of peripheral smears. Related hematology tests (e.g., serum iron levels, folic acid, B$_{12}$ levels, and G-6-PD) are also mentioned because they may be needed to assess a persistent and unexplained anemic state. Although platelets are formed by the bone marrow, these fragments of tissue are not really blood cells in the true sense of the words. Platelets are covered with tests of clotting factors in Chapter 13.

All the components of a CBC arise from stem cells in the bone marrow. Figure 2–1 shows how these stem cells can differentiate and mature into the reticulocytes, erythrocytes, and the five different kinds of leukocytes discussed in this chapter. Platelets, or thrombocytes, are discussed in Chapter 13 and immunoglobulins and T-lymphocytes in Chapter 14.

TABLE 2–1 Usual Tests Done Automatically by Cell Counters[a]

Hct	Hematocrit
Hgb	Hemoglobin
WBC	Leukocyte or white blood cells (differential requires separate test)
RBC	Erythrocyte or red blood cells
MCV	Mean corpuscular volume (RBC distributed width can also be calculated)
MCH	Mean corpuscular hemoglobin
MCHC	Mean corpuscular hemoglobin concentration
RDW	Red blood cell distribution width (not always reported)

[a]Can perform all tests on 1 mL of blood. Blood is collected in a vacuum tube with EDTA as anticoagulant (lavender top). Platelet counts may also be performed with some counters. See text for difference between a hemogram and a CBC.

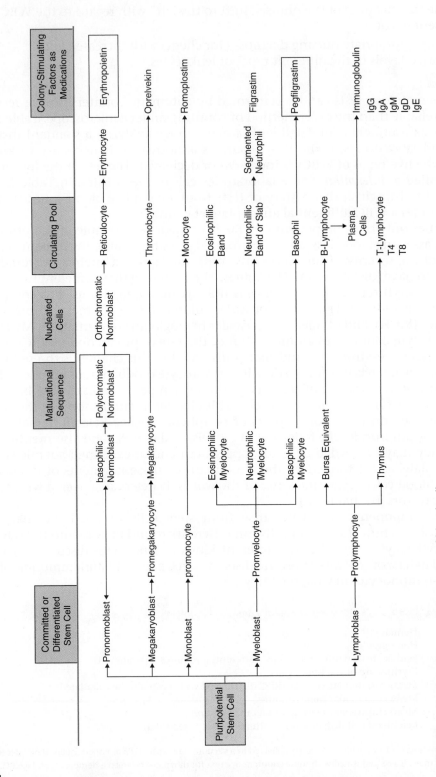

Figure 2-1 Formation and maturation of blood cells.

RED BLOOD CELL COUNT

The RBC count is a count of the number of RBCs per cubic millimeter (mm³) of blood. In addition to other less understood mechanisms, a hormone named *erythropoietin,* secreted mainly by the kidney, stimulates the production of RBCs by the red bone marrow. Tissue hypoxia causes an increased secretion of erythropoietin.

Preparation of Client and Collection of Sample

There is no special preparation of the client for this test, which requires 1 mL of venous blood. EDTA is used as the anticoagulant (lavender-topped vacuum tube).

REFERENCE VALUES FOR RBC COUNT	
Adult: Men	4.5–5.3 million (or 10^6)/mm³
Women	4.1–5.1 million/mm³
Pregnant women	Slightly lower
Newborn	5.5–6.0, gradually decreases
Children	4.6–4.8, varies with age

Note: Values increase at high altitudes.

Increased RBC (Polycythemia or Erythrocytosis)
Clinical Significance

Physiologic increases in RBC counts occur with a move to high altitude or after increased physical training. In both instances, the underlying reason is a response to an increased need for oxygen. At high altitude there is less oxygen in the atmosphere, so the bone marrow increases the production of RBCs. In the event of prolonged physical training, the increased muscle mass requires more oxygen.

The RBC count may be elevated for many pathologic reasons. One is a disease of unknown origin called *polycythemia vera*; the disease name implies that it is a true (vera) increase in RBC count. The increase in this case is not caused by an oxygen need, as it is in all other cases of polycythemia, which are termed *secondary polycythemia* or *erythrocytosis*. No general agreement has been reached regarding using the term *polycythemia* to indicate an increase in RBC count as well as other cells and *erythrocytosis* to designate an increase in RBC count alone. Two common clinical examples of secondary polycythemia, or more specifically erythrocytosis, are clients with chronic lung diseases and children with congenital heart defects who display cyanosis. The increased RBC count is an attempt to compensate for the chronic hypoxia brought on by the disease state.

In care for a client with an elevated RBC count, the nurse must differentiate primary from secondary polycythemia. In the event of primary polycythemia, medical treatment is geared to slowing the overactive bone marrow. Radioactive phosphorus was used for more than 40 years, but the usual current treatment of choice is phlebotomy to maintain a normal RBC count. (As polycythemia vera becomes more advanced, WBCs and platelets may also increase and thrombotic episodes may be severe. If the polycythemia or erythrocytosis is secondary to a state of chronic hypoxia, therapeutic measures are geared toward correcting the cause of the hypoxia. For example, the child with a congenital heart defect may undergo surgical treatment. For a client with chronic lung disease, hypoxia may not be treatable (see Chapter 6, on hypoxia).

Neonatal polycythemia, defined as an Hct above 65%, may be a response to hypoxia (active polycythemia) or due to factors that increase RBCs such as late cord clamping or blood transfusions (passive polycythemia). Treatment may involve partial exchange blood transfusion with normal saline (Armentrout & Huseby, 2003). A heel stick above 65% must be confirmed with a venipuncture sample.

Possible Nursing Diagnosis Related to Elevated RBC Count

Risk for Injury Related to Possible Formation of Venous Thrombi

One of the basic problems that occurs with polycythemia, regardless of the cause, is that the blood becomes more viscous, and this increased viscosity makes the client more susceptible to the formation of venous thrombi. A key goal for the client with polycythemia is to maintain adequate hydration. In some cases, it may be desirable to increase fluids to a set level, such as a minimum of 2,000 mL a day for an adult. Before assuming that fluids need to be increased, assess the overall status of the client, particularly the cardiovascular status. Both children with congenital heart defects and adults with chronic lung disease may often be on the verge of congestive heart failure. Confer with the physician to determine the optimal hydration state for individual clients. It is important that any client with polycythemia or erythrocytosis not become dehydrated. For example, it may be harmful for the client to avoid taking anything by mouth for an extended time before tests.

Encouraging Activity. The client with polycythemia needs as much activity as possible so that venous stasis does not contribute to the risk for venous thrombosis.

Decreased RBC

Clinical Significance

A low RBC can result from the following:

1. Abnormal loss of erythrocytes
2. Abnormal destruction of erythrocytes
3. Lack of needed elements or hormones for erythrocyte production
4. Bone marrow suppression

Anemia is a nonspecific term that can mean a decrease in the total number of RBCs, in the Hgb level of RBCs, or in both the number and the Hgb content of RBCs. Thus, if the RBC count is low, looking at Hgb levels is also important to classify the type of anemia. The classification of different types of anemia is covered in the section on erythrocyte indices.

It is not necessary for an RBC count to be used routinely to check for bleeding because the Hct can be performed more quickly. Refer to the section on Hct to see the nursing implications when the low RBC count is due to blood loss.

If the low RBC count is caused by a condition other than blood loss, then Hgb levels and a peripheral smear that identifies the shape and size of erythrocytes may be necessary to identify the type of anemia. Erythropoietin (EPO) assay may be done. Refer to the sections on Hgb and erythrocyte indices for related nursing diagnoses in different types of anemias.

HEMATOCRIT

The hematocrit or packed cell volume (Hct, PCV, or Crit) is a fast way to determine the percentage of RBCs in the plasma. When the serum is centrifuged, the WBCs and platelets rise to the top in what is called the *buffy coat*. Because the heavier RBCs are packed in the bottom, the Hct is sometimes also called the *packed cell volume* (PCV). The Hct is reported as a percentage because it is the proportion of RBCs to the plasma. Note that the results are based on the assumption that the plasma volume is normal. An Hct is useful as a measurement of RBCs *only if the hydration of the client is normal.*

Preparation of Client and Collection of Sample

Because the Hct can be performed on capillary blood, a client may undergo a finger stick (or heel stick for infants) rather than a venipuncture (see Chapter 1 for the procedure for heel and finger sticks). The first drop of blood is discarded. Enough blood is collected to fill a capillary tube supplied by the laboratory, and a small adhesive strip can be placed over the site. The stick method should be noted on the laboratory requisition because capillary values may be 5–10% higher than values by venipuncture. Do *not* squeeze the tissue to get capillary blood, because doing so adds tissue fluids, which dilute the sample.

REFERENCE VALUES FOR HCT	
Adult: Men	37–49%
Women	36–46%
Pregnant women	Decreases particularly in last trimester as serum volume increases—returns to pre-pregnancy values a few weeks after delivery.
Newborn	Up to 60%
Children	Varies with age

Note: Capillary blood may be 5–10% higher. Values increase in high altitudes.

Relation to Hemoglobin Levels

If the RBC count and Hgb are both normal, the Hct is about three times the Hgb. So a client whose Hct is 45% would be expected to have an Hgb level of about 15 g.

Increased Hematocrit

Clinical Significance

Because the Hct is a proportion (or percentage) of RBCs to plasma volume, any decrease in the volume of plasma causes an increase in Hct, even though the RBC count has not increased. For example, in a client with a burn, plasma can be lost in large amounts through damaged capillaries in the burned area. The loss of fluid from the vascular space makes the blood very concentrated, and hence the Hct may be as high as 60% or 65%.

If the client's hydration status is normal, an elevated Hct signifies a true increase in RBC count. Reasons for an increased RBC count (polycythemia) are discussed in the section on RBC count.

Possible Nursing Diagnosis Related to Elevated Hct

Deficient Fluid Volume

When caring for a client with an increased Hct, it is essential to find out if this is a reflection of (a) decreased plasma volume or (b) a true increase in RBC count. If all clinical assessments point to lack of volume, measures to increase the plasma volume are needed. For example, parenteral fluid replacement is an essential part of the treatment for a client with severe burns. In other, less severe situations, it may be sufficient to increase oral ingestion of fluids to overcome dehydration.

If the elevated Hct reflects an increased number of RBCs, additional fluids may be appropriate to decrease blood viscosity. The precautions for overhydrating a client with polycythemia are discussed in the section on increased RBC count, as is a nursing diagnosis related to the risk for the development of venous thrombi.

Decreased Hematocrit

Clinical Significance

A decreased Hct can be due to either (1) an overhydration of the client, which increases the plasma volume, or (2) a true decrease in the number of RBCs. The second reason for the low Hct is much more common. (See the section on RBC count for the causes of decreased numbers of RBCs.)

One of the important uses of the Hct is assessing the magnitude of blood loss. It is important for nurses to realize that a blood specimen for an Hct drawn immediately after a massive blood loss will probably be normal because both plasma and RBCs have been lost in equal proportions. Within a few hours after a bleeding episode, assuming the client has adequate fluid balance, the plasma volume returns to normal by a shift of some interstitial fluid into the plasma. The RBCs, however, cannot be replaced so quickly. The bone marrow takes about 7 days to make new cells, and those cells need another 4 days to mature. So a few hours after the bleeding episode, the plasma volume is back to normal and the Hct becomes low because the RBCs that were lost in the hemorrhage are still missing. *An Hct must always be interpreted in relation to the time the sample is drawn and to the probable hydration status of the client at the time.*

Possible Nursing Diagnoses Related to Decreased Hct

Risk for Excess Fluid Volume

In the rare situation in which a low Hct reflects an increased plasma volume, the client may show other signs and symptoms of excess fluid. Therapeutic measures may include a decrease in fluid intake. However, Hct is not a key assessment tool for volume expansion. (See the discussion on low serum sodium levels, Chapter 5, as a test for overhydration; see also Chapter 4, on osmolality.)

Risk for Activity Intolerance Related to Loss of Blood

Paleness of the skin and the conjunctiva are clues that there has been considerable blood loss. Checking for pallor of the conjunctiva is particularly helpful for assessing black clients. Because the plasma volume is usually replaced within a few hours after a bleeding episode, clients with low Hct may have normal blood pressures. If there is not enough fluid to shift in the vascular space to make up the loss, the blood pressure falls and the client shows signs of shock. However, if the blood loss is not severe enough to produce shock, the pulse may still give a clue to the magnitude of blood loss: The pulse increases when the client sits up—the "tilt" test. The pulse may become even more elevated if much exercise is attempted because the oxygen-carrying capacity of the blood is diminished. When the Hct is as low as 28%, the cardiac rate may be increased, even at rest. Monitoring the pulse before and after activity helps one assess the effect of the low Hct on the individual client.

Weakness and fatigue on exertion should be taken into account when planning activities. It may be better not to bathe the client, change the bed linens, and mobilize the patient all at the same time. If a low Hct continues to drop, a key nursing implication is to assess for signs of continued bleeding. A detailed description of nursing assessments for occult (hidden) bleeding is covered in Chapter 13, on clotting factors.

Differences Between Acute and Chronically Low Hematocrits. The effect of low Hct on the client depends not only on how low the Hct is but also on whether the loss is acute or chronic. If the Hct is low because of a sudden blood loss, signs of shock may quickly develop. A client with chronically low Hct may have only a few symptoms because the body has had time to adjust to the low number of RBCs. For example, clients undergoing renal dialysis often tolerate an Hct as low as 18%. (The low Hct in renal failure is partially due to a lack of the hormone erythropoietin, which is normally produced by the kidney.) A client with sickle cell anemia is another example of a person who may have a few symptoms related to an Hct as low as 18–20%. (In sickle cell anemia, the RBCs have an abnormal type of Hgb, which decreases the life of the cells.) The essential point to remember about interpreting the low Hct is to understand not only the reason for the low Hct but also whether the drop is acute or chronic.

Imbalanced Nutrition: Requirements for Iron and Protein

A client with a low Hct needs adequate iron and protein in the diet so that the bone marrow can manufacture additional RBCs. A client who has a lack of protein may produce less protein hormones such as erythropoietin. If oral intake is possible, the nurse may help the client choose foods that are high in protein and iron. Foods rich in iron are liver, egg yolk, lean beef, and prune juice. Iron derived from animal products, called *heme iron*, is readily available

(Continued)

Possible Nursing Diagnoses . . . (*Continued*)

for absorption. Iron from all other sources, called *nonheme iron*, is often not absorbed well because of dietary inhibitors. Food fortification to increase the consumption of bioavailable nonheme dietary iron has been effective in reducing the prevalence of iron deficiency anemia, particularly in young women and children. A dietitian can be useful to help plan optimal nutrition for clients with demonstrated deficiencies in iron or protein intake.

Deficient Knowledge Related to Iron Supplements

Once a client is deficient in iron, as happens with a chronic blood loss, it may be difficult to increase iron intake by diet alone. Sometimes iron supplements are prescribed. Clients need to be aware that iron supplements cause the feces to become dark greenish-black and that iron can be constipating. Iron is better absorbed in an acidic stomach, but some iron combinations are better tolerated with food. The client should not take antacids and iron together, because the iron is much less soluble in an alkaline medium. Other drugs, such as tetracycline and cholesterol-lowering drugs, also reduce iron absorption. The usual therapeutic plan is to continue iron supplements for about 3 months after the Hct is back to normal because the body takes this long to build up a reserve of iron. Clients are usually quite interested in knowing the change in Hct reading, and their inquiry can be a good occasion to explain why iron supplements are needed (Coyer & Lash, 2008). In the past, iron products were a leading cause of accidental poisoning in children. In 1997, the FDA proclaimed a regulation for unit-dose packaging for iron, and research showed this has been highly effective in presenting iron poisoning (Tenenbein, 2005).

Risk for Infection

Anemia with an accompanying iron deficiency may lessen the immunologic defenses of the client. Iron deficiency is often associated with other nutritional deficiencies that predispose the person to infections. Thus, measures to protect an anemic client from infection are warranted. (See Chapter 16, on infection control in clients at high risk.)

Alteration in Comfort

In addition to the fatigue and weakness discussed earlier, clients with anemia also are easily chilled. Extra blankets and warm clothing should be provided.

Risk for Alteration in Breathing Pattern

Dyspnea usually does not develop unless the Hct is quite low. When the Hct is low, the amount of oxygen to the tissue is reduced, but arterial blood gases are normal. Simply increasing the percentage of oxygen in the inspired air (FiO_2) does not solve the problem. For example, an anemic client with dyspnea would probably benefit more from a transfusion of RBCs than from O_2 administration. (See Chapter 6, on oxygen therapy, which may be needed for symptomatic relief.)

Risk for Alteration in Thought Processes

Some investigators believe that iron deficiency in children is accompanied by an impairment of intellectual performance and behavioral changes. Decreased work performance may occur in adults depending on the degree of the deficiency. Nurses should be aware of clients who are at high risk for chronic anemia and malnutrition because of the possible socioeconomic consequences of being unable to perform optimally at school or in the workplace.

Risk for Injury Related to Use of Blood Transfusions

If the Hct is less than 21%, a physician may order blood, usually in the form of packed cells, to replace the erythrocytes. Packed cells are used when the client needs the RBCs but not additional plasma. No set figure means the client needs blood. As discussed earlier, some clients have a chronically low Hct with few symptoms. Depending on the symptoms and on the individual circumstances, blood may be given before clients have an Hct as low as 25% or 30%. For example, if a client is going for surgery, it is important that the Hct not be too low—"too low" usually meaning less than 30%. Because blood transfusions can cause additional problems, such as allergic reactions or transmission of viruses, the physician may choose to let the body replenish erythrocytes normally whenever this is feasible. (See Chapter 14 for a discussion on transfusion reactions and nursing actions to prevent injury.) As a rough guideline, a unit of whole blood or packed cells raises the Hct about 3% in an adult.

HEMOGLOBIN

Hemoglobin is composed of a pigment (*heme*), which contains iron, and a protein (*globin*). If each erythrocyte has the normal amount of Hgb, the Hct is roughly three times the Hgb level. An Hct of 45% would indicate about 15 g of Hgb. It is not necessary to perform both tests to assess for bleeding. As already discussed, the Hct is a simpler test to monitor blood loss. If RBCs are abnormal in size or shape, or if Hgb is not being produced normally, the Hgb level cannot be estimated from the Hct. Hgb levels are necessary as part of the assessment for various types of anemia. (See the erythrocyte indices for an explanation of how the Hgb level is used with Hct and RBC tests to provide clear information about erythrocyte abnormalities.)

Preparation of Client and Collection of Sample

Venous blood is used for the test. EDTA (lavender-topped vacuum tube) is used as the anticoagulant in the collection tube. Hgb can also be assessed on blood collected with a finger stick.

REFERENCE VALUES FOR HGB	
Adult: Men	13.0–18.0 g/100 mL
Women	12–16 g/100 mL
Pregnant women	11–12 g/100 mL
Newborn	17–19 g/100 mL
	Average % of fetal hemoglobin
	1 day 77%
	3 wk 70%
	4 mo 23%
Children	14–17 g/100 mL, depending on age

Note: Values increase in high altitudes.

Increased Hemoglobin Level

Clinical Significance

Because a normal RBC already contains the optimum amount of Hgb, any increase in Hgb level must be evaluated in relation to the number and size of the erythrocytes. (See the discussion on erythrocyte indices for an explanation of how the Hgb level is used with the Hct and RBC count to determine if the erythrocyte is hypochromic [less color], normochromic, or [very rarely] hyperchromic.)

Decreased Hemoglobin

Clinical Significance

Because Hgb is a component of the RBC, all the conditions that cause a low RBC count also result in a low Hgb level. Some of the common conditions for a low RBC count are blood loss, hemolytic anemia, and any type of bone marrow suppression.

Hgb levels are low in clients who have abnormal types of Hgb, or hemoglobinopathies. RBCs with abnormal types of Hgb tend to be fragile and easily destroyed in the vascular system. The normal Hgb in adults is almost all adult Hgb (Hgb A) with only a very small amount (0–2%) of fetal Hgb (Hgb F). A process called *hemoglobin electrophoresis* can identify the specific type of abnormal Hgb that is present. More than 200 Hgbs can be identified, but only a few cause symptoms.

In thalassemia major, the client has an unusual amount of Hgb F and abnormalities in the synthesis of Hgb. In sickle cell anemia, the client has an abnormal Hgb called *sickle hemoglobin* (Hgb S). (See Chapter 18 for screening tests for sickle cell anemia and for thalassemia, which are both genetically determined.)

Possible Nursing Diagnoses Related to Decreased Hemoglobin

Most of the nursing diagnoses for a client with a low Hgb level are covered in the section on low Hct. Additional insights about the clinical significance of low Hgb levels are covered in the section on erythrocyte indices. (See the section on MCH and MCHC for nursing implications for hypochromic and normochromic anemias.)

It is possible to have a normal RBC count with a low Hgb level. For example, with iron deficiency anemia, the count may be near normal but each cell has less Hgb than normal. This is called *hypochromic* (less than normal color) anemia. The cells also tend to be *microcytic* (smaller than normal). Women in general need more iron than men because of the loss of iron in the menstrual flow, and women who have heavy flow may be prone to low Hgb levels. The demand for iron is increased in pregnancy. If a woman begins pregnancy with low iron reserves, she may become severely anemic as the pregnancy progresses. It is recommended that a pregnant woman be tested for Hgb levels at the beginning of pregnancy, about mid-pregnancy, and during the month before delivery. Because there is a normal drop in Hgb levels in the last trimester, due to the expanded plasma volume, some lowering in Hgb levels is "normal." This lowering is sometimes called the *physiologic anemia of pregnancy*. If the mother does not have enough stored iron to meet the demands of the fetus, iron supplements may be needed.

HOME TEST FOR HEMOGLOBIN

As discussed in Chapter 1, many FDA-approved test kits are available for purchase by consumers. The Anemia Meter Kit contains two lancets, alcohol wipes, gauze pad, adhesive bandage, and an "anemia meter" in a foil pouch. Results are available in 20 minutes. Consumers should discuss the results with their health care provider before they self-treat, as anemia can have many causes, as discussed in this chapter.

METHEMOGLOBIN

Methemoglobin is continuously being formed by the oxidation of heme iron to the ferric state. Normally, enzymes reduce the methemoglobin back to Hgb. Methemoglobin is not an oxygen carrier, so increased amounts of it can lead to cyanosis. The inability to reduce methemoglobin at a normal rate may be due to a congenital defect, but usually these clients have no symptoms (Hay et al., 2011). However, drugs such as sulfonamides, acetaminophen, dapsone, and benzocaine sprays can cause increased levels of methemoglobin that can lead to cyanosis and obvious signs of respiratory difficulty. Newborns are more susceptible to methemoglobinemia because they have less of the enzyme needed to reduce methemoglobin. Co-oximetry can be done on an arterial blood sample to determine the amount of dysfunctional hemoglobin. Usually, less than 1% of the total Hgb is methemoglobin. Cyanosis may occur when levels reach 15%. Methemoglobinemia creates a rust-colored blood specimen, Treatment may include ascorbic acid or methylene blue intravenously (McPhee, Papadakis, & Rabow, 2011). (See Chapter 6, on the effect of methemoglobin on oxygen saturation measurements.)

ERYTHROCYTE INDICES

To make the nonspecific term *anemia* more meaningful, it is necessary to see whether the individual RBCs are of normal size and whether they have the normal amount of Hgb. One can make the determinations by comparing the results of the Hgb, Hct, and RBC count. In laboratories that use automated counters—and all of them do now—the indices are automatically figured as part of the CBC. Nurses never need to calculate the indices, but the formula for each is given, because the formulas make it easy to explain the meaning of the results. In the examples used, the client has an Hct of 40%, an Hgb level of 13.5 g, and an RBC count of 4.5 million/mm^3. Note that with these figures, all the indices would, of course, be normal.

Preparation of Client and Collection of Sample

There is no need to draw additional blood because the indices are derived from the Hct, Hgb level, and RBC count.

Mean Corpuscular Volume

The MCV describes the mean or average size of the individual RBC in cubic micrometers (μm^3) or by volume in femtoliters (fL). The Hct percentage is multiplied by 10 and is divided by the RBC count to provide the MCV.

REFERENCE VALUES AND EXAMPLE FOR MCV

Reference values	$MCV = \dfrac{\text{Men } 78-100 \ \mu m^3 \text{ or fL}}{\text{women } 78-102 \ \mu m^3 \text{ or fL}}$
Formula	$MCV = \dfrac{\text{Hct (\%) 10}}{\text{RBC (millions/mm}^3)}$
Client example	$\dfrac{40 \times 10}{4.5} = 89 \mu m^3$

Note: Newborns and infants have higher values. Children have lower values. Some measure the MCV directly.

Change in the MCV Laboratories

Clinical Significance

The MCV is an indicator of the size of the RBCs. If the MCV is lower than 78 μm^3, the erythrocytes are *microcytic*, or smaller than normal. RBCs are microcytic in some types of anemia, such as iron deficiency anemia and lead poisoning. Thalassemia minor and thalassemia major (Cooley's anemia), which are genetic diseases, also cause microcytosis. (See Chapter 18, on screening tests for the thalassemias.) If the MCV is higher than 100 μm^3, the erythrocytes are *macrocytic,* or larger than normal. Macrocytic RBCs are characteristic of pernicious anemia and folic acid deficiencies. Macrocytosis is common in liver disease and is sometimes used as a marker of recent alcohol intake. An elevated MCV has been described as a predictor of mortality in clients with advanced cirrhosis. Excessive alcohol consumption often increases the MCV before there is liver damage. If the MCV is within normal reference range, the erythrocytes are *normocytic,* or of normal size. Anemia due to acute blood loss results in normocytic anemia.

The size of the RBCs is not enough to diagnose the reason for anemia, but with other indices (MCH and MCHC), anemia can be classified by size and color. Other tests, such as peripheral blood smear, can identify the characteristic cell shapes of various pathologic conditions.

Mean Corpuscular Hemoglobin

MCH is the amount of Hgb present in one cell. The result is reported by weight in picograms (pg). The weight of Hgb in the average cell is obtained by multiplying the Hgb level by 10 and dividing the result by the RBC count.

REFERENCE VALUES AND EXAMPLE FOR MCH

Reference values	$MCH = 25-35 \text{ pg}$
Formula	$MCV = \dfrac{\text{Hgb (b/100 mL)} \times 10}{\text{RBC (millions/mm}^3)}$
Client example	$\dfrac{13.5 \text{ g} \times 10}{4.5} = 30 \text{ pg}$

Mean Corpuscular Hemoglobin Concentration

The MCHC is the proportion of each cell occupied by Hgb. Because this is a proportion, the results are reported in percentages. To get the percentage, the Hgb is divided by the Hct and multiplied by 100.

REFERENCE VALUES AND EXAMPLE FOR MCHC	
Reference values	MCHC = 31–37%
Formula	$MCHC = \dfrac{Hgb\ (g/100\ mL)}{Hct} \times 100$
Client example	$\dfrac{13.5}{40} \times 100 = 33.8\%$

Changes in MCH and MCHC
Clinical Significance

These two parts of the erythrocyte indices (MCH and MCHC) are discussed together because both are ways to determine whether the erythrocytes are *normochromic* (normal color), *hypochromic* (less than normal color), or *hyperchromic* (more than normal color). Some institutions obtain only the MCH and not the MCHC. An MCHC less than 31% (or an MCH 0.25 pg) indicates that the erythrocytes have a decrease in Hgb concentration (hypochromic). Iron deficiency anemia is the most common type of hypochromic anemia. Chronic conditions that cause anemia may show some hypochromia, but they are usually not as marked as when there is a true deficiency of iron. Certain genetically caused anemias such as thalassemia (Cooley's anemia) cause hypochromia. With many types of anemia, the remaining cells have the normal amount of Hgb and hence are called normochromic. Hyperchromia (an abnormally high MCHC) is not seen except for a few rare conditions. As a rule, normal RBCs can hold only so much Hgb so the cells cannot be hyperchromic.

RED BLOOD CELL DISTRIBUTION WIDTH

The RBC distribution width (RDW) is calculated from the MCV and the RBC. Reference values are usually 11.5–14.5%. Only an increase in this index of variability is significant. The RDW as a numerical expression correlates with the degree of anisocytosis (unequal-sized cells). Clinicians may use the RDW to help differentiate various types of anemia. For example, in microcytic anemias, the RDW is increased with iron deficiency and beta thalassemia major but not with beta thalassemia minor. Macrocytic anemias caused by folate and B_{12} deficiencies show an increase in the RDW. The RDW should return to normal after appropriate treatment is begun for each type of anemia.

TABLE 2–2 Classification of Anemias by Erythrocyte Indices

Laboratory Results	Classification	Example of Common Pathologic Condition
MCV, MCH, and MCHC all normal	Normocytic, normochromic anemias	Acute blood loss, sickle cell anemia
Decreased MCV, decreased MCH, and decreased MCHC	Microcytic, hypochromic anemias	Iron deficiency, chronic blood loss, beta thalassemia
Increased MCV, variable MCH and MCHC	Macrocytic anemia	Vitamin B_{12} deficiency, folic acid deficiency*

*Another name for these macrocytic anemias is megaloblastic anemias. A peripheral blood smear will show oval macrocytes and hypersegmented neutrophils (Bain, 2005).

Possible Nursing Implications Related to Different Types of Anemia

It is important for the nurse to understand that abnormal erythrocyte indices are useful in classifying types of anemia, but they are not enough to establish a definite medical diagnosis. The history of the client, physical assessment findings, and other tests are needed to determine the cause of the anemia. Some general nursing diagnoses for clients with anemia are discussed in the sections on RBC, Hgb, and Hct. Other general nursing implications can be classified under the three categories of anemia. Table 2–2 lists the three categories and common pathologic conditions that could cause each type.

Microcytic, Hypochromic Anemias. Most likely, this type of anemia is due to an iron deficiency if other causes such as thalassemia minor are ruled out. The serum iron level can be measured, as can the iron-binding capacity and ferritin and transferrin levels discussed later. As discussed earlier, in the section on Hgb, it is difficult to correct an iron deficiency with diet alone. (See the section on Hgb for what to teach a client about iron therapy.) Because iron deficiency can occur due to chronic blood loss, men and postmenopausal women may be assessed for occult gastrointestinal bleeding. (See Chapter 13, on fecal occult blood testing, and Chapter 27, on sigmoidoscopy.)

Normocytic, Normochromic Anemias. The cause could range from acute blood loss to a chronic genetic problem such as sickle cell disease or other hemolytic disorders. With a normocytic anemia, iron supplements may not be needed, but the nurse should make sure that the client has adequate protein and iron in the diet because of the continuing need for an increased production of RBCs. If the anemia is of genetic origin, the nurse's role centers on helping the client and the family adjust to a chronic disease. (See Chapter 18, on genetic screening.) Anemia is but one sign of a larger pathologic problem.

Macrocytic Anemias. This type of anemia may be hypochromic, normochromic, or very rarely, hyperchromic. The two most common reasons for macrocytic anemias are vitamin B_{12} deficiency and folic acid deficiency. These two anemias are also called megaloblastic anemias. Megaloblastic refers to the appearance of a certain type of RBC precursor in the bone marrow and often in the bloodstream. (See the next section for two possible nursing diagnoses related to

> vitamin B_{12} and folic acid deficiencies.) Some drugs, such as zidovudine (an antiviral drug for HIV), cause macrocytosis. Macrocytosis occurs with cirrhosis, and alcohol abstinence reduces the increased MVC and RDW. Clients on metformin, an antidiabetic drug used in the treatment of Type 2 diabetes, may not absorb vitamin B_{12} well (Deglin, Vallerand, & Sanoski, 2011).

SERUM FOLIC ACID AND VITAMIN B_{12}

Both vitamin B_{12} and folate can be measured in the serum when the initial laboratory results show macrocytosis (elevated MCV), a low reticulocyte count (discussed later), and hypersegmented neutrophils. These tests are used to help in diagnosing a macrocytic anemia that may be due to dietary deficiency or malabsorption. Decreased folic acid and vitamin B_{12} levels are also being studied in relation to the development of Alzheimer's disease. Clients on metformin should have vitamin B_{12} and folic acid levels every 1–2 years (Deglin et al., 2011).

Preparation of Client and Collection of Sample

Check with the laboratory about food or drug interference. The test for folic acid requires 1 mL of serum. The test for vitamin B_{12} requires 12 mL of serum.

REFERENCE VALUES FOR FOLIC ACID AND VITAMIN B_{12}

Folic acid	3.1–17.5 ng/mL (aged may have lower values)
Vitamin B_{12}	>250 pg/mL (aged may have lower values)

Note: Some laboratories may measure the folic acid in red blood cells rather than in serum. Red blood cell values should be greater than 165 ng/mL (McPhee et al., 2011).

METHYLMALONIC ACID (MMA) AND HOMOCYSTEINE LEVELS

As noted earlier, the two most common reasons for macrocytosis are folic acid and vitamin B_{12} (cobalamin) deficiency. Two tests, other than direct measure of the vitamins, help differentiate the deficiency. Homocysteine accumulates with both deficiencies. (See Chapter 9 for more discussion on homocysteine.) Methylmalonic acid increases with B_{12} deficiency but not with folic acid deficiency. Also, MMA levels can detect early or subclinical B_{12} deficiency before serum B_{12} levels decrease. Laboratories may require serum, plasma, or urine samples for MMA levels. Check for reference values. Clients receiving B_{12} replacements may be monitored with MMA tests to ensure effective treatment. Urine levels may be measured for certain metabolic abnormalities (Wu, 2006).

Possible Nursing Diagnosis Related to Vitamin B$_{12}$ (Cobalamin) Deficiency

Deficient Knowledge Related to Need for Vitamin B$_{12}$

Because vitamin B$_{12}$ is present in all animal protein, a diet deficiency is rare. But mostly the problem is one of absorption. Vitamin B$_{12}$ deficiency is a rather common occurrence in the elderly, alcoholics, and clients who have undergone gastric surgery. Pernicious anemia (a type of macrocytic anemia) refers to a pathologic inability of the body to absorb vitamin B$_{12}$ because of the lack of the intrinsic factor in the stomach. (The Schilling test is a test for B$_{12}$ absorption; see Chapter 22.) About 90% of clients with pernicious anemia have autoantibodies to gastric parietal cells or to intrinsic factor (Candela & Meiner, 2004). Nurses can help clients understand that not all types of "tired blood" can be treated with over-the-counter vitamin and iron mixtures. Clients often do not understand that anemia is only a symptom. The underlying pathologic reason for the anemia must be determined to ensure its successful treatment. For example, if the macrocytic anemia turns out to be caused by pernicious anemia, the client needs vitamin B$_{12}$ for the rest of his or her life. So the nurse may be involved in helping the client and a member of the family learn to give injections. The importance of lifelong therapy must be emphasized to prevent relapses. Oral B$_{12}$ may be used instead of parenteral therapy. The dose is ten times higher when given orally (McPhee et al., 2011). Intranasal preparations of B$_{12}$ are also available (Deglin et al., 2011).

Possible Nursing Diagnosis Related to Folic Acid Deficiency

Imbalanced Nutrition Requirements for Folic Acid

Vitamin B$_{12}$ is present in all animal protein, so rarely do people in the United States develop a true deficiency. However, unless vegetables are fresh, folic acid deficiency can develop because most of the folic acid is destroyed by heat.

Pregnancy and the use of oral contraceptives are situations in which a macrocytic anemia may occur because of an increased need for folic acid in the diet. Recent studies have shown that an adequate intake of folic acid in childbearing women reduces the risk of neural tube defects. Nurses have been instrumental in educational programs to inform all women of childbearing age to consume 0.4 mg of folic acid daily. A 19% reduction in neural tube defects has occurred since the United States began folic acid food fortification in 1998. Although other factors may have contributed to this decline, the importance of folic acid supplementation has been demonstrated. Even now, not all women are aware of the need to also take the folic acid supplement before conception.

For clients who have erythrocyte indices that indicate some type of macrocytic anemia, the cause must be identified before supplementation is prescribed. Folic acid will reverse the anemia but not the other symptoms of pernicious anemia. Thus, neuropathy may continue to develop. About 2% of elderly people have undiagnosed pernicious anemia. Also, alcohol abuse may contribute to a macrocytic anemia. In such cases, diet teaching is of little avail until other issues are addressed.

SERUM IRON LEVELS, TOTAL IRON-BINDING CAPACITY, TRANSFERRIN SATURATION, AND SERUM FERRITIN LEVELS

These tests are not *routine* for all clients who may have iron deficiency. The screening tests of Hgb, Hct, and MCV combined with the medical history often are sufficient. The use of Hgb levels to detect iron deficiency may fail in some infants who do not yet show anemia. Therefore, researchers are investigating whether a test to identify Hgb in reticulocytes would be better for infants (Ullrich et al., 2005). Reticulocytes, discussed later in this chapter, are young RBCs that are in the bloodstream only for a day or two. The tests in this section are reserved for further evaluation of clients with microcytic, hypochromic anemia who do not respond to iron therapy. These tests are also used to evaluate iron metabolism and storage in diseases such as hemochromatosis, a genetic disorder that results in excessive iron deposits in organs.

Serum Iron Levels

Serum iron (Fe) levels can be measured directly. Because there is a diurnal variation in serum iron, with lower evening values, blood levels should be drawn in the morning. The client should not take any iron supplements for at least 24 hours before the test is performed.

Total Iron-Binding Capacity

Iron is transported in the bloodstream by transferrin, a plasma protein. Normally, about one-third of the available transferrin transports iron. The total iron-binding capacity (TIBC) is a measurement of the transferrin available to bind more iron. The TIBC is used with the serum iron to calculate transferrin saturation.

Transferrin Saturation

Transferrin saturation is not a direct measurement. It is calculated from the results of the serum iron and the TIBC. The formula is

$$\frac{\text{Serum iron}}{\text{TIBC}} \times 100 = \% \text{ of transferrin saturation}$$

Serum Ferritin Levels

Ferritin, the predominant iron storage protein, is directly related to the amount of iron storage in a healthy adult. However, illnesses such as infections, inflammations, and malignant diseases cause increased levels and thus may make ferritin level unreliable as an indicator of iron stores. If there are no chronic illnesses, serum ferritin determination is a very cost-efficient and reliable test for detecting iron deficiency. Malnutrition causes decreases, and thus ferritin levels, along with transferrin levels, are also used to assess protein depletion (see Chapter 10).

Preparation of Patient and Collection of Sample

Blood specimens for serum iron and TIBC are collected in *iron-free* tubes. Specimens for serum ferritin may be placed in either green- or lavender-topped tubes. Check

REFERENCE VALUES FOR IRON, FERRITIN, TIBC, TRANSFERRIN, AND ERYTHROCYTE PROTOPORPHYRIN

Serum iron	30–160 µg/dL (higher in men)
Serum ferritin	Normal 20–400 ng/mL
	Premenopausal women are in lower range
	Elderly may have iron deficiency erythropoiesis with ferritin levels as high as 75 ng/mL
Total iron-binding capacity (TIBC)	250–410 µg/dL
Transferrin saturation	20–50%

with the laboratory for amounts needed. Only iron must be drawn in the morning. An overnight fast is recommended.

Clinical Significance of Lack of Iron

Iron deficiency anemia results in a low serum iron level, an increased TIBC, and decreased transferrin saturation. In addition, the serum ferritin level is low (see Table 2–3). When there is no obvious cause of an iron deficiency, further investigations are necessary to identify the underlying pathologic condition. For example, iron deficiency anemia may be caused by an adenocarcinoma of the gastrointestinal tract, which often causes occult bleeding. (See Chapter 13, on hemoccult testing.)

Some risk factors include preterm or low-birth-weight infants and infants who are introduced to cow's milk before one year. School-age children should be screened if they have risk factors for anemia such as special health care needs or a background of poverty. Adolescent girls need screening every 5–10 years and then throughout their childbearing years. Extensive menstrual loss or known low iron intake would indicate the need for annual screening.

Clinical Significance of Iron Overload

Hemochromatosis (HFE gene), a common genetic disorder found particularly in Caucasians, causes iron overload. Mutations in the HFE gene can be identified. Nichols et al. (2006) noted that there is a complexity of relationships between iron absorption and binding, disease status, and HFE genotypes. Excess iron absorbed from food is deposited in various organs, such as the liver. Many people are unaware of the problem until serious damage is done to various organs. Therefore, some authorities, including the Iron Overload Disease Association, believe

TABLE 2–3 Changes in Laboratory Tests for Iron in Selected Diseases

	Iron Deficiency	Hemochromatosis	Hemosiderosis*
Serum iron	↓	↑	↑
TIBC	↑	↓	Normal
Ferritin	↓	↑	Normal to ↑
Transferrin saturation	↓	↑	↑

*Iron overload may be caused by iron poisoning or by multiple blood transfusions used to treat thalassemia (Chapter 18). See Wu (2006) for more details.

everyone should be screened for this disorder by the use of the transferrin saturation test and other tests as follow-up. Elevations of transferrin saturation, serum ferritin, and serum iron and a decrease in TIBC are characteristic of hemochromatosis. Once the disease is detected, periodic removal of blood (phlebotomy) can remove excess iron. Each pint of blood removes 200–250 mg of iron.

Hemosiderosis is caused by excessive iron intake or by multiple blood transfusions used to treat thalassemia. Clients may be given drugs to remove the excess iron. (See Chapter 18, on thalassemia.)

Possible Nursing Diagnosis Related to Lack of Iron

Imbalanced Nutrition: Related to Iron Deficiency

Nurses should be aware of the recommended daily requirements of iron for young children (15 mg), men (10 mg), and women of childbearing age (18 mg), as well as the specific needs during pregnancy and for the newborn. Diet teaching may help prevent deficiencies, but iron supplements may be needed, as discussed in the section on Hgb. Some iron supplements come with ascorbic acid to help absorption of the iron.

Possible Nursing Diagnosis Related to Iron Overload

Imbalanced Nutrition: Related to Iron Overload

Clients should avoid foods that are high in iron such as red meat and any medications that contain iron. Abstaining from alcohol is prudent to prevent any further liver damage. If the client has diabetes, the disease may be easier to control once iron levels are more normal. The American Liver Foundation (1-800-223-0179 or www.liverfoundation.org) has excellent educational material for the client with hemochromatosis.

GLUCOSE-6-PHOSPHATE-DEHYDROGENASE

Glucose-6-phosphate-dehydrogenase (G-6-PD) is one of many enzymes normally present in the erythrocytes. Some people have a lack of this enzyme because of a genetic defect. Hemolytic anemia may develop if the person is exposed to certain drugs, infections, or an acidotic state. Examples of drugs that cause hemolysis of erythrocytes in susceptible people are the sulfas and aspirin. The disease is also called favism because people with some variants of this X-linked disorder may have acute hemolytic anemia, 24–48 hours after eating fresh or dried fava beans. A peripheral blood smear, considered with the ethnicity of the client and clinical history, may give a provisional diagnosis before the assay gives confirmation (Bain, 2005). Several laboratory tests detect a deficiency of this enzyme.

Preparation of Client and Collection of Sample

There is no special preparation of the client. The test requires 9 mL of venous blood collected in a tube with a special anticoagulant (anticoagulant citrate dextrose [ACD]). Various laboratories may perform other types of tests that require only a few milliliters of blood with other anticoagulants. A screening test may be done before the quantitative measurement. An increased reticulocyte count falsely elevates G-6-PD.

REFERENCE VALUE FOR G-6-PD	
All groups	5–15 U/g Hgb

G-6-PD Deficiencies

Clinical Significance

The G-6-PD test may be used to determine if a hemolytic anemia is due to a lack of this specific enzyme. Other enzymes, such as pyruvate kinase, may also be deficient in the erythrocytes and cause anemia, but a lack of G-6-PD is more common. The lack of the enzyme is a sex-linked recessive trait carried on the X chromosomes, and mutations produce the variants that are identified (Hay et al., 2011). The effect is more pronounced in men. (See Chapter 18 for a discussion of genetic diseases.) Unless the person either is exposed to drugs that cause the hemolysis or has a severe infection or an acidotic state, he or she is typically unaware of the defect.

> ### Possible Nursing Diagnosis Related to G-6-PD Deficiency
>
> **Deficient Knowledge Related to Drugs and Foods to Avoid**
>
> A client who has a lack of G-6-PD must not be given any drugs that can cause hemolysis. Clients need health teaching about exactly which drugs are to be avoided. For example, many over-the-counter drugs contain aspirin. Certain foods, such as fava beans, are not tolerated if the defect is the Mediterranean variant. Different variants may cause different intolerances.

RETICULOCYTE COUNT

Reticulocytes are the less mature type of RBCs in the bloodstream. They are called reticulocytes because they show a fine network (reticulum) when stained. After about 4 days in the bloodstream, the cell loses this reticulum and becomes a mature RBC. The reticulocyte count (retic count) is valuable because it is a measurement of bone marrow function.

Preparation of Client and Collection of Sample

There is no special preparation of the client. The laboratory needs less than 1 mL of blood.

REFERENCE VALUES FOR RETIC COUNT	
Adult	0.5–2.5% of the total RBC count
Pregnant women	Slight increase
Newborn	Increased 3–5% first wk
Aged	Slight decrease

Increased Reticulocyte Count

Clinical Significance

An increase in the percentage of reticulocytes indicates that the release of RBCs into the bloodstream is occurring more rapidly than usual. Because this is a physiologic response to the need for more RBCs, the retic count may be as high as 10% after an acute blood loss. Such an increase is also expected when the appropriate treatment is begun for a specific type of anemia. For example, when a client with iron deficiency anemia is given iron supplements, the retic count may go as high as 32%. An increase in the retic count after therapy for anemia has begun is an encouraging sign that the bone marrow is responding to the treatment. Clients with sickle cell anemia usually have retic counts of 5–10% because of the increased destruction of RBCs and need constant replacement.

Decreased Reticulocyte Count

Clinical Significance

In certain macrocytic anemias (see the discussion under erythrocyte indices), cell development is arrested before the reticulocyte stage. For example, in pernicious anemia, the ineffective production of RBCs leads to a low retic count. A decrease in reticulocytes, particularly after a bleeding episode, indicates an abnormal response of the bone marrow. The client needs further medical evaluation to determine the reason for this lack of erythrocyte production.

ERYTHROPOIETIN ASSAY

Erythropoietin (EPO), a hormone produced primarily by the kidney, is the most important regulator of RBC production. Assays of this hormone may use several different methods.

Preparation of Patient and Collection of Sample

There is no special preparation of the patient. Conventional labs require 1 mL of venous blood.

REFERENCE VALUE FOR EPO

5–20 m/U/mL (children may have higher values)

Clinical Significance

An increased EPO, sometimes nearly double the normal value, is found in most types of anemia because the body is trying to increase the production of RBCs. One exception is the anemia of renal disease, because in this type of anemia, the kidneys have lost the ability to produce even normal amounts of EPO. EPO is available as a therapeutic injection, and nurses for a long time have been case managers for clients undergoing dialysis who receive this drug. Epoetin and darbepoetin are given subcutaneously or as an intravenous bolus (Deglin et al.,

2011). Paradoxically, these drugs can cause a more severe anemia by stimulating antibodies that cause pure red cell aplasia (PRCA). An increased EPO is found in polycythemia caused by hypoxia (secondary polycythemia) but is normal for polycythemia vera. Nursing diagnoses related to anemia and polycythemia are discussed earlier in this chapter, and nursing diagnoses for renal failure are presented in Chapter 4.

EPO URINE TEST AS DRUG SCREEN

As noted earlier in text, EPO has been manufactured to treat various types of anemia. Athletes, to improve endurance in competitive sports such as cycling, have misused these medications. A urine test, developed in time for the 2000 Olympics in Sydney, took advantage of the fact that the commercial EPO differs slightly from the natural hormone. Urine samples can be frozen for later testing. See Chapter 17, on the chain of custody for collecting samples for drug-abuse panels.

PERIPHERAL BLOOD SMEAR

The development of sophisticated, automated blood-cell analyzers has decreased the need for peripheral blood smears. Still, the blood smear remains a crucial diagnostic aid in various types of anemia, leukemia, lymphomas, thrombocytopenia, and thrombocytosis. In addition, a peripheral smear helps with the diagnosis of some bacterial infections and parasitic diseases (Bain, 2005). If necessary, a bone marrow aspiration or biopsy may be performed as a follow-up test for abnormal results (see Chapter 25). Some of the more common terms that may appear on laboratory reports are as follows:

Descriptive terms for RBCs

1. *Anisocytosis* means that the cells vary in size.
2. *Poikilocytosis* means that the cells are irregular in shape.
3. *Rouleaux formation* is a laboratory phenomenon in which RBCs stick to one another. (Note that this is the basis for the sed rate.)
4. *Basophilic stipplings* are a characteristic pattern of dark spots caused by some abnormalities of Hgb synthesis. This phenomenon is seen in lead poisoning and severe anemias.
5. *Howell–Jolly bodies* are small remnants of nuclear material found in certain hemolytic and megaloblastic anemias and after a splenectomy.

Descriptive terms for WBCs

1. *Atypical lymphocytes* (Downey cells) are characteristic of infectious mononucleosis, hepatitis, and other viral and allergic reactions. They are also present with certain malignant neoplasms of the bone marrow.
2. *Myelocytes* and *metamyelocytes* are two stages of immature leukocytes that are normally in the bone marrow, not in the bloodstream. Pathologic conditions in bone marrow production may cause the release of various immature forms into the bloodstream.

3. *Blasts* are primitive cells found in certain malignant neoplasms that involve the bone marrow.
4. *Döhle bodies* are small pear-shaped inclusions in the cytoplasm found in some malignant neoplasms, ingestion of toxic substances, and sepsis.

Descriptive term for platelets

1. *Thrombocytopathy* means abnormal-looking platelets. (See Chapter 13 for a discussion on platelet counts.)

ERYTHROCYTE SEDIMENTATION RATE OR SED RATE

The sed rate, or ESR, measures the speed with which RBCs settle in a tube of anticoagulated blood. The results are expressed as millimeters in an hour (mm/hr). An increase in plasma globulins or fibrinogen causes the cells to stick together (rouleaux formation) and thus to fall faster than normal. If the cells are smaller than normal (microcytic), they fall slower than normal; if they are larger than normal (macrocytic), they fall faster than normal. The laboratory takes into account any change in the size of the erythrocyte and corrects for this.

Because so many different conditions can cause an increase in globulins, fibrinogen, or other substances that can cause erythrocytes to clump together, the sed rate is a very nonspecific test. (See the discussion on C-reactive protein, Chapter 14, for another test of inflammation.) Both the sed rate and the C-reactive protein indicate a pathologic condition, but they do not identify the source. Sometimes the sed rate is explained as "showing how hot the fire (inflammation) is, but not where it is."

Preparation of Client and Collection of Sample

The test requires a minimum of 5 mL of anticoagulated blood. EDTA is used as the anticoagulant (lavender-topped vacuum tube).

REFERENCE VALUES FOR SED RATE

Westergren method

Adult: Men	0–17 mm/hr
Women	1–25 mm/hr
Pregnant women	44–114 mm/hr
Aged: *Men older than 50 years	1–20 mm/hr
Women older than 50 years	1–30 mm/hr
Children	1–13 mm/hr

Wintrobe method

Adult: Men	1–9 mm/hr
Women	1–20 mm/hr

*Upper limits may be even higher after age 65 years.

Increased Sed Rate

Clinical Significance

A marked increase in the sed rate during pregnancy is a normal occurrence because there is an increase in the globulin and fibrinogen levels during pregnancy. A pathologic reason for an increased sed rate is usually an inflammation or tissue injury. For sed rates greater than 100 mm (in the nonpregnant client, of course), the most likely causes are infections, malignant tumors, or collagen vascular diseases. Polymyalgia rheumatica and giant cell arteritis (temporal arteritis) represent a spectrum of a disease of unknown cause that affects older clients. Temporal arteritis can lead to visual loss if not diagnosed. A sedimentation rate helps determine the need for a temporal artery biopsy. The sed rate is often used to monitor the course of rheumatoid arthritis or pelvic inflammatory disease (PID) or infectious states in clients with acquired immune deficiency syndrome (AIDS). A micro-ESR is an inexpensive, easy bedside screening test for neonatal sepsis. Values increase with postnatal age (day of life plus 3 mm/hr). Up to 15 mm/hr is normal.

Possible Nursing Diagnosis Related to Elevated Sed Rate

Activity Intolerance

If the sed rate is used as a screening device, the results may not be useful in planning nursing care because an abnormal sed rate requires more testing to determine the underlying pathophysiologic condition. If the disease is known, the results of the sed rate are helpful in assessing the acuteness of the inflammatory process. For example, a client with rheumatoid arthritis may exhibit an increasing sed rate, which is one clue that the client may need therapeutic interventions to control the inflammation, as well as limitation of activity to allow inflamed joints to rest.

A decreasing sed rate is indicative of a lessening of the inflammatory response. The change in the sed rate should alert the nurse to confer with the physician about reevaluating limitations placed on a client who has rheumatoid arthritis. As another example, clients who take antibiotics for PID may undergo sed rates to determine if the pelvic inflammation is subsiding and thus if more activity is allowed.

Decreased Sed Rate

Clinical Significance

A low sed rate is usually not clinically significant. Clients with polycythemia vera, hypoalbuminemia, sickle cell anemia, or a deficiency in blood Factor V have decreased sed rates.

TOTAL WHITE BLOOD CELL COUNT AND DIFFERENTIAL

Two measurements of WBCs are commonly performed. One is the count of the total number of WBCs in a cubic millimeter of blood (WBC count). The other is the determination of the proportion of each of the five types of WBCs in a sample of 100 WBCs (differential). The first measurement, the WBC count, is an absolute number of so many thousand WBCs per cubic millimeter ($/mm^3$). The second measurement, the differential, is a percentage because it is a report of the proportion of each type of cell in a sample of 100. The precision of automated counters makes it easy to do an actual or absolute count of the various types of leukocytes. This absolute count is more useful than the differential. For example, if the total WBC count is 10,000/mm^3 with 2% bands (immature neutrophils) and 48% segmented or mature neutrophils, the absolute neutrophil count (ANC) per cubic millimeter is 5,000 (48% + 2% × 10,000). The ANC is useful for monitoring the effect of chemotherapeutic drugs that cause neutropenia.

It is important to understand that the differential is reported in percentages because an increase in the percentage of one type of cell always means a decrease in the percentage of another type, *even though* the absolute number for the second type of cell may not decrease. For example, a man has a normal WBC count of 10,000/mm^3, with a neutrophil count of 60% and a lymphocyte count of 30%. One can figure out that the man has 3,000 lymphocytes per cubic millimeter (10,000 total × 30%). If this man gets a severe bacterial infection, his total WBC may rise to 20,000/mm^3. In a severe bacterial infection, almost all the increase in WBC count is due to an increase in neutrophils. The differential count now shows 75% neutrophils and only 15% lymphocytes, but this does not mean the man has fewer lymphocytes. He has 15% of 20,000, or 3,000, lymphocytes per cubic millimeter, just as before. Only the proportions have changed.

REFERENCE VALUES FOR WBC DIFFERENTIAL

Adult: Men and Women Total WBC Count	4,500–11,000/mm^3 %	Absolute Count
Bands or stabs[a] (young neutrophils)	0–5	0–432
Segmented neutrophils or "polys" or "PMNs"	45–75	1,935–7,942
Eosinophils	0–8	0–756
Basophils	0–3	0–216
Lymphocytes	16–46	688–4,860
Monocytes	4–11	172–1,080

Differential adds to 100%[b]

Pregnant women	The leukocytosis of pregnancy (up to 16,000/mm^3) is due mostly to an increase in the neutrophils, with only a slight increase in lymphocytes. Labor causes a significant increase.
Newborn	On the day of birth, 18,000–40,000/mm^3, which drops to adult levels within 2 weeks. Reference values for differential have wide ranges depending on the time after birth. Neutrophils predominate for the first few days, but eventually lymphocyte predominance is seen.
Children	Until about age 3 or later, lymphocytes are more prominent than neutrophils. WBC counts up to 14,500/mm^3 may be in normal range depending on age. Consult a specific laboratory for relative values for the differential at different ages.
Aged	Some sources suggest the total WBC may decrease slightly with age.

[a]Bands may not be counted if automatic counter is used. To obtain bands, request a manual differential.

[b]If the laboratory uses certain automated instruments to count the WBC, some large cells may not take the stain properly. These large unstained cells (LUCs) may make up to 3% of the normal specimen. If there are more than 3% unstained cells, the laboratory performs a microscopic examination (peripheral smear) to identify the abnormal cells.

Increase in Neutrophils and Bands (Neutrophilia)

Clinical Significance

Neutrophils, classified as polymorphonuclear leukocytes (PMNs), seem to be the body's first defense against bacterial infection and severe stress. Normally most of the circulating neutrophils are in the mature form, which the laboratory can identify by the way the nucleus of the cell is segmented. Hence, some laboratories call mature neutrophils *segs* or segmented neutrophils; other names may be "polys" or PMNs. In contrast, the nucleus of the less-mature neutrophil is not in segments, but still in a band, so the lab calls these immature neutrophils *bands*. Another name for the bands is *stabs*, a name that comes from the German for rod. Notice that there are at least two names for mature neutrophils (segs, segmented neutrophils) and two names for immature neutrophils (bands or stabs). One way to recall the difference between bands and segmented cells is that bands are babies and segmented cells are seniors (Miller & Starks, 2010).

An increased need for neutrophils causes an increase in both the segs (mature neutrophils) and the bands (immature or young neutrophils).

When a client has appendicitis, one of the questions is: "Does the client have a shift to the left?" When laboratory reports were written by hand, the bands or stabs were written first on the left-hand side of the page. Hence, a "shift to the left" means that the bands or stabs have increased. Table 2–4 demonstrates what a shift to the left would look like in comparison to a normal differential in an *adult*.

Although, with a shift to the left, the lymphocytes appear to have decreased, as explained earlier, the differential is only a percentage. The total number of lymphocytes has not changed, but the neutrophils have increased. In bacterial infections, the total WBC does increase, and an examination of the differential enables one to determine that the increase is due to an increase in both immature and mature forms of neutrophils. Note that the WBC is just one aspect for

TABLE 2–4 Comparison of Normal Differential to a "Shift to the Left" in an Adult with an Acute Bacterial Infection[a]

	Stabs or Bands (%)	Segmented Neutrophils (%)	Eosinophils (%)	Basophils (%)	Lymphocytes (%)	Monocytes (%)
Normal differential— total WBC 5,000	3	61	4	1	26	5
"Shift to the left"[b]— total WBC 10,000	10↑	65	3	1	17	4

[a]In addition to the shift to the left, note that the absolute neutrophil count (ANC) has increased from 3,200 to 7,500, as determined by multiplying the total WBC count by the percentages of bands and segs (e.g., 64 × 5,000 = 3,200; 75 × 1,000 = 7,500).

[b]A newer term for "shift to the left" is bandemia. More than 10% bands is one of the criteria to diagnose sepsis (see Chapter 6, on lactic acid).

diagnosing appendicitis. Now scans such as CAT (computerized axial tomography) scans (CT) (Chapter 21) or ultrasound (Chapter 23) are routinely used (Zimmerman, 2008).

Possible Nursing Diagnoses Related to Increased Neutrophils

Risk for Infection and Spread to Others

When a client has an elevated neutrophil count, one of the first things to determine is whether the client has an infection. If so, should he or she be isolated to protect others? Although infection is not the only reason for an increased neutrophil count with a shift to the left, it should always be considered along with other factors. (See Chapter 16 for culture collections.) In the absence of any signs of infection, the nurse can assess whether there has been another assault to the body that has caused the bone marrow to increase the number of neutrophils.

Deficient Knowledge Related to Measures to Promote Recovery

The increase in neutrophils is actually a healthy response—a defense mechanism against an insult to bodily integrity. The nurse can help clients maximize their defense against assaults by promoting rest, adequate nutrition, and plenty of fluids. As the body successfully overcomes the assault, bacterial or otherwise, the neutrophil count falls back to normal. This falling neutrophil count is an objective assessment that therapeutic measures have been successful.

The term "shift to the right" is rarely if ever used to describe the alteration toward the other side of the neutrophil differential. A *shift to the right* may be used to imply that there are abnormal hypersegmented neutrophils, seen in some anemias and in liver disease. Sometimes a shift to the right is used to note a consistently high count of mature neutrophils that occurs in long-term infections.

Besides bacterial infections, an increase in neutrophils can be due to various inflammatory processes, physical stress, or tissue necrosis, such as that in myocardial infarction or in severe burns. As discussed in Chapter 12, there is increasing evidence that inflammation plays a role in the development of cardiovascular disease. Some researchers have suggested that a WBC count greater than 6,700 in postmenopausal women may be an independent risk factor for cardiovascular disease (Margolis et al., 2005). Newborns delivered by cesarean section have higher WBC counts than those delivered vaginally. Neutrophils are increased in granulocytic leukemia and in many other malignant diseases. Emotional stress can also increase the neutrophil count but usually not as dramatically as a physical stress. Some medications, such as lithium can cause leukocytosis (Deglin et al., 2011).

Decreased Neutrophil Count (Neutropenia) and Agranulocytosis

Clinical Significance

Although most bacterial infections cause an increase in the neutrophil count, some bacterial infections (e.g., typhoid, tularemia, or brucellosis) cause a decreased neutrophil count (neutropenia). (See Chapter 14, on serologic tests for infectious diseases.) Many viral diseases, such as hepatitis, influenza, measles, mumps, and rubella, also cause a decreased neutrophil count. (Most of these viruses cause lymphocytosis.) An overwhelming infection of any type may completely exhaust the bone marrow and cause neutropenia. Newborns, in particular, may deplete their bone marrow storage. Neutropenia may be an indicator of sepsis in the newborn. (See Chapter 16, on blood cultures.) Some drugs, particularly those used to treat cancer, can cause severe bone marrow depression. Radiation therapy, if it involves large areas of bone marrow, carries the risk of neutropenia. Antibiotics such as nafcillin, penicillins, and cephalosporins can induce neutropenia, as can psychotropic drugs such as clozapine, phenothiazines, and tricyclic antidepressants. Anakinra, an interleukin antagonist, slows the progression of rheumatoid arthritis but can cause neutropenia. So frequent monitoring is necessary (Deglin et al., 2011). Some adults may have a chronic benign neutropenia that is sometimes called *ethnic neutropenia* because it appears more often in blacks and Yemenite Jews.

The diagnosis of neutropenia in the pediatric population is fairly common. Most neutropenia observed in children is mild and occurs during viral infections. Most severe forms of neutropenia may be hereditary or caused by serious disease such as collagen vascular disease.

Agranulocytosis refers to a dramatic decrease in granulocytes (neutrophils, basophils, and eosinophils). The ANC will be 500 or lower. (A neutropenia of less than 1,000 is usually considered a critical or panic value.)

Possible Nursing Diagnoses Related to Decreased Neutrophil Count

High Risk for Infection

Clients with neutropenia (an absolute count of neutrophils less than 2,000) are prone to infections, and those with agranulocytosis (an absolute count less than 500) may have a rapid progression to a fatal sepsis (Thompson, 2009). Therefore, the nurse should carefully assess the WBC count to see any downward trends, and the client should be closely monitored for any signs of infection, such as sore throats, cough, or an occult rectal abscess. Fever may be the only symptom. (See Chapter 16, on tips for collecting cultures.)

Until 1983, reverse isolation was used for patients with neutropenia, but newer protocols based on research and the recommendations of the Centers for Disease Control and Prevention (CDC) emphasize meticulous handwashing as being the most important in protecting neutropenic clients from infection. Exposure to people with cold or other infectious diseases should be curtailed. Scrupulous personal hygiene must be maintained, and the environment must be controlled for bacterial and fungal sources such as fresh flowers or stagnant water. In addition, a "neutropenic diet" is served that avoids fresh fruit and raw vegetables (Leon & Pase, 2004). Granulocyte colony-stimulating factors (G-CSF), filgrastim or pegfilgrastim made by DNA recombinant technology, may be used to prevent severe neutropenia in clients receiving chemotherapeutic drugs (Katzung, Masters, & Trevor, 2009). For newborns, who sometimes have depletion of neutrophils, transfusions of neutrophils may be given to increase the storage pool.

Risk for Injury Related to Drugs That Cause Neutropenia

The nurse has the responsibility of checking the latest WBC count before giving drugs that may cause neutropenia. The nurse must confer with the physician, and the drug must be withheld if the neutrophil count drops below a certain number. For example, treatment with clozapine should be interrupted if the WBC drops to 3,000 or the granulocytes (neutrophils) drop below 1,500 (Deglin et al., 2011). The nadir is the point at which the WBC count drops to the lowest level after chemotherapy. Because in adults most WBCs are neutrophils, the change in neutrophils most affects the total count. However, neutropenia may be present even with a normal number of other types of WBCs, so the ANC discussed earlier is more useful.

For clients undergoing chemotherapy for cancer, the WBC count and ANC may be ordered daily. Some nurses become "chemotherapy specialists" and, under the supervision of a physician, take over the functions of cancer drug preparation and administration, client education, and monitoring of side effects, including the effects on the hematologic system.

Increased Eosinophil Count (Eosinophilia)

Clinical Significance

The actual function of the eosinophils is not clearly understood, but they are associated with antigen–antibody reactions. The most common reasons for an increase in eosinophils (eosinophilia) are allergic reactions such as asthma, hay fever, or hypersensitivity to a drug. Parasitic infestations, such as round worms, are another reason for an eosinophil increase. Other conditions in which eosinophils increase are certain skin diseases and neoplasms.

Eosinophilic pulmonary syndromes are a diverse group of disorders with pulmonary infiltrates and high eosinophil blood counts. Exposure to certain drugs may be the culprit, but often the cause is unknown (McPhee et al., 2011). Detection of eosinophils in sputum or broncho-alveolar lavage assists with diagnosis (see Chapter 16).

Decreased Eosinophil Count

Clinical Significance

Increased levels of adrenal steroids decrease the number of circulating eosinophils. For example, a decrease in eosinophils would be expected for a client with an allergy who begins corticosteroid therapy. Before the refinement of tests to measure corticosteroid levels directly, a drop in the eosinophil count after injection of adrenocorticotropic hormone (ACTH) (Thorn test) was an indirect measure of functioning adrenal glands. (See Chapter 15 for cortisol measurements.)

Possible Nursing Diagnoses Related to Eosinophilia

Deficient Knowledge Related to Avoidance of Allergens

If an increased eosinophil count has been attributed to a specific allergen, the nurse may be involved in helping the client learn to avoid the allergen. Otherwise, the eosinophil count may just be useful as an indication that the client is likely to have a history of allergies. This fact should then be taken into account in planning diets and assessing for allergic reactions to new drugs.

Possible Nursing Diagnoses . . . (Continued)

Risk for Injury Related to Infestation

If the elevated eosinophil count is due to a possible parasitic infestation, the nurse should question whether stool precautions are necessary. (See Chapter 16 for the collection of stool specimens for parasites.)

Changes in the Basophil Count

Clinical Significance of Increase in Basophils

The purpose of basophils in the bloodstream is not well understood. Few conditions seem to increase this relatively rare type of WBC. Leukemia and other pathologic alterations in bone marrow production may give rise to an increase in basophils.

Clinical Significance of Decrease in Basophils

Because the normal basophil count is considered to be 0–2%, a decline is not likely to be detected unless absolute counts are completed. Corticosteroids, allergic reactions, and acute infections all may lower the basophil rate.

Increased Lymphocyte Count (Lymphocytosis)

Clinical Significance

Lymphocytes are the principal components of the body's immune system, but only a small proportion of them circulate in the bloodstream. In the bloodstream, most are T lymphocytes (60–95%) rather than B lymphocytes (4–25%) or non-B or non-T lymphocytes (5–10%). The non-B–non-T lymphocytes are now called natural killer (NK) cells. To help assess immune deficiencies, such as AIDS, the laboratory must perform specialized tests of T lymphocytes. In the differential, all lymphocytes are grouped together. In adults, lymphocytes are the second most common type of WBC, after neutrophils. In children up to at least the age of 3 years, the lymphocytes are more numerous than the neutrophils. Even in older children, the percentage of lymphocytes nearly equals or even surpasses the percentage of neutrophils.

Lymphocytes increase in many viral infections, such as mumps or infectious hepatitis; they also increase with pertussis, with infectious mononucleosis, with some tumors, and often with tuberculosis. (See Chapter 14 for serologic tests for infectious mononucleosis.) *Chronic* bacterial infections cause an increase in lymphocytes. A common reason for marked lymphocytosis (80–90%) with blast cells is lymphocytic leukemia. Ninety percent of all leukemias, both acute and chronic, are lymphocytic. Acute lymphocytic leukemia is much more common in children, whereas chronic lymphocytic leukemia (CLL) is most common in older adults. CLL may cause a few symptoms and so may be detected when an older adult has routine blood work. The use of imatirinib often causes complete remission of CLL. Children also have a rather benign disease called *infectious lymphocytosis* in which the lymph count is quite high.

Possible Nursing Diagnoses Related to Lymphocytosis

Risk for Alteration in Health Maintenance

If the lymphocyte count is extremely high, the physician orders other tests to establish the possible existence of leukemia. The nurse needs to be aware of the specific type of leukemia diagnosed, because treatment measures and prognosis differ for different subcategories of the disease, and some types are curable, as noted earlier. The peripheral blood smear, maybe along with a bone marrow biopsy, is needed to differentiate clearly the type of abnormal white cells (see Chapter 25). Three potentially lethal complications in a leukemic client are (1) infection caused by the lack of normal WBCs, (2) hemorrhage caused by the lack of platelets, and (3) hyperuricemia caused by the increase of uric acid from cell destruction. (See Chapter 4 for a discussion about high serum uric acid levels in certain malignant diseases such as leukemia. See Chapter 13 for a discussion on low platelet counts, or thrombocytopenia.)

Risk for Injury Related to Infectious Process

If the lymphocyte count is not due to a malignant disease, the important question is whether the client has an infection that may be transmitted to others. Other measures, discussed under increased neutrophil counts, also apply because the nurse needs to help the person resist the assault that has triggered an immune response. The increased lymphocyte count is needed for a defense against a viral or chronic bacterial infection.

Decreased Lymphocyte Count (Lymphopenia)

Clinical Significance

Since the advent of the human immunodeficiency virus (HIV), a virus that affects T lymphocytes, much research has been done on the various types of T lymphocytes. Lymphocyte phenotyping uses flow cytometry to detect the many different types of lymphocytes. These subsets of lymphocytes are identified by their clusters of differentiation (CDs), which react to a cluster of monoclonal antibodies. For example, CD4 are the helper-inducer cells. (See the section on lymphocyte immunophenotyping.) AIDS causes a reduction in the total number of lymphocytes as well as changes in the ratios of the types of T lymphocytes. Adrenal corticosteroids and other immunosuppressive drugs also cause a decrease. Autoimmune diseases such as systemic lupus erythematosus commonly cause leukopenia and lymphopenia. Severe malnutrition also decreases the absolute number. Because increases in neutrophils occur for many reasons, decreased percentages of lymphocytes may often be explained by changes in the neutrophil count. Review the discussion in the beginning of this chapter if it is not clear why a marked increase in the percentage of neutrophils always causes a decrease in the percentage of lymphocytes, even though the absolute number of lymphocytes has not decreased.

Possible Nursing Diagnosis Related to Lymphopenia

Risk for Infection Related to Lack of Immunologic Protection

A client with a true (or absolute or actual) decrease in the number of lymphocytes is immuno-deficient. This client may need extensive protection from sources of infection. Also, if an immunodeficient client does get an infection, there may be few signs or symptoms that this assault is occurring. So the nurse needs to use careful assessment techniques to detect early infections in the absence of the classic signs such as fever. For example, clients undergoing chronic steroid therapy may have lower-than-normal levels of lymphocytes, so it should not be surprising that these clients sometimes have tuberculosis or other infections. Clients with AIDS are likely to have infections such as cytomegalovirus (CMV) (Chapter 14) or *Pneumocystis carinii* or *juveci* infection. (See Chapter 27, on bronchoscopy.) Since 1996, aggressive therapy with the newer antiretroviral therapy has markedly decreased these infections (McPhee et al., 2011).

Nurses can often help clients with chronic lowered resistance find ways to enhance their health by diet, rest, and all the measures too often overlooked as "simple" health habits. Sometimes the objective sign of a laboratory test can prompt the nurse to evaluate the total health of the client.

LYMPHOCYTE IMMUNOPHENOTYPING BY CLUSTER OF DIFFERENTIATION (CD)

The use of flow cytometry has made it possible to identify many types of lymphocytes. This identification of subsets of lymphocytes is most useful in the assessment of the immunologic status of a client. The lymphocytes are identified by their CD, each of which reacts with a cluster of specific antigens. The CD nomenclature was developed after some types of cells were already identified by other types of reagents, so laboratories may use other descriptions on laboratory reports. However, CD designations have become the common method for reporting results; many laboratories also include descriptive names. Wu (2006) lists CD1 to CD247 with detailed information about their uses.

Preparation of Client and Collection of Sample

Whole blood is collected. No special preparation of the client is required. Absolute cell counts require a CBC with differential on the same sample.

Clinical Significance

The reader is encouraged to review the immunology literature to find the most up-to-date use of lymphocyte phenotyping, as over 200 CDs have been identified (Wu, 2006).

The CD4 T-lymphocyte count has become important in the diagnosis and treatment of clients with HIV-1 infection. A CD4 count is a diagnostic case marker for AIDS. This test is also used as a criterion for initiating antiviral therapy for clients with HIV infection and for evaluating the response to therapy. (Also see viral loads in Chapter 14.)

CD3, the count of T lymphocytes, is used to assess the efficacy of OKT3 monoclonal antibody therapy in transplant recipients.

REFERENCE VALUES FOR LYMPHOCYTES

Cell Type	Mean (%)	Range (%)	Mean (cells/μL)	Range (cells/μL)
CD3 (T cells)	71	55–87	1,586	781–2,391
CD19 (B cells)	5	1–9	277	17–537
CD4 (Helpers)	43	24–62	1,098	447–1,750
CD8 (Suppressers)	42	19–65	836	413–1,260
CD4/CD8 Ratio	1.25	0.5–2.0		

Note: Flow cytometric analysis of peripheral blood lymphocyte subsets in children have shown that both the total and some subsets of T lymphocytes are higher in children up to the age of 3 years. Hay et al. (2011) note that CD4 declines to adult levels by about age 6 years.

Immunology laboratories can identify the percentage of stem cells related to the total WBCs in a blood sample. These hematopoietic progenitor (stem) cells are labeled CD34. Less than 0.05% is usually found. Lymphocyte immunophenotyping can also be done of bone marrow aspirates.

Increased Monocyte Count

Clinical Significance

Like basophils and eosinophils, monocytes are but a small percentage of the total WBC count. (Monocytes are present in tissues as macrophages.) Monocytes act as phagocytes in some chronic inflammatory diseases. A clinically significant increase of monocytes, for example, accompanies tuberculosis. Some protozoan infections such as malaria, as well as some rickettsial infections such as Rocky Mountain spotted fever, cause increases in the monocyte count. (See Chapter 14, on tests for rickettsial infections.) Monocytic leukemia, acute or chronic, also causes an increased monocyte count, but it is far less common than the lymphocytic type. Chronic ulcerative colitis and regional enteritis both cause an increased monocyte count, as do some collagen diseases. As a rule, the condition that causes increased monocytes is more likely to be a chronic condition, but further investigation for a specific pathologic condition is necessary to make the monocytic count useful in the clinical situation.

Questions

1. A client lost a large amount of blood during a mastectomy. An Hct drawn in the recovery room was 43%. It is now 12 hours after the operation, and the Hct just read is 37%. Which action by the nurse is appropriate?
   a. Take the client's blood pressure and call the physician immediately because the client is most likely bleeding again
   b. Slow down the rate of intravenous infusion of fluids until the physician can be notified because the client is probably overhydrated

    c. Consult the physician for further fluid orders because the client is probably slightly dehydrated

    d. Notify the physician of the lab report when rounds are made in a couple of hours because this drop in Hct is expected because of a fluid shift from the interstitial space

2. The test that is most frequently done to assess for loss of blood is the
   a. RBC count
   b. Hgb
   c. Hct
   d. CBC

3. The practice of being NPO for routine tests is likely to be detrimental for an adult female patient who has a
   a. Hemoglobin (Hgb) of 9 g/100 mL
   b. Red blood cell (RBC) count of 7 million/mm³
   c. Hematocrit (Hct) of 30%
   d. White blood cell (WBC) count of 3,000/mm³

4. As a rough guide, each unit of packed cells given to an adult raises the hematocrit about
   a. 3%
   b. 6%
   c. 9%
   d. 12%

5. Assuming that the erythrocyte indices are normal, the estimated hemoglobin (Hgb) level for a client whose Hct is 30% would be about
   a. 6 g
   b. 8 g
   c. 10 g
   d. 12 g

6. A female client has an Hgb of 11 g because of a continuing blood loss from a heavy menstrual flow. Which of the following nursing actions is the most appropriate?
   a. Encourage additional fluids to prevent thrombus formation
   b. Explain that increased physical activity stimulates increased production of red blood cells
   c. Assess dietary intake of protein and iron
   d. Prepare the client for the eventual need for blood transfusions to correct the anemia

7. Anemia caused by a recent blood loss would most likely be
   a. Microcytic (↓ MCV), hypochromic (↓ MCHC)
   b. Macrocytic (↑ MCV), normochromic (normal MCHC)
   c. Normocytic (normal MCV), hypochromic (↓ MCHC)
   d. Normocytic (normal MCV), normochromic (normal MCHC)

8. A low reticulocyte count would be expected for which one of the following clients?
   a. A client who has an untreated macrocytic anemia caused by vitamin B_{12} deficiency
   b. A client who has been receiving iron supplements for iron deficiency anemia
   c. A client who recently moved to a high altitude
   d. A client who had acute blood loss last week after a miscarriage

9. A 50-year-old client has rheumatoid arthritis that flares up occasionally. Her erythrocyte sedimentation rate (sed rate) is higher than it has been. The home care nurse is planning a visit to

evaluate the need for a change in care. In regard to this lab test, the nurse should consult with the physician about teaching the client to
a. Take additional fluids to prevent dehydration
b. Decrease fluid intake to prevent circulatory overload
c. Increase her activity to promote the full range of motion of all joints
d. Decrease her activity to promote the rest of joints, which are actively inflamed at present

10. A nurse practitioner in a women's health clinic, sees many clients of childbearing age. As part of her health teaching, she needs to inform the women that the risk of having a child with a neural tube defect is lessened if they have an adequate intake of
a. Vitamin B_{12}
b. Iron
c. Folic acid
d. Vitamin C

11. A client is receiving chemotherapy for treatment of cancer of the colon. His last white blood cell (WBC) count was 2,500/mm^3. On the basis of this laboratory report, a nursing care plan must include nursing interventions to
a. Protect from infection
b. Protect from stressful situations
c. Prevent stasis of circulation
d. Prevent dehydration

12. A client's white blood cell (WBC) count is 2,000, and the differential showed 40% neutrophils and 2% bands. The client's absolute neutrophil count (ANC) is
a. 1,640
b. 1,260
c. 840
d. 660

13. Eosinophil counts are usually elevated when the client
a. Has had an allergic reaction
b. Is undergoing corticosteroid therapy
c. Has a viral infection
d. Has a bacterial infection

14. A young woman is undergoing antibiotic therapy because of pelvic inflammatory disease (PID). The nurse checks the WBC count and differential to assess if the client has a shift to the left. Characteristic of a shift to the left is
a. An increase in stabs or bands (immature neutrophils)
b. A decrease in eosinophils
c. An increase in lymphocytes
d. A decrease in monocytes

References

Armentrout, D. C., & Huseby, V. (2003). Polycythemia in the newborn. MCN: American Journal of Maternal Child Health Nursing, 28(4), 234–239.

Bain, B. J. (2005). Diagnosis from the blood smear. New England Journal of Medicine, 353(5), 498–507.

Candela, L., & Meiner, S. (2004). Vitamin B_{12} deficiency: Issues in nursing care. *MED-SURG Nursing, 13*(4), 247–252.

Coyer, S. & Lash, A. (2008). Pathophysiology of anemia and nursing care implications. *MEDSURG Nursing, 17*(2), 77–84.

Deglin, J. H., Vallerand, A. H., & Sanoski, C. A. (2011). *Davis's drug guide for nurses* (12th ed.). Philadelphia: F. A. Davis.

Hay, W. W., Levin, M. J., Sondheimer, J. M., & Deterding, R. R. (Eds.). (2011). *Current pediatric diagnosis and treatment* (20th ed.). New York: McGraw-Hill.

Katzung, B. G., Masters, S. B., & Trevor, A. J. (Eds.). (2009). *Basic and clinical pharmacology* (11th ed.). New York: McGraw-Hill.

Leon, T. G., & Pase, M. (2004). Essential oncology facts for the float nurse. *MED-SURG Nursing, 13*(3), 165–171, 189.

Margolis, K. L., Manson, J., Greenland, P., Rodabough, R. J., Bray, P. F., Safford, M., et al. (2005). *Archives of Internal Medicine, 165*(5), 500–508.

Miller, J., & Starks, B. (2010). Deciphering clues in the CBC count. *Nursing 2010, 40*(7), 51–55.

Nichols, L., Dickerson, G., Phan, D., & Kant, J. (2006). Iron binding saturation and genotypic testing for hereditary hemochromatosis in patients with liver disease. *American Journal of Clinical Pathology, 125*(2), 236–240.

Tenenbein, M. (2005). Unit-dose packaging of iron supplements and reductions of iron poisoning in young children. *Archives of Pediatric and Adolescent Medicine, 159*(6), 593–595.

Thompson, N. (2009). Keeping neutropenic patients safe. How to protect patients and fight neutropenic fever. *American Nurse Today, 4*(3), 29–31.

McPhee, S. J., Papadakis, M. A., & Rabow, M. W. (Eds.). (2011). *Current medical diagnosis and treatment* (50th ed.). New York: McGraw-Hill.

Ullrich, C., Wu, A., Armsby, C., Rieber, S., Wingerter, S., Brugnara, C., et al. (2005). Screening healthy infants for iron deficiency using reticulocyte hemoglobin content. *Journal of the American Medical Association, 294*(8), 924–930.

Wu, A. H. (Ed.). (2006). *Tietz clinical guide to laboratory tests* (4th ed.). St. Louis, MO: Saunders Elsevier.

Zimmerman, P. (2008). Is it appendicitis? *American Journal of Nursing, 108*(9), 27–31.

Website

www.liverfoundation.org (Information on tests for iron overload.)

Answers

1. d, 2. c, 3. b, 4. a, 5. c, 6. c, 7. d, 8. a, 9. d, 10. c, 11. a, 12. c, 13. a, 14. a

Routine Urinalysis and Other Urine Tests

CHAPTER 3

- Collection of Urine Specimens 61
- Color of Urine 62
- Odor of Urine 62
- pH of the Urine 63
- Specific Gravity of the Urine 65
- Protein in the Urine (Proteinuria) 68
- Sugar in the Urine (Glycosuria) 70
- Ketones in the Urine 71
- Nitrites 72
- Leukocyte Esterase 73
- Examination of Urine Sediment (Microscopic Exam) 74
- Urinary Porphyrins 74
- Delta-Aminolevulinic Acid 76
- Urinary 5-Hydroxyindoleacetic Acid for Serotonin 76
- Collection of 24-Hour Urine Specimens 77

OBJECTIVES

1. State three important nursing considerations in obtaining the urine for routine urinalysis and for random testing.

2. Recognize findings on a routine urinalysis report that may have pathologic significance.

3. Summarize important points about the various types of dipsticks and other reagents used by the nurse for urine testing.

4. Explain when periodic tests of urine pH, specific gravity, protein, glucose, and ketones may be useful in planning and modifying nursing goals.

5. Describe what should be taught to a client about any 24-hour urine collection.

6. Give examples of common tests and the types of preservatives used for 24-hour urine specimens.

Because a routine urinalysis is indeed routine for almost every client, the nurse needs to understand fully the meaning of each component of urinalysis. All these tests are screening tests that may indicate the need for a more thorough assessment. All of the tests can be completed quickly with the use of chemically impregnated paper strips that can be dipped into a urine specimen. In some situations, the nurse may use this "dipstick" method as one part of the assessment. It is important to make sure that the materials for testing are fresh (note the date on the container) and that the directions are followed exactly. Some strips must be read within a certain time limit, and specific directions should always be included with the testing equipment. Because color changes are the basis for the results of the dipstick test, good light is needed, and personnel need to be examined for color blindness. (See Chapter 1 on testing by nurses.)

Specific techniques for each component of the urinalysis are covered in this chapter. Table 3–1 is a summary of reagent strips for urinalysis.

Table 3–1 Reagent Strips for Urinalysis

Substance Tested and Tips on Interpreting	Further Discussion in Addition to Chapter 3
pH—Colors range from orange through yellow and green to blue to cover the entire range of urinary pH. Make sure not to let urine remain on test strip, or the acid reagent from neighboring protein may run over and make the pH acidic or more acidic.	Chapter 6 on respiratory and metabolic alkalosis and acidosis
Protein—Detects as little as 5–20 mg albumin/dL. May be false positive with alkaline urine. Does not test for Bence Jones protein.	Chapter 10 on protein electrophoresis
Glucose—Enzyme method specific for glucose only. So need reduction method (Clinitest) for any other types of sugar. May be affected by ascorbic acid. Large quantities of ketone may depress color.	Chapter 8 on tests for galactosemia
Ketone—Provides results as small, moderate, and large. Reacts with acetoacetic acid and acetone but not β-hydroxybutyric acid. PKU or L-dopa can cause false positive.	Chapter 8 for serum ketone tests
Bilirubin—Sensitive to 0.2–0.4 mg bilirubin/dL. Icotest tablets are more sensitive. May be affected by chlorpromazine, phenazopyridine, ethoxazene, or ascorbic acid.	Chapter 11 for tests of bilirubin
Occult blood—More sensitive to hemoglobin and myoglobin than intact erythrocytes. Complements the microscopic exam. Affected by ascorbic acid and some infections that produce peroxidase.	Chapter 13 for detecting occult bleeding
Nitrites—Any pink color suggests urinary infection, but a negative result does not provide sufficient proof of the absence of bacteria, because some bacteria do not produce nitrites. Nitrates are also affected by ascorbic acid. High specific gravity may also inhibit nitrates.	Chapter 16 on urine cultures
Leukocytes—Positive test for leukocyte esterase suggests urinary tract infection. Avoid contamination by vaginal secretions.	Chapter 16 on urine cultures
Urobilinogen—False positive with porphobilinogen, P-amino-salicylic acid, or azo dyes, such as phenazopyridine, found in sulfisoxazole or phenazopyridine.	Chapter 11 for more on urobilinogen
Ascorbic acid—If ascorbic acid is as high as 25 mg/dL, the strip turns purple. Alerts that glucose, nitrite, occult blood, and bilirubin may not be accurate because of interference from ascorbic acid.	

Note: Complete information on all testing products is available by contacting companies that make diagnostic kits. Reagent strips in various combinations are available for consumers.

The last part of this chapter presents the correct procedure for collecting 24-hour urine specimens. The final table lists the usual substances tested with 24-hour specimens, whether any preservatives are needed, and where the test is covered in detail in later chapters.

COLLECTION OF URINE SPECIMENS

For a routine urinalysis, the laboratory needs at least 10 mL of urine. However, for the macroscopic urinalysis, done with a dipstick, less urine is sufficient. The microscopic urinalysis does require a little more urine. The perineal area in women or the end of the penis in men should be cleaned before the urine is collected. For a female client, collecting midstream urine lessens the contamination of the urine from vaginal secretions or menstrual flow; use of a vaginal tampon also helps in this respect. For infants, wiping with a sterile wipe may stimulate voiding or a collection bag can be attached to the genitalia. A cotton ball in a diaper can be used for quick collection of urine for dipstick testing.

If *culture and sensitivity* are to be completed in addition to the routine urinalysis, the urine has to be in a sterile container. In that case, collecting a clean-catch

REFERENCE VALUES FOR ROUTINE URINALYSIS	
Macroscopic urinalysis with a dipstick	
pH	5–9 with a mean of about 6 (depends on diet)
Specific gravity	
Adult	Range of 1.001–1.035. Random sample usually about 1.015–1.025
Infant to 2 years	Range of 1.001–1.018
Aged	May have a lower range because of decreasing concentrating ability
Protein	Usually negative; a few healthy people may have orthostatic proteinuria
Sugar	Usually negative; may be trace in normal pregnancy. Lactosuria common in last trimester
Ketone	Should be negative
Nitrites and leukocyte esterase (LE)	Both should be negative
Bilirubin	Negative
Urobilinogen	0.1–1.0 Ehrlich units/dL
Microscopic urinalysis	
Microscopic sediment[a]	
Crystals	Usually have little clinical significance (see discussion)
Casts	Most are pathologic; a few hyaline casts are considered normal
WBCs	Should be only a few white blood cells in the urine (less than 4–5 per high-power field)
RBCs	Only an occasional red blood cell is expected (less than 2–3 per high-power field)

[a]Performed if protein, blood, nitrites, or LE are positive. See Table 3–5 for significance of epithelial cells and other sediment.

urine sample may necessitate the use of an antiseptic solution as well as cleansing of the area. Limited research exists on whether the collection technique makes a difference in symptomatic women. Urine for culture and sensitivity is discussed in Chapter 16.

If the client is instructed to bring in a urine specimen from home, any small clean jar with a tight-fitting nonrusty lid may be used. The first voided specimen in the morning is ideal for routine urinalysis because the urine is concentrated, and any abnormalities will be more pronounced in the screening tests.

Urine specimens need to be examined within 1 hour. Urine that is left standing too long becomes alkaline because bacteria begin to split urea into ammonia. Visualization of microscopic casts and the test for protein are inaccurate if the urine has undergone a conversion to a high pH (i.e., if it has become alkaline). Urine should be refrigerated if the specimen cannot be sent to the laboratory within 1 hour.

COLOR OF URINE

Normally the color of urine, from light yellow to dark amber, depends on its concentration. *Urechrome* is the name of the pigment that gives urine the characteristic yellow color. When the reason for a color abnormality is not known, the laboratory must perform a chemical analysis to determine the cause. Usually the nurse or the client first notices that something is wrong with the urine color. Such changes should always be called to the attention of the physician and recorded in the nurse's notes.

A number of things can cause a change in the color of urine. If the client is known to be taking a medication that causes color changes in the urine, this information should be written on the laboratory slip. It is also important that clients be told about expected color changes in the urine so they do not become unnecessarily concerned. For example, phenazopyridine, a drug used as a urinary tract analgesic, causes the urine to turn orange. Table 3–2 lists some drugs that can change the color of urine. Some foods, such as beets or rhubarb, may cause color changes in the urine, as do some dyes used in food. Purulent matter in the urine gives urine a cloudy appearance. Blood makes the urine dark and "smoky" looking. Pseudomonas infections of the bladder may give the urine a greenish color. Bilirubin turns the urine a dark orange liquid that foams on shaking. (The other reason that urine may foam is the presence of large amounts of protein.)

ODOR OF URINE

Old urine has the very characteristic smell of ammonia because bacteria split the urea molecules into ammonia. If a freshly voided urine specimen has a foul odor, there may be a urinary tract infection (i.e., bacteria are converting urea to ammonia in the bladder).

A foul odor in freshly voided urine, however, may also be due to drugs or food. Asparagus gives a distinct smell to the urine. The unusual odor should be charted and called to the laboratory's attention for any needed further investigations. Some metabolic abnormalities caused by genetic defects can cause a peculiar odor in the urine of newborns. (See Chapter 18 on tests for genetic defects.)

Table 3-2 Drugs That Can Color Urine

Generic Name and Brand Name of Drug	Color Produced in Urine
Amitriptyline	Blue-green (rare)
Cascara	Red in alkaline urine, red-brown in acid urine
Chloroquine	Rusty yellow or brown
Chlorzoxazone	Orange or purple-red (rare)
Deferoxamine	Red
Iron preparations	Dark brown or black on standing
Levodopa	Dark brown on standing, red or brown in hypochlorite toilet bleach
Methocarbamol	Brown, black, or green on standing
Metronidazole	Dark brown on standing (rare)
Nitrofurantoin	Brown, yellow
Phenazopyridine	Orange-red
Phenothiazines	Pink-red, red-brown
Phenytoin	Pink, red, red-brown
Quinine and derivatives	Brown to black
Riboflavin	Intense yellow
Rifampin	Red-orange
Sulfasalazine	Orange-yellow in alkaline urine
Triamterene	Pale blue fluorescence

Note: Compiled from various sources. See www.mayoclinic.com for more examples of medications and conditions that change the color of urine.

pH OF THE URINE

Higher pH means toward the alkaline side, and *lower pH* means toward the acid side. Normally the pH of urine tends to be lower, or acidic, largely because of diet. Meat and eggs contribute much of the acid metabolic wastes, whereas most fruits and vegetables, including citrus fruits, contribute to an alkaline urine. Thus a meatless diet would be one reason why the pH of urine may be higher than usual.

Most bacteria that cause urinary tract infections, with the exception of *Escherichia coli*, make urine alkaline because the bacteria split urea into ammonia and other products. The urea-splitting properties of many bacteria also explain why urine left standing at room temperature for more than 1 hour usually turns alkaline from bacterial contamination.

Urine pH varies in different types of acidosis and alkalosis. All forms of acidosis cause a strongly acid urine because the body is trying to compensate for the acidotic state by excreting hydrogen ions. If the acidotic problem is renal in origin, however, the kidneys may not be able to secrete large amounts of hydrogen ions, so the urine is not strongly acid. One might expect that in alkalosis the urine would become alkaline because the body would tend to retain hydrogen ions to compensate for the alkalotic state. Yet the pH of the urine often remains acid, even with severe types of alkalosis, because the kidneys are obligated to excrete hydrogen ions if potassium ions are not available. The relations among potassium levels, acid–base balance, and urine and blood pH levels are discussed in detail in Chapter 6 on blood gases.

Possible Nursing Diagnosis Related to pH Testing

Deficient Knowledge Related to Measures to Control Urine pH

Usually changes in the pH of urine are not very important because the pH fluctuates with food and with the metabolic state of the client. Sometimes, however, it may be necessary to see that the urine remains alkaline or acid. For example, if a client has a tendency to form uric acid or cystine stones, it may be desirable to keep the urine alkaline or the pH at least as high as 6.5. Sometimes medications are given to achieve an alkaline urine. The nurse may need to teach the client to monitor the pH of the urine to see that it remains alkaline. This teaching is made easy by means of the dipstick method.

In other situations it may be desirable that the urine pH remains strongly acid (about 5.5). The two common clinical justifications for not letting the urine ever be alkaline are the following:

1. Alkaline urine promotes the growth of certain organisms in the urine.
2. Alkaline urine promotes the formation of calcium phosphate renal stones in susceptible people. Calcium oxalate stones are not affected by urine pH.

For example, people with quadriplegia are prone to the formation of renal stones because of the higher calcium content in the urine that results from a lack of mobility. Such clients are also prone to urinary tract infections because of urinary stasis caused by loss of bladder control. Increasing the acidity of the urine may help prevent both infections and calcium stones. Clients are told to drink cranberry juice several times a day to increase the acidity of their urine. Milk products may be limited, as may citrus fruits, which leave an alkaline ash. However, vitamin C tablets help acidify the urine. Research has found that specific compounds in cranberries inhibit the adherence of *E. coli* to the surface of the bladder. See Chapter 16 for more discussion.

Recommendations to prevent renal stones focus on preventive measures of ample hydration, avoidance of infection, and proper emptying of the bladder. In addition, some evidence supports that in men with recurrent calcium oxalate stones and hypercalciuria, a normal calcium diet combined with a restricted intake of animal protein and salt provides greater protection against renal stones than does the traditional low-calcium diet.

Testing the pH of Vaginal Secretions

Dipsticks may also be used on vaginal secretions. The vaginal secretions are usually acidic, but the presence of amniotic fluid makes an alkaline reaction. The pH is a test to assess if the amniotic "bag of waters" has broken.

Dipsticks for the pH of Gastric Contents

The pH of the gastric contents is strongly acid, whereas the contents below the pylorus are alkaline. A dipstick test of secretions from a long gastrointestinal tube, such as a Cantor, helps assess if the tube has progressed through the pylorus. Although children tend to have a higher gastric pH as compared to adults, research has shown that the pH test and the color of the aspirate can be used for proper feeding tube placement when an x-ray is not feasible (Westhus, 2004). The pH of gastric secretions is useful in monitoring the effectiveness of medications, such as cimetidine, given to reduce gastric acidity. (See Chapter 13 on combination pH and occult blood tests for gastric contents.)

SPECIFIC GRAVITY OF THE URINE

The urine specific gravity is a measure of the density of urine compared with the density of water, which is 1.000. The higher the number, the more concentrated is the urine, unless there are abnormal constituents in the urine. Adults have a wide range from very dilute to very concentrated. In infants, the upper limits for specific gravity are much lower than the adult limits because the immature kidneys are not able to concentrate urine as effectively as mature kidneys. Often nurses may measure specific gravity as part of an assessment of fluid balance, using a urinometer, or a refractometer, or dipsticks as discussed earlier.

Two Methods for Testing Specific Gravity

Urinometer

An older method to test specific gravity uses a float called a *urinometer* or *hydrometer*. The float has been calibrated to the 1.000 mark when floating in distilled water at 68–72°F (20.2–22.4°C).

A test tube is filled with 20 mL of urine, and the float is placed into the liquid. The higher the density of the urine, the more the float rises in the urine. The calibrated mark on the float that the urine covers is the specific gravity reading. Reading the marks exactly is sometimes difficult because the numbers are very small and close together. However, a reading of 1.011 or 1.012 is acceptable, because only wide variations are clinically significant.

Refractometer

The refractometer looks like a small telescope. Only a drop of urine is needed. This drop is placed on a slide at the end of the scope, and the refractor is held up to a light. The instrument must be kept level. The density of the particles in the urine determines the direction of the beam of light through the eye of the scope. The refractor is calibrated to translate the refractive index into the standard way of reporting the specific gravity. For example, if the light beam is at the 1.026 mark, this figure is recorded as the specific gravity of the urine.

The refractor has an added advantage of measuring the protein content in the same drop of urine. The protein measurements are on the right side of the scale. Knowledge about the presence of protein in the urine is important in measuring specific gravity because protein in the urine makes specific gravity falsely high.

REFERENCE VALUES FOR SPECIFIC GRAVITY	
Adult	Range of 1.001–1.040 with random samples of about 1.015–1.025
Infant to 2 years	1.001–1.018
Aged	May have a decrease in concentrating power so that upper limits are lowered

Increase in Specific Gravity

Clinical Significance

The specific gravity is falsely high if glucose, protein, or a dye used for diagnostic purposes is in the urine. All these abnormal constituents increase the density of the urine. If they are not present, the high specific gravity means the kidneys are putting out very concentrated urine, for which there are two reasons: (1) the client is lacking in fluids or (2) there is an increased secretion of antidiuretic hormone (ADH), which causes a decrease in urine volume. Trauma, stress reactions, and many drugs cause increased ADH secretion.

If the urine does not contain protein, glucose, or dyes, a high urine specific gravity most often indicates that the client needs additional fluids. It is much rarer that a high specific gravity would be caused by an increased secretion of ADH.

Nurses should understand, however, the nature of a phenomenon called *surgical diuresis*. In a client who has experienced considerable stress, such as a major surgical procedure, the urine specific gravity is higher than normal because additional fluid is being held in reserve in the vascular system because of the presence of extra ADH and other hormones. As the stress lessens, ADH and other hormones, such as the glucocorticosteroids, return to normal levels, and the fluid that was held in reserve is then excreted. This excretion of extra urine a few days after an operation is sometimes referred to as surgical diuresis. It is important for nurses to understand the nature of this kind of fluid retention so that they do not overload clients with fluids because the specific gravity is a little higher than normal.

Possible Nursing Diagnosis Related to Increased Specific Gravity

Deficient Fluid Volume

A specific gravity that continues to increase or that remains high when stress is not an overriding factor is a clear indication that the client is not achieving adequate fluid intake. In acutely ill clients, this condition necessitates medical orders for increased intravenous infusion of fluids. In the nursing home setting or for clients with chronic problems, it may be up to the nurse to devise ways to provide the client with oral fluids. A specific gravity that drops back to normal is an objective evaluation that the client is no longer dehydrated. Specific gravity readings are more objective than charting "concentrated" urine. However, color of urine may be significant. Mentes, Wakefield, and Culp (2006) discussed the use of a color chart developed by Armstrong and colleagues to monitor the hydration status of nursing home residents.

The nurse also needs to be aware of clients who could be dehydrated because of a shift into a "third space." The normal two spaces are intracellular fluid and extracellular fluid compartments. A third space is any fluid collection that is physiologically useless, such as edema or ascites. "Third spacing" creates the potential for hypovolemia and decreased renal output.

Decreased Specific Gravity
Clinical Significance

A low specific gravity is indicative of dilute urine. Dilute urine is normal if the client has consumed a considerable amount of fluids. Diuretics cause a large urine output with a low specific gravity. Chapter 4 contains a discussion of tests for serum and urine osmolality. These tests are much more accurate in determining the actual dilution or concentration of the urine as compared with the dilution or concentration of the plasma. Specific gravity readings are only crude indicators of fluid imbalances in serious conditions.

Sometimes a client has a *fixed specific gravity* around 1.010. (This reading is usually pronounced as "ten-ten" because "one-point-zero-one-zero" is much harder to say.) A fixed specific gravity does not change even when the client becomes dehydrated. This continuously low specific gravity indicates that the kidneys have lost the ability to concentrate urine. The fixed specific gravity is always about 1.010 because this value is the density of the plasma.

Another rare reason for a continuously low specific gravity is a deficiency of ADH. If not enough ADH is being secreted by the posterior pituitary gland, the kidneys excrete too much water. This condition is called *diabetes insipidus*. See Chapter 4 on serum osmolality.

Possible Nursing Diagnoses Related to Decreased Specific Gravity

Risk for Excess Fluid Volume

Often a careful assessment of the client's total fluid intake uncovers the explanation for a low specific gravity. If the intake is larger than normal, it may be necessary to evaluate the possibility that the client is in danger of a fluid overload. For example, clients may be receiving intravenous fluids in addition to oral intake. Intake and output records and daily weights help assess any fluid overload.

Risk for Alterations in Health Maintenance

A persistently low specific gravity when the fluid intake is not high is a serious sign that necessitates medical evaluation. A low specific gravity of a routine early morning specimen indicates the need for a thorough assessment of the renal system and an evaluation of ADH secretion if the physician deems it necessary. People with fixed low specific gravities (1.010) may have difficulty getting medical insurance because they are considered at high risk for future renal problems.

A client who is known to have a fixed specific gravity of 1.010 needs to be kept well hydrated so that the kidneys can effectively remove waste products. As kidney disease progresses, fluid restrictions and other interventions may be needed. The two common tests for renal function, BUN and creatinine, and the possible nursing diagnoses related to each are covered in Chapter 4.

PROTEIN IN THE URINE (PROTEINURIA)
Qualitative Method

Most often protein in the urine is checked by the dipstick method. This method does not detect the presence of abnormal proteins such as the globulins and the Bence Jones protein of myelomas. For most screening purposes, however, the dipstick method is adequate (see Table 3–1 for one type of dipstick). Nurses often use it for testing for albumin in the urine of prenatal clients. People with diabetes are prone to renal disease, so they may undergo yearly checks for microalbumin, which is discussed later in this section. If there is a need to check the urine for protein other than albumin, the laboratory uses other agents such as sulfosalicyclic acid. The dipsticks are designed to be used with acid urine, so there may be a false positive for protein if the urine is highly alkaline. Time is not critical in reading the results. Note the exact color chart for each particular brand.

REFERENCE VALUES (QUALITATIVE METHOD) FOR PROTEIN IN URINE	
Trace	As little as 25 mg/dL[a]
1+	30 mg/dL
2+	100 mg/dL
3+	300 mg/dL
4+	More than 2,000 mg/dL

[a]See discussion on microalbuminuria for identifying very early nephropathy.

Microalbuminuria

Normally the urine contains less than 1.0 mg/dL of albumin, but as noted above, the standard dipsticks for urinalysis begin showing a trace of albumin only when levels are about 25 mg/dL. Clients who are spilling small amounts of albumin that cannot be detected by the older method of testing are said to have microalbuminuria. The term was coined to mean a small amount of albumin, not a small molecule of albumin.

A dipstick using a semiquantitative immunoassay can detect albumin excretion as low as 1.0 mg/dL. The laboratory may report a microalbumin-to-creatinine ratio. This test has become important in detecting very early diabetic nephropathy. People with type 1 diabetes (see Chapter 8 on the new classifications of diabetes) should be tested annually after they reach puberty or after they have had the disease for 5 years. Clients with type 2 diabetes should be tested at diagnosis and then on an annual basis (www.diabetes.org). The presence of microalbuminuria calls for interventions to help prevent a decrease in renal function. If glucose control is not optimal, the client needs help in achieving tight glucose control (see Chapter 8). Also, the amount of protein in the diet needs to be evaluated, as high levels of protein may be harmful. In the United States, many people consume much more protein than the recommended daily allowance of 0.8 g of protein per kilogram of weight. For clients who have microalbuminuria, the American Diabetes Association recommends that clients have no more than the RDA.

Albumin-to-Creatinine Ratio

In addition to dipstick test, a 12- or 24-hour urine specimen may be sent to the laboratory to assess the small amount of albumin that is being excreted by the kidneys. A ratio greater than 300 mg of albumin/1 g of creatinine for someone without diabetes signals chronic kidney disease. For people with diabetes who have as little as 30 mg albumin/1 g creatinine should receive treatment by a nephrologist (Castner, 2010).

Drugs to control hypertension may be needed. The use of drugs that inhibit the angiotensin-converting enzyme (ACE inhibitors) has been shown to delay progression of renal disease in clients with diabetes. Evidence exists that these drugs can significantly slow progression of kidney disease in people with diabetes, even when blood pressure is normal. ACE inhibitors to treat microalbuminuria are also effective in nondiabetic renal disease.

Clinical Significance

Severe stress can cause proteinuria, but this is usually a temporary occurrence. Clients should not be tested during acute febrile episodes, during urinary infections, or after the administration of drugs that can cause renal damage. Heavy exercise may also cause transient proteinuria. Persistent protein in the urine is a common characteristic of renal dysfunction. Almost all types of kidney disease cause mild (up to 500 mg a day) to moderate (up to 4,000 mg a day) protein leakage into the urine. Some people have proteinuria that is called *orthostatic* or *postural* because it occurs only when the person is in the upright position. Usually no renal abnormalities are associated with this apparently benign condition. Preeclampsia and toxemia of pregnancy cause massive loss of protein in the urine. In what is called the *nephrotic syndrome*, which may be the end result of many diseases that cause renal dysfunction, the protein loss is as much as 4,000 mg a day. Albumin is the primary protein lost in all these conditions. Myelomas and certain other malignant tumors cause large protein losses, too, but because these proteins are abnormal, it is necessary for the laboratory to use special quantitative methods to determine the presence of these proteins. (See Chapter 10 on urine protein electrophoresis.)

Possible Nursing Diagnoses Related to Proteinuria

Alteration in Health Management

Persistent protein in the urine is an indication for further assessment of the renal system. Also, proteinuria, detected by the inexpensive urine dipstick, can independently indicate patients at greater risk for coronary heart disease and stroke (Madison et al., 2006). The nurse may be the one to explain to the client how to collect a 24-hour specimen. If the proteinuria is due to renal dysfunction, other laboratory tests should be completed to assess the degree of impairment. (See Chapter 4.) A client with diabetes who tests positive for microalbuminuria may need help in achieving optimal glucose control (see Chapter 8), tight blood pressure control, and restrictions in protein intake (see Chapter 10). Lifestyle modifications related to smoking and cholesterol (see Chapter 9) may also be needed.

Alteration in Health Management for Pregnant Clients

For a pregnant client, a check for protein in the urine is a routine part of each prenatal visit. If repeated dipsticks with a clean-catch specimen show proteinuria, a quantitative analysis is performed. In pregnancy, a 24-hour urine collection for protein should not contain more than 500 mg. In the event that the pregnant client begins to show protein in the urine, it is important to assess carefully for hypertension and edema. Proteinuria, hypertension, and edema have been the classic triad for preeclampsia. In pregnant women with chronic hypertension, proteinuria is associated with adverse neonatal outcomes independent of the development of preeclampsia. See Chapter 18 for an update on preeclampsia.

GLUCOSE IN THE URINE (GLYCOSURIA)

There are two different methods of screening for glucose in the urine:

1. Dipsticks change color in the presence of glucose because of the reaction of an enzyme, glucose oxidase.
2. Clinitest tablets use the reducing properties of cupric oxide to cause a color change in the presence of glucose and other sugars.

Increased Glucose in the Urine (Glycosuria)

Clinical Significance

Glucose in the urine signifies either (a) hyperglycemia (see Chapter 8 for a detailed discussion of the causes of hyperglycemia) or (b) a decreased renal threshold for glucose.

The *renal threshold* for glucose is usually about 160–190 mg/100 mL in the blood; in other words, no glucose is spilled into the urine until the blood glucose rises above this level. Various situations may alter the renal threshold for glucose. For example, in pregnancy the renal threshold for glucose may be lowered so that small amounts of glycosuria may be present and are usually not considered abnormal. Lactosuria is common in the third trimester. Clients receiving hyperalimentation have glycosuria if the intravenous solution (which has very concentrated glucose) is infused faster than the pancreas can produce insulin.

> ## Possible Nursing Diagnosis Related to Glycosuria
>
> ### Risk for Deficient Fluid Volume
>
> A high concentration of glucose in the blood acts as an osmotic diuretic, so water is excreted as the glucose spills into the urine. The presence of glycosuria, from any cause, alerts the nurse that the client needs additional fluid intake and could undergo severe dehydration if the glycosuria is allowed to continue. (See Chapter 8 for a discussion on hyperglycemic hyperosmolar nonketotic coma [HHNK].) If the glycosuria is due to hyperalimentation therapy, the physician may eliminate the spilling of glucose in two different ways: (1) slow down the rate of the concentrated glucose solution or (2) order insulin to help the body use the large load of glucose.
>
> In a client with diabetes, a continued spilling of glucose leads not only to severe dehydration but also to ketonuria and eventually to ketoacidosis, as the ketone bodies build up in the serum. The nurse needs to be aware that the presence of a positive acetone with a positive glucose indicates a need for immediate medical intervention. (See the discussion on ketoacidosis in Chapter 8 and on metabolic acidosis in Chapter 6.)

KETONES IN THE URINE

Ketones are metabolic end products of fatty acid metabolism. When the body does not have sufficient glucose to use for energy, the excretion of ketones increases. The three ketone bodies in the urine are acetone, acetoacetic acid, and β-hydroxybutyric acid. Test strips and tablets check only for acetone and acetoacetic acid, but this is sufficient because a change in the small amount of acetone signifies the same degree of change in the other ketones. Acetoacetate and acetone can also be measured in the serum (see Chapter 8).

As in the tests for glucose, acetone can be tested either with a dipstick or with a tablet. Both methods show a deepening purple color when acetone is present. The scale indicates small, moderate, or large amounts of acetone. Symptomatic ketosis occurs at levels of about 50 mg/dL or when the client has moderate acetone in urine testing. Urine containing phenylketones (PKU; Chapter 18) or L-dopa metabolites may give false-positive results.

REFERENCE VALUES FOR KETONES	
Normal urine should not contain enough ketones to give a positive reading.	
Small	20 mg/dL
Moderate	30–40 mg/dL
Large	80 mg/dL or greater

Presence of Ketones in Urine

Clinical Significance

The presence of ketones in the urine signifies that the body is using fat as the main source of energy. Fats are used when glucose is unavailable to the cells. Glucose may not be available because it is not being transported to the cells, as in diabetes, or because glucose is lacking in the body because of starvation, vomiting, fasting, or an all-protein diet. The American Diabetes Association recommends that clients test for ketones when their blood glucose level is more than 300 mg/dL (www. diabetes.org).

Possible Nursing Diagnoses Related to Ketones in Urine

Risk for Injury Related to Development of Diabetic Acidosis

If the client is known to have diabetes, ketonuria (a positive acetone by testing) indicates that the insulin and glucose balance is not satisfactory. An abundance of glucose is in the bloodstream, but it is unavailable to the cells. A client with diabetes and a positive acetone has switched to using fats as the primary source of energy because the lack of insulin prohibits the transport of glucose to the cells. As the ketones accumulate, they use up the bicarbonate buffer (see Chapter 6), and ketoacidosis can develop. Extra fluids help the body eliminate excess ketones. (See Chapter 8 for more information about ketoacidosis and other treatments needed.)

Imbalanced Nutrition: Requirements of Glucose

If the acetone is positive because of a starvation state, the positive ketone is associated with a negative glucose in the urine and normal blood glucose. A search must be made for other reasons why the cells do not have glucose. Questions to be asked would be

1. Has the client had a reduced amount of food?
2. Has there been a lot of vomiting?
3. Is the client trying to lose weight by being on an all-protein diet?

Depending on the circumstances, the client needs glucose in some form so that fats and proteins do not continue to be the primary source of energy. The client also needs extra fluids so that the ketones can be excreted by the kidneys. Clients on tube feedings that are very high in protein may show ketones in the urine unless they also receive adequate glucose in the feeding, along with plenty of water to rid the bloodstream of the ketones.

NITRITES

Most species of bacteria, such as those of the family Enterobacteriaceae, if present in the urine, cause the conversion of nitrates, which are derived from dietary metabolites, to nitrites. Thus a dipstick for nitrites is a check for urinary infections. A negative nitrite test or negative culture does not provide proof that the urine is free of all bacteria, particularly if there are clinical symptoms to the contrary. Some bacteria do not produce nitrites. Note that the nitrite test is usually combined with the leukocyte esterase (LE) test discussed next. See Table 3–3 for examples of individual tests discussed in other chapters.

Preparation of Client and Collection of Sample

Optimal results are obtained by using a first morning urine sample that has been "incubating" in the bladder for 4 hours or more. The urine should be collected by a

Table 3–3 Examples of Individual Tests on Urine Discussed in Other Chapters

Test	Reference Value	Specimen	Information About Test
Bence Jones protein light chains	Negative	First morning specimen	Chapter 10, on urine electrophoresis
Human chorionic gonadotropin (HCG)	Negative (unless pregnant)	First morning specimen	Chapter 18
Tests for occult blood	Negative	Random	Chapter 13, on tests to detect bleeding. Note microscopic exam is more sensitive test
Ketones	Negative	Random	Chapter 8
Bilirubin	Negative	Random	Chapter 11
Urobilinogen	Up to 1.0 Ehrlich units/2 h	2-h specimen (1–3 PM)	Chapter 11
Nitrites	No pink color	Clean-catch or mid-stream specimen	This chapter and Chapter 16, on urine cultures
Leukocyte esterase	Negative	Random, clean-catch	This chapter and Chapter 16, on urine cultures

clean-catch midstream technique (see Chapter 16 on clean-catch urine specimens), and it should be tested within an hour of voiding. As an alternative to the clean-catch method, the client may wet the strip by holding it in the urinary stream.

REFERENCE VALUES FOR NITRITES	
Nitrate reagent	Turns pink if bacteria are present. The pink color is *not* quantitative in relation to the number of bacteria present. Ascorbic acid or a high specific gravity may invalidate the results. Blood or other pigments in the urine can interfere with the color changes.
Cultures	Usually growth of 100,000/mL is considered evidence of a bacterial infection. (See Chapter 16 on culture reports.)

A specialized dipstick for nitrites can also be used for a culture. Immediately after the strip is read, it is put into a transparent bag. The dipstick has two miniaturized culture areas that support both gram-positive and gram-negative bacteria. If the dipstick is to be cultured, it must not be touched. The dipstick in the bag is put into an incubator for a minimum of 18 hours. Results are ready within 18–24 hours. Various companies make diagnostic culture kits (see Chapter 16).

LEUKOCYTE ESTERASE

The LE test identifies enzymes found in granulocytes, histiocytes, and *Trichomonas* species. The test detects 5–15 white blood cells (WBCs) per high-power field and, thus, has an advantage over the microscopic examination because the LE test detects both lysed and intact cells. The combination of LE with the nitrite test (discussed earlier) provides a sensitive screen for predicting urinary tract infections. It was found that the combination of the two tests had 95% sensitivity and 85% specificity for detecting urinary tract infections in women with dysuria. In young children, these tests are less sensitive (Hay et. al, 2011). Enhanced urinalysis may be done, using a hemocytomer, to evaluate the number of WBCs in uncentrifuged urine. Getting an uncontaminated urine sample in infants and young children may require a suprapubic aspiration (Dulczak & Kirk, 2005). For pregnant women, the LE test may be used to test for infection in the amniotic fluid. Test kits containing LE and nitrites are available for consumers.

Preparation of Client and Collection of Sample

Dipsticks for LE are used the same way as other reagent strips for urinalysis. Concentrated urine is most satisfactory for testing. The dipstick is read at 2 minutes by comparing with a color chart and noting trace to + + +. Color changes that occur after 2 minutes have no diagnostic value. Ascorbic acid and some antibiotics may interfere with the test.

REFERENCE VALUES FOR LE

A result matching any color block designated by a + sign indicates the presence of increasing amounts of leukocytes in urine. A "trace" reading should be retested with a fresh urine specimen. Positive results for LE and nitrites may be followed up with a urine culture (see Chapter 16).

EXAMINATION OF URINE SEDIMENT (MICROSCOPIC EXAM)

The urine sediment is centrifuged and examined microscopically for crystals, casts, red blood cells (RBCs), WBCs, and bacteria or yeast. Table 3–4 contains a brief summary of the meaning of each of these findings. Laboratories only do a microscopic examination on special request unless the routine urinalysis is positive for protein, blood, nitrites, or WBC esterase. A routine urinalysis done by using chemical dipsticks may be called a macroscopic exam. If occult blood is suspected, the microscopic analysis is better for detection than the dipsticks. If urine is collected with a syringe and needle from the port of a Foley catheter, the needle should be removed before the urine is squirted into the specimen cup. Pushing the urine through the needle may damage cells and casts. Red cell casts dissolve within 20 minutes.

URINARY PORPHYRINS

Porphobilinogen, coproporphyrins, and uroporphyrins are intermediaries in the synthesis of heme, which is part of Hgb and of several enzymes. Delta-aminolevulinic acid (Δ-ALA) is an important enzyme for the formation of porphobilinogen. Abnormalities of porphyrin metabolism may be either genetic or caused by drug

Table 3–4 Summary of Microscopic Exam of Urine	
WBCs	Normally there should not be more than a few white blood cells in the urine (4–5 per high-power field). Infections or inflammations anywhere along the urinary tract cause an increase of WBCs in the urine.
RBCs	Normally there should be only an occasional red blood cell in the urine (2–3 per high-power field). An increased number of RBCs in the urine indicates bleeding somewhere in the urinary system, which may be caused by renal disease, trauma, or a bleeding disorder. The American Urological Association recommends a referral if there are more than 3 RBCs for 2 out of 3 microscopic exams (Rao et al., 2010). In women, it is important to make sure that the urine was not contaminated by the menstrual flow. Insertion of a tampon and a collection of midstream urine are ways to prevent this contamination.
Crystals	Most crystals have little clinical significance. If the client is taking drugs that may cause crystallization in the urine, such as some of the sulfa drugs, this finding may be clinically important.
Casts	A few hyaline casts are considered normal, but all other casts need to be evaluated by the physician. Unlike crystals, casts are suggestive of kidney disease. Casts are a compacted collection of protein, cells, and debris that are formed in the tubules of the kidneys. Those that form in the distal tubule have a narrow caliber. Those that form in the collecting tubules tend to be very broad. Broad granular casts are sometimes called *renal failure casts* because they indicate renal destruction. The width and composition of the cast is important in the diagnosis of and prognosis for renal disease.
Bacteria or yeast	Often the presence of a few bacteria or yeasts is indicative only of contamination from the perineal area, but a culture and sensitivity may need to be performed if a large number of bacteria are noted on routine screening. Chapter 16 discusses the nursing implications for obtaining a urine specimen for a culture and sensitivity or for a smear. See the tests for nitrites and leukocyte esterase discussed in this chapter.
Epithelial cells	Squamous epithelial cells, usually from the vagina or urethra, do not have much significance. Large numbers may signify contamination by secretions. Renal tubular epithelial cells are associated with renal disease. Transitional epithelial bladder cells may be normal or could signify a possible neoplasm (McPhee, Papadakis, & Rabow, 2011).

intoxication, usually lead. Several tests can be completed to demonstrate an abnormality in the metabolism of heme. Because the porphyrins are precursors of the pigment (heme), the urine may be burgundy or pink when exposed to black light.

Preparation of Client and Collection of Sample

Coproporphyrin and uroporphyrin usually require a 24-hour urine specimen with a preservative. Testing for porphobilinogen is performed on a random urine specimen, consisting of 10 mL of freshly voided urine. Specimens should be protected from light.

REFERENCE VALUES FOR PORPHYRINS	
Coproporphyrin	50–250 mg/day
Uroporphyrin	0
Porphobilinogen	0

Abnormal Porphyrins

Clinical Significance

Elevations of these tests are indications of one of the porphyrias, which are several different diseases that may be acute or chronic. The disease may be difficult to diagnose because it mimics so many other conditions. At present, treatment is symptomatic. Acute intermittent porphyria, the most common, can be precipitated by barbiturates and other drugs. Because some types of porphyria are genetic diseases, studies should also be performed on relatives of affected clients.

DELTA-AMINOLEVULINIC ACID

Δ-ALA is an enzyme needed for the proper conversion to porphobilinogen in the metabolic formation of heme. Although Δ-ALA is not present in the urine of healthy people, it is present in lead intoxication. Also, Δ-ALA may be elevated in certain kinds of genetic deficiencies of porphyrin metabolism (the porphyrias). This test was commonly performed for lead exposure and poisoning but is no longer recommended for this purpose.

However, this test may be useful to assess the effectiveness of chelation therapy (Wu, 2006). See Chapter 17 on lead poisoning.

Preparation of Client and Collection of Sample

A 24-hour urine sample should be collected (see instructions at the end of this chapter). Specimen should be protected from light. Various methods require different preservatives.

REFERENCE VALUE FOR D-ALA
1–7 mg/day

URINARY 5-HYDROXYINDOLEACETIC ACID FOR SEROTONIN

Glands in the gastrointestinal tract secrete the hormone serotonin. Carried in the platelets, serotonin is a vasoconstrictor that is especially important to small arterioles after tissue injury. It is also a regulator of smooth muscle contraction, such as in peristalsis. The chief metabolite of serotonin, excreted in the urine, is 5-hydroxyindoleacetic acid (5-HIAA). Certain tumors, called *carcinoid tumors,* of the argentaffin cells in the gastrointestinal tract may begin to secrete abnormal amounts of serotonin. Hence, a measurement of the amount of 5-HIAA in the urine is a help in diagnosing carcinoid tumors. (McPhee et al., 2011).

Preparation of Client and Collection of Sample

The client must not eat foods such as bananas, tomatoes, plums, avocados, eggplant, or pineapples because all these foods contain a large amount of serotonin.

Because many drugs may also affect the test results, the nurse must check with the laboratory about specific drug interactions. The urine is collected in a special container with 10 mL of hydrochloric acid (HCl) or boric acid. Follow the procedure for a collection of 24-hour specimen (discussed at the end of this chapter).

REFERENCE VALUES FOR 5-HIAA	
24-Hr screening test	Negative
Quantitative test	2–9 mg/day—women lower than men

Clinical Significance

An elevated level of 5-HIAA in the urine is evidence of increased serotonin, which may be caused by carcinoid tumors. These tumors may be either benign or malignant. Note that tumors in other organs may sometimes produce serotonin. (See Chapter 15 on ectopic hormone production by tumors.) The symptoms of serotonin excess may include cyanotic episodes, flushing of the skin, diarrhea, abdominal cramps, and bronchial constriction. The nurse should note and record any type of symptoms that occur during the time the client is undergoing studies for a possible carcinoid tumor. The principal clinical manifestations of the syndrome are due to biologically active agents released by the tumor. In addition to the release of serotonin, bradykinin, histamine, and adrenocorticotropic hormone (ACTH), other substances are released. Treatment involves surgical removal of the tumor. These tumors are usually slow growing, and drug therapy may be used. Platelet serotonin is the most sensitive and consistently increased marker for long-term monitoring for most types of carcinoid tumors. Blood levels may be needed when urine samples are normal or borderline (Wu, 2006).

COLLECTION OF 24-HOUR URINE SPECIMENS

These collections are useful only if *all* the urine is collected for 24 hours. Even if "just one specimen" is discarded, the test is not valid. The nurse must make sure that the client fully understands the importance of saving all the urine. Because of the problem with incomplete urine collections, laboratories sometimes check the creatinine present in the urine to validate that the urine is representative of a full 24 hours. Assuming the client does not have renal problems, a creatinine value below the normal range for age and body weight suggests an incomplete collection.

To begin the 24-hour urine collection, the client voids and *discards* the urine so that the urine from the previous night is not included. Then all the urine for the next 24 hours is saved and put into a large collection bottle. If a client voids and discards the urine at, say 8:20 AM, the test ends at 8:20 AM the next day. The client should do a final voiding as close to 8:20 AM as possible so that the last urine in the bladder can be included. The urine specimen should be sent to the laboratory as soon as possible. The times for beginning and ending the urine collection should be noted on the requisition.

The laboratory supplies the collection bottle, along with any preservative needed. (See Table 3–5 for common 24-hour urine specimens and the preparations

Table 3–5 24-Hour Urine Specimens

Substance Tested	Reference Values (day = 24-hr day)	Preservative Needed	Information About Test
Aldosterone	5–19 mg/day	Boric acid	Chapter 15
Amylase	24–76 U/mL	None	Chapter 12—may do for only 2 hr
Calcium	≤300 mg/day	Need 10 mL of HCl	Chapter 7
Catecholamines Epinephrine Norepinephrine	<20 mg/day <100 mg/day	Need 10 mL of HCl (pH kept 2–3)	Chapter 15
Coproporphyrin	50–250 mg/day Children <80 lb; 0–75 mg/day	5 g of Na carbonate	This chapter
Creatinine	15–25 mg/kg body weight	None	Chapter 4
Creatinine clearance	Male: 95–135 mL/min Female: 85–125 mL/min	None	Need serum creatinine (Chapter 4)
Delta-aminolevulinic acid	1–7 mg/day	None	See this chapter and Chapter 17
5-HIAA	2–9 mg/day (women lower than men)	10 mL of HCl	See this chapter
Lead	≤120 mg/day	None	Make sure lead-free container (Chapter 17)
Phosphate	1 g/day—varies with intake	10 mL of HCl	Chapter 7
Potassium	25–125 mEq/day	None	Chapter 5
Pregnanediol	Men: < 1 mg/day Women: 1–8 mg/day	Refrigerate	Chapter 15
Protein	<150mg/day	None	See quantitative and qualitative tests in this chapter and notes for pregnancy
Sodium	40–220 mEq/day	None	Chapter 5
Urea nitrogen	6–17 g/day	None	Chapter 4
Uroporphyrin	0–30 mg/day	5 g of Na carbonate	See this chapter
Vanillylmandelic acid	Up to 9 mg/day	12 mL of HCl	Chapter 15

Note: Most laboratories prefer all 24-hour urine specimens iced. Check with the laboratory for the specific technique used and reference values.

needed.) Clients need to be told if there is a preservative, so that no direct contact occurs with a toxic solution. The laboratory should also notify the nurse or the client if certain drugs or foods invalidate the test. (See the discussions in the various chapters on specific points for each test.) If a preservative is not used, a few specimens, such as those for hormones, must be refrigerated. Usually refrigeration is preferred for most urine tests, but the nurse should validate this requirement with the laboratory. The rationale for refrigeration is to inhibit bacterial growth, which may interfere with some tests.

For toddlers, when a diaper is used at night, a 12-hour specimen may have to suffice. For infants, urine may be collected in disposable paste-on collection bags. Rarely, it may be necessary to insert a Foley catheter to obtain a 24-hour urine collection from a child. The danger of a urinary tract infection is a disadvantage.

Questions

1. A specimen of urine for a routine urinalysis should be
   a. At least 60 mL
   b. Put into a sterile container
   c. An early morning specimen, if possible
   d. Sent to the laboratory as a stat procedure

2. Which of the following tends to make the urine pH higher?
   a. Meat
   b. Eggs
   c. Cranberry juice
   d. Citrus juices

3. A client has just been taught how to perform blood glucose checks for her newly diagnosed diabetes. She asks the clinic nurse what other tests she should carry out if her blood glucose level is more than 300 mg/dL. The nurse responds by instructing the client to follow up an elevated blood glucose level by performing a urine dipstick for
   a. Glucose
   b. Specific gravity
   c. Protein
   d. Ketones

4. In interpreting the meaning of specific gravity of a urinalysis for a child younger than 2 years, it is important for the nurse to realize that in a child this young, the maximum specific gravity is
   a. Much lower than for an adult
   b. Higher than for an adult
   c. Essentially the same as the adult range
   d. Fixed at 1.010

5. Which of the following clients demonstrates the concept of a "fixed" specific gravity?
   a. A client whose specific gravity is 1.025 on three early morning urine specimens
   b. A client whose specific gravity is 1.010 on a random urine specimen
   c. A client whose specific gravity remains about 1.008 while he is taking diuretics
   d. A client whose specific gravity was 1.010 during a prolonged period of fluid restriction

6. A client is asked to obtain a urine specimen before arising to rule out orthostatic or postural
   a. Glycosuria
   b. Ketonuria
   c. Proteinuria
   d. Hematuria

7. The nurse in a prenatal clinic has just tested a client's urine and found it to be 0.5% for glucose and 3+ for protein by the dipstick method. There will be a 30- to 40-minute delay before the client sees the physician. She says she is "feeling okay," so she wishes to have her appointment rescheduled. Which action by the nurse would be the most appropriate?
   a. Reschedule her appointment for another day because glucose and protein in the urine are not uncommon in the third trimester of pregnancy
   b. Say nothing about the urine test but insist that she wait to see the physician because the clinic schedule is always full
   c. Take a nursing history from the client and tell her the glucose in her urine needs investigation by the physician because she may be diabetic
   d. Take her blood pressure, check her ankles, and explain why it is necessary to make these assessments to help the physician evaluate the seriousness of the proteinuria. Emphasize that it is important for the client to wait to see the physician

8. A male client 15 years of age, has had type 1 diabetes for more than 5 years. He has had yearly urine dipstick tests for albumin. He asks the nurse why the physician has ordered a new test, a "microalbuminuria." The most accurate reply by the nurse would be: "The microalbuminuria test is
   a. A 24-hour urine test to check for very small particles of albumin."
   b. A more sensitive test than the regular dipstick test. Tiny amounts of albumin can be detected."
   c. The same test you have been having each year. The name just denotes a new technique."
   d. A procedure that compares the albumin in your urine with the microalbumin in your blood."

9. The client is a 19-year-old college freshman who is quite obese. She has come to the campus health clinic because she feels very tired. A routine complete blood count and urinalysis are normal except for a trace of acetone. (Urine glucose was negative.) Based on these laboratory findings, which questions by the nurse will most likely help detect the reason for the abnormal ketones?
   a. Have you been eating a lot of fats lately?
   b. Have you been under a lot of stress?
   c. Is there a history of diabetes in your family?
   d. Have you been on a strict reducing diet lately?

10. A client is in the last trimester of her pregnancy. Dipstick tests for nitrites and leukocyte esterase in the urine were positive. Her specific gravity was normal. These positive reactions are evidence of
    a. Preeclampsia
    b. Normal dietary metabolites of protein
    c. Possible urinary tract infection
    d. Possible lack of ascorbic acid in her diet

References

Castner, D. (2010). Understanding the stages of chronic kidney disease. *Nursing 2010, 40* (5), 25–31.

Dulczak, S., & Kirk, J. (2005). Overview of the evaluation, diagnosis, and management of urinary tract infections in infants and children. *Urologic Nursing, 25*(3), 185–192.

Hay, W. W., Levin, M. J., Sondheimer, J. M., & Deterding, R. (Eds.). (2011). *Current diagnosis and treatment: Pediatrics* (20th ed.). New York: McGraw-Hill.

Madison, J. R., Spies, C., Schatz, I. J., Masaki, K., Chen, R., Yano, K., et al. (2006). Proteinuria and risk for stroke and coronary heart disease during 27 years of follow-up: The Honolulu Heart Program. *Archives Internal Medicine, 166*(8), 884–889.

McPhee, S. J., Papadakis, M. A., & Rabow, M. W. (Eds.). (2011). *Current medical diagnosis and treatment* (50th ed.). New York: McGraw-Hill.

Mentes, J. C., Wakefield, B., & Culp, K. (2006). Use of a urine color chart to monitor hydration status in nursing home residents. *Biological Research for Nursing, 7*(3), 197–2003.

Rao, P., Gao, T., Pohl, M., & Jones, J. (2010). Dipstick pseudohematuria: Unnecessary consultation and evaluation. *Journal of Urology, 183*(2), 560–565.

Westhus, N. (2004). Methods to test tube feeding placement in children. *MCN: American Journal of Maternal Child Health Nursing, 29*(5), 282–287.

Wu, A. H. (Ed.). (2006). *Tietz clinical guide to laboratory tests* (4th ed.). St. Louis, MO: Saunders.

Websites

www.diabetes.org (Information on tests for diabetes.)
www.mayoclinic.com (Information on other medications that change the color of urine.)

Answers

1. c, 2. d, 3. d, 4. a, 5. d, 6. c, 7. d, 8. b, 9. d, 10. c

Renal Function Tests

- Blood Urea Nitrogen or Serum Urea Nitrogen   83
- BUN-to-Creatinine Ratio   84
- Urinary Urea Nitrogen and Nitrogen Balance   88
- Creatinine Levels in Serum   88
- Creatinine Clearance Test   90
- Estimation of Glomerular Filtration Rate (GFR)   91
- Cystatin C and Beta-2-Microglobulin   91
- Serum and Urine Osmolality   92
- Uric Acid (Serum and Urine)   96

OBJECTIVES

1. Compare and contrast the factors that affect blood urea nitrogen (BUN) and serum creatinine levels.
2. Explain the rationale for checking BUN or serum creatinine levels before administration of certain antibiotics.
3. Describe the nursing diagnoses that are appropriate when a client has markedly elevated BUN and serum creatinine levels.
4. Given the values for urinary urea nitrogen and the client's intake of protein, calculate the nitrogen balance to determine if dietary adjustments are warranted.
5. Compare the usefulness of urine osmolality to the measurement of urine specific gravity.
6. Given various changes in serum and urine osmolality, plan appropriate nursing interventions.
7. Prepare a teaching plan that helps a client with high serum uric acid levels to decrease the possibility of renal stones.
8. Describe the role of the nurse in preparing clients for creatinine clearance tests.

Some of the tests discussed in this chapter are used only for renal assessment, whereas others have several purposes. For example, serum creatinine levels, urine creatinine levels, and the creatinine clearance tests are all used only to evaluate renal function, and only renal dysfunction changes the result. However, BUN, also used primarily to assess renal function, can be affected by other factors and may be used to assess deficient fluid volume. The urinary urea nitrogen is used to assess nitrogen balance. Tests for serum and urine osmolality are useful not only in assessing renal function but also for assessing fluid requirements and fluid imbalances. The discussions of urine osmolality should be read after one has read about specific gravity measurements in the previous chapter. One test covered in this chapter, uric acid, is not really a test for renal dysfunction, but uric acid is likely to be elevated in severe renal dysfunction. Therefore, the discussion on uric acid fits into a general discussion about renal dysfunction, even though it is not used as an assessment tool for the severity of the dysfunction.

BLOOD UREA NITROGEN OR SERUM UREA NITROGEN

The BUN test measures the amount of urea nitrogen in the blood or serum. Urea, a waste product of protein metabolism, is formed by the liver and carried in the blood to the kidneys for excretion. Because urea is cleared from the bloodstream by the kidneys, the BUN can be used as a test of renal function. However, protein breakdown, dehydration, overhydration, and liver failure all invalidate the BUN as a test for renal dysfunction.

Preparation of Client and Collection of Sample

There is no special preparation of the client. The laboratory needs 1 mL of blood or serum for the test.

REFERENCE VALUES FOR BUN	
Adult	8–25 mg/dL Values may be slightly higher in men than in women
Pregnant women	Values may decrease about 25%
Newborn	Values tend to be slightly lower than adult ranges
Aged	Values may be slightly increased because of lack of renal concentration

Increased BUN
Clinical Significance

Diseased or damaged kidneys cause an elevated BUN because the kidneys are less able to rid the blood of the waste product urea. Even if the kidneys are not diseased or damaged, conditions in which renal perfusion is decreased result in an increase of urea in the blood. Thus a client in shock or one in congestive heart failure may have higher-than-normal BUN levels caused by poor circulation to the kidneys. A client who is severely dehydrated may also have an elevated BUN level because of the lack of volume to excrete waste products. Because urea is an end product of protein metabolism, a diet high in protein, such as tube feedings, may cause some increase in the BUN level. Bleeding into the gastrointestinal tract also causes an elevated BUN because digested blood is a source of protein. For example, loss of 1,000 mL of blood into the gastrointestinal tract may elevate the BUN to 40 mg/dL.

BUN-TO-CREATININE RATIO

Because creatinine is changed only by renal dysfunction, a comparison of the BUN with the serum creatinine is useful. A client with a BUN of 15 mg might have a serum creatinine level of about 1.0 mg. If the client becomes dehydrated or has increased protein (such as with gastrointestinal bleeding), the BUN increases, whereas the creatinine does not; so the ratio of 15:1 would be increased in dehydration or in protein breakdown. However, the ratio of BUN to creatinine would be less than 15:1 in low protein intake, overhydration, or severe liver failure, which reduces the BUN but not the creatinine level. BUN-to-creatinine ratios may range from 6:1 to 20:1.

Use of BUN or Creatinine to Monitor Nephrotoxic Drugs

BUN and creatinine levels are also used to monitor clients who are receiving drugs known to be potentially nephrotoxic, such as antibiotics classified as aminoglycosides. Some of the aminoglycosides are gentamicin, tobramycin, and netilmicin. Before administering a drug that is known to be potentially nephrotoxic, nurses should look at the client's BUN and creatinine levels. If either level is higher than the reference range, they should withhold the drug until consulting a physician. Because aminoglycosides tend to also be toxic to the eighth cranial nerve, assessments of auditory and vestibular functions are ways to monitor for neurotoxicity. Impaired hearing or dizziness is more likely to occur if the drug is continued when there is renal dysfunction. Measurements of the levels of drugs in the serum are completed so that a therapeutic level can be maintained. (See Chapter 17 for a discussion about the measurement of serum levels of aminoglycosides such as gentamicin.) It is important to keep the client well hydrated when aminoglycosides are used because they are excreted almost unchanged in the urine.

Possible Nursing Diagnoses Related to Increased BUN

Risk for Deficient Fluid Volume

Because an increased BUN may be caused by anything that causes poor renal perfusion or renal dysfunction, it is important to look at the BUN in relation to the pathologic process for the individual client. If the BUN is due to poor renal perfusion, the focus is on increasing renal flow. For example, if the client is dehydrated this must be corrected. However, if the elevated BUN reflects actual renal damage, fluids may have to be restricted or increased, depending on the phase of acute renal failure. The client is most likely to have severe fluid and electrolyte imbalances during the oliguric–anuric phase and the late diuretic phase. The nurse must monitor the necessary fluid requirements and keep accurate intake and output (I&O) records. Table 4–1 compares glomerular filtration rate (GFR) in various stages of renal disease. Note that the BUN-to-creatinine ratio may help identify dehydration rather than renal disease. Also see the discussion on serum and urine osmolality for other assessments of a deficient fluid volume.

If the elevated BUN can be traced to a great increase in protein in the diet, a reduction of protein or an increase of fluid intake or both helps the kidney eliminate the excess urea. For example, increased fluids are needed with high-protein supplements.

Nutritional Imbalances: Requirements of Sodium, Potassium, and Protein

As kidney disease advances, fluid, electrolyte, and hormonal imbalances create the need to constantly review the nutritional needs of the client. Anemia requires the use of EPO (Chapter 2) and attention to the need for additional iron in the diet. Sodium and potassium are excreted by the kidneys. Sodium may have to be restricted, and supplemental potassium is contraindicated in a client who has progressive renal dysfunction. (See Chapter 5 on hyperkalemia and hypernatremia.) Usually protein in the diet is not restricted for mild renal insufficiency, but one would question a high-protein diet, which would tend to increase the BUN even more. The protein level may have to be adjusted to maintain lean body mass and still not cause a high BUN. Once the client is on dialysis, the dietary restrictions may be lessened. Inadequate nutrition, as measured by serum albumin levels (Chapter 10), is associated with higher mortality rates. In chronic kidney disease, the kidneys become less capable of producing activated vitamin D and excreting phosphorous, leading to decreased serum calcium levels and increased phosphorus levels. Both events stimulate parathyroid hormone production that can lead to a complex bone disease if not treated early (Legg, 2005). See Chapter 7 for a discussion on treatments for low calcium and high phosphorus in renal disease.

Children and adolescents with renal failure present additional nutritional problems because of the needs of their growing bodies. Few infants are given fluid restrictions. Infants may be experiencing life-threatening hyperkalemia (high potassium level), even though the BUN is not greater than 35 mg/dL.

Impairment of Skin Integrity

Azotemia means an increase of nitrogenous waste products in the serum. *Uremia* is the broader name given to the toxic condition in which the kidneys are not able to excrete urea and other substances such as potassium, creatinine, and organic acids. In the days before the advent of peritoneal and renal dialysis, clients with high levels of BUN would have a condition called *uremic frost*, which consisted of urea crystals that were being excreted through the sweat glands. Fortunately, urea levels can be lowered now with dialysis before clients experience toxic uremia. However, itching is often a problem, and the potential for skin breakdown is always present.

Risk for Injury Related to Weakness and Possible Confusion

Clients with a mild gradual increase in BUN level may not have many symptoms. The level of BUN that causes symptoms in clients varies tremendously. As BUN levels continue to rise, the client is likely to experience fatigue, muscle weakness, and some nausea and vomiting. There may be a decline in mental awareness, drowsiness, or confusion. Nurses need to assess the mental and physical capabilities of any client with an increased BUN level to ensure safe care. Clients who may be slightly confused or unsteady on their feet need careful watching. Hypertension and arrhythmias may limit activity, so blood pressure and pulse must be closely monitored. Some noted that many of the most troublesome symptoms of uremia are really those of anemia, and the use of erythropoietin injections to raise the Hct may eliminate fatigue, dyspnea, angina, and depression. (See Chapter 2 on erythropoietin assays.)

(Continued)

Possible Nursing Diagnoses . . . *(Continued)*

Alterations in Health Maintenance Related to Need for Readjustment of Medications

Clients with elevated BUN and creatinine levels may need modifications in their drug regimen. For example, clients with diabetes need less insulin as their renal function decreases. Other common drugs that have a prolonged effect in clients with compromised renal function include digoxin, phenothiazines, meperidine, and several antibiotics. Clients in Stage 4 (see Table 4–1) may be taking 11 or more drugs daily. Information about the stage helps in teaching the client about what drugs and herbs to avoid. Clients should check with a renal specialist before beginning any new medications (Campoy & Elwell, 2005). Other medication teaching may involve information about the angiotensin-converting enzyme (ACE) inhibitors used to protect the kidney from further damage (Castner, 2010). Also, clients may need information about over-the-counter drugs, such as ibuprofen or naproxen, that may have an adverse effect on damaged kidneys.

Risk for Infection Related to Alterations in the Immune System and Phagocytosis

Clients undergoing chronic dialysis have an increased risk for infection not only because of the invasive devices used but also because of a decrease in lymphocytes and alterations in the functioning ability of lymphocytes, monocytes, and neutrophils. Nursing interventions to protect the client from infection are a high priority. (See Chapter 2 on lymphocytes, monocytes, and neutrophils and ways to enhance resistance to infection.)

Alteration in Bowel Elimination Related to Constipation

Clients with chronic renal disease often have problems with constipation because of restricted fluid intake and lack of exercise. Increasing fiber in the diet may be limited because many high-fiber foods are high in potassium and phosphorus. Usually, these clients do need stool softeners on a regular basis, and the sodium and calcium in these products are not sufficient to warrant concern. (See Chapter 7 for a discussion on high phosphorus and magnesium levels and the danger of some laxatives for clients with renal failure.)

Risk for Disturbance in Self-Esteem and Self-Concept

The psychological needs of the client usually decrease if the client has a type of acute renal failure that is reversible. However, many types of renal damage are not reversible. As renal function becomes compromised, many pathologic changes occur. These changes and the need for alterations in lifestyle can be devastating to the client and their significant others. Depression, anxiety, and a feeling of powerlessness may develop as clients consider possible options such as home or hospital hemodialysis, peritoneal dialysis, or an eventual renal transplant. The nurse can find the coping methods previously used by the clients for major life changes and help them use the successful methods for the present crisis. A psychiatric nurse or a social worker may also be used for support. Sometimes clients with chronic renal failure interpret emotions in physical rather than phychological terms, such as saying they feel tired rather than sad. A nurse may screen for emotional problems by asking specific questions such as "How often have you felt sad in the past 4 weeks?" The quantifiable responses such as "none," "some of the time," or "all of the time" can indicate whether further intervention is warranted (Thomas-Hawkins & Zazworsky, 2005).

Anxiety Related to Treatment Options

Nurses need to make sure clients get all the information they need about treatment options. From the early stages of Stage 3 (Table 4–1), a nephrology team should be consulted to explain treatment options to the client and to help delay the progression as much as possible. By Stage 4, clients need even more detailed preparation for Stage 5, which will mean dialysis, a transplant or a choice for palliative care. Research supports the importance of early evaluation, intervention, and education to decrease morbidity and mortality in chronic renal disease (Dinwiddie, Burrows-Hudson, & Peacock, 2006).

Table 4–1 Staging Chronic Renal Disease with GFR	
Stage 1	Kidney damage (90–130)*
Stage 2	Mildly decreased GFR (60–89)
Stage 3	Moderately decreased GFR (30–59)
Stage 4	Severely decreased GFR (15–29)
Stage 5	Kidney failure GFR (less than 15)—dialysis or transplant

*Number is based on mL/min/1.73 m².

See the National Kidney Foundation website (www.kidney.org) for more information on staging renal disease.

Decreased BUN

Clinical Significance

Just as dehydration may cause an elevated BUN, overhydration causes a decreased BUN. An increase in antidiuretic hormone (ADH) is a pathologic reason for dilute plasma. Increases in plasma volume, such as in pregnancy, reduce the BUN level. A marked decrease in protein breakdown also tends to lower the BUN. Usually a BUN that is slightly lower than the reference values has little clinical significance. Because urea is synthesized by the liver, severe liver failure causes a reduction of urea in the serum. Yet the inability of the liver to form urea results in an increase in other nitrogenous products, such as ammonia, so tests for ammonia levels are much more clinically significant in liver dysfunction than are lowered BUN levels. (See Chapter 10 on ammonia levels.)

Possible Nursing Diagnosis Related to Decreased BUN

Risk for Excess Fluid Volume

Because a decreased BUN raises the possibility of expanded plasma fluid volume, some attention should be given to the overall hydration status of the client. Yet the test by itself is not helpful in identifying plasma dilution. (See the section on serum osmolality in this chapter and Chapter 5 on serum sodium as tests for plasma dilution.)

URINARY UREA NITROGEN AND NITROGEN BALANCE

The urinary urea nitrogen can be measured and compared with the amount of protein ingested to determine the nitrogen balance of the client. There is about 1 g of nitrogen in each 6 g of protein, and the loss of nitrogen is about 4 g from stool and insensible loss. Based on these facts, the following formula has been devised:

$$\text{N balance} = \frac{\text{Protein intake (g)}}{6.25} - (\text{24-hour urinary urea nitrogen} + 4)$$

A value less than 0 indicates a negative nitrogen balance as shown in the following example:

$$\text{N balance} = 50/6.25 - (6 + 4) = -2$$

A negative nitrogen balance is an indication that the client needs a greater protein intake (see Chapter 10). Nitrogen balance determinations are frequently used to evaluate the effectiveness of total parenteral nutrition.

Preparation of Client and Collection of Sample

See Chapter 3 on the method for collecting 24-hour urine specimens. No preservation is needed. The dietitian usually accesses protein intake. The nurse must accurately record all food intake.

REFERENCE VALUE FOR URINARY UREA

6–17 g of urinary nitrogen in 24 hr

REFERENCE VALUE FOR NITROGEN BALANCE

0 or greater   (see earlier discussion for formula)

CREATININE LEVELS IN SERUM

Creatinine is the waste product of creatine phosphate, a high-energy compound found in skeletal muscle tissue. The measurement of serum *creatinine* is useful in evaluating any type of renal dysfunction in which a large number of nephrons have been destroyed.

Preparation of Client and Collection of Sample

The laboratory needs 1 mL of venous blood. High doses of ascorbic acid or barbiturates may distort the results. Ketone bodies and cephalosporin antibiotics may elevate the results.

REFERENCE VALUES FOR SERUM CREATININE	
Adult: Men 　　　Women	0.6–1.5 mg/dL 0.6–1.1 mg/dL Values tend to be slightly higher for men because of their larger muscle mass.
Pregnant women	Values are reduced in pregnancy, presumably because creatinine clearance is markedly increased.
Newborn	Lower than children
Children	0.2–1.0 mg/dL. Slight increases with age because values are proportional to body mass.

Table 4–2 Relationship of Creatinine Levels to Estimated Amount of Nephron Loss

Creatinine Level	Estimated Loss of Nephron Function
Normal creatinine (0.6–1.5 mg/dL)	Up to 25% loss
Creatinine level >1.5 mg/dL	>50% nephron function loss
Creatinine level of 4.8 mg/dL	As much as 75% nephron function loss
Creatinine level of –10 mg/dL	90% loss of nephron function—end-stage kidney disease

These figures are rough estimates. Wu (2006) noted that a 50% reduction in GFR doubles the serum creatinine level.

Increased Creatinine Level

Clinical Significance

The only pathologic condition that causes a clinically significant increase in serum creatinine level is damage to a large number of nephrons (Table 4–2). Unlike the BUN, the serum creatinine level is not affected by protein metabolism and is only minimally affected by the hydration state of the client.

As discussed in the section on BUN, a change in the BUN-to-creatinine ratio may be useful in pinpointing the primary factor that needs correction. Because the creatinine is not increased until at least one-fourth of the nephrons are nonfunctioning, it is usually not elevated in diminished renal reserve as is the BUN. Thus clients with an increased creatinine are most likely to have potentially severe renal impairment. Like the BUN, serum creatinine is used to detect potential renal damage when nephrotoxic drugs, such as the aminoglycoside antibiotics, are used. Serum creatinine levels are also routinely measured for all dialysis clients and for clients who have had renal transplants. Some renal transplant units prefer to monitor a rise in the serum concentration of beta-2-microglobulin, a serum protein, as the earliest indicator of renal transplant rejection. See Chapter 10 for another use of beta-2-microglobulin. Because creatinine levels rise and fall more slowly than BUN levels, creatinine levels are preferred for long-term assessment of renal function.

Possible Nursing Diagnoses Related to Increased Creatinine

See section on BUN.

Decreased Creatinine Level

Clinical Significance

A decreased serum creatinine level may indicate atrophy of muscle tissue. However, if skeletal muscle problems are suspected, the serum creatine is used. Note also that the creatine kinase (CK) is an important enzyme test for muscular disease. (See Chapter 12 on CPK or CK.)

CREATININE CLEARANCE TEST

The creatinine clearance test is used as an indication of GFR. The test compares the serum creatinine level with the amount of creatinine excreted in a volume of urine for a specified time. The time may be 2, 12, or 24 hours. At the beginning of the test, the client empties his or her bladder, and this urine is discarded. Thereafter, all the urine voided during the specified time period is collected. (See Chapter 3 on 24-hour urine collections. No preservative is needed.)

Sometime during the test period, a blood sample is drawn to determine the serum creatinine level. The rate of creatinine clearance is thus determined by the following formula:

$$\frac{\text{Urine creatinine} \times \text{Urine volume}}{\text{Creatinine clearance rate}} = \text{Creatinine in serum}$$

expressed in milliliters per minute per 1.72 m² of body surface.

REFERENCE VALUES FOR CREATININE CLEARANCE	
Adult: Men	95–135 mL/min Varies with the amount of lean body mass, so muscular men are usually in the upper limits of the range.
Women	85–125 mL/min
Pregnant women	May be as high as 150–200 mL/min.
Premature and newborn infants	35–65 mL/min
Children (older than 1.5 years)	55–85 mL/min
Aged	Values diminish with age, even if no renal disease exists. Glomerular filtration rate declines about 10% per decade after 50 years of age.

Decreased Creatinine Clearance

Clinical Significance

A decreased creatinine clearance rate is an indication of decreased glomerular function. In preeclampsia, the creatinine clearance drops as it does with renal impairment. However, the lesions on the kidney for preeclampsia are reversible, so there are no long-term problems unless there were problems before the pregnancy. Creatinine clearance rate is a more sensitive indication of renal dysfunction than serum creatinine alone because the serum creatinine may remain normal until the creatinine clearance is less than half the normal. Creatinine clearance is also used to evaluate the progression of renal disease. A minimum creatinine clearance of about 10 mL/min is necessary to maintain life without the use of renal or peritoneal dialysis.

The results of the creatinine clearance test, together with other assessments of renal dysfunction, help determine the long-term plans for the client. Clients may have repeated creatinine clearance tests because changes in the results may be more clinically significant when compared over a period of time.

ESTIMATION OF GLOMERULAR FILTRATION RATE (GFR)

The estimated GFR by a formula is a relatively accurate reflection of kidney function, so laboratories may report a calculated GFR. The formula, derived from a study called Modification of Diet in Renal Disease (MDRD), uses the plasma creatinine, the serum urea nitrogen, serum albumin, and age, race, and gender to calculate the GRF, whereas the Cockcroft–Gault formula uses plasma creatinine, weight, gender, and age. Both the formulas are available at www.kidney.org/professionals and www.nephron.com.

> ### REFERENCE VALUES FOR ESTIMATED GFR
>
> GFR Non-African American >60 mL/min
>
> GFR African American >60 mL/min

Clinical Significance

The estimated GFR is useful for identifying clients who may have Stage 3, 4, or 5 chronic kidney disease. However, the estimated GFR is not able to identify Stage 1 and 2 as noted in Table 4–1.

Repeated values between 30 and 59 usually mean Stage 3. However, the nurse should be aware that clients over 65 years often have values in this range. This is one reason why some medication dosages may need to be less in the elderly.

Values between 15 and 29 usually mean that kidney function is far below normal, and values less than 15 indicate very severe renal impairment. Follow-up testing and medical interventions are needed if the client is not already known to have chronic renal disease.

CYSTATIN C AND BETA-2-MICROGLOBULIN

Cystatin C, a protein produced at a constant rate by all nucleated cells, may be useful as a marker of renal function because diet, muscle mass, or inflammation do not change blood levels (Wu, 2006). Plasma or serum samples may be used. Adults usually have about 0.5–1.0 mg/L, with higher levels occurring with age. Shlipak et al. (2005) found cystatin C a stronger predictor of death and cardiovascular events than creatinine, in elderly people. Another marker of renal function is beta-2-microglobulin, discussed in Chapter 10.

SERUM AND URINE OSMOLALITY

The osmolality of serum, urine, or any other fluid depends on the number of active ions or molecules in a solution. The osmolality of a solution reflects the total *number* of osmotically active particles in the solution, without regard to the size or weight of the particles. In laboratory reports, osmolality is expressed in milliosmoles per kilogram of water (mOsm/kg water).

Although nurses do not need to know how to calculate milliosmoles, they may find it helpful to understand conceptually the meaning of a milliosmole (mOsm). A milliosmole is 1/1,000 of an osmole. *Osmoles* are a standard of measurement based on the freezing point of a solution: As the number of osmotically active particles in a solution increases, the freezing point decreases. For example, a lower temperature is needed to freeze a salt solution than to freeze plain water. As a standard of measurement, one osmole is the amount of a particular solute that lowers the freezing point of 1 kg of water 1.86°C. With a standard measurement of osmoles and of milliosmoles for clinical studies, the precise concentration of active solutes in the serum and urine can be calculated. Although sodium is the principal constituent of serum osmolality, urea nitrogen is also one of the major factors in urine osmolality.

Serum Osmolality

Sodium, BUN, and blood glucose levels are important factors in determining serum osmolality. In severe dehydration, serum osmolality increases. Chapter 5 discusses hypernatremia as a type of hyperosmolar dehydration, and Chapter 8 discusses hyperglycemic hyperosmolar nonketotic (HHNK) dehydration. An estimate of serum osmolality may be obtained from the laboratory values of sodium, potassium, BUN, and blood glucose, as shown in Table 4–3. The osmolality calculated from laboratory values may be as much as 9 mOsm less than the measured one. This difference between the measured and the estimated is called the *osmolal* or *osmole gap*. Unmeasured substances such as methanol or ethanol increase this gap even greater, because each 0.10 mg/dL of ethanol raises the serum osmolality about 22 mOsm. Thus, a serum osmolality may be useful for screening for alcohol ingestion. Chapter 17 discusses the direct measurement of blood alcohol levels.

Urine Osmolality

Urine osmolality, like specific gravity, is a measurement of the concentration of the urine. (See Chapter 3 on the specific gravity of urine.) Urine osmolality reflects the

Table 4–3 Estimation of Serum Osmolality from Laboratory Values Formula

2(Na) + BUN/2.8 + Blood glucose/18

Example of normal reference values

2(135) + 12/2.8 + 110/18

270 + 4.29 + 6.11 = 280 mOsm[a]

[a]*Osmolal gap*. This gap is the difference between the estimated (calculated) and the measured serum osmolality. A gap of more than 9 mOsm provides a clue to unusual solutes such as alcohol.

total number of osmotically active particles in the urine, without regard to the *size* or *weight* of the particles. As a result, high sugar concentrations, proteins, or dyes do not disproportionately raise urine osmolality as they do the specific gravity of the urine. The urine osmolality test has at least three other advantages over the specific gravity:

1. The temperature variable is controlled with the osmolality determination, so the results are more accurate.
2. Because the osmolality test is a more sensitive measurement, a small change in the amount of solutes is evident with the osmolality test, but not with the specific gravity.
3. The urine osmolality can be compared with the serum osmolality to provide a more definitive idea of the fluid balance or imbalance.

The disadvantages of the osmolality test are that it cannot be completed immediately by the nurse as can the specific gravity and it is more expensive.

Preparation of Client and Collection of Sample

There is no special preparation of the client for the test. Depending on the type of machine used, the laboratory can perform an osmolality on as little as 2–5 mL of serum or urine.

REFERENCE VALUES FOR SERUM AND URINE OSMOLALITY	
Serum osmolality	Range 280–296 mOsm/kg water. Usually about 285 (290 mOsm = 1.010 specific gravity)
Urine osmolality	Extreme range of 50–1,400 mOsm/kg water, but average is about 500–800 mOsm (800 mOsm = 1.022 specific gravity). Newborns have low urine osmolality. After an overnight fast (14 hr), the urine osmolality should be at least three times the serum osmolality.

Increased Urine Osmolality

Clinical Significance

A high urine osmolality, when the serum osmolality is normal or increased, indicates that the kidneys are conserving water (Table 4–4). As the serum osmolality rises, because of the presence of abnormal solutes or due to hemoconcentration, the urine osmolality should also rise: The higher the number of milliosmoles in the urine, the more concentrated is the urine. This is the expected physiologic response to a lack of fluids for metabolic needs.

A less-than-normal serum osmolality and a high urine osmolality do not constitute a normal physiologic response. For some reason the plasma remains dilute. An increased level of the ADH causes a dilution of the plasma and a more concentrated urine. This syndrome is called syndrome of inappropriate ADH (SIADH) secretion. Medications, trauma, or stress reactions may cause an increased production of ADH, but this reaction is usually transitory. Advanced age may increase susceptibility to an increased secretion of ADH (McPhee, Papadakis, & Rabow, 2011). Fluids may need to be restricted for SIADH.

Table 4-4 Clinical Implications of Changes in Osmolality

Serum Osmolality (280–296 mOsm)	Urine Osmolality (500–800 mOsm)	Clinical Significance
Normal or increased	Increased	Fluid volume deficit
Decreased	Decreased	Fluid volume excess
Normal	Decreased	1. Increased fluid intake or 2. Diuretic use
Increased or normal	Decreased (with no increase in fluid intake)	1. Kidneys unable to concentrate urine or 2. Lack of ADH (diabetes insipidus)
Decreased	Increased	Syndrome of inappropriate secretion of ADH (SIADH) can be caused by stress, trauma, drugs, or malignant tumor.

Note: See discussion in the text under high and low urine osmolality for more details on clinical significance and possible nursing diagnoses. Note that alcohol can increase serum osmolality. See Table 4–3 for note on osmolal gap.

Possible Nursing Diagnoses Related to Increased Urine Osmolality

Risk for Deficient Fluid Volume

A very high urine osmolality means that the client is dehydrated. A moderately high urine osmolality is probably also due to a lack of fluids, as long as it is not due to fluid retention resulting from an increased ADH level. The urine osmolality should be used as only one part of the database about the fluid balance of the client. Other factors, such as clinical signs of dehydration, total intake and output, weight gain or loss, and the pathologic state of the client, must all be taken into account. The serum osmolality, if available, helps to determine the amount of dehydration present. The type and method of fluid replacement depend on the cause and severity of fluid loss.

Risk for Excess Fluid Volume

If the client's retention of fluids is possibly due to an increased level of ADH, extra fluids may not be warranted, even though the urine osmolality is high. For example, in a client who is recovering from an operation, concentrated urine may be normal for 2 or 3 days after the operation, because ADH is holding some extra fluid in the plasma. As the stress level decreases, hormone levels return to normal, and the extra fluid is released. This is sometimes called surgical diuresis. A similar diuresis occurs after other kinds of stress such as extensive burns. A comparison of serum and urine osmolality may be helpful in differentiating a slightly increased urine osmolality due to fluid retention from one that continues to increase because of a basic lack of fluids. It is important neither to overload clients with fluids nor to let them become dehydrated. Nurses can use the serum osmolality as one objective measurement.

Low Urine Osmolality

Clinical Significance

Urine osmolality should always be higher than serum osmolality unless there is a known reason for the excretion of dilute urine, such as increased fluid intake or the use of diuretics (Table 4–4). In the case of either, the serum osmolality is expected to be within normal range as the excess fluid is excreted. What is not expected is a continuing low urine osmolality when the serum osmolality begins to increase. With the client in a dehydrated state, the urine osmolality should be quite high. If the serum osmolality is normal and the urine osmolality remains about 280 mOsm/kg water, this set of conditions indicates an inability to concentrate urine, which may be an early sign of renal damage. Or it may be caused by a lack of secretion of ADH, which causes the client to have very dilute urine all the time. This pathologic lack of ADH is called *diabetes insipidus* (DI). DI may be caused by some pathology of the brain (central DI) or if the kidney becomes resistant to ADH (nephrogenic). Nephrogenic DI is less common and is usually related to lithium use or hepercalcemia in adults (Simmons, 2010). A client with central DI will need replacement of ADH, which is usually given intranasal as desmopressin (Deglin, Vallerand, & Sanoski, 2011).

Possible Nursing Diagnoses Related to Low Urine Osmolality

Risk for Fluid Volume Imbalances

Because dilute urine is expected in clients undergoing diuretic therapy, the main nursing concern is to monitor fluid balance so that not too much fluid is lost. A low urine osmolality is also expected if the goal is to increase fluids to make the urine dilute. Urine osmolality can be an objective evaluation that an increased fluid intake is having the desired results. (Recall that a client who is not getting enough fluids has a consistently high urine osmolality.)

Risk for Alteration in Urinary Elimination

Eventually with renal dysfunction, the urine osmolality may remain the same as the plasma level, which is about 290 mOsm/kg water. Chapter 3 explained that a "fixed" urine specific gravity is always about 1.010, because this is the specific gravity of the plasma. The comparison of urine and plasma osmolalities is a more sensitive measurement of this same concept. Nursing implications for clients with an inability to concentrate urine include a careful assessment of the amount of fluids they need to excrete waste products. Dehydration must be avoided.

Deficient Knowledge Related to Replacement of ADH

Much more rarely, a decreased urine osmolality may be related to a lack of ADH, in which case nurses would observe that the client is excreting huge amounts of urine. The treatment of choice is intranasal desmopressin acetate (DDAVP), a synthetic analogue of ADH. The medication is usually given as an intranasal spray or as a tablet. Intravenous and subcutaneous preparations are also available (Deglin et al., 2011). Desmopressin may also be used to treat nocturnal enuresis in children (Hay et al., 2011). Nurses may be responsible for teaching the client how to take the drug and how to observe for any side effects or complications.

URIC ACID (SERUM AND URINE)

Uric acid is the end product of purine metabolism. Purines, which are in the nucleo-proteins of all cells, are obtained from both dietary sources and the breakdown of body proteins. The kidneys excrete uric acid as a waste product.

The exact level of uric acid that is considered pathologic is controversial. In recent years, it has been generally recognized that the so-called normal ranges of uric acid are quite wide. In light of this ambiguity and because uric acid levels show day-to-day and seasonal variations in the same person, clinicians usually order several uric acid levels over a period of time. Urine uric acid levels may also be used to evaluate gout or determine overexcretion of uric acid.

Preparation of Client and Collection of Sample

An overnight fast is needed. To perform the test, the laboratory needs 1 mL of serum, which has to be sent immediately to the laboratory. It may be useful to ask about a dietary history of intake of purine-rich foods. For urine specimens, the laboratory may require use of an alkaline preservative in the 24-hour urine collection bottle. (See Chapter 3 on client instructions for 24-hour collections.)

REFERENCE VALUES FOR SERUM URIC ACID	
Adults: Men 　　　Women	3.6–8.5 mg/dL 2.3–6.6 mg/dL
Pregnant women	In early pregnancy, the levels fall about one-third but rise to nonpregnant levels by term.
Children (10–18 years): Boys 　　　　　　　　Girls	2.0–5.5 mg/dL 2.0–4 mg/dL Striking rise in boys 12–14 years coincides with puberty. Rise in girls may occur at 12 years.
Aged: Men older than 40 years 　　　Women older than 40 years	2–8.5 mg/dL 2–8.0 mg/dL Rise in women is related to menopause.

Uric acid levels tend to vary from day to day and from laboratory to laboratory.

REFERENCE VALUE FOR URINE URIC ACID	
250–750 mg/24-hr specimen	Influenced by purine content in diet (see Table 4–5)

Increased Uric Acid Level (Hyperuricemia)

Clinical Significance

Although gout, a disease much more common in men than women, is the specific disease associated with consistently high serum uric acid levels, several other conditions commonly cause hyperuricemia:

1. The most common is renal impairment because the kidneys normally excrete uric acid. However, because the level of the uric acid increase does not correlate with the severity of the renal disease, serum uric acid is not used as a test of renal function. (The BUN and creatinine tests are the two basic blood tests for renal function.)

2. A variety of drugs, such as thiazides and some other diuretics, can cause an abnormal elevation in serum uric acid by impairing uric acid clearance by the kidneys.

3. In preeclampsia and particularly in eclampsia, serum uric acid levels are quite high, partially because of the reduced GFR.

4. Another common reason is abnormal cell destruction, such as that associated with neoplasms. In neoplastic disease, chemotherapy or radiation therapy may further elevate serum uric acid levels because of the accelerated destruction of cells. Allopurinol, which prevents uric acid elevation, is sometimes started 24 hours before chemotherapy.

5. With prolonged fasting or chronic malnutrition, uric acid levels are higher than normal, because of the breakdown of cells.

Table 4–5 Examples of Foods High in Purines

Liver	Lentils
Sardines	Mushrooms
Anchovies	Spinach
Kidneys	Asparagus
Sweetbreads	

Possible Nursing Diagnoses Related to Increased Uric Acid Levels

Alteration in Comfort Related to Joint Pain

Because some clients have asymptomatic hyperuricemia, the basic nursing assessments for pain are not always a clue that there is a problem with uric acid. The symptoms of gout are caused by deposits of urate crystals in the joint. For clients with gout, the warning symptom may be discomfort from the bedspread resting on a toe or swelling and pain in one joint. Usually, the pain becomes intense and requires frequent pain medication until the gout is brought under control.

Alteration in Fluid Requirements

Whatever the reason for the high uric acid level, the danger is that uric acid, in the form of urates, crystallizes in an acidic urine and forms renal stones. In the absence of a contraindication, clients with high levels of serum uric acid need a liberal intake of fluids to prevent renal stones. "Liberal intake of fluids" should be put into specific terms, such as enough fluid to maintain a urine output of 2,000 mL/day. The specific gravity test (Chapter 3) is useful to evaluate whether the urine is dilute enough.

(Continued)

Possible Nursing Diagnoses Related . . . (Continued)

Deficient Knowledge Related to Any Dietary Modification

Dietary restrictions are usually not emphasized because drugs are used to reduce persistently high levels of serum uric acid. However, foods that are high in purines (such as sardines, anchovies, and organ meats) should probably be completely eliminated from the diet (Table 4–5); the nurse can also find out whether other meats, poultry, or fish should be restricted in their total amounts. Alcohol is to be avoided because it inhibits urate excretion. It is important that clients with high levels of serum uric acid have adequate nutrition, because fasting or starvation diets cause more of an increase in serum acid levels. Any needed weight reduction must be accomplished gradually. Maintaining adequate nutrition for a client undergoing chemotherapy may be very difficult; failure to do so may compound the serum uric acid problem.

Deficient Knowledge Related to Medications

Depending on the level of the serum uric acid and the underlying pathophysiologic condition, the physician may order:

- For acute attacks:

1. Colchicine, which does not seem to affect uric acid metabolism but does decrease urate crystal deposition
2. A nonsteroidal anti-inflammatory drug (NSAID), as an alternative to colchicine

- For maintenance therapy:

1. Uricosuric agents, which promote the elimination of urate salts, such as probenecid or sulfinpyrazone.
2. Drugs that interfere with the production of uric acid levels, such as allopurinol.
3. Febuxostat, a nonpurine selective inhibitor of xanthine oxidase, may be an alternative to allopurinol (Becker et al., 2005). This hypoallergenic drug is the first new drug for gout in many years.

Clients need to be taught the specifics about the drug ordered for them because maintenance therapy will probably be continued for years or even for life (Deglin et al., 2011).

In addition to hydration and medications, a third factor may be helpful in decreasing the possibility of renal stones from hyperuricemia: an alkaline urine. Normal urine has an acid pH because cheese, eggs, bread, meat, fish, poultry, and some fruits and vegetables contribute to acid waste products. An acidic urine, pH as low as 5.5, may contribute to urate crystallization (McPhee et al., 2011). Because one cannot routinely achieve alkalinization of the urine without severe dietary restrictions, medication such as sodium bicarbonate or potassium citrate may be used to make the urine pH higher or closer to the alkaline side.

The effectiveness of either dietary modifications or drug treatments should be periodically evaluated by testing the pH of the urine. This is easily performed by using the dipstick method described in Chapter 3. Nurses should teach clients to test their own urine.

Decreased Serum Uric Acid Level
Clinical Significance

Decreased levels usually reflect an increase in plasma volume, such as with SIADH or the effect of drugs. Renal tubular defects and liver disease also can decrease serum uric acid levels. Idiopathic hypouricemia commonly is transient. There are no specific clinical symptoms with low uric acid levels.

Questions

1. A client with congestive heart failure has a slightly elevated BUN. What is the most likely explanation for the abnormal BUN?
   a. Plasma dilution caused by aldosterone increase
   b. Increased protein breakdown caused by stress
   c. Poor renal perfusion
   d. Impaired liver function

2. Because some antibiotics may be nephrotoxic, BUN and creatinine levels should be checked before the administration of antibiotics classified as which of the following?
   a. Aminoglycosides, such as gentamicin
   b. Cephalosporins, such as cephapirin
   c. Penicillins, such as penicillin G
   d. Tetracyclines, such as doxycycline

3. The client's laboratory reports show a BUN of 75 mg and a creatinine level of 6.0 mg. (Reference values for the hospital are BUN 8–25 mg/dL and creatinine 0.6–1.5 mg/dL.) Which nursing action would be appropriate based on the laboratory information?
   a. Take vital signs every 2 hours
   b. Question whether potassium should be continued in the intravenous solution
   c. Encourage the intake of protein foods in the diet
   d. Encourage more active ambulation

4. A client is having a 4-hour creatinine clearance test begun this morning. He has just emptied his bladder. For this test, what should he be instructed to do?
   a. Save a urine sample each time he urinates so this can be compared with serum creatinine levels drawn every 30 minutes
   b. Save all the urine voided in the next 4 hours after he is given a dose of creatinine intravenously
   c. Continue to take nothing by mouth while the urine is being collected as a 4-hour specimen
   d. Save all urine for 4 hours and expect to have blood drawn once for a serum creatinine level

5. For testing for renal function and fluid balance, urine osmolality is a superior test to urine specific gravity because urine osmolality
   a. Can be performed faster on the clinical unit
   b. Detects the presence of specific electrolytes
   c. Is not changed much by glucose, protein, or radiographic dyes
   d. Requires less urine

6. When SIADH occurs in response to severe stress, which of the following is the laboratory reports for serum and urine osmolality most likely to reflect?
   a. A slight increase in serum and urine smolality
   b. A slight decrease in serum osmolality and an increase in urine osmolality
   c. A slight decrease in serum and urine osmolality
   d. A slight increase in serum osmolality and a decrease in urine osmolality

7. A client has a serum osmolality of 290 mOsm/kg and a urine osmolality of 1,400 mOsm/kg. On the basis of this information, the nurse should assess this client for effects of which of the following?
   a. Fluid overload
   b. Fluid volume deficit
   c. Lack of antidiuretic hormone
   d. Renal dysfunction

8. A urine osmolality of 300 mOsm/kg or a specific gravity of 1.010 on a first-morning-voided urine specimen is an indication that the client needs to be further assessed for which of the following?
   a. Fluid volume deficit
   b. Circulatory overload
   c. Renal dysfunction
   d. Nothing (this is a normal finding)

9. Higher-than-normal serum uric acid levels are likely for which one of the following?
   a. A client, age 8 years, who is undergoing chemotherapy for leukemia
   b. A client, age 63 years, who has rheumatoid arthritis
   c. A client, age 21 years, who has pelvic inflammatory disease
   d. A client, age 34 years, who is 2 months pregnant

10. Which of the following foods are highest in purine content?
    a. Dairy products
    b. Organ meats
    c. Grains
    d. Citrus fruits

11. What are the two measures, other than drug therapy, that help reduce the possibility of the formation of uric acid renal stones?
    a. Forcing fluids and keeping urine alkaline
    b. Exercise and consuming liberal amounts of fluids
    c. Exercise and keeping urine acid
    d. Forcing fluids and keeping urine acid

References

Becker, M. A., Schumacher, H. R., Wortmann, R. L., MacDonald, P. A., Eustace, D., Palo, W. A., et al. (2005). Febuxostat compared with allopurinol in patients with hyperuricemia and gout. *New England Journal of Medicine, 353*(23), 2450–2461.

Campoy, S., & Elwell, R. (2005). Pharmacology & CKD. *American Journal of Nursing, 105*(9), 60–72.

Castner, D. (2010). Understanding the stages of chronic kidney disease. *Nursing 2010, 40*(5), 25–31.

Deglin, J. H., Vallerand, A. H., & Sanoski, C. A. (2011). *Davis's drug guide for nurses* (12th ed.). Philadelphia: F. A. Davis.

Dinwiddie, L. C., Burrows-Hudson, S., & Peacock, E. (2006). Stage 4 chronic kidney disease. *American Journal of Nursing, 106*(9), 40–52.

Hay, W. W., Levin, M. J., Sondheimer, J. M., & Deterding, R. (Eds.). (2011). *Current diagnosis and treatment: Pediatrics* (20th ed.). New York: McGraw-Hill.

Katzung, B. J., Masters, S. B., & Trevor, A. J. (2009). *Basic and clinical pharmacology* (11th ed.). New York: McGraw-Hill.

Legg, V. (2005). Complications of chronic kidney disease. *American Journal of Nursing, 105*(6), 40–50.

McPhee, S. J., Papadakis, M. A., & Rabow, R. W. (Eds.). (2011). *Current medical diagnosis and treatment* (50th ed.). New York: McGraw-Hill.

Shlipak, M. G., Sarnak, M. J., Katz, R., Fried, L. F., Seliger, S. L., Newman, A. B., et al. (2005). Cystatin C and the risk of death and cardiovascular events among elderly persons. *New England Journal of Medicine, 352*(20), 2049–2060.

Simmons, S. (2010). Flushing out the truth about diabetes insipidus. *Nursing 2010, 40*(1), 55–59.

Thomas-Hawkins, C., & Zazworsky, D. (2005). Self-management of chronic kidney disease. *American Journal of Nursing, 105*(10), 40–49.

Wu, A. H. (Ed.). (2006). *Tietz clinical guide to laboratory tests* (4th ed.). St. Louis, MO: Saunders.

Websites

www.kidney.org (Information on all renal tests.)
www.nephron.com (Information on tests for glomerular filtration rate.)

Answers

1. c, 2. a, 3. b, 4. d, 5. c, 6. b, 7. b, 8. c, 9. a, 10. b, 11. a

Four Commonly Measured Electrolytes

- Interpreting Serum Electrolyte
  Reports   103
- Measurement by Milliequivalents   104
- Chemical Electrical Neutrality   105
- Anion Gap   106
- Serum Sodium   107
- Urine Sodium   114
- Serum Potassium   114
- Urine Potassium   120
- Serum and Urine Chloride   121
- Serum Bicarbonate or Carbon
  Dioxide, Total   123

OBJECTIVES

1. State which of the four commonly measured electrolytes show wide variation in different age groups and in pregnancy.
2. Differentiate between milligrams (mg), milliequivalents (mEq), and milli-moles (mmol) in relation to measurements of electrolytes in the serum and in replacement therapy.
3. Give examples of how the serum cations and anions are kept in electrical neu-trality by the kidney and by shifts into and out of cells.
4. Explain the effect of water deficit and water overload on serum sodium levels.
5. Describe nursing assessments that might help identify clients with increased and decreased serum sodium levels.
6. Identify possible nursing diagnoses for clients with hypernatremia and hyponatremia.
7. Explain why serum potassium levels may not accurately reflect total body potassium levels.
8. Describe the nursing assessments that might help identify clients with increased or decreased serum potassium levels.
9. Identify possible nursing diagnoses for clients with hyperkalemia and hypokalemia.
10. Explain the clinical significance of the relationship of serum chloride to serum bicarbonate.

Although many electrolytes are in the blood, when electrolytes (or "lytes") are ordered as a laboratory test, the test is for the four common ones discussed in this chapter. A shorthand method of reporting lytes on a client's chart is

$$\frac{140 \mid 103}{4 \mid 27}$$

Sodium and chloride are the two values on the top, and potassium and bicarbonate are on the bottom. Laboratory evaluations of these four basic electrolytes are critical in the assessment of fluid and electrolyte balance as well as acid–base balance.

This chapter focuses primarily on the serum levels of the first three electrolytes and on the urine levels of sodium and potassium. Because the reference values for these three electrolytes are essentially the same for all populations after the newborn period, it is expedient for nurses to memorize them. Only bicarbonate is substantially changed according to age and pregnancy.

Bicarbonate is discussed in the next chapter in relation to acid–base balance and arterial blood gases. The discussion explains why some laboratories may report serum bicarbonate levels with a test called the "CO_2 content."

The three less commonly measured electrolytes—calcium (Ca^{2+}), magnesium (Mg^{2+}), and phosphate (PO_4^-)—are covered in Chapter 7.

INTERPRETING SERUM ELECTROLYTE REPORTS

When interpreting the reports of serum electrolytes, one must always keep in mind that the laboratory report reflects only *serum* levels. It may not be an accurate reflection of the body's total electrolyte level. Generally, the level of electrolytes in the serum is very close to the electrolyte levels in the interstitial fluid. However, interstitial fluid does not have the plasma proteins found in serum. Because the electrolytes can shift readily from plasma to interstitial fluid, or vice versa, the extracellular fluid remains similar in substances other than the plasma proteins.

However, the electrolyte compositions of extracellular (serum and interstitial) fluid and intracellular (cell) fluid are strikingly different. Sodium (Na^+) and chloride (Cl^-) are the two principal electrolytes in the extracellular fluid, whereas potassium (K^+), magnesium, and phosphate are the principal intracellular ions (Table 5–1). Shifts of electrolytes do occur between the cells and the extracellular fluid, but not in large amounts. So the measurement of only serum levels cannot always accurately reflect the status of the electrolytes in the individual cells. For example, during a pathologic state, such as acidosis, more potassium will shift out of the cells because more hydrogen (H^+) ions are moving into the cell. Thus the serum level may seem normal or even high, yet the cells are becoming deficient in their main electrolyte, potassium.

Serum sodium and chloride levels rarely reflect the total sodium or chloride content in the body because a change in these levels causes a corresponding change in the volume of the plasma. Sodium and chloride are responsible for most of the osmotic pressure in extracellular fluids. So if the sodium and chloride ions increase in the plasma, they retain more water in the plasma. Hence the concentration of sodium is still reported as 135–145 mEq and the chloride as

Table 5-1	Composition of Electrolytes in Serum, Interstitial Fluids, and Cells	
Fluid	**Principal**	**Electrolytes**
■ **EXTRACELLULAR**		
Serum	Na^+	Sodium
	Cl^-	Chloride
	HCO_3^-	Bicarbonate
Interstitial	Almost the same as plasma (note no plasma proteins)	
■ **INTRACELLULAR**		
Cellular	K^+	Potassium
	Mg^{2+}	Magnesium
	PO_4^-	Phosphate

100–106 mEq, both *per liter of fluid*. More sodium and chloride (i.e., more salt) in the plasma hold more water in the vascular system and eventually in the interstitial spaces (edema).

MEASUREMENT BY MILLIEQUIVALENTS

Electrolytes are reported in milliequivalents (mEq) rather than in milligrams (mg). The reason is that milligrams measure only the weight of the chemical element, and equal weights do not mean equal chemical activity. For example, it takes 39 mg of potassium to equal 23 mg of sodium in a measurement of chemical activity based on a common standard (Table 5–2). The standard of equivalents is based on how many grams of an element or compound liberate or combine with 1 g of hydrogen. Because it takes 23 g of sodium to liberate 1 g of hydrogen, the equivalent weight of sodium is 23 g. A *milliequivalent,* the term used in laboratory reports, is one-thousandth (1/1,000) of an equivalent. If it takes 23 g to make 1 equivalent, 23 mg equals 1 mEq.

The important point to remember about the standard of equivalents and milliequivalents is that 1 mEq of one element always has the same chemical activity as

Table 5-2	Conversion of Milligrams to Milliequivalents
Measurement of Weight	**Measurement of Chemical Activity**
23 mg of sodium (Na^+)	1 mEq
39 mg of potassium (K^+)	1 mEq
36 mg of chloride (Cl^-)	1 mEq
30 mg of bicarbonate (HCO_3^-)	1 mEq

■ **PROBLEM 1**
1,000 mg of sodium = _____ mEq
Solution: 1,000 / 23 = 43 mEq

■ **PROBLEM 2**
40 mEq of potassium = _____ mg
Solution: 40 × 39 = 1,560 mg

1 mEq of another element. If milligrams or grams are used to measure the amount of electrolytes in diets or medications, the amount of electrolyte milliequivalents must be converted to discuss the physiologic effect of the drugs or diet. For example, a diet of 1,000 mg of sodium (not sodium chloride) would provide about 43 mEq of sodium. This figure is derived from the fact that it takes 23 mg of sodium to make 1 mEq: 1,000 mg/23 mg = 43 mEq. A more detailed discussion about sodium and salt is covered in the section on sodium. Usually sodium is measured in milligrams.

Potassium is the other electrolyte that may sometimes be measured in milligrams in medication or diet prescriptions. A diet that contains 1,560 mg of potassium supplies 40 mEq of potassium (it takes 39 mg of potassium to equal 1 mEq: 1,560 mg + 39 = 40 mEq). Medications, such as potassium chloride, may be marked in both milligrams and milliequivalents.

CHEMICAL ELECTRICAL NEUTRALITY

All electrolytes in the serum carry either negative charges (*anions*) or positive charges *(cations)*. These negative and positive charges must always be in perfect balance so that the serum remains neutral. The electrical neutrality of the serum is essential in understanding why certain electrolytes may be lost or retained in the serum, even though this upsets acid–base balance.

One way for the body to always maintain an equal number of positive and negative ions in the serum is shifting of electrolytes from the cells or vice versa. For example, when bicarbonate (HCO_3^-) levels are reduced in the serum, other negative ions must replace the missing negative bicarbonate ions. To keep the electrical balance in the serum neutral, chloride can shift out of the cells. This *chloride shift* occurs in the transport of carbon dioxide. Another example involves the relationship of the positive ions potassium and hydrogen. When the level of serum potassium falls, there is an increased shift of potassium out of the cells to keep the serum potassium normal. As potassium comes out of the cell, hydrogen diffuses into the cell to replace the loss of positive ions intracellularly. This shifting of electrolytes from plasma to cells and vice versa is actually a more complex situation, because the kidneys are also working to remove any excess ions from the bloodstream.

Because sodium, hydrogen, and potassium are all positive ions, a change in one means a change in the others. In the distal tubules of the kidney, sodium is usually reabsorbed in exchange for either potassium or hydrogen ions. If there is an abundance of hydrogen ions to excrete, the kidney does not excrete many potassium ions. However, if the potassium level in the serum is low, the kidneys have to continue to excrete hydrogen ions even when the hydrogen is needed to maintain the acid–base balance of the serum. The relation of increased potassium levels to acidosis, as well as that of decreased potassium levels to alkalosis, is discussed in the section on potassium.

When the sodium ion is reabsorbed by the kidney, a negative ion of either chloride or bicarbonate must also be reabsorbed. If one of these two negative ions is low in the serum, more of the other must be absorbed to maintain the proper amount of anions (negative ions). This inverse relation between chloride and bicarbonate is an important consideration in some types of metabolic acid–base imbalances.

ANION GAP

Table 5–3 shows the amount of positive ions (Na$^+$ and K$^+$) compared with the amount of negative ions (Cl$^-$ and HCO$_3^-$). For the two cations (positive ions) and two anions (negative ions) that are measured in the serum, there seem to be more positive ions than negative ions, because some of the anions are not measured. This difference between the number of cations and the number of measured anions is called the *anion gap*. Actually, this gap (of 14 mEq in Table 5–3) is made up of unmeasured anions such as sulfates, phosphates, and organic acids. Usually these unmeasured anions are about 10–20 mEq, depending on the particular references used by a laboratory. The anion gap is extensively used for quality control in the laboratory as a check that there is no error in the measurement of electrolytes.

The clinical importance of the anion gap is that it is increased in the types of metabolic acidosis in which organic or inorganic acids are increased in the bloodstream. This increase in the anion gap is helpful in identifying the type of acidosis present. If there is no change in the unmeasured anions in metabolic acidosis, the decreased bicarbonate level (a negative ion) is replaced by an increased serum chloride level (another negative ion). Decreases in the anion gap can occur because of a reduction in unmeasured anions, such as albumin, or an increase in unmeasured cations, such as potassium, calcium, magnesium, and lithium (McPhee, Papadakis, & Rabow, 2011).

By this point, the reader may be a little bewildered by so many references to acid–base balance when this chapter is supposed to be on electrolytes. Electrolyte disturbances and acid–base imbalances are so intimately connected that it is hard to learn about one and not the other. Following the summary of acid–base balances in the next chapter, Table 6–6 provides general guidelines of how each electrolyte is changed in the four different types of acid–base imbalance. The concept of the anion gap is also explored in Chapter 6, in the discussion on the three types of metabolic acidosis.

Preparation of Client and Collection of Sample

Usually, all four electrolyte tests are routinely carried out, but sometimes only one is ordered, particularly the potassium. It is especially important that the blood sample not be traumatized because hemolysis of cells makes the potassium report inaccurate. (Recall that potassium is an intracellular ion.) A 0.5-mL sample is obtained by means of venipuncture and collected in a tube without additives. The client does not need to be fasting. Portable analyzers that use capillary blood are also available for point-of-care testing.

Table 5–3 Anion Gap				
Positive Ions (Cations)		**Negative Ions (Anions)**		**Unmeasured Anions**
Sodium	140 mEq	Chloride	103 mEq	Phosphates
Potassium	4 mEq	Bicarbonate	27 mEq	Sulfates Organic acids
Total	144 mEq	Total	130 mEq	(gap of 14 mEq)
		144 − 130 = gap of 14 mEq[a]		

[a]If laboratories do not use potassium in the equation, the anion gap is usually 7–16 mEq rather than 10–20 mEq.

REFERENCE VALUES FOR COMMON ELECTROLYTES

Sodium (Na$^+$)	136–145 mEq/L
Potassium (K$^+$)	3.5–5.1 mEq/L (higher in newborns)
Chloride (Cl$^-$)	98–107 mEq/L
Bicarbonate (HCO$_3^-$) (measured as CO$_2$ content)	
Adult	21–30 mEq/L
Pregnancy	19–20 mEq/L (see P$_{CO_2}$ levels in Chapter 6 for explanation of the reason for lower bicarbonate levels in pregnancy). During the puerperium, the serum bicarbonate again increases and the chloride decreases slightly (DeCherney et al., 2007).
Infant	20–26 mEq/L
Children	Slightly lower than references for adults

Note: All four electrolytes may be reported in millimoles per liter (mmol/L) rather than mEq if the SI is adopted by a laboratory. There is no change in basic numbers for these four electrolytes (see Chapter 1 on SI units).

SERUM SODIUM

Sodium has the highest concentration of all the electrolytes measured in the serum; yet changes in its level are not commonly seen, because its concentration is always related with fluid balance. Because sodium is the primary factor in maintaining osmotic pressure in the extracellular fluid, changes in sodium are hidden because "water goes where salt is." So one must always interpret a change in serum sodium levels in relation to possible fluid overload or dehydration. A rough estimate of plasma osmolality (discussed in Chapter 4) can be calculated from the sodium level by multiplying the sodium level by 2. A normal serum sodium of 140 mEq/L times 2 would equal a normal plasma osmolality of about 280 mOsm/kg water.

The serum level of sodium is not totally dependent on diet because the kidneys can conserve sodium when necessary. The hormone aldosterone causes a conservation of sodium and chloride and an excretion of more potassium. The 2010 Dietary Guidelines recommend reducing sodium intake to less than 2,300 mg a day for healthy adults age 50 years or younger. For individuals older than 50 years, or individuals with diabetes, chronic kidney disease, and high risk for hypertension, or African Americans, the goal should be 1,500 mg or less (*www.cnpp.usda.gov*). Nurses can help clients adjust their diets to these new guidelines by informing them that it takes a few weeks to get used to less sodium (Wheeler, 2010).

It is necessary to measure sodium, not just sodium chloride, in the diet because sodium is present in forms other than salt. For example, monosodium glutamate is added to many foods in the American diet. Most American diets can be substantially reduced in sodium by avoiding very salty foods and not adding extra salt to foods at the table. One gram of sodium chloride is about 0.6 g of chloride and about 0.4 g, or 17 mEq, of sodium (400 mg/23 mg = 17 mEq). Table 5–4 lists the amount of sodium in different proportions of salt and food substances. Table 5–5 describes the meaning of sodium labels for food.

REFERENCE VALUES FOR SODIUM

Newborn, cord blood	126–166 mmol/L
Infant	139–146 mmol/L
Child	138–145 mmol/L
Adult	136–145 mmol/L
Older adult (after age 90)	132–146 mmol/L

Reference values are from Wu (2006).

Hemodilution in pregnancy may cause slight drop in adult values.

Note that serum sodium decreases by 1.6 mmol/L for every 100-mg rise in serum glucose.

Table 5–4   Relative Sodium Content of Foods

Foods with about 500 mg sodium (22 mEq)	¼ scant tsp salt (40% of salt is sodium) ¾ tsp monosodium glutamate ½ boullion cube 1 cup (240 mL) tomato juice Average serving of cooked cereal 1 hotdog 1 ½ oz (42 g) ham
Foods with about 250 mg sodium (11 mEq)	1 oz (28 g) canned tuna ⅔ cup (158 mL) buttermilk 5 salted crackers
Foods with about 200 mg sodium (9 mEq)	1 slice bread 2 slices bacon 3 oz (84 g) shrimp ½ oz (14 g) cheese 1 tbsp (15 mL) catsup

Note: The American Heart Association has a wealth of literature on low-sodium diets.

Table 5–5   Meaning of Sodium Labels for Food

"Sodium free"	Less than 5 mg of Na^+ per serving
Very low sodium	35 mg or less of Na^+
Low sodium	140 mg or less of Na^+
Reduced sodium	Processed to reduce usual level of Na^+ by at least 25%
Light or lite in Na^+	At least 50% less than the salted type
Unsalted	Processed without salt

Note: Also teach clients to note the actual sodium content for specific foods (Table 5–4).

Rinsing canned vegetables can reduce sodium (Morin, 2010).

Increased Serum Sodium Level (Hypernatremia)

Clinical Significance

An increase in the serum sodium level becomes apparent only when there is not sufficient water in the body to balance the increasing sodium level. Because sodium has an osmotic action, an increase in serum sodium pulls water into the

Table 5-6 Clinical Situations Commonly Associated with Serum Sodium Abnormalities

■ **HYPERNATREMIA**—serum Na increased (↑) 145 mEq/L
Dehydration is the most frequent cause
Overuse of intravenous saline solutions
Exchange transfusion with stored blood
Impaired renal function

■ **HYPONATREMIA**—serum Na decreased (↓) 135 mEq/L
Excessive water—"dilutional" hyponatremia
Loss of sodium by vomiting, diarrhea, gastrointestinal suctioning, or sweating
Use of diuretics, diabetic acidosis, Addison's disease, or renal disease, which all cause increased loss of sodium via urine

Note: See text for explanation of why fluid volume changes are usually the underlying cause for changes in serum sodium levels.

vascular system from the interstitial spaces and the cells. When the laboratory test for *serum* sodium level is elevated, the client is depleted in water, not only in the extracellular compartment but also in the cells (Table 5–6). Thus many cases of an increase in *total body* sodium do not cause an increased *serum* sodium level. For example, clients with congestive heart failure have sodium retention caused by the action of the hormone aldosterone. However, the retention of sodium means an equal retention of water, so the serum sodium level remains about 140 mEq per *liter* of fluid.

For the serum sodium level to be increased on a laboratory report, it is necessary that either (1) there is a large increase in sodium *without* a proportional increase in water or (2) there has been a loss of a large amount of water *without* a proportional loss of salt. Under most circumstances, increasing sodium intake without increasing water intake is not likely because an increased sodium intake makes a person very thirsty. If the client is receiving intravenous fluid, such as normal saline solution, it may be possible to overload with sodium. Intravenous solutions of normal saline contain 0.9% sodium chloride, that is, 0.9 g of salt in 100 mL or 9 g in 1,000 mL. This percentage is 154 mEq of sodium and 154 mEq of chloride per liter. Also, the use of a concentrated sodium chloride solution rather than sterile water as a diluent for intravenous medications can lead to hypernatremia in infants or small children. Infants who receive exchange transfusions with stored bank blood may become hypernatremic because stored blood has high sodium levels. An intravenous infusion of dextrose 5% in water is given to prevent overload of sodium.

The much more common reason for an increased serum sodium level is a loss of a large amount of water without a proportional loss of sodium. For example, diarrhea or vomiting may cause a severe decrease in total body water, particularly in infants. Not all dehydration results in an increased sodium level, however, because just as much sodium may be lost as water; this loss of equal amounts of sodium and water is called *isotonic dehydration*, and is the type that occurs in most infants hospitalized for a deficient fluid volume caused by vomiting or diarrhea. In dehydration caused by a loss of water or a lack of water intake, the sodium loss is not proportional, and hence the dehydration is *hypertonic*. Even in the early stages of hypertonic dehydration, the serum sodium level is not elevated because water is pulled from the interstitial spaces to keep the sodium at a normal dilution in the serum.

A serum sodium level that begins to rise above normal is a sign of a serious deficit of water that has extended to the cellular level. Another term for this type of dehydration is *hyperosmolar dehydration*. The serum is increased in osmolality, not because of a total sodium increase, but because of a total body water deficit.

Possible Nursing Diagnoses Related to Hypernatremia

Deficient Fluid Volume

The initial symptom of hypernatremia is likely to be thirst, which, if the person is unconscious, confused, or very young, is a subjective symptom that is not communicated to the nurse. Also, the thirst response, the body's primary signal for the need for more fluids, becomes blunted with age (Mentes, 2006). Other clinical assessments that correlate with a high serum sodium level include elevated temperature; dry, sticky mucous membranes; and little or no urine output. The specific gravity of urine is high if the kidneys are still able to concentrate urine. The hematocrit (Hct) is increased when the water deficit is severe. In infants, a high-pitched cry and depressed fontanels are other signs of severe water deficit. Hyperactive reflexes and irritability may lead to seizures with high sodium levels (Given, 2010).

In adults, each 3 mEq of serum sodium above the usual reference range represents a deficit of about 1 L of fluid. Thus, a serum sodium level of 157 mEq would be about 12 mEq above the reference range of 135–145 mEq. This excess indicates a deficit of about 4 L of fluid. Because 1 L of water weighs 1 kg (2.2 lb), a loss of 4 L means a weight loss of nearly 9 lb (4 kg). In a small child, the loss of even a liter of fluid would constitute severe dehydration because a loss of 2.2 lb may be 10% of the total weight of the child. The most accurate measurement of the amount of water deficit is the client's loss of weight. Daily weights should be part of the nursing assessment for any clients experiencing fluid losses.

Assisting with Treatments. For hypernatremia caused by a water deficit, the therapeutic interventions focus on replacing the lost water. If oral intake is not possible, physicians order intravenous fluids to hydrate the client. A typical order for hypernatremia may be dextrose 5% with 0.45% sodium chloride (Sweeney, 2010). Fluid deficits need to be corrected gradually, particularly in infants. A decrease in serum sodium more than 0.5–1.0 mEq/L an hour may cause cerebral edema, seizures, and severe injury to the central nervous system (CNS) (Hay et al., 2011). Fluid orders may have to be changed every few hours depending on the response of the client and the results of serial sodium levels. If the dehydration was caused by gastrointestinal problems, food is gradually added back to the diet. The BRAT diet (bananas, rice cereal, applesauce, and tea or toast) is easy on the gastrointestinal tract.

Preventing Sodium Overload. Often the nurse may be able to prevent hypernatremia caused by water deficit by careful observation of clients at risk. For instance, clients who are not taking enough oral fluids may become water deficient. Those who are receiving normal saline solutions (0.9% NaCl) should be checked for any signs of hypernatremia. Intravenous solutions for maintenance are usually only one-half normal saline (0.45% NaCl) or even one-fourth normal saline (0.25% NaCl). Normal saline solutions (0.9% NaCl) are not used for maintenance solutions unless the client has hyponatremia. Infants who receive blood exchange usually have a peripheral line for infusion of dextrose 5% in water (D_5W), because the stored blood is high in sodium.

Excess Fluid Volume Related to Excess Sodium

When both sodium and water are retained in excessive amounts, the symptoms are different from when sodium is in excess. The signs and symptoms of increased total body sodium levels are weight gain, elevated blood pressure, dyspnea, and pitting edema (the common signs of fluid retention). In adults, edema becomes apparent only after about 3 L of water is retained; this amount of water retention would mean 3 kg (6.6 lb) of weight gain before the edema shows. Thus weight gain is the most sensitive detector of early fluid retention.

Deficient Knowledge Related to Need for Sodium Restriction

A client with both sodium and water retention is often prescribed diuretics or a low-sodium diet. Also, clients with hypertension usually eat low-sodium diets. About 30% of clients with hypertension can benefit from a 500-mg sodium diet, but because compliance is difficult, a more moderate goal is usually set. A diet of 500 mg is very restrictive. It allows only 22 mEq of sodium a day (500 mg ÷ 23 mg = 22 mEq). A teaspoon of salt has 2,000 mg of sodium or 87 mEq. (See Table 5–5 on the meanings of sodium labels.)

The effectiveness of sodium restriction is determined by the absence of fluid retention or a reduction in blood pressure and *not by the serum sodium level*. Nurses may need to go over this point several times with clients. It may be difficult for clients to see a need to restrict sodium and salt intake when the laboratory report is "normal" for sodium. The American Heart Association has excellent teaching material about low-sodium diets.

Decreased Serum Sodium Level (Hyponatremia)

Clinical Significance

Like serum sodium increases, serum sodium decreases are not accurate reflections of total body sodium levels because sodium is usually lost with water. The more common reason for a low serum sodium is an excess of water in the body. The water excess can be caused by giving salt-free intravenous fluids. Intravasation, an over-absorption of large volumes of water into the vascular system, can be a complication from diagnostic procedures or surgery where a large amount of water is instilled in a body cavity such as the bladder or uterus. The excess fluid absorbed into the vascular system can drop sodium to a dangerous level. Also, in stress and severe illness, there may be an increased production of antidiuretic hormone (ADH), which causes an increase in total body water. The syndrome of inappropriate ADH (SIADH) secretion can also be caused by various drugs such as antidepressants and psychotropics (McPhee et al., 2011). Compulsive water drinking by mentally ill clients can cause hyponatremia or water intoxication. Most cases of water excess are usually terminated by an increased urine output, which restores the sodium and water balance. (See Chapter 4 on serum and urine osmolality.)

Although a real water excess is the more common reason for a low serum sodium level, actual sodium depletion can also be a cause of a low serum sodium level. Ordinarily, the hormone aldosterone conserves sodium, but a continual loss of sodium with only water replacement and no sodium replacement eventually leads to true sodium depletion. For example, a client who is taking diuretics and consuming a restricted sodium diet may experience massive sodium depletion from the body. Excessive sodium loss also occurs in

1. Some types of renal failure, in which there is "salt wasting."
2. Diabetic acidosis, in which polyuria contributes to a great loss of sodium. For each 100-mg increase of serum glucose, the serum sodium decreases by 1.6–2.0 mmol/L.
3. Vomiting and diarrhea, particularly in young children, if gastrointestinal losses are replaced only with water.
4. Vigorous exercise, in which perspiration can deplete sodium.
5. Deficiency of adrenal corticosteroids (Addison's disease). The severe hypotension of an addisonian crisis occurs because the total body sodium is not enough to keep fluid in the vascular system. (See Chapter 15 on cortisone tests.)
6. Cerebral salt-wasting syndrome (CSWS) sometimes occurs after acute central nervous system injury or surgery. One of the ways to distinguish this from SIADH is that the client has volume depletion with the low sodium level (Jimenez et al., 2006).

Possible Nursing Diagnoses Related to Hyponatremia

Excess Fluid Volume Related to Water Intoxication

Although this discussion differentiates the symptoms of hyponatremia (low sodium level) caused by fluid excess from those caused by a true sodium deficit, the clinical signs and symptoms usually are not so clear-cut.

When the low serum sodium level is due to just an excess of body water, the client has a weight gain equal to the amount of excess liters retained. For example, a client undergoing routine maintenance administration of intravenous fluids should not be gaining weight because the caloric intake is minimal. (A bottle of 1,000 mL of dextrose 5% contains only 50 g of dextrose.) In fact, an adult client who is undergoing maintenance use of intravenous fluids of dextrose 5% usually loses about half a pound a day. If the client is gaining weight at all, this weight has to be water. A gain of a pound means the retention of more than 500 mL of fluid. (Every nurse should memorize the fact that a liter of water weighs 1 kg (2.2 lb), or a pound for every pint.)

The other symptom of water excess is an increased urine output. If the water excess continues and if the kidneys cannot eliminate the excess water, the water diffuses into the interstitial spaces and eventually into the cells. The edema that develops is generalized; it is not contained in dependent areas such as the feet. So, for example, the face may look a little puffy. Edema of brain cells causes nausea and vomiting and eventually convulsions when the serum sodium is as low as 120 mEq. Many cases of compulsive water drinking in mentally ill clients are not detected until a seizure occurs. Psychogenic polydipsia may result in an intake of 10 L of fluid a day.

Careful nursing assessment of the intake and output records, as well as of weight gains, for clients who are susceptible to fluid overload can do much to prevent severe water intoxication. For example, elderly clients may have an increase in ADH that makes them more susceptible to hyponatremia (McPhee et al., 2011).

Imbalanced Nutrition Related to Sodium Depletion

Nurses need to be aware of clients who may be experiencing true depletion of sodium, because this type of low serum level can often be prevented if early symptoms of sodium depletion are noticed. For example, clients undergoing nasogastric suctioning can lose large amounts of sodium if very large amounts of water rather than normal saline solution are used to irrigate the nasogastric tube. Repeated tap water enemas in the elderly may also cause hyponatremia, as can large doses of diuretics. With mild to moderate depletions of sodium, the serum sodium level remains within the normal reference range while the urine sodium becomes low. (See the next section on urine sodium levels.) As the total sodium becomes low, the client has anorexia, apathy, and sometimes a sense of impending doom. Confusion may occur, particularly in elderly clients. Muscle cramps, weakness, and diarrhea reflect the lack of sodium for normal muscle contractions. Eventually the low serum sodium leads to hypotension and shock because there is a loss of osmotic pressure in the vascular system. Infants, although they may be lethargic, may not have symptoms until the sodium level is low enough to cause cerebral edema and seizures.

Assisting with Sodium Replacement. The therapeutic measures for true sodium depletion are geared toward replacing both sodium and lost fluid. Usually the intravenous solution used for replacement is normal saline solution (0.9% NaCl), although in extreme cases, a hypertonic (3% NaCl) saline solution may be used. For example, in life-threatening cerebral edema, which may occur with cerebral salt wasting, hypertonic solutions may be used (Tocco, 2010). Nurses must carefully monitor clients who are receiving hypertonic intravenous fluids, because too rapid an infusion of a hypertonic solution is very dangerous. The hypertonic solution not only can cause hemolysis of red blood cells but also can pull a large amount of fluid into the vascular space, leading to circulatory overload. The hypertonic solutions of salt are rarely used now. Either normal saline solution (0.9% NaCl) or Ringer's lactate (another isotonic solution) can supply enough sodium to safely make up the deficiency.

Deficient Knowledge Related to Specific Need for Replenishing Sodium

Because the body can conserve sodium, it is not necessary to instruct clients to eat high-sodium foods over a long period. Yet clients who may become sodium depleted because of vomiting, diarrhea, or vigorous exercise should drink salty replacement fluids such as broths instead of water alone. For infants, special formulas of electrolytes are used to replace gastrointestinal losses. Athletes who perform vigorous exercises know to replace lost fluids with special oral electrolyte preparations that are commercially available. In the past, salt tablets were often used by people who engaged in intense physical activity; it is now generally recommended to replace salt more gradually by dietary increases or salty fluids. One cup (240 mL) of tomato juice has 486 mg of sodium (see Table 5–8).

As mentioned, the U.S. diet usually contains more than enough sodium, but sometimes clients may follow too restricted a sodium diet. For example, nurses may need to assess the dietary habits of elderly clients to make sure that their sodium restrictions are not too severe, particularly if they begin taking diuretics. Children with cystic fibrosis lose extra sodium in their sweat. (See Chapter 18 on the sweat test for CF.) Clients who take lithium must also have plenty of sodium in their diet. (See Chapter 17 on lithium toxicity.) If the serum sodium is too low, the body retains too much lithium.

URINE SODIUM

Normally, the amount of sodium excreted in the urine varies with sodium intake. Increased amounts of aldosterone in the serum may cause a decreased secretion of urine sodium. (See Chapter 15 on serum and urine aldosterone levels, which may also be ordered.) Conversely, a decreased level of aldosterone activity causes an increased loss of sodium in the urine. Diabetic acidosis, SIADH, and diuretics also cause an increased loss of sodium. Various types of renal failure may cause either increased losses or retention of sodium. Poor perfusion to the kidney (prerenal azotemia) may lead to a low urine sodium, whereas acute tubular necrosis may cause a high urine sodium level.

Preparation of Client and Collection of Sample

See Chapter 3 on 24-hour urine collections. No special preservative is needed. The diet of the client should be noted as to the amount of sodium intake.

REFERENCE VALUES FOR URINE SODIUM

40–220 mEq/24 hr or 30 mEq/L (diet dependent)

Full-term infants have sodium clearance of about 20% of adult values.

SERUM POTASSIUM

Potassium is primarily an intracellular ion, but the small amount in the serum is essential for normal neuromuscular and cardiac function. Small changes in serum potassium level can have profound effects on cardiac muscle. Current guidelines for potassium are noted in Table 5–7. These levels, higher than previously recommended, should be met by a variety of foods, not by supplements. Daily intake is important because the kidneys continue to excrete 40–80 mEq/day, even when there is no intake. Evidence from a study called Dietary Approach to Stop Hypertension (DASH) led to recommendations for more potassium in the diet. See the earlier discussion in which clients should have a sodium diet as low as 1,500 mg daily. The DASH diet, high in fruits and vegetables and low in sodium, helps prevent and treat hypertension (McPhee et al., 2011).

Although potassium can also be lost in gastrointestinal drainage, the kidneys excrete almost all the potassium. The renal mechanism for potassium ion excretion is shared with another positive ion, hydrogen. Either a potassium or a hydrogen ion is excreted when a sodium ion is reabsorbed by the kidney. This relationship

Table 5–7 Recommended Daily Potassium Intake

Children 1–3	3,000 mg
4–8	3,800 mg
9–13	4,500 mg
Adults	4,700 mg

See Dietary Guidelines for Americans, 2010, of the Center for Nutrition Policy and Promotion (www.cnpp.usda.gov/dietaryguidelines.htm) for information on the new dietary guidelines.

partially explains why potassium levels are increased in acidosis and decreased in alkalosis. The shifting of potassium and hydrogen ions into and out of the cells in acid–base imbalances also contributes to marked changes in potassium levels. (See Chapter 6 on acid–base balances.)

Pseudohyperkalemia can be caused by fist clenching during phlebotomy, so the client should not clench the fist when blood is drawn. Thrombocytosis falsely elevates potassium levels, so an elevated platelet count should be recorded. Storage of the sample will also elevate potassium levels.

REFERENCE VALUES FOR SERUM POTASSIUM	
Newborn, cord blood	5.6–12.0 mmol/L
Infant	4.1–5.3 mmol/L
Child	3.4–4.7 mmol/L
Adult	3.5–5.1 mmol/L

Note: Plasma values will be about 0.1 mmol/L lower (Wu, 2006).

Hemodilution of pregnancy may cause a slight drop in the values.

Increased Serum Potassium Level (Hyperkalemia)

Clinical Significance

The most common cause of an increased serum potassium level (hyperkalemia) is inadequate renal output (Table 5–8). Thus, hyperkalemia is always a problem in the oliguric phase of renal failure unless potassium intake is limited. (See Chapter 4 for the distinction between renal insufficiency and renal failure.)

The intake of too much potassium in medications can also cause an increased serum potassium level. An overdose from oral supplements of potassium is unlikely, but the danger is real with intravenous use of potassium in high concentrations. Other medications, such as penicillin K, which contains potassium ions, can cause hyperkalemia if renal output is not adequate. (See Chapter 4 on BUN and creatinine levels as assessments of renal function.)

Because potassium is primarily an intracellular ion, anything that causes massive cell destruction increases the serum potassium level. Thus, massive tissue injury

Table 5–8 Clinical Situations Commonly Associated with Serum Potassium Abnormalities

■ **HYPERKALEMIA**—serum K^+ increased (↑) 5.0 mEq/L (or above 6.5 in newborns)
Renal failure
Too-rapid intravenous infusion of K^+ replacement
Initial reaction to massive tissue damage
Associated with metabolic acidosis (see Chapter 6)

■ **HYPOKALEMIA**—serum K^+ decreased (↓) 3.5 mEq/L
Diuretics
Inadequate intake when NPO, vomiting, or receiving K^+-free IV feedings
Large doses of corticosteroids
Aftermath of tissue destruction or high stress
Associated with metabolic alkalosis (see Chapter 6)

Note: See the text and references at the end of this chapter for further details.

Table 5–9 Examples of Medications That Can Cause Hyperkalemia

Drug Classifications	Examples of Drugs
Ace inhibitors	Lisinopril and 9 others
Angiotensin receptor blockers	Losartan and 6 others
Hormonal contraceptive	Ethinyl estradiol/drospirenone
Potassium sparing diuretics	Amiloride Eplerenone Spironolactone Triamterene
Nonsteroidal anti-inflammatory drugs	Ibuprofen

Note: See Deglin, Vallerand, & Sanoski (2011) and Katzung, Masters, & Trevor (2009) for more information.

or a burn causes the release of potassium from damaged cells. Although the serum potassium level may increase after cellular damage, the actual total body potassium is decreased. Thus, the hyperkalemia that occurs with a burn or an injury is followed by hypokalemia.

Because aldosterone and other steroids cause a retention of sodium and an increased excretion of potassium, conditions in which hormones are decreased may cause an increased serum potassium level. For example, in Addison's disease, malfunctioning of the adrenal cortex reduces the corticosteroid level. Serum sodium levels are decreased, and serum potassium levels may be increased. (See Chapter 15 on laboratory tests for cortisone.)

Hyperkalemia is often associated with metabolic acidotic states. In acidosis, the kidney must excrete more hydrogen ions, which means less secretion of potassium ions by the renal selection mechanism. In addition, an abundance of hydrogen ions in the serum means that some of these ions go into the cells, which drive potassium out of the cells. Thus, in acidotic states, the total body potassium is not increased, but more potassium ions are present in the serum. Serum potassium rises about 0.6 mEq/L for every 0.1 decrease in blood pH. If the acidotic state is due to diabetic ketoacidosis, the lack of insulin compounds the problem of hyperkalemia because potassium needs insulin, as does glucose, to be transported into the cell. (See Chapter 8 on ketoacidosis.)

Possible Nursing Diagnoses Related to Increased Potassium Levels (Hyperkalemia)

Risk for Injury Related to Effect of Hyperkalemia on Heart and Other Muscles

Probably the most important thing to remember about checking for symptoms of increasing serum potassium levels is that many of the symptoms are nonspecific. Potassium is important to nerve and muscle function, but so are most of the other electrolytes. Early symptoms of hyperkalemia may be irritability, nausea, diarrhea, and abdominal cramping. Later symptoms may include skeletal muscle weakness. The muscle weakness can progress to a flaccid-type paralysis with difficulty in speaking and breathing.

Hyperkalemia is usually an emergency situation because a high serum potassium level can cause cardiac arrhythmias that can lead to cardiac arrest: The heart stops in diastole.

Because the clinical signs of hyperkalemia can be confused with other conditions (hypokalemia can also cause paralysis), the level of serum potassium must be assessed by the laboratory report, not by physical symptoms alone. Remember that the serum laboratory test may not reflect the total body potassium. The electrocardiogram (ECG) is a very sensitive indicator of intracellular potassium, even when the serum potassium still seems normal. Nurses need to be able to identify hyperkalemia on an ECG strip. High-peaked T waves and a prolonged QRS interval are typical findings for hyperkalemia.

Assisting with Medical Interventions. Although there is no specific antidote for hyperkalemia, several different medications may be used to treat a high serum potassium level:

1. Sometimes calcium gluconate is given intravenously to lessen cardiac toxicity. Calcium may be particularly useful if the calcium levels were initially low or borderline. Calcium is not used if the client is taking digitalis, because digitalis and calcium have a synergistic effect on the heart. Calcium gluconate is generally preferred over calcium chloride because clients with hyperkalemia often have hyperchloremia. Calcium calms the irritable myocardium and has a positive inotropic effect.
2. Sodium bicarbonate may be given intravenously if acidosis is present. As the pH of the blood returns to normal, potassium shifts back into the cells. Also, when the pH is normal, the kidney can secrete more potassium ions because there is no demand to excrete so many hydrogen ions.
3. Intravenous solutions with 50% glucose and insulin help promote the reentry of potassium into the cells, even for clients who do not have diabetes.
4. Sodium polystyrene sulfonate, given orally or by enemas, is a sodium–potassium exchange resin (Deglin et al., 2011).
5. Inhaled beta-2 agonists such as albuterol also enhance a shift of potassium to cells (Hay et al., 2011).
6. For a client with chronically high potassium levels caused by renal failure, treatment includes peritoneal dialysis or hemodialysis.

Deficient Knowledge Related to Sources of Potassium

The nurse needs to find out whether the hyperkalemia is likely to be a chronic or recurring situation. If so, the client needs to be taught to read the labels on foods and medications to determine whether they are high in potassium. For example, most salt substitutes are composed of large amounts of potassium. Instant coffee and other prepared foods may have potassium as one of the ingredients.

Teaching about eliminating potassium from the diet may also have to be carried out. To reinforce client behavior, a contract may be written between the nurse and the client to keep potassium levels low through diet adherence. Potassium levels can be one evaluative tool of effective teaching. (Table 5–10 lists foods particularly high in potassium.)

Risk for Injury Related to Subsequent Development of Hypokalemia

If the high serum levels of potassium are caused by metabolic shifts in acidosis, the potassium shifts back into the cells when the pH returns to normal, and clients may have a serum deficit. Also, if the serum potassium level increases because of cell damage, the potassium lost from injured cells results in a total body deficit. Always consider the possibility that the hyperkalemia of today could result in hypokalemia tomorrow.

Decreased Serum Potassium Levels (Hypokalemia)

Clinical Significance

Because potassium is not conserved well in the body, an inadequate intake results in a low serum level. However, as the daily need of potassium for an adult is only about 80 mEq (3 g), insufficient oral intake is usually not the cause for a low potassium level unless the person is not taking anything at all by mouth. Even in fasting states, the serum potassium level may not drop immediately, because the breakdown of cells for energy causes the release of potassium.

More commonly, hypokalemia results from an excessive loss of potassium. Any loss of fluid from the gastrointestinal tract causes a loss of potassium. The most common cause of hypokalemia worldwide is diarrhea. Almost all diuretics cause an increased excretion of potassium, except spironolactone, amiloride, and triamterene. Certain hormonal changes also contribute to an excessive excretion of potassium. The corticosteroids cause sodium retention and potassium excretion. Certain tumors may produce hormones that act much like the steroids and thus increase potassium excretion. (See Chapter 15 on ectopic hormone production.) Drugs that cause excessive beta-sympathetic stimulation, such as epinephrine, can cause a transient hypokalemia (Deglin et al., 2011).

An alkalotic serum pH (pH>7.4) is another reason for a lowered serum potassium level. In alkalosis, hydrogen ions shift out of the cell in an attempt to lower the pH of the serum to normal. When hydrogen shifts out of the cell, more potassium shifts into the cell to replace the missing positive ions. Conversely, a low serum potassium level also contributes directly to the development of an alkalotic state because, when serum potassium levels are low, the kidneys must excrete more hydrogen ions in exchange for the reabsorption of sodium by the distal tubule. So either alkalosis may be the cause of hypokalemia, or hypokalemia may contribute to the development of metabolic alkalosis. The role of hypokalemia in the development of metabolic alkalosis is covered in Chapter 6, in the section on bicarbonate changes in acid–base balance.

Possible Nursing Diagnoses Related to Hypokalemia

Altered Cardiac Output Related to Development of Arrhythmias

Hypokalemia can cause bradycardia or paroxysmal tachycardia, premature ventricular contractions (PVCs), and other arrhythmias. However, abnormalities in cardiac rhythm are extremely unusual in clients without underlying cardiac disease even when the potassium is below 3.0 mEq/L. Potassium levels are usually not allowed to drop below 4.0 mEq for clients with cardiac problems. For clients taking digitalis, hypokalemia is quite dangerous because the toxic effects of digitalis are more likely to occur when the serum potassium level drops quickly. The typical ECG in a client with hypokalemia has prominent U waves, and the T waves are flat with eventual ST depression.

Risk for Injury Related to Development of Muscle Weakness

Nurses need to be aware of clients who may be having extra losses of potassium so they can assess for potential hypokalemia. Although certain clinical symptoms are caused by hypokalemia, these symptoms can also be caused by other clinical abnormalities. Clients with a low serum potassium level may have anorexia, muscle weakness, a decrease in bowel sounds, and abdominal distention due to decreased peristalsis (ileus). Ileus and lethargy are key symptoms of hypokalemia in newborns. Flaccid paralysis may develop with more severe hypokalemia, as well as with hyperkalemia, because both potassium imbalances alter the resting potential of muscle cells. Low serum potassium levels may make respiratory effort difficult.

Assisting with Potassium Replacement. Depending on the severity of the hypokalemia, potassium may be replaced in three ways: (1) intravenously, (2) by oral supplements, or (3) by diet.

Risk for Injury Related to Use of Intravenous Potassium

Potassium chloride is never given directly by intravenous push, no matter how severe the deficiency. Usually, no more than 40 mEq of potassium is added to 1,000 mL of intravenous fluids, although sometimes as much as 80 mEq is added to a liter. Clients should usually not be given more than 10 mEq in an hour, although some authorities say 20 mEq/hr is safe in severe deficiencies (Deglin et al., 2011). If the intravenous solution with the potassium must be slowed down because of a burning sensation, the solution must be made more dilute or a central catheter should be used. Potassium in high concentrations is irritating to the vein wall.

Any client who is receiving potassium must have adequate urinary output. In adults, "adequate" means at least 30 mL/hr. Newborns should produce 1 mL of urine per kilogram per hour. Thus, a newborn who weighs 4 kg (8.8 lb) should produce about 4 mL/hr of urine. In older children, 1–2 mL/kg per hour is a minimum output. The urinary output should always be assessed before potassium is added to an intravenous infusion. Once the intravenous infusion is begun, nurses must continue to make sure that urinary output remains adequate. Otherwise, hyperkalemia can develop rapidly.

Deficient Knowledge Related to Oral Potassium Supplements

Oral preparations of potassium chloride may come marked in various strengths, such as 10% or 20% solutions, or as so many milligrams per teaspoon. On the bottle, however, the dosage in milliequivalents is also given, and this is the dosage form that should be used. One teaspoon of potassium chloride elixir is not as precise as 20 mEq. Every client should be told the dosage exactly in milliequivalents, not simply to take a certain amount by volume.

The oral preparations of potassium come in various forms of elixirs, capsules, and tablets, some that fizz when mixed with juice. Most potassium supplements also contain chloride, which may be a needed replacement in metabolic alkalosis (see Chapter 6). The most important problem with oral supplements of potassium is the gastrointestinal upsets they can cause; therefore, nurses should teach clients not to take potassium supplements on an empty stomach. Liquids should be diluted. Orange juice is a good vehicle because it has a high potassium level. Overdoses of oral potassium supplements are not common, but it is important that the urinary output always be adequate.

Potassium replacement can also be accomplished with a relatively inexpensive salt substitute that contains potassium chloride. Many salt substitutes contain more than 50 mEq of potassium per teaspoon (4 mL). The client should consult the physician about the use of salt substitutes.

(Continued)

Possible Nursing Diagnoses . . . (Continued)

Deficient Knowledge Related to Dietary Sources of Potassium

The dietary intake of potassium is usually about 40–80 mEq for adults. For clients who take diuretics or who, for other reasons, need a higher intake of potassium, it may be wise to assess their dietary habits to see if they can gain extra potassium by dietary intake. Table 5–10 shows the amount of potassium in some common foods. By including potassium-rich foods, clients may be able to reduce or eliminate the need to take potassium supplements. The serum potassium levels for clients undergoing long-term diuretic therapy should be checked periodically to make sure dietary intake of potassium is adequate to balance an increased potassium loss.

URINE POTASSIUM

The amount of potassium in the urine varies with the diet. It also varies with an increased amount of serum aldosterone or cortisol, which causes an increased excretion of potassium. Renal failure causes a decreased excretion of potassium. The primary use of a 24-hour urine potassium is to assess hormonal functioning and to determine if hypokalemia is of renal or nonrenal origin. Excretion of less than 20 mEq/day in the presence of hypokalemia is evidence that the hypokalemia is not from renal loss. (See Chapter 15 on aldosterone and cortisol levels.) Urine potassium levels are also sometimes used in research studies as one indication of the stress level of the body.

Preparation of Client and Collection of Sample

See Chapter 3 for 24-hour urine collections. No preservative is needed.

Table 5–10 Foods High in Potassium and Corresponding Sodium Content

Potassium at Least 10 mEq or More by Serving	Sodium (mg)
Avocado, ½	5
Banana, 1 medium	1
Cantaloupe, 1 cup	19
Dates, 10	1
Figs, 5	10
Molasses, 2 tbsp	3
Orange juice, 1 cup	2
Potato, 1 baked	2
Prunes, 10 (high calories)	9
Salt substitutes (varies, but may be 30–40 mEq in a tsp)	Varies; check label
Soybeans, ½ cup	2
Tomato juice, canned, 1 cup	486 (can look for low-sodium type)

Note: The American Heart Association (www.heart.org) has patient information cards as well as pamphlets about potassium content in foods.

> ## REFERENCE VALUE FOR URINE POTASSIUM
>
> 25–125 mEq/24 hr (varies with diet)

SERUM AND URINE CHLORIDE

Chloride, the principal negative ion in the extracellular fluid, is important, in combination with sodium, for maintaining osmotic pressure in the serum. A loss or a gain of chloride is often due to the factors that also cause a loss or gain of sodium. Chloride is found in a variety of foods, usually in combination with sodium. A diet restricted in sodium also causes a reduction of chloride intake but not to an inadequate level. The kidneys selectively secrete chloride or bicarbonate ions, depending on the acid–base balance. In some types of renal failure, chloride excretion may be impaired. Chloride can be measured in the urine with sodium and potassium as part of a 24-hour specimen (see Chapter 3).

> ## REFERENCE VALUES FOR SERUM CHLORIDE
>
> | | |
> |---|---|
> | Newborn, cord blood | 96–106 mmol/L |
> | Infant, 0–30 days | 98–113 mmol/L |
> | Older adult (after age 90) | 98–111 mmol/L |
> | All other age groups | 98–107 mmol/L |
>
> Reference values are from Wu (2006).
>
> The value falls very little during hemodilution of pregnancy.

> ## REFERENCE VALUES FOR URINE CHLORIDE
>
> | | |
> |---|---|
> | Adult | 110–250 mEq/24 hr |
> | Child | 15–40 mEq/24 hr |
> | Infant | 2–10 mEq/24 hr |

Increased Serum Chloride Level (Hyperchloremia)

Clinical Significance

Hyperchloremia is a term that is rarely used clinically. An increase in chlorides in the serum is not a primary focus because the increase must always be evaluated in relation to (1) an increase in sodium levels or (2) a decrease in the serum bicarbonate level.

Aldosterone, a mineral corticosteroid, causes retention of both sodium and chloride. In most cases, a proportional increase in water retention makes the electrolytes in the serum appear not to be increased. For the sodium and chloride levels to be elevated, there must be a deficit of water or a large intake of sodium chloride. Because, in these situations, the chloride level parallels the rise or fall of the sodium level, the sodium level is used to monitor fluid deficits.

In some clinical situations, the rise in chlorides may be even greater than the rise in sodium levels. In some types of renal failure, the kidneys are unable to excrete chlorides properly; this inability leads to a type of acidosis called *renal hyperchloremic acidosis*. Chlorides may also be greatly increased in the bloodstream if large amounts of normal saline solution (0.9% NaCl) are infused over several days. "Normal saline" is not really normal in relation to the sodium and chloride content of the serum, even though it is classified as an isotonic solution. Normal saline contains 154 mEq of sodium ions and 154 mEq of chloride ions per liter. This is a little higher than the serum level of 135–145 mEq for sodium ions and a great deal higher than the 100–106 mEq for serum chloride.

Possible Nursing Diagnoses Related to Increased Chloride Levels

Because changes in chloride levels always take place in combination with changes in other electrolytes, assessments depend on nurses' understanding of the reason for the increased chloride level. For example, if the chloride level is related to an increased sodium level, the nursing diagnoses for sodium are to be followed. If the increased chloride level is causing or was caused by acidosis, the symptoms exhibited are those of acidosis. (Care of clients with metabolic acidosis is covered in the section on bicarbonate levels in Chapter 6.)

Chloride levels are increased in some types of acidosis because the chloride is needed to replace the loss of another negative ion, bicarbonate, from the serum. If the metabolic acidosis is due to an increase of other negative ions, such as ketoacids, the chlorides are not increased—and may actually decrease—because of diuresis. The changes in the bicarbonate level, in the chloride level, and in the unmeasured negative ions (the anion gap) give useful information about what is causing the acidotic state. The most important thing to remember about the relation between a high serum chloride level and acidosis is that if the chlorides are higher than normal, this condition causes a drop in the serum bicarbonate level because there is room for only a set amount of negative ions. If the serum bicarbonate level drops first, chlorides may be increased to keep the correct number of negative ions in the serum. Increased chloride levels can be either a cause or a result of metabolic acidosis.

Decrease in Serum Chloride Level (Hypochloremia)

Clinical Significance

Decreases in the serum chloride level are commonly due to loss from vomiting, gastric suction, diarrhea, and the use of diuretics.

Because sodium, hydrogen, and potassium ions are usually lost with the chlorides, a chloride drain is only part of a larger problem. For example, the loss of chlorides from the serum means that more bicarbonate must be retained to replace the lack of negative ions, thus contributing to the development of metabolic alkalosis. The loss of potassium or hydrogen ions also contributes to the development of metabolic alkalosis. Conversely, alkalotic states can cause a low chloride level. In metabolic alkalosis, the bicarbonate level in the serum increases, so the other principal negative ion, chloride, must decrease in the bloodstream. (By now the inverse relation between the negative ions bicarbonate and chloride should be clearly apparent.)

As explained in Chapter 6, clients with chronic lung disease often have high serum bicarbonate levels to balance an increased P_{CO_2} in the bloodstream. This chronically elevated serum bicarbonate level also causes a decreased serum chloride level. This condition would be considered a normal compensation in clients with chronic lung disease.

Possible Nursing Diagnosis Related to Decreased Chloride Levels

Imbalanced Nutrition Related to Chloride Losses

Nurses need always to be aware of clients who may be losing abnormal amounts of chlorides, so that replacement therapy can begin before alkalotic states develop. For example, clients who are undergoing gastrointestinal suctioning are losing not only chlorides but also potassium and hydrogen ions. All three losses contribute to the development of metabolic alkalosis. Because potassium supplements contain chloride, the use of potassium chloride is one way that lost chlorides are replaced. If necessary, the physician may order normal saline solution (0.9% NaCl) to be given intravenously to replace large chloride losses. The use of oral electrolyte solutions for infants or salty broths for adults to replace sodium losses has already been mentioned. Nurses must always keep in mind that a loss of electrolytes usually involves several electrolytes and never just chlorides alone.

SERUM BICARBONATE OR CARBON DIOXIDE, TOTAL

Serum bicarbonate levels are routinely part of both electrolytes and arterial blood gases. Note that the carbon dioxide (CO_2) combining power or total carbon dioxide is often used as an indirect measurement of serum bicarbonate. This indirect measurement is usually about 2 mmol/L or mEq/L more than the actual bicarbonate level, which makes up 95% of the total CO_2 combining power. The carbon dioxide is different from P_{CO_2}, which is a measure of blood gas. (Both are discussed in Chapter 6.) Because changes in serum bicarbonate level always signify some changes in acid–base balance, the relation between bicarbonate and carbonic acid is important. A bicarbonate-to-carbonic acid (as measured by the Pa_{CO_2}) ratio of 20:1 is the most important buffer in the serum. The 20:1 ratio is fundamental to understanding the clinical significance of changes in serum bicarbonate levels. The next chapter includes a summary of this ratio and a discussion of how serum bicarbonate levels decrease and increase in acid–base imbalances.

Questions

1. The home care nurse is making a visit to an elderly client who is taking digoxin and a diuretic for treatment of congestive heart failure (CHF). The nurse should be the most concerned about which of the following laboratory results? A serum level of
   a. Na^+ = 130 mmol/L
   b. K^+ = 3.0 mmol/L

    c. $Cl^- = 95$ mmol/L
    d. $HCO_3^- = 29$ mmol/L

2. When the total amount of serum Na^+ and K^+ ions (cations) are compared with the total amount of serum Cl^- and HCO_3^- ions (anions), there are fewer anions. This "anion gap" is due to which of the following facts?
   a. There are always more cations (positive ions) than anions (negative ions) in the serum
   b. Some anions, such as organic acids, are not measured
   c. The electrical balance is not always neutral in acid–base imbalances
   d. The loss of electrolytes decreases the total number of anions in the serum

3. When a client has an abnormal serum sodium (Na^+) report, the most useful nursing assessment to help explore the reason for the sodium imbalance would be which of the following?
   a. Dietary intake pattern of salt and sodium-containing foods
   b. Intake and output records and daily weights
   c. Vital signs during the past 24 hours
   d. Record of all medications given

4. A laboratory report of an increased serum sodium level would most likely be part of the clinical findings for a client
   a. With severe congestive heart failure who has pitting edema of the ankles
   b. Undergoing corticosteroid therapy for several months for rheumatoid arthritis
   c. Having diarrhea and unable to take fluids by mouth
   d. Receiving maintenance intravenous fluids of dextrose 5% in 0.2% sodium chloride for several days after an operation

5. A laboratory report of a slightly low serum sodium (Na^+) is least likely for which of the following conditions?
   a. Diet containing no more than 2.3 g (100 mEq) of sodium daily
   b. Maintenance intravenous solutions of 5% dextrose in water (D_5W) for several days
   c. Drinking large amounts of water after strenuous exercise
   d. Use of a diuretic that is an aldosterone-blocking agent

6. A characteristic assessment expected for a client with a high serum sodium (Na^+) level caused by a water deficit would include
   a. Hypertension
   b. Thirst
   c. Weight gain
   d. Subnormal temperature

7. A characteristic assessment for a client with a low serum sodium (Na^+) level caused by total body sodium depletion would be
   a. Confusion
   b. Hypertension
   c. Weight gain
   d. Flaccid paralysis

8. An increase in serum sodium (Na^+) levels is usually an indication that the client needs which of the following?
   a. Less sodium in the diet
   b. Less fluid intake
   c. More fluid intake
   d. Both sodium and water restrictions

9. Which of the following clients is the least likely to have an elevated serum K+ level?
   a. A client who is experiencing renal failure
   b. A client who suffered extensive burns today
   c. A client who is in metabolic alkalosis
   d. A client who has Addison's disease

10. A low serum potassium (K+) is most likely to be a problem for
    a. A client who is undergoing long-term diuretic therapy with thiazides
    b. A client who has mild morning sickness
    c. A client who is undergoing chemotherapy as part of treatment of leukemia
    d. A client who has a severe respiratory infection and who is not taking much fluid

11. Which of the following signs or symptoms is the most suggestive of hyperkalemia?
    a. Paralytic ileus (lack of bowel sounds)
    b. Peaked T waves on the cardiac monitor
    c. Skeletal muscle cramps
    d. Depressed T waves on the cardiac monitor

12. A client scheduled for a laparoscopic cholecystectomy tomorrow has a serum K+ of 2.3 mEq. (She has been taking thiazide diuretics.) The nurse is to monitor the potassium replacement, which the client is to receive intravenously. Which of these guidelines about potassium is correct?
    a. Urine output should be at least 100 mL/hr
    b. No more than 10–20 mEq of KCl should be given in an hour
    c. No more than 10 mEq of KCl should be added to 1,000 mL of intravenous fluids
    d. KCl is given IV push only in extreme cases in which the serum K+ is less than 2.5 mEq

13. The physician has prescribed a potassium chloride (KCl) supplement to be taken in liquid form three times a day. The nurse should instruct the client to
    a. Dilute the KCl in water, but not in juice
    b. Never take the KCl at the same time as any other medicine
    c. Not take the KCl on an empty stomach
    d. Keep the KCl in the refrigerator

14. Which item does not contain at least 10 mEq of potassium?
    a. Orange juice, 1 cup
    b. Cranberry juice, 1 cup
    c. Instant coffee, 3 g
    d. Potato, 1 baked

15. Which one of the following clients is the least likely to have low serum chloride (Cl-) levels?
    a. A client who has an elevated serum bicarbonate (HCO3-) level caused by ingestion of baking soda
    b. A client who has had severe vomiting
    c. A client who is taking loop diuretics and is on a low-sodium diet
    d. A client who is experiencing renal failure

References

DeCherney, A. H., Nathan, L., Goodwin, T. M., & Lauter, N. (Eds.). (2007). *Current obstetric & gynecologic diagnosis & treatment* (10th ed.). New York: McGraw-Hill.

Deglin, J. H., Vallerand, A. H., & Sanoski, C.A. (2011). *Davis's drug guide for nurses* (12th ed.). Philadelphia: F. A. Davis.

Given, S. B. (2010). Hypernatremia. *Nursing2010, 40*(10), 72.

Hay, W. W., Levin, M. J., Sondheimer, J. M., & Deterding, R. (Eds.). (2011). *Current diagnosis and treatment: Pediatrics* (20th ed.). New York: McGraw-Hill.

Jimenez, R., Casado-Flores, J., Nieto, M., & Garcia-Teresa, M. (2006). Cerebral salt wasting syndrome in children with acute central nervous system injury. *Pediatric Neurology, 35*(4), 261–263.

Katzung, B. G., Masters, S. B., & Trevor, A. J. (Eds.). (2009). *Basic and clinical pharmacology* (11th ed.). New York: McGraw-Hill.

McPhee, S. J., Papadakis, M. A., & Rabow, M. W. (Eds.). (2011). *Current medical diagnosis and treatment* (50th ed.). New York: McGraw-Hill.

Mentes, J. (2006). Oral hydration in older adults. *American Journal of Nursing, 106*(6), 40–50.

Morin, K. (2010). The scoop on salt. *MCN, 35*(5), *299.*

Sweeney, J. (2010). Managing hypernatremia. *Nursing2010, 40*(9), 63.

Tocco, S. B. (2010). Cerebral salt wasting: An overlooked cause of hypernatremia. *American Nurse Today, 5*(3), 34–36.

Wheeler, M. L. (2010). The salt challenge. *Diabetes Forecast, 63*(10), 11.

Wu, A. H. (Ed.). (2006). *Tietz clinical guide to laboratory tests* (4th ed.). St. Louis, MO: Saunders Elsevier.

Websites

www.cnpp.usda.gov (Center for Nutrition Policy and Promotion of Dietary Guidelines)
www.heart.org (Information on diets low in sodium and high in potassium.)

Answers

1. b, 2. b, 3. b, 4. c, 5. a, 6. b, 7. a, 8. c, 9. c, 10. a, 11. b, 12. b, 13. c, 14. b, 15. d

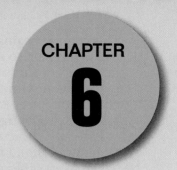

Arterial Blood Gases and Related Tests

CHAPTER

6

- Purpose of Blood Gases   128
- Summary of Acid–Base Balance   128
- Arterial Blood Gases in General   131
- pH of the Blood   133
- Partial Pressure of Carbon Dioxide $Paco_2$ 135
- Serum Bicarbonate and Total Carbon Dioxide Content   139
- Partial Pressure of Oxygen Pao_2 145
- Oxygen Saturation Sao_2 148
- Co-Oximetry or Multiwave Oximeters   150
- Blood Lactate   151

OBJECTIVES

1. Demonstrate the four-step sequence in interpreting the meaning of arterial blood gas (ABG) reports to determine the four primary acid–base imbalances.
2. Explain how the buffering system, the lungs, and the kidneys maintain the serum bicarbonate–carbonic acid ratio of 20:1.
3. Describe the nurse's role when ABGs are drawn.
4. Explain how reference values for blood gases are altered in pregnancy and in the newborn period.
5. Explain the physiologic basis for the symptoms of acidosis and alkalosis, both metabolic and respiratory in origin.
6. Identify possible nursing diagnoses for clients with decreased and increased $Paco_2$ (respiratory alkalosis and acidosis).
7. Identify the possible nursing diagnoses for clients with increased or decreased serum bicarbonate levels (metabolic alkalosis and acidosis).
8. Explain how electrolytes alter and are altered by changes in the acid–base balance.
9. Explain the concept of the anion gap in relation to the various kinds of metabolic acidosis.
10. Explain why high concentrations of oxygen may be dangerous for a client with a low Pao_2 and a high $Paco_2$.
11. Compare and contrast how Pao_2 and $Paco_2$ levels are used by the nurse to assist with treatment of respiratory problems.
12. Describe the basic pathologic process that produces increased lactic acid in the serum.

This chapter begins with an introductory section about acid–base imbalances. Several tables help to show the fundamental differences in the four primary acid–base imbalances. After this general discussion, pH, $Paco_2$, and bicarbonate tests are presented because of their significance in acid–base imbalances. The last part of the chapter discusses Pao_2 and oxygen saturation and measurement of lactic acid as an assessment of dangerous hypoxia at the cellular level.

Each laboratory measurement is discussed as a separate test so that the reader can better understand the clinical significance of both increases and decreases in each value. As in other chapters, possible nursing diagnoses for each change in laboratory tests are discussed after the clinical significance.

PURPOSE OF BLOOD GASES

The P before the o_2 and co_2 stands for the partial pressure of the gases, and the a denotes arterial. The respiratory gases include nitrogen, oxygen, carbon dioxide, and water vapor. Dalton's *law of partial pressure* states that the total pressure exerted by a mixture of gases is the sum of the individual partial pressure. Table 6–1 shows the percentage of gases in the blood and how this determines the partial pressure of each.

Blood gases are used to determine the respiratory status or the acid–base balance of the client. If the primary focus is to evaluate the respiratory status of the client, then the Pao_2, $Paco_2$, and pH levels, as well as the oxygen saturation, are the most important to evaluate. If the primary focus is to evaluate a metabolic acid–base imbalance, the Pao_2 has little significance. By looking first at the pH, then the $Paco_2$, and finally the bicarbonate level, one can figure out whether the acidosis is respiratory or metabolic in origin. In some confusing clinical situations, clients may have a combination of acid–base disorders, but this chapter focuses on the four basic types. Table 6–2 summarizes the way to interpret blood gas results to determine the primary acid–base imbalance. The last part of this chapter discusses hypoxic states that are not directly related to acid–base imbalances.

SUMMARY OF ACID–BASE BALANCE

The normal pH of arterial blood is between 7.35 and 7.45, with 7.4 taken as the average. Varying from this narrow range can be disastrous. Many chemical reactions in the body do not function normally if the pH of the blood is not in the normal range. If the pH is less than 7.35, the condition is called *acidosis*. If the pH is

Table 6–1 Four Gases in Arterial Blood at Sea Level		
Gas	**Percentage of Gas**	**Partial Pressure (mm Hg)**
Nitrogen (not measured)	75.5	574
Oxygen	13.0	99—venous drops to 40 mm Hg
Carbon dioxide	5.3	40—venous rises to 46 mm Hg
Water vapor (not measured)	6.2	47
Totals	100.00	760

Note: The total pressure exerted by a mixture of gases is the sum of the individual partial pressures. At altitudes above sea level, the partial pressures of gases are less because the total atmospheric pressure is less than 760 mm Hg.

Table 6–2 Four Steps to Determine the Four Primary Acid–Base Imbalances

Step 1: Look at pH	Is the pH >7.45? If so, the client is alkalotic. Go to Step 2. Is the pH <7.35? If so, the client is acidotic. Go to Step 3.
Step 2: When the pH is elevated	Is the $Paco_2$ <40 mm Hg? If so, the alkalosis is respiratory in origin. Is the $Paco_2$ >40 mm Hg or in the normal range? If so, the alkalosis is not respiratory in origin. Look for metabolic causes. Go to Step 4.
Step 3: When the pH is decreased	Is the $Paco_2$ >40 mm Hg? If so, the acidosis is respiratory. Is the $Paco_2$ <40 mm Hg or normal? If so, the acidosis is metabolic in origin. Go to Step 4.
Step 4: Looking at the bicarbonate in relation to the pH	Note that in metabolic acidosis, both the pH and the bicarbonate levels are decreased. In metabolic alkalosis, both the pH and the bicarbonate are elevated. (See Table 6–4 for compensation.)

Note: Lawes (2009), Pruitt (2010), and Swiderski and Byrum (2007) include several case studies as practice for determining acid–base imbalances by looking at laboratory reports in a systematic manner.

greater than 7.45, it is called *alkalosis*. As demonstrated in Table 6–2, if the increased or decreased pH is due to a marked change in $Paco_2$, the acid–base imbalance is respiratory in origin; all other acid–base imbalances are considered metabolic.

Understanding how $Paco_2$ and bicarbonate (HCO_3^-) function in the buffering system of the body is necessary if one is to be able to interpret the meaning of abnormal blood gas values. Buffer systems act as chemical sponges, which can give off or absorb hydrogen ions. There are minor buffers in the bloodstream, such as hemoglobin (Hgb), phosphates, and proteins, but these are not measured in evaluating the acid–base balance. The main buffer system is the bicarbonate–carbonic acid buffer system. The carbonic acid level is measured indirectly with $Paco_2$ level and the bicarbonate level with an indirect bicarbonate level as the total carbon dioxide content. This bicarbonate–carbonic acid buffer system is often referred to as the *20:1 ratio*, which means 20 parts of bicarbonate for 1 part of carbonic acid.

Note that although the carbonic acid level is not measured directly, it can be calculated because it is always 3% of the $Paco_2$. Hence a $Paco_2$ of 40 mm Hg indicates 1.2 mEq of carbonic acid in the serum, which must be balanced by 20 parts of bicarbonate or 24 mEq (Table 6–3). As long as this ratio is maintained, whether it is 40:2

Table 6–3 Three Laboratory Tests That Measure the Bicarbonate–Carbonic Acid Buffer System

$CO_2 + H_2O$	$\rightleftarrows$	H_2CO_3	$\rightleftarrows$	H	+	HCO_3^-
↓		↓		↓		↓
Carbon dioxide measured by $Paco_2$ (40 mm Hg) Test 2		Carbonic acid not measured directly but is always 3% of $Paco_2$ or 3% × 40 mm Hg = 1.2 mEq		Concentration of hydrogen ions measured by pH (7.35−7.45) Test 1		Bicarbonate level measured by serum bicarbonate (24 mEq) Test 3
$Paco_2$ controlled by lungs				Hydrogen, bicarbonate, and other electrolytes controlled by kidneys		

Test 1: pH; Test 2: $Paco_2$; Test 3: serum bicarbonate

Note: A bicarbonate level of 24 mEq and $Paco_2$ of 40 mm Hg (carbonic acid of 1.2 mEq) is the desirable 20:1 ratio that maintains the pH of serum between 7.35 and 7.45. See text on the use of total CO_2 content as an indirect measure of the bicarbonate level.

or 10:0.5, the pH of the blood stays in the normal range. Thus, if the carbonic acid level changes, the kidneys try to compensate by changing the bicarbonate level. For example, because a $Paco_2$ of 34 mm Hg reflects a carbonic acid level of 1 mEq (34 × 3% = 1.02), the bicarbonate level must drop to 20 mEq to keep a 20:1 ratio. If the bicarbonate level changes, the lungs change the $Paco_2$ and carbonic acid level, but this type of compensation is limited because the lungs must continue to function for oxygen exchange.

Only the lungs control the regulation of $Paco_2$. In the bloodstream, carbon dioxide combines with water to form carbonic acid. If more $Paco_2$ is retained, the condition results in more carbonic acid and hence the person tends toward acidosis. If more carbon dioxide is expired (hyperventilation), there is less carbonic acid in the bloodstream and the person tends toward alkalosis. By this mechanism, the lungs can shift the pH of the blood in just a few minutes.

The kidneys are also instrumental in the regulation of the pH of the bloodstream. The kidneys not only constantly excrete hydrogen ions but also control the serum bicarbonate level and retain or excrete sodium, potassium, and chloride ions. For substantial corrective shifts, it may take the kidneys several days to restore the pH to normal.

If all these regulatory mechanisms—buffer systems, lungs, and kidneys—are not successful in restoring the pH, the condition progresses with varying speeds to acidosis, leading to coma and death, or alkalosis, with irritability, tetany, and sometimes death. As a general rule, acidotic states are usually more life-threatening than alkalotic states.

By looking at three laboratory tests, one can usually determine whether the acid–base imbalance is respiratory or metabolic in origin. Table 6–4 shows the laboratory findings for each of the four basic types of acid–base imbalance *before* compensation occurs and how compensation changes the laboratory tests. In the actual clinical situation, because the client may have more than one imbalance, a chart does not always pinpoint the origin of the difficulty.

Table 6–4 Changes in pH, $Paco_2$, and HCO_3 and the Compensatory Mechanisms in Acid–Base Imbalances

	pH	$Paco_2$	HCO_3^-	Compensation
Respiratory alkalosis	↑	↓	Normal until compensation	Kidneys eventually reduce HCO_3^-. Take a few days to complete.
Metabolic alkalosis	↑	Normal unless lungs compensate	↑	Lungs try to increase $Paco_2$ slightly. Can do it quickly.
Respiratory acidosis	↓	↑	Normal until kidneys compensate	Kidneys eventually retain more HCO_3^-. Take a few days to complete.
Metabolic acidosis	↓	Normal until lungs compensate	↓	Lungs usually reduce $Paco_2$. Can do it quickly.

Note: See text for full explanation. Note that (1) in respiratory alkalosis and respiratory acidosis, the pH and the $Paco_2$ vary inversely; (2) in metabolic alkalosis and metabolic acidosis, the pH and the HCO_3^- rise or fall together; (3) the kidneys try to compensate for respiratory imbalances, but the compensation takes several days; and (4) the lungs try to compensate for metabolic imbalances, and their compensation is accomplished in a few minutes, but it is limited.

Table 6–5 Common Reasons for Acid–Base Imbalances

Primary Acid–Base Imbalance	Description of Imbalance	Common Reasons for Imbalance
Respiratory alkalosis	Decrease in $Paco_2$ caused by hyperventilation	Anxiety, fever, pain, hypoxia, improperly adjusted respirator
Respiratory acidosis	Increase in $Paco_2$ caused by hypoventilation	Chronic lung disease that causes CO_2 retention Respiratory depression from drugs or anesthesia
Metabolic alkalosis	Increase in serum bicarbonate (HCO_3^-) caused by increased intake of bicarbonate or increased loss of chlorides, hydrogen, or potassium ions	Vomiting or gastric suctioning, which causes loss of hydrogen, chloride, and potassium ions Ingestion or infusion of soda bicarbonate
Metabolic acidosis	Decrease in serum bicarbonate level caused by excess acid production, loss of bicarbonate, or increase in serum chloride levels	Excess acids such as ketone bodies in diabetic acidosis or lactic acid in cardiac arrest Loss of bicarbonate via intestines Increase in serum chloride level—renal failure

Note: See text for explanation and McPhee, Papadakis, and Sanoski (2011) for more details.

Table 6–4 makes the fundamental difference between respiratory and metabolic acid–base imbalances easy to see. If there is a marked increase or decrease in $Paco_2$, the acid–base imbalance is respiratory in origin. Otherwise, the imbalance is metabolic, and the change in the bicarbonate level has shifted the pH. Table 6–5 summarizes the common reasons for each type of acid–base imbalance.

If the acidosis or alkalosis is metabolic in origin or if the respiratory problem is chronic enough for the kidneys to be involved, it is also important to look at the laboratory tests for electrolytes. (Refer to Chapter 5 review: (1) the inverse relation between chloride (Cl⁻) and the bicarbonate ions, (2) the concept of anion gap, and (3) why hyperkalemia is associated with acidotic states and hypokalemia with alkalotic states. Chapter 3 describes the changes in urine pH in the different types of acidosis and alkalosis.) Table 6–6 shows the usual electrolyte abnormalities for each of the four primary types of acid–base imbalances.

ARTERIAL BLOOD GASES IN GENERAL

Preparation of Client and Collection of Sample

A physician or other clinician skilled in arterial puncture must collect the blood sample, which can be drawn from the radial, brachial, or femoral arteries. In most hospitals, only physicians are allowed to perform femoral punctures, whereas nurses with special training may perform radial or brachial punctures.

The site must be disinfected and allowed to dry. Clients need to be told that the puncture is momentarily painful. If they are very afraid of the procedure or if the attempt to obtain a specimen is prolonged, clients may hyperventilate because of anxiety, which can thus alter test results. If arterial blood samples are needed

Table 6-6 Possible Changes in Electrolytes and Urine pH for Acid–Base Imbalances

	Sodium (Na⁺)	Potassium (K⁺)	Chloride (Cl⁻)	Urine pH
Respiratory alkalosis	Usually not changed	Low if alkalosis persists	Increased when HCO_3^- decreases for compensation	High if chronic problem
Metabolic alkalosis	Usually not changed	Low	Low	High or, para-doxically, pH may continue low
Respiratory acidosis	Usually not changed	Increased	In compensation, the increase in HCO_3^- causes decrease in Cl⁻.	Low. Many H⁺ ions excreted
Metabolic acidosis	Total Na⁺ is low if diuresis occurs as in diabetic acidosis. Serum levels may be normal in some states.	May be high, although cellular deficit of K⁺. Serum potassium raises about 0.6 mEq/L for each 0.1 decrease in pH.	May increase to replace lost HCO_3^-. If unmeasured anions are high, Cl⁻ may decrease or be normal.	Very low pH, as kidneys try to excrete H⁺ ions

Note: See Chapter 5 for discussion on electrolytes and anion gap and Chapter 3 for urine pH.

frequently, clients usually have an arterial catheter in place. Nurses usually obtain specimens from an arterial line. In neonates, arterial sampling can be performed with an umbilical catheter.

After being collected in an airtight, heparinized syringe, the blood must be packed in ice for transport to the laboratory. The airtight container and the ice help prevent loss of gases from the sample. Special care units may have facilities for testing the sample immediately in the unit. It is necessary to expel all air bubbles within 2 minutes and put the sample on ice if the test is not completed within 10 minutes of collection.

The amount of blood needed for ABGs depends on the technique used. Although some blood gas analyzers can test less than 0.5 mL of blood, accuracy is more assured with a minimum of 3 mL. If a prepackaged ABG kit is not available, 0.5–1.0 mL of heparin can be used to coat the inside of a glass syringe. Too much heparin with a small sample causes inaccurate results.

After the sample is drawn, continuous pressure should be applied to the puncture site for at least 5 minutes if the radial artery is used and 10 minutes for the femoral. If the client has any bleeding problems, the pressure dressing should be taped on and left for several hours.

It is important to record on the laboratory slip whether the client was receiving oxygen at the time the sample was drawn, because there may be quite a difference in Pao_2 if the client is undergoing oxygen therapy as opposed to breathing room air. The nurse should record how long the client has been receiving a specific amount of oxygen, such as "25 minutes on 2 L by nasal cannula." If the client is undergoing assisted ventilation, the settings for the respirator should be recorded in case changes have to be made later. The temperature of the client should also be noted because a fever increases metabolic rate.

If arterial blood cannot be obtained, capillary blood samples may be used. The area should be warmed for 5 minutes before the sample is taken. The warmed ear site is used in children and adults, whereas the warmed heel is used for infants. (See Chapter 1 for the heel stick technique.)

Point-of-Care Testing for ABGs

Point-of-care (POC) tests are available for ABGs. One study on the use of POC testing for ABGs in the pediatric cardiac catheterization suite showed a turnaround time (TAT) of 2.55 minutes, while the TAT for the central laboratory ranged from 2 to 21 minutes (Golden et al., 2010).

REFERENCE VALUES FOR BLOOD GASES*		
	Arterial	**Venous**
pH	7.35–7.45	7.31–7.41
Pao_2	80–100 mm Hg	35–40 mm Hg
$Paco_2$	35–45 mm Hg	41–51 mm Hg
HCO_3^-	21–28 mmol/L	22–29 mmol/L
Base excess	–2 to +2 mmol/L	
Oxygen saturation	<97%	

*All reported values are corrected to 37°C (body temperature) unless otherwise specified.

See each individual item for reference values in various age groups.

pH OF THE BLOOD

The pH test measures the alkalinity or acidity of the blood. For chemical solutions, a pH of 7 is the neutral point; greater than 7 is alkaline, and less than 7 is acid. For blood pH, the neutral point is 7.4. It is critical that blood pH remain within a narrow range because many enzymes and other physiologic processes do not function normally when the pH is altered.

REFERENCE VALUES FOR pH	
Adult	7.35–7.45 (arterial)
	7.30–7.41 (venous)
Newborn	7.3–7.4 (arterial)

Note: See specialty texts for fetal blood sampling. For fetal scalp blood sampling, if the pH is above 7.25, the fetus is usually not compromised. Fetal umbilical samples are about 7.24 ± 0.07 for arterial samples and 7.32 ± 0.06 for venous samples in term nulliparous pregnancies (DeCherney et al., 2007).

Increased pH of Arterial Blood (Alkalosis)

Clinical Significance

An increased serum pH indicates that the client is in a state of alkalosis. To determine whether the alkalosis is respiratory or metabolic in origin, it is necessary to look at the $Paco_2$ and the serum bicarbonate level. If the alkalosis is respiratory in origin, the $Paco_2$ is markedly decreased. If the alkalosis is metabolic in origin, the serum bicarbonate level is markedly elevated. The common clinical situations that cause these changes and the reference values are discussed in the sections on $Paco_2$ and serum bicarbonate tests.

Possible Nursing Diagnoses Related to Alkalotic States

Risk for Injury Related to Neuromuscular Irritability and Possible Tetany

Specific nursing implications depend on whether the alkalosis is respiratory or metabolic in origin. Some general symptoms of both types of alkalosis include tingling in the extremities or nose, facial twitching, light-headedness, muscle tremors, and tetany. The neuromuscular irritability in alkalotic states occurs because calcium is less soluble in an alkaline medium. Many of the symptoms of alkalosis are those of hypocalcemia. (See Chapter 7 on hypocalcemia.) Clients must be protected from falls and assessed for convulsive movements.

Altered Breathing Pattern

In respiratory alkalosis, the respiratory rate is high because hyperventilation is the cause of the alkalosis. Factors that cause hyperventilation and possible nursing interventions are discussed in the section on $Paco_2$ levels. In metabolic alkalosis, the respiratory rate is normal to slightly depressed, with slow and shallow breaths. The depressed respiration in metabolic alkalosis is an attempt by the lungs to retain more $Paco_2$ to balance the increased serum bicarbonate level. The effect on the breathing pattern is of minimal importance, as discussed in the section on increased bicarbonate levels.

Decreased pH of Arterial Blood (Acidosis)

Clinical Significance

A decreased serum pH indicates that the client is in a state of acidosis. To determine whether the acidosis is respiratory or metabolic in origin, it is necessary to look at the $Paco_2$ and the serum bicarbonate level. In respiratory acidosis, the $Paco_2$ is increased; in metabolic acidosis, the serum bicarbonate level is lower than normal. Each type of acidosis is covered in the discussion about $Paco_2$ and serum bicarbonate levels. Note in Table 6–7 that newborns with low Apgar scores tend to have a proportionately low pH.

Possible Nursing Diagnoses Related to Acidotic States

Risk for Injury Related to Change in Level of Consciousness

Specific nursing implications depend on whether the acidosis is respiratory or metabolic in nature. General symptoms for both types of acidosis include headaches, weakness, lethargy, and confusion. The level of consciousness is depressed as the acidotic state worsens. Unless the acidotic state is corrected, drowsiness leads from a stuporous state to coma and eventually to death.

Altered Breathing Patterns

As with alkalotic states, the respiratory patterns are opposites for the two types of acidosis. In respiratory acidosis, the respiratory rate is decreased because hypoventilation is the cause of respiratory acidosis. An ineffective breathing pattern is the focus of care. In metabolic acidosis, the respiratory rate is faster and deeper than normal (Kussmaul's respirations) because the lungs are trying to compensate for the decreased serum pH by expiring more carbon dioxide. Because the rate is a compensatory one, the breathing pattern is not a focus of care.

Table 6–7 Relationship of Apgar Scores to pH Level in Newborn

Sign	Score 0	Score 1	Score 2
Heart rate	Absent	<100 beats/min	>100 beats/min
Respiratory rate	Absent	Low, irregular, hypoventilate	Good, crying lustily
Muscle tone	Flaccid	Some flexion of extremities	Active motion, well flexed
Reflexes	No response	Cry, some motion, grimace	Vigorous cry
Color	Blue, pale	Body pink, hands and feet blue	Completely pink

APGAR SCORE	ESTIMATE OF pH
≥7	7.27
≤6	7.22

Note: Apgar score is a simple and practical method to assess the overall physical status of the infant immediately after delivery. It is assessed 1 minute and 5 minutes after birth. Although it is usually assumed that this score reflects the degree of neonatal asphyxia, DeCherney et al. (2007) caution that recent studies suggest that there is poor correlation between Apgar scores and the degree of acidosis, particularly in premature infants. Asphyxia should be diagnosed only after cord blood determinations (Hay et al., 2011).

PARTIAL PRESSURE OF CARBON DIOXIDE ($Paco_2$)

The $Paco_2$ test measures the partial pressure of carbon dioxide in the arterial blood. As noted earlier, when carbon dioxide is transported in serum, some of it is combined with water to form carbonic acid ($H_2CO_3^-$), which dissociates into bicarbonate (HCO_3^-) and hydrogen (H^+) ions. The actual carbonic acid level in the serum is not measured, but it can always be determined by multiplying the $Paco_2$ by 3%. A $Paco_2$ of 40 mm Hg is 1.2 mEq of carbonic acid ($40 \times 3\%$). Because the end result is an increase in the amount of free hydrogen ions, an increase in $Paco_2$ causes blood pH to drop to less than 7.35.

REFERENCE VALUES FOR $Paco_2$	
Adult	35–45 mm Hg (arterial) 41–51 mm Hg (venous) Values are slightly lower in women.
Pregnant women	Values may be 30 mm Hg by the end of the second trimester. 30–37 mm Hg is normal for pregnancy because of hyperventilation. The kidneys compensate by excreting more bicarbonate, so the pH of about 7.4 is maintained.
Altitude	At higher altitudes the atmospheric pressure is lower, so the $Paco_2$ is proportionately reduced. (See discussion of Pao_2 values.)

Increased $Paco_2$ (Hypercarbia or Hypercapnia)

Clinical Significance in Respiratory Acidosis

An increased $Paco_2$ indicates that the normal amount of carbon dioxide is not being expired. Any situation that causes hypoventilation, such as drug overdose that results in respiratory depression, causes an elevated $Paco_2$. Higher-than-normal $Paco_2$ levels are also present in certain chronic lung conditions in which the exchange of carbon dioxide and oxygen is impaired. Clients with chronic obstructive pulmonary disease (COPD) may have both hypoxia and hypercarbia (elevated $Paco_2$), although the latter is not always associated with hypoxia. Some acute lung dysfunctions, such as pneumonia, may cause hypoxia but not an elevated $Paco_2$. Hypoxia does not always lead to a retention of carbon dioxide, for two basic reasons. First, carbon dioxide diffuses more readily across alveolar surfaces than does oxygen, so an impairment of respiratory function results in a decrease in Pao_2 before the $Paco_2$ changes. Second, hypoxia is a stimulus for breathing. If the lungs can respond to the low oxygen level by increasing the respiratory rate, the carbon dioxide level may stay normal or drop below normal because of the hyperventilation.

The type of hypoventilation that causes an increased $Paco_2$ can be transitory and self-limiting, such as when the breath is held. The resultant high level of $Paco_2$ cannot be maintained because it becomes an overpowering stimulus for taking a breath—one cannot commit suicide by holding one's breath. Clients with chronic lung disease who have high carbon dioxide levels no longer use carbon dioxide as a stimulus for breathing. Instead, hypoxia becomes the primary stimulus for breathing, and the kidneys compensate for the gradual increase in $Paco_2$ by increasing the serum bicarbonate level. The normal blood pH is maintained as long as the kidneys can keep the 20:1 ratio of bicarbonate to carbonic acid. It takes the kidneys several days to compensate for increasing $Paco_2$, so a quick increase in $Paco_2$, or acute respiratory failure, leads to respiratory acidosis.

In acute respiratory acidosis the HCO_3^- will be increased about 1 mEq/L for every 10 mm Hg increase in $Paco_2$. However, in chronic respiratory acidosis, HCO_3^- will be increased about 5 mEq/L for every 10-mm Hg increase, which will become compensated respiratory acidosis (Pruitt, 2010).

Clinical Significance in Metabolic Alkalosis

In metabolic alkalosis, the $Paco_2$ is usually more than 40 mm Hg because the lungs are attempting to reestablish the bicarbonate–carbonic acid ratio by increasing the carbonic acid to match the increased serum bicarbonate. This compensatory hypoventilation is not effective because the respiratory rate cannot be depressed appreciably without causing hypoxia.

Possible Nursing Diagnoses Related to Hypercapnia

Altered Sensory–Perceptual Awareness Related to Change in Level of Consciousness

Nurses must always be aware of the early signs of increasing $Paco_2$ levels. The term *CO₂ narcosis,* another name for respiratory acidosis, gives a clue that carbon dioxide can be a central nervous system depressant. Early signs of increased $Paco_2$ may be headache, dizziness, and confusion. The confusion may progress to decreasing levels of consciousness until the patient is comatose. The treatment of respiratory depression may include assisted ventilation until the underlying pathophysiologic condition can be treated. Nursing interventions are geared toward improving respiratory status. Frequent ABGs help to monitor the improvement of the client and ensure that carbon dioxide levels are not increasing.

The seriousness of an elevated $Paco_2$ can be evaluated only in relation to the amount of compensation that has occurred. For example, clients with chronic lung disease may have a higher-than-normal $Paco_2$ with a higher-than-normal bicarbonate level and a resulting normal pH. Chronic hypercapnia is usually well tolerated. However, a drug that depresses the respiratory center or a respiratory infection may throw such compensated clients into respiratory acidosis, or CO_2 narcosis.

Risk for Injury Related to Use of Oxygen and Sedatives in Clients with Chronic Obstructive Pulmonary Disease

High doses of oxygen can be lethal for clients who have a chronically high $Paco_2$ because hypoxia has become the respiratory stimulus for the client. The medullary center no longer responds to high levels of $Paco_2$, which is normally the primary stimulus for respiration, because the chronically elevated $Paco_2$ has made the center insensitive to carbon dioxide as a stimulus for breathing. The only stimulus for breathing is hypoxia. This obliteration of the hypoxic drive is not the sole explanation for CO_2 retention. Administration of oxygen may result in vasodilation of arteries with change in the normal ventilation to perfusion match (a V/Q mismatch). Another theory, the Haldene effect, refers to the fact that when more oxygen is carried by hemoglobin (Hgb), there is less room for CO_2. For clients with advanced emphysema, a Pao_2 of 55–60 mm Hg is "normal." The clients' color may improve as the hypoxia is eliminated, but respirations become slower and slower because the client no longer has a stimulus to breathe. If these clients are not stimulated to breathe, $Paco_2$ rises even higher, and they may die from respiratory acidosis. Supplemental oxygen could be given at night to clients who have stable but severe COPD, to prevent a fall of Pao_2 with sleep.

Very small doses of drugs, such as morphine or some sedatives, can depress respiration to a serious degree, because the response to hypoxia is depressed. (See the discussion of Pao_2 on ways to assess and intervene for hypoxia in clients with acute or chronic respiratory problems.)

Decreased Paco$_2$

Clinical Significance in Respiratory Alkalosis

Just as hypoventilation leads to an increased Paco$_2$, hyperventilation leads to a decreased Paco$_2$. (The terms *hypocarbia* and *hypocapnia* are sometimes used.) Often, hyperventilation is due to severe anxiety. Hysterical or semihysterical people tend to breathe rapidly and deeply, with a lot of sighing. Physical conditions, such as fever, pain, or hypoxia, also can cause hyperventilation. No matter what the stimulus, the end result is that if enough carbon dioxide to lower the Paco$_2$ is expired, the client experiences respiratory alkalosis.

Some people may have a slightly low Paco$_2$ most of the time, but usually this form of chronic hyperventilation is not noticed until the client has an acute anxiety attack. It is unusual to see compensation for respiratory alkalosis, because severe hyperventilation typically does not last long enough for the kidneys to begin to excrete extra bicarbonate. An exception, however, is a client using a respirator: An improperly adjusted respirator can be responsible for hyperventilation that continues over a long time. Mechanical ventilation that creates hypocapnia and high levels of oxygen in the blood may result in reduced cerebral blood flow.

Clinical Significance in Metabolic Acidosis

A lower-than-normal Paco$_2$ can be a compensatory mechanism for metabolic acidosis. For example, clients in diabetic acidosis use up much of the bicarbonate buffer in their bloodstream to buffer the ketone bodies. The lungs try to restore the 20:1 ratio by reducing the Paco$_2$ and hence the carbonic acid part of the ratio (Kussmaul's respirations), but this compensation cannot offset the severe metabolic acidosis.

Possible Nursing Diagnoses Related to Hypocapnia

Anxiety Related to Neuromuscular Irritability

Most of the symptoms that result from a lowered Paco$_2$, which can be alarming to the client and to the nurse, can be explained by the effect of an alkaline pH on serum calcium levels. Because calcium is less soluble in an alkaline medium, less ionized calcium is available when the blood pH rises above normal. Hence the client has symptoms of hypocalcemia. (See Chapter 7 for the symptoms of hypocalcemia.) There may be tingling of the fingers, twitching, muscle tremors, carpopedal spasms, and even tetany. The person may feel light-headed and dizzy. If the hyperventilation is less severe and more of a chronic problem, the person may have only symptoms such as chronic exhaustion or diffuse weakness.

Nurses in emergency departments or outpatient clinics are the ones most likely to see clients who are seeking treatment because of hyperventilation. Recognizing that the client is hyperventilating is easy, but assessing whether it is due to anxiety or to physical causes may not be so easy. Ruling out fever, pain, or hypoxia as the reason for the hyperventilation is important. (If the hyperventilation is due to an underlying metabolic acidosis, there will be no symptoms of alkalosis because the pH remains acid from the metabolic problem.)

Anxiety Related to Unknown Factors

If the hyperventilation is due to functional anxiety, nursing interventions can be instrumental in stopping the hyperventilation. The client needs to be reassured that slower breathing will decrease the symptoms. Breathing into a paper bag helps to increase the $Paco_2$ level. The nurse needs to maintain a calm, soothing environment so that the client can gain control and reduce the feeling of anxiety. Hyperventilation may be a recurring problem that warrants a referral for counseling to help the client learn ways to deal with anxiety. If the anxiety level is high, the physician may order drugs to reduce the anxiety. Sometimes the client may need to be taught the proper method of diaphragmatic breathing. The long-term goal is to help the client deal with the anxiety and to see how the anxiety has caused the breathing problem.

Ineffective Breathing Pattern Related to Hypoxia and Other Causes

The nurse needs to be aware of other situations in which hyperventilation may occur. For example, a client in labor may not be performing her breathing exercises correctly and thus may experience respiratory alkalosis. Also, clients using respirators need careful monitoring to make sure that the ventilation rate is not too fast. If hyperventilation is due to a stimulus such as fever, therapeutic measures to reduce the fever eliminate the hyperventilation. The most likely cause of respiratory alkalosis, other than anxiety, is hypoxia. (See the discussion of Pao_2 levels.) Paper bag rebreathing can reduce oxygen levels sufficiently to endanger hypoxic clients.

SERUM BICARBONATE AND TOTAL CARBON DIOXIDE CONTENT

Bicarbonate functions as an important buffer in the bloodstream. To keep the pH in the bloodstream between 7.35 and 7.45, the bicarbonate in it is kept at a 20:1 ratio to carbonic acid. The section on $Paco_2$ explained how changes in $Paco_2$ cause changes in bicarbonate level. Also, because bicarbonate and chloride are both negative ions in the serum, an increased retention of serum chloride means less retention of bicarbonate. Thus, serum bicarbonate measurements are useful in both acid–base imbalances and electrolyte imbalances, and they are, therefore, a routine part of laboratory tests for either electrolytes or arterial blood gases.

Direct and Indirect Methods to Measure Bicarbonate

Several different laboratory methods measure serum bicarbonate level. Some laboratories may perform direct measurements of the bicarbonate and report it as such. One indirect method involves measuring the total carbon dioxide content of the serum and calculating the bicarbonate level from this figure. An older method involves measuring the carbon dioxide combining power of the serum.

Nurses do not need to understand the technicalities of how these various tests are performed, but it is important to use the reference values that correspond to the exact method used by a specific laboratory. There is less standardization of bicarbonate measurement than with the other electrolytes. If a laboratory report does not have an item marked *bicarbonate*, look for *total carbon dioxide content* or *carbon dioxide capacity*, which reflects the bicarbonate component of the blood. This carbon dioxide content is different from the $Paco_2$ in a blood gas measurement.

Meaning of "Base Excess" or "Base Deficit"

Most laboratories also measure the total buffer base of the body and report this as a *base deficit* or a *base excess*. The *buffer base* refers to all the buffer ions in the serum, including not only bicarbonate but also phosphates, Hgb, and plasma proteins. The total buffers are usually about 50 mEq/L, but the laboratory reports only so many minus or plus milliequivalents. The normal would be a –2 mEq to a +2 mEq. For example, a –3 mEq means a *base deficit*, which correlates to a decrease in bicarbonate levels. A result of more than 2 mEq signifies a *base excess*, which correlates with an increased bicarbonate level.

REFERENCE VALUES FOR BICARBONATE[a]	
Adult	Arterial 21–28 mmol/L or mEq/L* Venous 22–29 mmol/L or mEq/L*
Pregnant women	Falls early in pregnancy by an amount consistent with the fall in $Paco_2$. A $Paco_2$ of 34 mm Hg is balanced with a bicarbonate of about 20 mEq to keep the pH about 7.4.
Newborn	20–26 mEq/L (Premature infants may have even lower reference values.)
Children	Slightly lower references than those for adults
Base excess or base deficit	–2 to +2 mEq/L

[a]Bicarbonate levels measured by carbon dioxide content show variation in results.

*See Chapter 4 on difference in mEq and mmol for electrolytes.

Increased Serum Bicarbonate Level (Base Excess)

Clinical Significance in Metabolic Alkalosis

The loss of hydrogen, potassium, and chloride ions all contribute to the development of metabolic alkalosis. First, any loss of hydrogen ions causes a proportional increase in the bicarbonate side of the bicarbonate–carbonic acid buffering system. Second, as discussed in Chapter 5, when potassium is low in the serum, the kidneys are unable to excrete bicarbonate normally. Third, when chloride, a negative ion, is decreased in the bloodstream, another negative ion is needed to keep the positive and negative ions balanced in the serum. Thus, the kidneys cause a retention of bicarbonate to replace the missing chloride.

The most common reason for an increase in the bicarbonate level is a loss of gastric contents. Clients who vomit or who have nasogastric suctioning without proper potassium chloride (KCl) replacement are prone to have high bicarbonate levels. Clients taking diuretics may also lose abnormal amounts of chloride and potassium and thus experience metabolic alkalosis.

An increase in the serum bicarbonate level can also occur with the ingestion of large amounts of sodium bicarbonate. As a home remedy, clients may take baking soda (soda bicarbonate), which is systemically absorbed. Commercial antacids are usually not systemically absorbed, so they do not cause alkalosis, but they may contribute to metabolic alkalosis if there is inadequate renal function. Alkalosis can also occur from overdosage with intravenous soda bicarbonate to treat acidosis. In the past, sodium bicarbonate was considered one of the primary drugs for cardiac arrest. Now the American Heart Association (www.heart.org) considers it acceptable only for types of acidosis that are bicarbonate responsive. Bicarbonate is not recommended for most cardiac arrests, which are most likely hypoxic lactic acidosis. (See the discussion of lactic acid at the end of this chapter.)

Clinical Significance in Respiratory Acidosis

An increased serum bicarbonate level is a compensatory mechanism for the elevated $Paco_2$ of a client with chronic lung disease. The increased bicarbonate level is necessary to keep the pH of the serum normal.

Possible Nursing Diagnoses Related to Increased Bicarbonate Levels

Risk for Injury Related to Neuromuscular Irritability

Usually clients with metabolic alkalosis do not have many symptoms directly related to the acid–base imbalance. Their respiration may be slow because their lungs are trying to compensate by conserving carbon dioxide. The change in respiratory rate is usually too slight to be clinically significant. Observable symptoms are related to the decreased solubility of calcium in an alkaline pH. As with respiratory alkalosis, clients may experience neuromuscular irritability, tingling in the fingers, twitching of the nose or lips, and even tetany or convulsions if the alkalosis is not corrected. Safety measures should be instituted.

Risk for Altered Cardiac Output Related to Arrhythmias

Because hypokalemia is associated with metabolic alkalosis, the client must be monitored for cardiac arrhythmias and will most likely need both potassium and chloride replacement (Table 6–5). Nursing implications for potassium chloride administration are covered in Chapter 5. The client may be given isotonic solutions intravenously to replenish the loss of chlorides. Fruit juices and broth may be given in less severe depletions of chloride and potassium.

Deficient Knowledge Related to Danger of Sodium Bicarbonate

If the client has a history of increased intake of soda bicarbonate, stopping the ingestion is usually enough to correct the base excess. Clients need to be taught that baking soda is not a desirable antacid because it is absorbed into the bloodstream.

Decreased Serum Bicarbonate Level (Base Deficit)

Clinical Significance in Metabolic Acidosis

Unless the client has a low $Paco_2$, and thus a low serum bicarbonate level as compensation, a decrease in the serum bicarbonate level is an indication that the client has metabolic acidosis. The severity of the acidotic state depends on how low the blood pH has dropped. The decrease in serum bicarbonate level that occurs in metabolic acidotic states can be due to

1. Utilization of the bicarbonate to buffer acids, such as excessive lactate, ketone bodies, or other toxic metabolites, that contain hydrogen ions (the most common type of metabolic acidosis seen clinically)
2. A primary loss of bicarbonate
3. An increase in serum chloride level

Increased Production of Acids. In a normal state of health, as acids are produced or introduced into the body, they are neutralized by the bicarbonate–carbonic acid buffering system and eventually excreted by the kidneys. With a sudden increase in acids in certain pathologic states, the kidneys do not have enough time to excrete the acids or enough bicarbonate to neutralize them.

1. In diabetic acidosis, the acids produced are the ketone bodies.
2. In shock, the tissue hypoxia results in an excessive buildup of lactic acid (see test for lactic acid at the end of this chapter).
3. In renal failure or in severe dehydration, the kidneys can no longer excrete hydrogen ions or acids such as the phosphates and sulfates.
4. In cardiac arrest, there is an immediate buildup of lactic acid (as well as a high $Paco_2$, so the client has both respiratory and metabolic acidosis).
5. Aspirin overdose floods the system with an acid. (Initially, the acetylsalicylic acid [ASA] acts as a respiratory stimulant that causes respiratory alkalosis, but the end result may be acidosis.)

Concept of Anion Gap. The lactates, phosphates, ketone bodies, and other acids that can cause metabolic acidosis are negative ions (anions) in the bloodstream. So an increase in these acids increases the anion gap, which is the amount of unmeasured negative ions or anions in the bloodstream (see Chapter 5). It is determined by comparing the total amount of positive ions in the serum (primarily sodium and potassium) with the total amount of negative ions in the serum (primarily chloride and bicarbonate). When the total positive and the negative ions are compared in the bloodstream, there is a gap because one type of negative ion, namely, the acids, is not measured. Usually, the unmeasured acids account for about 10–20 mEq of the total negative ions (Wu, 2006).

In metabolic acidosis, the increase in the negative ions of ketoacids, lactate, phosphate, sulfate, or other acids makes the anion gap larger because more unmeasured negative ions are present in the bloodstream. The anion gap may be as high as 25 mEq/L in severe ketoacidosis or lactic acidosis. The anion gap is useful in differentiating this first type of metabolic acidosis from the other two types because in them there is no increase in the acids that comprise the unmeasured negative ions and, therefore, no increase in the anion gap. The mnemonic MUDPILES can be used to recall frequent causes of an elevated anion gap due to metabolic acidosis (see Table 6–8).

Primary Loss of Bicarbonate. A primary loss of bicarbonate can occur with gastrointestinal losses below the pylorus because the intestinal tract and pancreatic

	Table 6–8 Frequent Causes of Elevated Anion Gap
M	Methanol
U	Uremia
D	Diabetic ketoacidosis
P	Paraldehyde
I	Iron and isoniazid
L	Lactic acidosis
E	Ethanol or ethylene glycol
S	Salicylates

Note: See Madden (2008) for discussion on the use of this mnemonic in pediatric poisoning. Also see Chapter 5 for more details on the anion gap.

secretions are rich in bicarbonate. (As a rule, gastrointestinal losses above the pylorus, such as vomiting or gastric suctioning, tend to cause alkalosis because of the loss of hydrogen, potassium, and chloride ions. So alkalosis is related to vomiting and acidosis to diarrhea. However, dehydration from either vomiting or diarrhea is likely to result in acidosis because of the inability of the kidney to excrete acid byproducts.) The primary loss of bicarbonate (a negative ion) leads to an increased chloride level to keep the positive and negative charges balanced in the serum. The anion gap does not increase.

Increase in the Serum Chloride Level. A primary increase in the serum chloride level means that another negative ion, bicarbonate, must be proportionally decreased. The lowering of serum bicarbonate level keeps the electrical charges of the serum electrolytes balanced, but it causes acidosis because the buffering ability of the serum is decreased.

This third type of metabolic acidosis (hyperchloremic acidosis) is a much less common clinical occurrence than the first two types. High doses of chlorides in intravenous infusions may raise the serum chloride level. Also, some types of renal failure result in an inability to excrete chloride ions properly.

Possible Nursing Diagnoses Related to Decreased Serum Bicarbonate Levels

Risk for Injury Related to Altered Sensory Perceptions and Level of Consciousness

It is important for nurses to recognize early symptoms of acidosis, because severe acidosis can be life threatening. When a client has a lowered serum bicarbonate level that is causing metabolic acidosis, one of the key symptoms is hyperventilation. This deep and rapid respiration (Kussmaul's respirations) is an attempt to restore the 20:1 bicarbonate–carbonic acid ratio by decreasing the carbonic acid in the blood. (Recall that 3% of the $Paco_2$ is carried in the

(Continued)

Possible Nursing Diagnoses . . . (Continued)

blood stream as carbonic acid.) These fast and deep respirations may look like the client has "air hunger," but they really reflect an attempt to expire extra $Paco_2$. This increased respiratory rate may be one of the first clues that the pH is dropping. As the pH drops lower, the client begins to exhibit signs of confusion, lethargy, and eventually coma. (A diabetic coma is a form of severe metabolic acidosis.) Newborn infants can experience severe metabolic acidosis if they are not kept warm and given sufficient calories. Acidosis can develop immediately, such as with a cardiac arrest, or slowly, as in a client with renal failure. Some clients with diabetes who do not take their insulin may go into a coma within a day or so. A young child with diabetes may go into acidosis very quickly, whereas an adult with diabetes may not experience ketoacidosis until after several days have elapsed. The important thing is to know the type of situation that can lead to metabolic acidosis so that any changes can be detected early.

The most important goal of treatment is to eliminate the cause of the acidosis. A cold-stressed newborn must be warmed and fed. A client with diabetes requires insulin so that glucose, rather than fats, can be used as the primary source of energy. Clients in shock must have increased oxygen perfusion at the cellular level to replace the anaerobic metabolism that has caused a buildup of lactic acid (see lactic acid measurement at the end of this chapter).

Risk for Injury Related to Intravenous Use of Sodium Bicarbonate

Although the goal of treatment is to eliminate the cause of the acidosis, the client may need sodium bicarbonate administered intravenously to bring the serum pH back to normal immediately. Sodium bicarbonate may be given in direct intravenous push or in a continuous intravenous infusion. Other drugs should not be mixed with the bicarbonate solution because they may precipitate in an alkaline pH. For example, calcium precipitates in a strongly alkaline pH.

The respiratory rate is one objective assessment of the effectiveness of therapy. When clients with acidosis are given sodium bicarbonate, the hyperventilation decreases as the pH of the blood returns to normal. Sometimes the client may be given enough sodium bicarbonate to produce rebound metabolic alkalosis. Monitoring laboratory tests can prevent this. In an acute emergency, such as a cardiac arrest, it is essential that someone, usually the nurse, keep a detailed record of all the medications given to the client.

Fluid and Electrolyte Imbalance Related to Acidosis

Close monitoring of the intake and output for clients in acidosis is essential to prevent severe dehydration and further electrolyte imbalances. During acidotic states, more hydrogen ions go into the cells, and potassium ions are forced out. Hyperkalemia is associated with acidotic states. The potassium that leaves the cells is eventually excreted by the kidneys so that the aftermath of metabolic acidosis is a depletion of total body potassium. As discussed earlier in the section on anion gap, chloride levels increase in some types of acidosis. Sodium may also be depleted, particularly in diabetic acidosis in which diuresis has been a prominent feature. A nurse caring for a client who is recovering from metabolic acidosis must be aware of all the nursing implications for changes in each of these electrolytes, each of which is discussed in Chapter 5.

PARTIAL PRESSURE OF OXYGEN (Pao_2)

The Pao_2 measures the amount of oxygen dissolved in the blood. The partial pressure is calculated by multiplying the amount of gas in a solution (%) by the total pressure (mm Hg [millimeters of mercury]). Hence the laboratory reports the Pao_2 as "so many millimeters of mercury (mm Hg)." In a healthy young person, arterial blood may have about 13% oxygen dissolved in the plasma. At sea level, the Pao_2 is 13% × 760 mm Hg, or 98.8 mm Hg. As can be seen by the reference values, breathing pure oxygen, moving to a high altitude, or simply aging makes quite a difference in the partial pressure of oxygen in the bloodstream.

REFERENCE VALUES FOR Pao_2	
Adult	80–100 mm Hg while breathing room air. May be greater than 225 mm Hg if breathing 40% oxygen (with normal lungs).
Newborn	60–70 mm Hg are usually given as maximum reference values, or 40–60 mm Hg in some laboratories.
Aged[a]	The Pao_2 drops about 3–5 mm Hg for each decade after 30 years of age. After 70 years of age, a Pao_2 of about 85 mm Hg is the maximum reference value.
Location	In high altitudes, such as Denver, where the atmospheric pressure is 670 mm Hg, the maximum reference value for a person younger than 30 years is about 87 mm Hg.

[a]The relation between age and Pao_2 can be approximated by the formula

$$Pao_2 = 104 - [age \times 0.27]$$

Increased Pao_2

Clinical Significance

The only clinical situation that creates a high Pao_2 is the administration of high doses of oxygen. One hundred percent oxygen may increase the Pao_2 to more than 500 mm Hg. Whether high oxygen pressures in the blood can alter certain bodily conditions, such as aging, is a controversial subject that is being explored.

Possible Nursing Diagnosis Related to Increased Pao_2

Risk for Injury Related to Prolonged Use of High Levels of Oxygen

Retinopathy of prematurity (ROP), formerly called retrolental fibroplasia, is associated with prolonged exposure to high blood concentrations of oxygen. Oxygen alone was once thought to be the culprit for retrolental fibroplasia, but recent studies indicate that high blood oxygen levels are but one of the factors in ROP. Prolonged use of oxygen for clients of all ages can cause drying of the airways and even permanent lung damage. In adults, oxygen toxicity in the lungs is related not to its concentration or to the Pao_2 but to the partial pressure of inspired oxygen.

(Continued)

> ## Possible Nursing Diagnosis . . . (*Continued*)
>
> The nurse should question any order for the prolonged use (>8 hours) of 100% oxygen. In severe and complicated cases of hypoxia, the client may have to receive high concentrations of oxygen for an extended period. Frequent monitoring of blood gases is necessary to evaluate whether the oxygen therapy is satisfactory and whether lower concentrations of oxygen can be used. The general rule is to use the lowest possible amount of inspired air, that is, oxygen (Pao_2), to keep the Pao_2 no more than 90 mm Hg unless special circumstances, such as carbon monoxide intoxication, require higher Pao_2 levels. Toxicity to oxygen rarely develops if the Fio_2 is kept less than 40%. (See the section on elevated $Paco_2$ for the special dangers of oxygen therapy for some clients with obstructive disease.)

Decreased Arterial Pao_2

Clinical Significance

Many different conditions can cause hypoxia, which is usually defined as Pao_2 of less than 60 mm Hg in adults. With atelectasis or emphysema, there may be ventilation to blood flow abnormalities so that oxygen does not reach the bloodstream. Hypoventilation, such as in a client who has taken a respiratory depressant, causes hypoxia. Anatomic defects, such as when arterial and venous blood intermix, cause hypoxia. In essence, any situation that interferes with CO_2–O_2 exchange leads to a lowered Pao_2.

Because the $Paco_2$ may be elevated, normal, or decreased with a decreased Pao_2, it is important to look at the laboratory reports for both $Paco_2$ and pH when evaluating the clinical significance of a low Pao_2. With many types of hypoxia, the $Paco_2$ may remain normal because carbon dioxide can diffuse much more readily than oxygen can across alveolar surfaces. If the hypoxia state is causing marked hyperventilation, the $Paco_2$ may actually drop below normal. For example, with pneumonia, both the Pao_2 and the $Paco_2$ may be lower than normal. The infection in the lungs interferes with oxygen exchange more than with carbon dioxide exchange. The hypoxia leads to hyperventilation in an attempt to increase oxygen. The hyperventilation causes more expiration of carbon dioxide, so the $Paco_2$ becomes lower than normal (respiratory alkalosis). In respiratory depression, such as that caused by general anesthesia, lowered Pao_2 levels cannot stimulate increased respiration, so the $Paco_2$ level rises (respiratory acidosis). In chronic lung disease, hypoxia may occur alone or with an increase in $Paco_2$ as the lung damage becomes worse. The clinical significance of hypoxia, compounded by hypercapnia (high $Paco_2$), is quite different from that of hypoxia alone, as noted earlier.

> ## Possible Nursing Diagnoses Related to Hypoxia or Decreased Pao_2 Levels
>
> ### Altered Tissue Perfusion Related to Hypoxia
>
> The nurse may be instrumental in preventing serious complications from hypoxia by detecting it before cyanosis occurs, which is a late symptom of hypoxia. Peripheral cyanosis that occurs

in the nailbeds reflects poor peripheral perfusion, but not necessarily an extremely low Pa_{O_2}. Tissue hypoxia is not synonymous with arterial hypoxia. Central cyanosis is best assessed by looking at the tongue. In adults, the Pa_{O_2} is less than 50 mm Hg by the time central cyanosis occurs. The blue of central cyanosis denotes at least 5 g of unoxygenated Hgb in the arterial blood—or more than one-third of the total Hgb in the blood. The nurse needs to look for early symptoms of hypoxia, such as tachycardia and restlessness. By the time this one-third or more of the Hgb is unsaturated, the client may be in distress. Lack of oxygen to the myocardium can alter cardiac output and produce arrhythmias.

Assessing for Cyanosis in Dark-Skinned Clients. Because cyanosis is difficult to assess in dark-skinned clients, nurses must become familiar with the client's precyanotic color. When cyanosis is suspected, nurses can press on the skin to produce pallor. In cyanotic tissue, the color returns slowly by spreading from the periphery to the center. Also the lips and the tongue become ashen gray in a black client with cyanosis.

Risk for Injury Related to Use of Oxygen

When oxygen is ordered for a client with hypoxia, nurses must make sure that the safety and the comfort of the client are maintained. Clients and family need clear instructions about the danger of smoking. Discontinuing oxygen for just a few minutes may cause a considerable drop in the Pa_{O_2} of some clients, and it may take as long as 20 minutes to restore the previous level. Because hypoxia can contribute to the development of severe cardiac arrhythmias, 100% oxygen may be given before and after suctioning. However, rather than providing hyperoxygenation by increasing the inspired oxygen concentration, one can use a double-lumen oxygen insufflation catheter to continue the flow of oxygen during endotracheal suctioning. The nurse may also use the pulse oximeter, discussed later, to determine whether oxygen therapy can be interrupted for oral temperatures, feedings, or other procedures. Some clients with a chronically low Pa_{O_2} may have home oxygen, so they need instructions on the safety measures needed for long-term oxygen therapy. The most objective assessment of the need for continual oxygen therapy is the blood gas report. A client using a ventilator may have blood gases drawn frequently to assess if the ventilator is properly adjusted. (See the section on elevated Pa_{O_2} for the danger of a prolonged high Pa_{O_2}.) Clients who have chronic hypoxia may often be undergoing oxygen therapy at home. The goal is usually to keep the oxygen saturation above 90% or a Pa_{O_2} of 60 mm Hg, which is slightly higher than the standard criteria of 88% or 89% or a Pa_{O_2} of 55 mm Hg for reimbursable oxygen therapy. Clients who have a partial pressure of oxygen (Pa_{O_2}) of 56–59 mm Hg or saturation of oxygen (Sa_{O_2}) of 89% in arterial blood may be reimbursed for home oxygen therapy if they have certain cardiac conditions or Hct above 56%. However, they must have a second oxygen test 3 months after therapy has begun (McPhee et al., 2011). Clients may need to try several methods of oxygen delivery to determine what is therapeutic and cost effective.

Impaired Gas Exchange Related to Factors Other Than Simple Hypoxia

For some clients with hypoxia, oxygen may not be the primary need. For example, if the hypoxia is due to mucous plugs blocking some of the airways, coughing, deep breathing, and maybe suctioning need to be instituted. If hypoxia is due to an acute condition, such as an asthmatic attack, hydration and bronchodilation are as important as oxygenation. When

(Continued)

> **Possible Nursing Diagnoses . . . (Continued)**
>
> a client is allowed to stay in one position, not all areas of the lungs are equally ventilated, so some unoxygenated blood goes back to the left atrium. This is called *physiologic shunting*. By changing the client's position frequently, physiologic shunting does not add to the problem of hypoxia. However, if the hypoxia is due to poor cardiac output, changing positions often may be tiring to the client and not a top priority. It is important to understand the reason for the hypoxic state so that nursing measures are geared to help the client use oxygen effectively and conserve energy so that oxygen need is not increased.
>
> The possible nursing implications for clients with a low Pao_2 and a high $Paco_2$ are covered in the section on $Paco_2$. It is essential for the nurse to understand the danger of giving high concentrations of oxygen to clients who have hypoxia coupled with a chronically increased $Paco_2$. Recall that a client with chronic emphysema who has an elevated $Paco_2$ and a "normal" Pao_2 of 50–60 mm Hg is using the hypoxia as a stimulus for breathing. As noted earlier in the section on use of oxygen therapy, even though supplemental oxygen can cause retention of CO_2 in some clients with COPD, it causes only a minimal decrease in respiratory rate and tidal volume in others. The only drug therapy that has been demonstrated to improve COPD is supplemental oxygen (McPhee et al., 2011).
>
> **Anxiety Related to Dyspnea**
>
> Some clients, such as those with lung cancer or other destructive lung diseases, may have continual problems with dyspnea because their Pao_2 is chronically low and oxygen therapy is of limited use. Specific items taught to help restore control and power over the shortness of breath (SOB) include controlled breathing through pursed lips, relaxation techniques, work simplification measures, and breathing techniques to use in activities of daily living.

OXYGEN SATURATION (Sao_2)

Because the Pao_2 measures the amount of dissolved oxygen in the blood, not the amount of oxygen carried by the Hgb, one must determine the oxygen saturation of the blood to evaluate its total carrying capacity. If the Hgb is carrying the normal amount of oxygen, the oxygen saturation is close to 100%. The oxygen saturation of the Hgb is affected by the partial pressure of oxygen, by the temperature, by the pH, and by the chemical and physical structure of the Hgb itself. Unless there is substantial change in the last three factors, the oxyhemoglobin dissociation curve can be used to compute the oxygen-carrying capacity of the blood.

Decrease in the Oxygen Saturation

Clinical Significance

Shunting of blood from the venous to the arterial system causes decreased oxygen saturation. The oxygen saturation is also low with carbon monoxide poisoning because carbon monoxide combines with Hgb more than 200 times faster than oxygen does. The additional information from the oxygen saturation test is usually part of the assessment of a client who is having cardiac catheterization

> ## REFERENCE VALUES FOR OXYGEN SATURATION
>
> 96–100% (arterial sample)
>
> Comparison with Pao_2 values (normal pH and temperature):
>
> 98% = Pao_2 of 100 mm Hg
>
> 95% = Pao_2 of 80 mm Hg
>
> 89% = Pao_2 of 60 mm Hg
>
> 84% = Pao_2 of 50 mm Hg
>
> 35% = Pao_2 of 20 mm Hg
>
> *Note:* Venous blood has about 70–75% oxygen saturation.

studies (see Chapter 26). The oxygen saturation is a measurement of the reserve of oxygen in the Hgb that can be used to replenish the oxygen dissolved in the plasma (i.e., the Pao_2 measured as the blood gas). As noted in the reference values, decreases in oxygen saturation correlate with a decrease in Pao_2, although not in a linear manner. Table 6–9 shows a comparison of Pao_2, Spo_2, and Sao_2 and Spo_2 is discussed next.

Use of Pulse Oximeter to Monitor Oxygen Saturation (Spo_2)

Although blood gases, with oxygen saturation as one component, are the most accurate way to assess for hypoxemia, the pulse oximeter, less costly and more convenient, has become an important tool for nurses to use in many clinical settings. Using a pulse oximeter has been called taking the "fifth vital sign."

Pulse oximeters are noninvasive devices that estimate the oxygen saturation of arterial blood by measuring the amount of light absorbed by Hgb in red blood cells. A light-emitting sensor sends beams of light through the tissue, and a light-detecting sensor records the amount of light absorbed by the oxygenated Hgb. (The pulse oximeter is called a *pulse* oximeter because it senses arterial blood by pulsation.) A computer converts the absorption rate to a percentage of oxygen saturation, which is displayed on a digital readout along with the pulse rate. Recent advances include built-in indicators of arterial flow that display the strength of the blood flow and a pulse bar that indicates the relative strength of the pulse. Most pulse oximeters store information that can be printed as a hard copy.

Table 6–9 Methods of Measuring Oxygen Levels

Pao_2	Partial pressure of oxygen measures tissue oxygenation and can be used to diagnose hypoxia in the tissues. Normal is 80–100 mm Hg
Sao_2	Partial pressure of arterial blood gases measures arterial saturation to diagnose hypoxemia. Normal is 96–100%.
Spo_2	Pulse oximeter estimates arterial oxygen saturation. A fit, healthy person should have an Spo_2 of 97–99% on room air.

In addition to large units that combine blood pressure measurements with pulse oximetry readings, there are very small portable oximeters that can fit in a nurse's pocket.

Preparation of Patient

The pulse oximeter probes must be placed on a site with good circulation. Fingers, earlobes, toes, and the bridge of the nose are all possible sites. Some probes are disposable and must be taped in place. Nondisposable probes use clips. Before attaching the probe to a client, test the functioning of the machine by attaching the probe to a healthy person. If possible, let the client hear the alarm so that he or she will be prepared for the sound. Reassure him or her about what steps might be taken if oxygen saturation is too low. Also let the client know that if the probe becomes dislodged, the alarm will go off.

Technical difficulties with the equipment and inadequate blood flow to the extremity can cause false alarms. Changes in the Hgb levels and the presence of contrast medium (see Chapter 21) may also produce inaccurate readings. Carbon monoxide bound by Hgb will falsely elevate the oxygen saturation reading as will methemoglobinemia (Chapter 2), an adverse effect of some drugs. Specific methemoglobin concentrations can be measured by a multiwave CO-oximeter. Current research has found that ambient light does not significantly affect pulse oximetry readings (Valdez-Lowe, Ghareeb, & Artinian, 2009).

A study comparing ABGs and pulse oximetry with clients who had sickle cell disease demonstrated that the pulse oximetry was less invasive and as accurate unless the client was critically ill or had carboxyhemoglobin.

If a capnograph is an addition to the pulse oximeter, special airway adapters are used to measure end tidal CO_2.

REFERENCE VALUE OF PULSE OXIMETER (Spo_2)

Neonates

Neonates' blood contains fetal hemoglobin, which releases less oxygen to body tissues, so their Spo_2 levels should be above 95%.

Adults should have levels between 97% and 99% but levels as low as 92% may be acceptable for some conditions (Mininni et al., 2009).

Arterial hypoxemia has been defined as less than 90% while on room air.

CO-OXIMETRY OR MULTIWAVE OXIMETERS

CO-oximetry or multiwave oximeters use four different wavelengths to measure four types of Hgb—oxyhemoglobin, deoxyhemoglobin, methemoglobin, and carboxyhemoglobin—as a percentage of the total Hgb or in terms of grams per deciliter (g/dL). In contrast, the pulse oximeter discussed earlier uses just two wavelengths of reflected light to estimate the percentage of saturated Hgb or oxyhemoglobin. Also, the routine blood gas analysis for partial pressure of oxygen does not detect methemoglobin or carboxyhemoglobin.

A new eight-wavelength pulse oximeter is available that measures methemoglobin and carboxyhemoglobin in addition to the usual measurement of oxygen saturation and pulse rate (Barker et al., 2006). This may expand oxygenation monitoring in certain settings, but currently CO-oximetry testing is done in a centralized laboratory. Smaller laboratories may have to send specimens to a centralized laboratory.

Preparation of Client and Collection of Sample

Whole blood is collected in a green tube. Blood should be collected before oxygen therapy is started. Because the half-life of carbon monoxide is only 4–5 hours after exposure, blood should be drawn as soon as possible.

REFERENCE VALUES FOR CO-OXIMETRY-PERCENTAGE OF TOTAL HEMOGLOBIN	
Carboxyhemoglobin	Nonsmokers 0.5–1.5%
	Heavy smokers 8–9%
Methemoglobin	Less than 1%

Clinical Significance

An increase in carboxyhemoglobin occurs in carbon monoxide (CO) poisoning. The resulting tissue ischemia can lead to organ failure and death. Carbon monoxide poisoning is the leading cause of death by poisoning in industrialized countries, so nurses need to educate clients about this danger (Rosenthal, 2006). Faulty furnaces, motor vehicles, stoves, and gas heaters are the common culprits. Exposure to methylene chloride, which is found in paint stripper fumes, can also cause carbon monoxide poisoning because this chemical is metabolized to CO in the liver. Treatment includes the use of 100% oxygen and, if necessary, intubation with mechanical ventilation. Lactic acidosis may be present as discussed later. Clients who are severely affected need to be moved to a facility that has a hyperbaric oxygen chamber (Smith, 2006).

The causes and treatment of methemoglobin are discussed in Chapter 2. Cyanosis develops when the level is about 15%. Clients with suspected methemoglobin need prompt treatment.

BLOOD LACTATE

Lactic acid is produced by anaerobic glycosis and is a normal byproduct of strenuous exercise. Dangerous levels of lactic acid can develop from pathologic conditions that cause prolonged hypoxia. Sepsis from a bacterial infection can lead to septic shock and death. So guidelines from the Surviving Sepsis Campaign recommend the use of measures to recognize early sepsis and intervention to normalize the hypoxia and buildup of lactic acid (Dellinger et al., 2008). The key is a blood lactate test that measures if the infection is serious enough to interfere with oxygen at the tissue level. A blood lactate is drawn at the same time as the blood culture in the emergency department (ED).

Goal-directed resuscitation for sepsis has been reported to reduce mortality when applied in the ED. Research findings support the use of blood lactate levels rather than the continuous $Scvo_2$ measurements that may monitor hypoxia (Jones et al., 2010).

Liver disease can also cause a buildup. (Lactic acidosis is the first type of metabolic acidosis discussed in the section on decreased serum bicarbonate levels.) Lactic acidosis can develop in a short time and almost immediately with a cardiac arrest. It can also coexist with other types of acidosis such as those brought on by diabetes, dehydration, or renal failure. It can be idiopathic in a seriously ill client and can be fatal within a short time. Some clients, especially those with poor renal failure, may develop lactic acidosis when they take metformin, a drug used to treat diabetes. This drug should be withheld before radiographs with contrast medium (Chapter 20) or other situations where renal function may be compromised. Lactic acidosis may also be a threat for clients who are on some of the antiretrovirals used to treat human immunodeficiency virus (HIV) (Deglin, Vallerand, & Sanoski, 2011).

Preparation of Client and Collection of Sample

Venous or arterial blood is collected in either a gray-topped or a green-topped container, depending on the laboratory method. Note on the laboratory slip whether the blood is arterial or venous, because values differ. The specimen should be packed in ice and analyzed within 15–30 minutes after collection.

Gross hemolysis depresses results. Falsely low values occur with high lactic dehydrogenase (LDH) levels. Elevations of lactate may occur with exercise, epinephrine, alcohol, glucose, and sodium bicarbonate infusions. Values may increase 20–50% after meals (Wu, 2006).

REFERENCE VALUES FOR LACTIC ACID OR BLOOD LACTATE		
Venous	1.5–2.2 mEq/L	(0.5–2.0 mEq/or mmol/L)

Point-of-Care (POC) Lactate Test

A handheld portable whole-blood lactate analyzer can be used as a POC test. This test can be useful in places where clinical decisions are hampered by lack of clinical resources. A study by Moore et al. (2008) found that a whole-blood lactate test done by POC predicted with 81% accuracy a sevenfold higher mortality in clients with sepsis in a population in Uganda.

Questions

1. In a client with no previous metabolic acid–base imbalances, hyperventilation results in which of the following?
   a. ↓ $Paco_2$ and ↓ pH of serum
   b. ↓ $Paco_2$ and ↑ pH of serum
   c. ↑ $Paco_2$ and ↑ pH of serum
   d. ↑ $Paco_2$ and ↓ pH of serum

2. In a client with chronic lung disease, the kidneys can compensate for an elevated $Paco_2$ by which of the following?
    a. Retaining additional HCO_3^- (bicarbonate)
    b. Excreting more Na^+ and K^+ ions
    c. Excreting carbonic acid
    d. Retaining H^+ ions to balance the $Paco_2$

3. When a client has blood drawn from the radial artery for arterial blood gases (ABGs), the nurse should
    a. Pack the blood sample in ice for transport to the laboratory
    b. Keep pressure on the puncture site for at least 1 minute
    c. Transfer the blood sample to a heparinized test tube
    d. Draw a second sample in 10 minutes

4. A client is admitted with ketoacidosis. The nursing student reports to the RN that on admission, the client's respirations are rapid (30 per minute) and seem very deep. The RN should do which of the following?
    a. Recheck the respirations because it is unusual to have such a high rate with a ketoacidosis
    b. Check for signs of infection because this is probably causing the increased rate
    c. Notify the physician that the client is having dyspnea
    d. Ask the students about their understanding of acid–base balance

5. Which of the following assessments by the nurse supports the possibility that a client is going into metabolic acidosis?
    a. Twitching
    b. Irritability
    c. Slow, shallow breaths
    d. Difficulty being aroused

6. A 7-lb newborn has an Apgar score of 7 (the normal is 10). He lost points for heart rate, respiratory rate, and color. The meperidine given to his mother before delivery has resulted in the newborn having a slight
    a. Metabolic alkalosis (bicarbonate excess)
    b. Respiratory alkalosis (low $Paco_2$)
    c. Metabolic acidosis (bicarbonate deficit)
    d. Respiratory acidosis (high $Paco_2$)

7. In a normal pregnancy, blood gases are which of the following?
    a. The same as in the nonpregnant state
    b. A lower $Paco_2$ and a lower HCO_3^-
    c. A higher $Paco_2$ and a higher HCO_3^-
    d. A lower $Paco_2$ and a higher HCO_3^-

8. High concentrations of oxygen may be dangerous for a client with a chronically elevated $Paco_2$ because the client
    a. May experience respiratory distress because of oxygen toxicity
    b. Has hypoxia as a stimulus for breathing
    c. Depends on the $Paco_2$ as a stimulus for breathing
    d. Has a high $Paco_2$, not a low Pao_2

9. Respiratory alkalosis (low $Paco_2$) could result from which one of the following situations?
    a. Hypoxia
    b. Hypokalemia

    c. Hypothermia

    d. Opioid overdose

10. Which one of the following clients should be observed for possible signs of tetany if the calcium levels are borderline normal?

    a. A client who had a cardiac arrest yesterday

    b. A client who tends to hyperventilate when she is anxious

    c. A client who was hypotensive after her delivery today

    d. A client who is in respiratory distress

11. A college student, age 18 years, is in the emergency department. She says she is having an "anxiety" attack. She complains of feeling light-headed and "shaky" all over. Which action by the nurse would be most appropriate in this situation?

    a. Have the client practice taking rapid, deep breaths

    b. Provide a pamphlet on anxiety attacks

    c. Have the client identify what has made her so anxious now

    d. Ask the client to breathe into a paper bag

12. Which type of loss from the gastrointestinal tract contributes to the development of metabolic alkalosis (high serum bicarbonate)?

    a. Draining fistula from pancreatic cyst

    b. Gastric suctioning

    c. Diarrhea

    d. Ileostomy drainage

13. Which one of the following conditions causes a decrease in serum bicarbonate (HCO_3^-) level?

    a. Prolonged increase in $Paco_2$

    b. Increased serum chloride level

    c. Markedly increased serum sodium level

    d. Increased serum potassium level

14. A child has lost an abnormal amount of chlorides because of vomiting. The loss of chlorides contributes to which of the following?

    a. Respiratory alkalosis (low $Paco_2$)

    b. Respiratory acidosis (high $Paco_2$)

    c. Metabolic alkalosis (base excess)

    d. Metabolic acidosis (base deficit)

15. A client was admitted to the hospital with severe vomiting associated with pregnancy. She has been unable to retain any meals or liquids. Her dehydrated and near-starvation state may lead to which of the following?

    a. Metabolic acidosis (base deficit)

    b. Metabolic alkalosis (base excess)

    c. Respiratory acidosis (high $Paco_2$)

    d. Respiratory alkalosis (low $Paco_2$)

16. A 6-lb 2-oz (2.7-kg) newborn had a normal Apgar score. A half-hour after birth, her rectal temperature is 96.8°F (36.3°C). She must burn extra calories because she is cold stressed. Unless she is warmed and fed, she is likely to experience which of the following?

    a. Metabolic acidosis (base deficit)

    b. Respiratory acidosis (high $Paco_2$)

    c. Metabolic alkalosis (base excess)

    d. Respiratory alkalosis (low $Paco_2$)

17. The anion gap is increased (i.e., the unmeasured negative ions are increased) in which one of these types of acidosis?
    a. Primary loss of serum bicarbonate
    b. Increase of lactic acid
    c. Increase of chlorides
    d. Increase of CO_2

18. A client has been receiving sodium bicarbonate intravenously for metabolic acidosis. The nursing assessment that indicates the sodium bicarbonate has restored the blood pH to normal is which of the following?
    a. Blood pressure is in normal range
    b. Urine output has increased
    c. Irritability and muscle spasms decreased
    d. Respirations have returned to normal

19. Blood gases drawn on a client reveal a normal Pao_2, a slightly low $Paco_2$, and a slightly high pH. Which of the following clients would most likely have these blood gas results?
    a. A client who has chronic emphysema
    b. A client who is in diabetic ketoacidosis
    c. A client who is recovering from anesthesia and has received a considerable amount of muscle relaxants
    d. A client who has been using breathing exercises during her labor contractions

20. An elderly man has been admitted with a diagnosis of respiratory acidosis caused by a chronic lung condition. In his laboratory data, which of the following would be indicative of his acid–base difficulty? (Assume some compensation has occurred.)
    a. High blood pH, low $Paco_2$, high HCO_3^-
    b. Low blood pH, high $Paco_2$, high HCO_3^-
    c. High blood pH, low $Paco_2$, low HCO_3^2
    d. Low blood pH, high $Paco_2$, low HCO_3^-

21. A young man is on a ventilator because of a drug overdose. Which of the following sets of blood gases would be an indication that the respirator needs to be set at a lower rate?
    a. $Paco_2$ 60 mm Hg, Pao_2 100 mm Hg, pH 7.32; HCO_3^- 28 mEq
    b. $Paco_2$ 40 mm Hg, Pao_2 80 mm Hg, pH 7.42; HCO_3^- 25 mEq
    c. $Paco_2$ 30 mm Hg, Pao_2 98 mm Hg, pH 7.56; HCO_3^- 26 mEq
    d. $Paco_2$ 45 mm Hg, Pao_2 110 mm Hg, pH 7.42; HCO_3^- 29 mEq

References

Barker, S. J., Curry, J., Redford, D., & Morgan, S. (2006). Measurement of carboxyhemoglobin and methemoglobin by pulse oximetry: A human volunteer study. *Anesthesiology, 105*(5), 892–897.

DeCherney, A. H., Nathan, L., Goodwin, T. M., & Lauter, N. (Eds.). (2007). *Current obstetric & gynecologic diagnosis & treatment* (10th ed.). New York: Lange Medical Books/McGraw-Hill.

Deglin, J. H., Vallerand, A. H., & Sanoski, C. A. (2011). *Davis's drug guide for nurses* (12th ed.). Philadelphia: F. A. Davis.

Dellinger, R. P., Levy, M. M., Cartlet, J. M., Bion, J., Parker, M. M., Jaeschke, R., et al. (2008). Surviving Sepsis Campaign:

International guidelines for management of severe sepsis and septic shock. *Critical Care Medicine, 36*(4), 1394–1396.

Golden, A. B., Hill, J. A., O'Riordan, M. A., Sandhaus, L. M. (2010). Point-of-care gas analysis in the pediatric cardiac catheterization suite: A clinical outcome study. *Journal of Near-Patient Testing & Technology, 9*(2), 108–110.

Hay, W. W., Levin, M. J., Sondheimer, J. M., & Deterding, R. (Eds.). (2011). *Current diagnosis and treatment: Pediatrics* (20th ed.). New York: McGraw-Hill.

Jones, A. E., Shapiro, N. I., Trzeciak, S., Arnold, R. C., Claremont, H. A., Kline, J. A., et al., (2010). Lactate clearance vs central venous oxygen saturation as goals of sepsis therapy. *JAMA, 303*(6), 739–746.

Lawes, R. (2009). Body out of balance: Understanding metabolic acidosis and alkalosis. *Nursing* 2009, *39*(11), 50–54.

Madden, M. (2008). Responding to pediatric poisoning. *Nursing 2008, 38* (8), 52–55.

McPhee, S. J., Papadakis, M. A., & Rabow, M. W. (Eds.). (2011). *Current medical diagnosis and treatment* (50th ed.). New York: McGraw-Hill.

Mininni, N. C., Marino, M. L., Kohler, W., & Stephan, M. J. (2009). Pulse oximetry: An essential tool of the busy med-surg nurse. *American Nurse Today, 4*(9), 34–36.

Moore, C. C., Jacob, S. T., Pinkerson, R., Meyanja-Kizza, H., Reynolds, S. J., Scheld, V. V. (2008). Point-of-care lactate testing predicts mortality of seer sepsis in a predominantly HIV type 1-infected patients population in Uganda. *Clinical Infectious Disease, 46*(2), 215–222.

Pruitt, B. (2010). Interpreting ABGs. *Nursing 2010, 40*(7), 31–35.

Rosenthal, L. D. (2006). Carbon monoxide poisoning. *American Journal of Nursing, 106*(3), 40–46.

Smith, D. H. (2006). Methylene chloride inhalation. *Nursing 2006, 36*(6), 88.

Swiderski, D., & Byrum, D. (2007). Are you an ABG ace. *American Nurse Today, 2*(4), 18–21.

Valdez-Lowe, C., Ghareeb, S. M., & Artinian, N. T. (2009). Pulse oximetry in adults. *American Journal of Nursing, 109*(6), 52–59.

Wu, A. H. (Ed.). (2006). *Tietz clinical guide to laboratory tests* (4th ed.). St. Louis, MO: Saunders Elsevier.

Website

www.heart.org (Information on use of bicarbonate in cardiac arrest.)

Answers

1. b, 2. a, 3. a, 4. d, 5. d, 6. d, 7. b, 8. b, 9. a, 10. b, 11. d, 12. b, 13. b, 14. c, 15. a, 16. a, 17. b, 18. d, 19. d. 20. b, 21. c

Three Less Commonly Measured Electrolytes and Vitamin D

CHAPTER

7

- Serum Calcium 158
- Urinary Calcium 166
- Vitamin D Levels 167
- Serum Phosphorus or Phosphates 168
- Urinary Phosphorus or Urine Phosphates 171
- Serum Magnesium 172
- Magnesium Load Test with 24-Hour Urine Collection 175

OBJECTIVES

1. Explain the relation between parathyroid hormone (parathormone) and serum and urine levels of calcium and phosphorus.

2. Identify nursing assessments useful in detecting hypercalcemia or hypocalcemia.

3. Plan appropriate nursing interventions to decrease the harmful effects of hypercalcemia.

4. Analyze clinical situations to determine which clients are likely to have changes in serum phosphorus or calcium levels.

5. Identify potential nursing diagnoses for clients with calcium and phosphorus imbalances.

6. Prepare teaching plans for clients who must decrease or increase calcium and phosphorus intake.

7. Identify nursing assessments useful in detecting serum and magnesium excess and deficiency.

8. Identify potential nursing diagnoses for clients with magnesium excess or deficiency.

9. Describe the latest guidelines for vitamin D requirements.

Both calcium and phosphorus serum levels are controlled by parathyroid hormone (parathormone or PTH). The end results of an increased secretion of PTH are an increased serum calcium level and a decreased serum phosphorus level. Although the serum calcium level often varies inversely with the phosphorus level caused by this hormonal control, both calcium and phosphorus may be increased or decreased together in other clinical situations. Calcium and phosphorus are discussed in separate sections, but the reader needs to be aware that both tests are useful in assessing an imbalance of either electrolyte. In addition, urinary tests for both may give additional information about their overall metabolism. Methods of testing for calcium and phosphorus in the urine are discussed after each section on the electrolytes. Vitamin D levels are discussed after the section on calcium.

Magnesium is less well understood than the other two electrolytes. It is known that a marked increase in serum magnesium has been shown to decrease the release of PTH and that aldosterone causes a decrease in serum magnesium as it does for potassium. The section on magnesium discusses the relationship of magnesium with calcium and potassium in deficiency states.

Unlike the more commonly measured electrolytes discussed in Chapter 5 (Na$^+$, K$^+$, Cl$^-$, HCO$_3^-$), the three electrolytes in this chapter are not always measured in milliequivalents (see Chapter 5 for a definition of milliequivalent). Because a particular laboratory may use either *milligram* or *milliequivalent*, reference values using both systems are presented. In addition, some laboratories may use the SI units discussed in Chapter 1. For Na, K, Cl, and HCO$_3$, the SI and milliequivalent figures are the same. But for Ca, P, and Mg, the SI figures are different from the milliequivalent figures.

SERUM CALCIUM

Calcium (Ca^{2+}), a positively charged ion, circulates in the bloodstream both in the free, or ionized, state and bound to plasma proteins. Some authorities strongly recommend measurement of the ionized calcium rather than the total, but this is a more difficult and time-consuming procedure. The bound calcium, carried chiefly by albumin, is about half of the total calcium in the bloodstream. Because most laboratories measure the total calcium level, not just the ionized calcium, a change in serum albumin level means a change in the total serum reference values. A decrease of 1 g of albumin means that the serum total calcium level is about 0.8 mg less. Because the free, or ionized, calcium affects neuromuscular function, a low calcium level caused by a low albumin level does not cause symptoms of hypocalcemia. Factors that cause decreased serum albumin levels are discussed in Chapter 10.

The amount of calcium in the serum is quite small compared with that present in the teeth and bones. The bones contain a tremendous reservoir of calcium that can be used if needed to keep the serum calcium level normal. Two hormones control serum calcium levels. Calcitonin, a hormone secreted by the thyroid gland, protects against a calcium excess in the serum. PTH, secreted by the parathyroid gland, keeps a sufficient level of calcium in the bloodstream; an increase in PTH not only increases serum calcium levels but also decreases phosphorus levels. Thus, for many types of serum calcium imbalance, it is important to evaluate the serum phosphorus level, too. The relation between phosphorus and calcium is discussed in detail in the section on serum phosphorus levels.

Calcium is obtained from several food sources, of which milk products are the best: 1 cup (240 mL) of milk, for example, contains 236 mg of calcium. Other sources that contain a fairly large amount of calcium include vegetables such as turnip greens, collard greens, white beans, and lentils (Table 7–1). Intestinal cells need vitamin D, a unique vitamin made entirely in the body from cholesterol and a photochemical reaction, to absorb calcium. Thus, sunlight and a diet adequate in fat are important to ensure proper levels of vitamin D. Protein is also required for the proper utilization of calcium. Chronic nutritional deficiencies of calcium, vitamin D, and protein eventually result in lowered serum calcium levels. Yet, because

Table 7-1 Examples of Foods High in Calcium or Phosphorus

Food in 100-g Portions	Calcium (mg)	Phosphorus (mg)
Swiss cheese	925	563
Cheddar cheese	750	478
Brick cheese	730	455
American cheese	697	771
Turnip greens	246	58
Almonds	234	504
Collard greens	203	63
Beans, white	144	425
Milk (100 g = scant 1/2 cup [120 mL])	118	93
Frankfurter	32	603
Bologna	32	581
Peanuts	69	401
Whole wheat flour	41	372
Liver	8	352

of the vast reservoir of calcium in the bones, dietary deficiencies do not often cause lowered serum calcium levels.

The recommended calcium intake varies across the life span, as shown in Table 7–2. Calcium supplementation to a total intake of about 1,500 mg a day has been shown to inhibit age-related bone loss in postmenopausal women. In 1984, only one calcium supplement was on the market. After the National Institutes of Health (NIH) issued a report about osteoporosis and calcium, the market was flooded with products boasting their calcium content. Research on the efficacy of calcium with vitamin D supplementation has shown a small but significant improvement in hip bone density in healthy postmenopausal women, but the risk of hip fractures was not reduced and the risk of kidney stones increased (Jackson

Table 7-2 Recommended Calcium Intake Across the Life Span

Age	Calcium Intake (mg)
1–3 years	700
4–8 years	1,000
9–18 years	1,300
19–50 years	1,000
>51 years (for males)	1,000
>51 years (for females)	1,200
Pregnant/lactating female < 18 years	1,300
Pregnant/lactating female older than 19 years	1,000

Note: See www.iom.edu and www.cnpp.usda.gov.

et al., 2006). Excess calcium is excreted in the urine. The measurement of urinary calcium is covered after the discussion on serum calcium levels.

Preparation of Client and Collection of Sample

A fasting specimen is desirable. One milliliter of serum is collected in a redtop tube. Always check if the serum albumin level is decreased, as explained in the footnote of serum calcium reference values.

REFERENCE VALUES FOR SERUM CALCIUM (TOTAL)[a]	
Adult	Tends to be slightly higher in men 9.0–10.5 mg/dL, or 2.2–2.6 mmol/L
Pregnant women	Falls gradually to a level at term about 10% below nonpregnant level; consistent with the fall in albumin
Newborn	7.4–14 mg/dL or 3.7–7 mEq
Children	Is slightly higher in children—may be up to 12 mg

[a]Each 1-g drop in serum albumin decreases the total calcium by 0.8 mg, and each 0.1 drop in pH below 7.4 decreases the total calcium by 0.01 mg.

Ionized Calcium

A little over 40% of the total serum calcium is ionized, or "free." A measurement of this physiologically active calcium costs more than a routine total calcium but may be beneficial for conditions such as hyper- or hypoparathyroidism (see Chapter 15). Acidosis causes an increase in the ionized portion of calcium, and alkalosis a decrease. The clinical significance of this is discussed under the section on hypocalcemia.

Preparation of Client and Collection of Sample

Three milliliter of whole blood should be collected in a plastic syringe with dry heparin and packed in wet ice for immediate delivery to the laboratory. The use of a cork keeps the sample under anaerobic conditions and eliminates the need to adjust the pH of the sample (Wu, 2006).

REFERENCE VALUES (WHOLE BLOOD)[a]	
Adult	4.6–5.10 mg/dL or 1.15–1.27 mmol/L

[a]Reference values for serum and plasma are slightly lower.

Increased Serum Calcium Level (Hypercalcemia)

Clinical Significance

As with many other tests, dehydration gives a falsely high reading of serum calcium level. An increased level of PTH causes a persistently elevated serum calcium level. Because adenomas of the parathyroid gland can cause the gland to produce additional amounts of PTH, the physician may order several other tests, including

Table 7-3 Common Causes of Hypercalcemia and Hypocalcemia

■ **HYPERCALCEMIA** (serum Ca^{2+} levels > 10.5 mg/dL, or see values for specific laboratory)
False rise caused by dehydration
Hyperparathyroidism (serum phosphorus level decreased)
Malignant tumors
Immobilization
Thiazide diuretics
Vitamin D intoxication (serum phosphorus level increased)

■ **HYPOCALCEMIA** (serum Ca^{2+} levels < 8.5 mg/dL, or see values for specific laboratory) Infants have levels lower than 8 or 7.5 mg/dL
False decrease caused by low albumin levels
Hypoparathyroidism (serum phosphorus level increased)
Early neonatal hypocalcemia
Chronic renal disease (serum phosphorus level increased)
Pancreatitis
Massive blood transfusions
Severe malnutrition (serum phosphorus level decreased)
Symptoms of hypocalcemia when client is alkalotic although total serum calcium is normal (see text)

Note: Serum phosphorus levels help with interpretation of serum calcium levels.

an assay of PTH levels to rule out the possibility that a parathyroid tumor is responsible for hypercalcemia. Often the client may have no symptoms even though the laboratory report shows a higher-than-normal serum calcium level. Hyperparathyroidism, the most common cause of hypercalcemia, is treated by surgical removal of some of the parathyroid glands. Surgery is the treatment of choice because even clients with mild calcium elevation and no symptoms are at risk for renal failure, osteoporosis, and cardiovascular disease (Quillen, 2006).

There are several other common reasons for the serum calcium level being higher than normal (Table 7–3). The most common is the release of calcium in metastatic bone disease as bone is destroyed. Metastatic hypercalcemia occurs most often in breast, lung, and prostate cancers (Thompson, 2010). Also, some of the hormonal changes in malignant states may contribute to raising the serum calcium level. Some tumors produce PTH-like substances. (See Chapter 15 for a discussion on ectopic hormone production.) About 25% of the clients with multiple myeloma have hypercalcemia (Mangan, 2006). Long-term immobilization may result in increased serum calcium levels because the lack of normal bone stress causes the release of calcium from bone. Thiazide diuretics are another reason for hypercalcemia. Excessive milk intake (at least 3 quarts [2.8 L] of milk a day) is a less frequent cause of hypercalcemia. Vitamin D intoxication can also result in hypercalcemia.

Possible Nursing Diagnoses Related to Hypercalcemia

Imbalanced Fluid Requirements Related to Risk for Injury from Formation of Renal Stones

An increased serum calcium level almost always means increased calcium excretion by the kidneys. Thus, insofar as a high concentration of calcium in the urine may lead to the formation of

(Continued)

Possible Nursing Diagnoses . . . (*Continued*)

renal stones (*calculi*), it is very important that a client with hypercalcemia stay well hydrated. Some authorities suggest that the urine volume needs to be greater than 2,500 mL in 24 hours. Health teaching for the client at home should include information on how to make sure the urine is never concentrated; the client must be aware of the importance of drinking fluids at bedtime and also during the night. A home care nurse can help make out a schedule for the client or a member of the family to follow.

Calcium is more likely to precipitate in an alkaline urine. Yet, because the urine pH is normally acidic (≈6), precipitation may not be a threat unless a urinary tract infection develops, which may make the urine alkaline. Measures, such as the intake of cranberry juice, to change an alkaline urine to acidic are discussed in Chapter 3.

For emergency treatment of hypercalcemia, forced diuresis with intravenous normal saline solution is usually used because calcium excretion improves when sodium supplementation is provided. The standard saline solution infusion rate is 200–300 mL/h. The nurse must monitor daily weights and intake and output records to avoid overload. Furosemide may be given. Thiazide diuretics are avoided with hypercalcemia because they exacerbate the condition.

Risk for Injury Related to Slowing of Reflexes

The client with an increased serum calcium level may demonstrate some slowing of reflexes. Because increased serum calcium levels decrease the permeability of nerve cell membranes to sodium, the depolarization process is affected, and the nerve fibers have a decreased excitability. This condition may result in some lethargy or a general sluggish feeling. Other possible problems are anorexia and constipation. Confusion may develop.

Risk for Altered Cardiac Output

An elevated serum calcium level also tends to slow the heart, and arrhythmias may develop. If the client is taking digoxin, a high serum calcium level may be particularly dangerous because it potentiates the effect of digoxin.

Risk for Injury and Impaired Mobility Related to Development of Pathologic Fractures

If the hypercalcemia is a result of loss of calcium from the bones, the client becomes very susceptible to fractures. These types of fractures are referred to as *pathologic fractures* because the bone is made fragile by a pathologic process. Clients who are prone to pathologic fractures must be handled very gently. The nurse must be alert to any vague symptoms of bone pain. Sometimes just turning in bed can cause a fracture. If the client can walk, weight bearing can help minimize loss of calcium from the weight-bearing bones. A walker or other supportive device is essential for safety. Walking helps maintain skeletal integrity.

Deficient Knowledge Related to Therapy for Hypercalcemia

Treatment for hypercalcemia depends on the underlying cause (e.g., surgery for hyperparathyroidism). However, in a hypercalcemic crisis, dialysis may be appropriate (Quillen, 2005).

Several drugs may be used to reduce high serum calcium levels after rehydration with saline solution and diuresis with furosemide (Katzung, Masters, & Trevor, 2009). With all these drugs, the client must remain well hydrated at all times, including during the night.

1. Bisphosphonates, given orally or intravenously, cause a decrease in bone resorption. A newer drug in this class, zoledronic acid, has proven to be very effective for the hypercalcemia of malignancy (Deglin, Vallerand, & Sanoski, 2011). The nurse should monitor serum creatinine levels (Chapter 4) as well as serum levels of calcium, phosphate, and magnesium.
2. Calcitonin is a synthetic preparation of the hormone produced by the thyroid gland. Clients with Paget's disease may take calcitonin injections daily over a long period of time. Often the nurse must teach the client how to perform the injections at home. Allergic reactions can occur.
3. Plicamycin, an antineoplastic drug, is also sometimes used to reduce high serum calcium levels in clients with malignant neoplasms. A single dose may reduce elevated serum calcium levels for several days. However, thrombocytopenia, along with many toxic side effects, may result from the use of this drug.
4. Glucocorticosteroids, such as prednisone and some others, reduce serum calcium levels, but they may take 7–10 days to do so. The nurse and the client must be aware of the potential side effects of the use of corticosteroids. (See Chapter 15 on hormones.)
5. Gallium nitrate infusions are approved for management of hypercalcemia in malignancy.

Imbalanced Nutrition: Related to Possible Dietary Restrictions

For hypercalcemia related to malignant conditions, it is usually not necessary to avoid foods high in calcium. For hyperparathyroidism, the major cause of hypercalcemia, surgery is curative. For vitamin D intoxication, and some chronic types of hypercalcemia, restriction of calcium and vitamin D may be warranted.

Table 7–1 gives examples of foods high in calcium.

Impaired Skin Integrity

An uncommon but potentially very serious skin necrosis can occur in clients with end-stage renal disease or with other diseases that alter calcium and phosphorus metabolism. This abnormal skin calcification (calciphylaxis) is also called uremic small vessel disease or uremic gangrene syndrome. Meticulous wound care, pain management, and measures to prevent sepsis are important to prevent mortality (Beitz, 2004; Schmitz & Reyes, 2009).

Decreased Serum Calcium Level (Hypocalcemia)
Clinical Significance

Because much of serum calcium is bound to albumin, it is important to make sure that the lowered calcium level is not due to a lowered serum albumin level.

Just as *hyper*parathyroidism causes *hyper*calcemia, *hypo*parathyroidism causes *hypo*calcemia, because PTH controls serum calcium levels. Hypoparathyroidism, or a lack of PTH, can be due to accidental damage to the parathyroid glands during operations on the thyroid. The hypocalcemia from surgical removal of the parathyroid glands may be more severe than from other causes of hypoparathyroidism.

Early neonatal hypocalcemia is a clinical condition experienced by some infants in the first 24–48 hours of life. Neonatal hypocalcemia may occur either early, in the first 2 days of life, or later, in the first week or two. Early onset is associated with prematurity, sepsis, respiratory distress, and maternal diabetes. Late-onset hypocalcemia has been linked to a high intake of phosphates in feedings (Hay et al., 2011).

Hypocalcemia is also commonly seen in clients with renal failure when elimination of acid phosphates is impaired. The increase in phosphates in the serum causes a decreased calcium level because of the inverse relation between these two levels. (See the beginning of the chapter for an explanation of this interrelation caused by PTH control.) Also in chronic renal disease, because the kidneys are unable to finish the process of making vitamin D chemically active, calcium absorption is impaired. The tubules of the kidneys are responsible for the final active form of vitamin D, which functions as calcitrol, a hormone necessary for calcium absorption. Vitamin D is the only vitamin known to be converted to a hormonal form. Children who have chronic renal disease may have rickets because of the lowered serum calcium level.

Serum calcium level also can be lowered because calcium is being deposited in tissues. In pancreatitis, the fatty acids that are released can bind up calcium. The pancreas may actually become calcified in areas of necrotic tissue. In massive blood transfusions, the serum calcium level may drop because the calcium ions in the blood are bound by the citrate the blood bank uses as an anticoagulant. The liver removes the citrate from the circulation, but it may not be able to do so fast enough when a large amount of blood is infused.

Severe malnutrition may eventually lead to hypocalcemia, but, because of the vast reserves of calcium in the bones, a calcium-deficient diet does not immediately cause a drop in serum calcium levels. Hence, a pregnant or lactating woman who does not consume enough calcium continues to have a normal serum calcium level as she loses calcium from the teeth and bones. Children and elderly people who have calcium-deficient diets usually retain normal serum calcium levels, too. But rickets develops in children, and osteomalacia, or softening of the bones, develops in older people. Osteoporosis, a health problem for many postmenopausal women, may be related to a lack of calcium intake that existed for many years.

Severe malnutrition that includes a lack of vitamin D and protein eventually causes a lowered serum calcium level when calcium cannot be released from the bones or teeth.

The nurse should bear in mind the effect of pH on calcium solubility. In alkalotic states, even though the total serum calcium does not change, the amount of ionized calcium is less because calcium is less soluble in an alkaline medium. A decrease in the ionized portion of serum calcium causes symptoms of hypocalcemia even though the laboratory test looks normal. (Recall that the serum calcium level measures both bound calcium and ionized calcium.)

When a client is in an acidotic state, the total serum calcium level may be low, but the client has few symptoms because more calcium is in the ionized state. When the pH returns to normal, there is less ionized calcium, and the symptoms of hypocalcemia become apparent. Thus, acidotic states may mask true hypocalcemia.

Possible Nursing Diagnoses Related to Hypocalcemia

Risk for Injury Related to the Development of Tetany

The symptoms of hypocalcemia vary depending on how low the serum calcium level drops and on how abruptly it drops. Hypocalcemia causes muscle twitching and cramps, which may lead to generalized muscle spasms called *tetany*. These cramps in the muscles are due to the neuromuscular irritability from the lack of calcium ions. In a client with a low serum calcium level, tapping of the jaw causes a facial spasm (Chvostek's sign). Some clients, particularly women, may exhibit this sign even though the calcium level is normal. Another assessment of low serum calcium levels is to look for carpopedal spasms (spasms in the hands and feet). Spasms may be elicited when the arm becomes a little ischemic. For example, when the nurse takes the blood pressure, the client's hand may twitch when the cuff is left inflated for a couple of minutes (Trousseau's sign). Subtle signs of neuromuscular irritability caused by hypocalcemia, such as a twitching of the nose, may be overlooked unless the nurse is aware that any neuromuscular irritability should be watched for in a client who may experience hypocalcemia. In the newborn, the symptoms may include twitching or convulsions. The symptoms of hypocalcemia often coincide with those of hypoglycemia in the newborn. (See Chapter 8 for a discussion on hypoglycemia in the newborn.)

Because clients with the potential for hypocalcemia may have a convulsive state, the nurse must be prepared for such a possibility. Calcium gluconate for intravenous administration should be on an emergency cart. After operations on the thyroid or parathyroid gland, an ampule of calcium gluconate is usually kept at the bedside. Clients at risk for hypocalcemia usually have their serum calcium levels measured daily. Untreated hypocalcemia can lead to laryngeal spasms and death.

Special Emphasis for Symptoms of Hypocalcemia in Alkalosis. If a client is having symptoms of tetany because less calcium is in an ionized state, the client is not given calcium as treatment. In alkalosis, the symptoms arise from a lack of ionized calcium, not from a true lack of calcium. When the pH returns to normal, the calcium is once again ionized in the correct amount for neuromuscular functioning. (The possible nursing implications for the client in alkalosis are covered in Chapter 6.)

Risk for Injury Related to Replacement of Calcium

The treatment of hypocalcemia depends on the underlying cause. For prevention of tetany and convulsions, the serum calcium level must be raised quickly to normal. If the signs of tetany are severe, the physician orders calcium to be given intravenously. Several different salts of calcium are available for direct intravenous push (Deglin et al., 2011). The medication may give the client a feeling of warmth because of the vasodilation that occurs along with a drop in the blood pressure or arrhythmias for which the client must be monitored.

In less acute situations—when the client is having few symptoms—calcium may be added to intravenous fluid. Because calcium precipitates in an alkaline medium, calcium salts can never be added to intravenous fluids with an alkaline pH. Most dextrose and saline solutions are acid in pH, but this point must be carefully checked because an intravenous infusion may also contain sodium bicarbonate.

(Continued)

Possible Nursing Diagnoses ... (Continued)

Because calcium has a profound effect on the heart, some physicians may choose to have the client use a cardiac monitor the entire time calcium is being replaced. This precaution is most likely if the client is also taking digoxin because calcium increases the possibility of digitalis toxicity.

Deficient Knowledge Related to Use of Oral Calcium Supplements

For mild hypocalcemia, and in chronic states, the client may be given various oral preparations of calcium salts. An inexpensive source of calcium is some antacids. Chewable tablets are favored by some. Newborns may be given oral supplements, once feedings are tolerated. Metabolites of vitamin D, such as calcifediol or calcitriol, are used to increase serum calcium levels in certain metabolic disorders. The use of vitamin D supplements requires careful monitoring of serum calcium levels because vitamin D has a cumulative effect.

Imbalanced Nutrition: Requirement For Calcium

Calcium requirements are best met by having adequate calcium in the diet. So the nurse must assess the dietary habits of individual clients to determine whether their calcium intake is adequate. If the client does not like milk or cheese (which, as dairy products, are among the best sources of calcium), powdered milk can be added to many dishes without changing their taste. A tablespoon of powdered milk contains nearly 50 mg of calcium (Table 7–1). Foods high in oxalates and phosphates, such as spinach, rhubarb, and asparagus, tend to decrease calcium absorption. Also, a lack of protein decreases calcium utilization, but a diet with excess protein wastes calcium. Elderly clients may have a decrease in gastric hydrochloric acid, which decreases calcium absorption.

Deficient Knowledge Related to Phosphate Binders

Another way to help raise the serum calcium level is to reduce the amount of phosphate intake. (The relationship of high phosphorus levels with low serum calcium levels is discussed in the section on phosphorus.)

URINARY CALCIUM

Preparation of Client and Collection of Sample

All urine for 24 hours is collected in a special bottle that contains 10 mL of hydrochloric acid (HCl). The hydrochloric acid keeps the pH of the urine low (pH 2–3) because calcium tends to precipitate in an alkaline medium. The client consumes the usual diet. Any increased intake of protein by the client should be noted because more calcium is excreted on a high-protein diet. (See Chapter 3 for general instructions about 24-hour urine collections.)

REFERENCE VALUES FOR URINARY CALCIUM	
Adult	50–300 mg/dL, depending on dietary intake
Children	About 5 mg/kg of body weight if on normal dietary intake of calcium

Clinical Significance

Normally up to 99% of the calcium filtered by the kidneys is reabsorbed. An increased urinary calcium level is usually due to an elevated serum calcium level, but some patients have idiopathic hypercalciuria. The amount of calcium being excreted in the urine may differ for various types of hypercalcemia, so the 24-hour urine collection may give extra diagnostic clues. For example, a highly elevated urine calcium does not usually accompany primary hyperparathyroidism because the increased amount of PTH promotes additional reabsorption of calcium. In other types of hypercalcemia, such as with malignant tumors, the urine calcium level may be as high as 800 or 900 mg in 24 hours. In conditions in which there is a low serum calcium level, such as in primary hypoparathyroidism, the urinary excretion of calcium is very low.

VITAMIN D LEVELS

Vitamin D, the sunshine vitamin, is really a hormone that is essential for the absorption of calcium and phosphorus and is used to a lesser degree compared to magnesium. In children, a severe deficiency leads to rickets, and in adults a deficiency leads to osteomalacia. More recently, research has identified that even a small insufficiency of vitamin D may cause various health problems. Although most of the studies that show a correlation with disease states are observations, there is increasing evidence that vitamin D may be beneficial in reducing some auto-immune disease, cancer and cardiovascular (Holick, 2009).

Preparation of Client and Collection of Sample

There is no special preparation of the client for this test, which requires 1.5 mL of venous blood in a gold-colored tube.

REFERENCE VALUES FOR TOTAL VITAMIN D, 25 HYDROXY (OH) LEVELS 1	
Normal range	Above 30 ng/mL
Insufficiency	10–30 ng/mL
Deficiency	Less than 10 ng/mL
Excess	Above 150 ng/mL

Note: Reference values are based on information from Holick (2009).

Increases in Vitamin D Levels

Clinical Significance

Vitamin D toxicity may cause symptoms such as nausea, anorexia, weakness, and constipation. Laboratory results will show hypercalcemia, hypercalciuria, and hyperphosphatemia. An increase in sunshine exposure does not cause an increase in the active form of vitamin D. The role of supplements in causing vitamin D toxicity is currently under investigation, as even large doses of ergocalciferol (D3) have been reported as causing toxicity (Stephenson & Peiris, 2009).

Decreases in Vitamin D Levels

Clinical Significance

Clients who have severe deficiency will most likely have a more complicated pathology that needs to be addressed. For those with an insufficiency, vitamin D supplements will be prescribed. Several types of oral and intravenous preparations are available (Deglin et al., 2011).

Note that the newest guidelines for vitamin D are 600 IUs from age 1 to 70, including during pregnancy. After age 70, the recommended daily allowance is 800 IUs. Visit the website www.iom.edu for additional information.

SERUM PHOSPHORUS OR PHOSPHATES

Laboratories may report phosphorus levels as phosphorus (P) or phosphate (PO_4) levels, as phosphorus is one component of phosphate. Whereas potassium is the main intracellular *cation*, phosphorus is the main intracellular *anion*. So phosphorus is in bone tissue and skeletal muscle, and phosphates regulate many enzymatic actions critical for energy transformations. Because phosphorus has a close relation to calcium, the phosphorus level is usually more useful as a diagnostic tool when evaluated in relation to the serum calcium level.

The phosphate electrolyte is the only electrolyte that is markedly different in values for children and adults. (The bicarbonate ion discussed in Chapter 5 does have slight variations with age.) The marked increase in phosphate ions in young children is partially explained by the increased amount of growth hormone present until puberty.

The recommended dietary allowance for phosphorus, except in infancy and during lactation, is a one-to-one ratio to calcium. Thus, an adult requires about 800 mg of phosphorus a day. In infants and lactating women, the need for calcium exceeds the need for phosphorus. In most U.S. diets, however, the intake of phosphorus is probably twice that of calcium: The average calcium intake may be about 700 mg, whereas the average phosphorus intake is about 1,500 mg. This higher phosphorus intake occurs for two reasons. First, phosphorus is abundant not only in dairy products but also in many natural foods. Second, many food additives contain substantial amounts of phosphates. Processed meat, cheese, and soft drinks are three sources that are quite high in phosphates. Table 7–1 lists other foods that are high in calcium or phosphates.

Like calcium, phosphorus is controlled by PTH. Increases in the level of PTH cause a decrease in the serum level of phosphorus and an increased secretion of phosphorus by the kidneys.

Additional phosphates are excreted by the kidneys. Some phosphate is also excreted in the feces. Drugs, such as aluminum hydroxide, can increase fecal excretion of phosphates.

Preparation of Client and Collection of Sample

One milliliter of serum is needed. Fasting state is required. Because increased carbohydrate metabolism lowers serum phosphorus levels, the client should not have intravenous solutions of glucose running before the test. If an intravenous infusion of glucose is being administered, record it on the laboratory slip. The serum needs to be sent to the laboratory as soon as possible because the laboratory must quickly separate the serum from the cells.

REFERENCE VALUES FOR SERUM PHOSPHORUS	
Adult	3.0–4.5 mg/dL or 1.0–1.4 mmol/L
Pregnant women	Slightly lower in pregnancy
Newborn	5.7–9.5 mg/dL; may be higher in premature infants and for a few days after birth
Children	4–6 mg; levels decline with maturity
Aged	May be slightly lower in the aged

Increased Phosphate Level (Hyperphosphatemia)
Clinical Significance
The clinical significance of an elevated phosphorus level is always evaluated in relation to the serum calcium levels to get a clear idea of what may be a very complicated pathologic process (Table 7–4):

1. When the phosphorus level is elevated and the serum calcium level is low, hypoparathyroidism may be the reason. The lack of PTH decreases the renal excretion of phosphates.

2. In some types of renal dysfunction, the kidneys cannot excrete phosphate ions. A high phosphate level in the serum then depresses the serum calcium level through several hormonal actions. High phosphate levels may be associated with an increased risk for infection, so hyperphosphatemia in dialysis clients needs aggressive management (Plantiga et al., 2008).

3. Diseases of childhood may sometimes involve an increase in the production of growth hormone and an increase in the serum phosphate levels. In such a case, the serum calcium level is not elevated.

Table 7–4 Common Reasons for Changes in Serum Phosphate Levels

■ **HYPERPHOSPHATEMIA** (serum phosphorus > 4.5 mg/dL in adult)
Hypoparathyroidism (serum Ca^{2+} decreased)
Renal failure (serum Ca^{2+} decreased)
Increased growth hormone
Vitamin D intoxication (serum Ca^{2+} increased)
Phosphate intoxication from sodium phosphate enemas

■ **HYPOPHOSPHATEMIA** (serum phosphorus < 2.6 mg/dL in adult)
Hyperparathyroidism (serum Ca^{2+} increased)
Diuresis
Malabsorption, or malnutrition (serum Ca^{2+} decreased)
Carbohydrate loading or refeeding syndrome
Antacid abuse

Note: Serum calcium (Ca^{2+}) helps in interpretation.

4. If the phosphates in serum are elevated because of vitamin D intoxication or the excessive intake of milk, the serum calcium level also is most likely elevated.

5. In certain malignant conditions, the serum phosphate level may either remain normal or be somewhat elevated when serum calcium is elevated.

6. Overuse of phosphate enemas, especially in elderly people, can elevate serum phosphate level and decrease serum calcium level.

Possible Nursing Diagnoses Related to Increased Phosphate Levels

Imbalanced Nutrition: Requirement for Calcium and Phosphorus

If the underlying problem is due to hypoparathyroidism, replacement with calcium and vitamin D corrects the problem. If the phosphorus and calcium levels are both elevated, clients may be instructed to moderately reduce calcium and phosphorus in their diet by limiting dairy products (see the discussion of hypercalcemia diets). If the serum phosphorus level is increased and the serum calcium level is normal or decreased, the dietary restriction of dairy products must be countered by calcium supplements. It is difficult to reduce the serum phosphorus level with diet alone because phosphorus is abundant in many more foods than is calcium. Some medications also may contain large amounts of phosphates. For example, sodium phosphate enemas are contraindicated if hyperphosphatemia is possible.

Deficient Knowledge Related to Use of Phosphate Binders

If the phosphorus level is high and the calcium level is low, as often happens in renal failure, the client needs information about the medication used to reduce the phosphate level. Aluminum hydroxide gels (Alu-Caps or Aludrox), given by mouth, unite with the phosphates present in food to form insoluble aluminum phosphate. These insoluble phosphate compounds are then excreted in the feces. Constipation may become a problem. Magnesium hydroxide also binds phosphates, but the additional magnesium intake is contraindicated in renal failure. Aluminum hydroxide is continued even after dialysis is started because dialysis cannot efficiently reduce serum phosphate levels.

A newer drug that binds phosphate, sevelamer, avoids any concerns about toxicity from aluminum (Deglin et al., 2011).

Decreased Serum Phosphorus Level (Hypophosphatemia)

Clinical Significance

Moderate hypophosphatemia can result from a variety of conditions (Table 7–4):

1. Hyperparathyroidism results in a high serum calcium level and a low phosphorus level.

2. Diuretics may cause a low phosphorus level.

3. Phosphates can be lost in large amounts in some types of renal diseases, although phosphate retention is more common.

4. Drugs that bind phosphate, such as aluminum or magnesium gels, can cause phosphate deficiency. However, diets are usually high in phosphates, so this pharmacologic binding of antacids is usually not a concern.

5. Malabsorption syndromes may eventually lead to low serum phosphorus levels.

Other clinical conditions in which serum phosphorus concentrations may decrease are alcoholic withdrawal, diabetes mellitus, the recovery diuretic phase after severe burns, hyperalimentation therapy, and nutritional recovery syndrome. Low levels of serum phosphate, magnesium, and potassium can occur as early as 12 hours after rapid refeeding, because more glucose and these electrolytes enter cells (Yantis & Velander, 2009).

Possible Nursing Diagnoses Related to Decreased Phosphorus Levels

Risk for Injury Related to Neuromuscular Deficits

It is hypothesized that lowered serum phosphorus levels produce central nervous system symptoms such as irritability and confusion. Hence, nurses must be aware that clients with any altered electrolyte may not be able to function normally; safety precautions become important. Plasma phosphate levels can plunge rapidly when a malnourished client resumes a normal diet.

Risk for Injury Related to Replacement Therapies

Therapy for low serum phosphate levels may include administration of phosphate salts in oral or intravenous form. Because clients likely to experience low phosphorus levels may also experience low potassium and low magnesium levels, the nurse must be familiar with all the replacements being used.

Imbalanced Nutrition: Related to Decreased Phosphorus

If the client can tolerate oral feedings, milk is a good source of phosphorus. Long-term health teaching about phosphorus intake usually is not necessary because in a conventional diet, phosphates are abundant. The concern for a client who has a low serum phosphorus level is to correct the often complex metabolic problem that has caused the deficiency in the serum.

URINARY PHOSPHORUS OR URINE PHOSPHATES

Preparation of Client and Collection of Sample

All urine is collected over a 24-hour period. There is no need for a preservative in the bottle, and the urine does not have to be kept cold. (Note that for urine calcium, a preservative is needed. When both calcium and potassium are to be collected, the preservative does not interfere with the test for phosphorus.)

REFERENCE VALUE FOR URINARY PHOSPHORUS	
All groups	0.4–1.3 g in 24 hours; varies with intake; average is 1 g in 24 hours

Clinical Significance

Urinary phosphorus levels usually reflect the amount of both organic and inorganic phosphates in the diet. Because PTH decreases renal reabsorption of phosphorus, hyperparathyroidism causes an increased urinary phosphorus level 70–75% of the time. The urinary phosphorus test is most often used when there is a complex metabolic problem, such as an endocrine disturbance or malnutrition problems, and when a very complete investigation of all electrolyte disturbances must be performed to monitor the progress of the client.

SERUM MAGNESIUM

Primarily an intracellular ion, magnesium (Mg^{2+}) appears in the bloodstream only in very small amounts. The bulk of magnesium is combined with calcium and phosphorus in the bones. Magnesium is essential for neuromuscular function and for activation of some enzymes. Changes in serum magnesium levels affect other serum ions, too, such as potassium, calcium, and phosphorus. Thus, magnesium deficiency is not usually seen alone. Evidently the body can store magnesium because deficiencies usually develop in chronic conditions and not in acute conditions.

Daily requirement for magnesium is 420 mg for men and 320 mg for women. Supplements are not usually recommended for healthy adults who can meet their requirements by a diet that includes whole grain foods, nuts, and a variety of fruits and vegetables (www.cnpp.usda.gov/).

Magnesium is excreted primarily by the kidneys. The hormone aldosterone causes an increased excretion of magnesium as it does of potassium. Compared with the facts known about potassium, much is still to be learned about how magnesium functions in the body. (See Chapter 5 for a detailed discussion of the effect of aldosterone on potassium levels.) Magnesium is given not only for replacement but also as therapy for preeclampsia, preterm labor, and an expanding array of medical conditions, including ischemic heart disease and arrhythmias. Unlike potassium, magnesium supplements are not likely to cause a dangerous clinical state unless the client has impaired renal function. However, intravenous magnesium sulfate in pregnancy is a high-alert medication and overdosages continue to occur (Simpson, 2006).

Preparation of Client and Collection of Sample

The client should be fasting. One milliliter of serum is needed. Calcium gluconate may interfere with some test methods. Hemolysis of the specimen must be avoided because magnesium is primarily an intracellular ion. Lowered albumin levels cause lower magnesium levels.

REFERENCE VALUES FOR SERUM MAGNESIUM	
Adult	1.8–3.0 mg/dL or 0.8–1.2 mmol/L
Pregnant women	Gradual fall of about 10–20%
Children	1.54–1.86 mEq/L
Aged	No reported difference

Note: Values are highly method specific.

Increased Serum Magnesium Level (Hypermagnesemia)

Clinical Significance

Renal failure is the most common reason for magnesium excess because the kidneys are unable to excrete magnesium normally. If renal output is not adequate, an increased magnesium level may result from the administration of medications containing magnesium, such as milk of magnesia (Table 7–5). Also, severe cases of hypermagnesemia have been reported because of incorrect use of magnesium replacements.

Obstetric clients may receive magnesium parenterally as treatments of the hypertensive disorders of pregnancy and for premature labor (DeCherney et al., 2007). The therapeutic level of magnesium for treatment of toxemia in pregnancy is in the 2.5–5.0 mEq/L range. Institutional protocols concerning the frequency of drawing blood for serum magnesium levels differ when the obstetric client is having magnesium sulfate infused. Simpson and Knox (2004) noted that a thorough assessment is more important than laboratory values because toxic and therapeutic levels vary within and between individuals. For a pregnant woman having eclamptic seizures, magnesium sulfate may be prescribed as an intravenous bolus followed by a continuous infusion that is not discontinued until 24 hours after delivery.

Decreased Serum Magnesium Level (Hypomagnesemia)

Clinical Significance

A decrease in serum magnesium is usually due to a chronic problem involving a low intake of dietary magnesium over a period of time (Table 7–5). For example,

Table 7–5 Common Reasons for Changes in Serum Magnesium Level

■ **HYPERMAGNESEMIA** (serum Mg^{2+} level > 2 mEq/L)
Renal failure
Intravenous administration of $MgSO_4$

■ **HYPOMAGNESEMIA** (serum Mg^{2+} level < 1.5 mEq/L)
Chronic malnutrition (e.g., alcoholism)
Diarrhea or draining gastrointestinal fistulas
Diuretics
Diabetes
Hypercalcemia or other complex metabolic disorders
Refeeding syndrome

people who use alcohol as the primary source of calories may become deficient in magnesium. Deficiencies may also result from impaired absorption, such as that associated with a draining intestinal fistula or loss from heavy use of diuretics. Clients with deficiency of magnesium and potassium have many similar etiologies (McPhee, Papadakis, & Rabow, 2011). Clients with diabetes, especially whose diabetes is not well controlled, may also be having magnesium deficiency. Sometimes the cause of low serum magnesium is idiopathic. Urinary magnesium may provide earlier evidence of a deficiency than does a serum level.

Possible Nursing Diagnoses Related to Increased Magnesium Levels

Risk for Injury Related to Altered Neuromuscular Functioning

Higher-than-normal levels of serum magnesium produce sedation, depression of the neuromuscular system, and reduction in blood pressure. If a mother was given $MgSO_4$, the newborn may have lethargy and respiratory depression. Whether the excess magnesium is due to renal failure or intravenous therapy for toxemia, an excess of magnesium can lead from muscle weakness to muscle paralysis, so that deep tendon reflexes are weak or absent. In severe hypermagnesemia (>10 mEq/L), paralysis of voluntary muscles produces flaccid quadriplegia and respiratory failure. Severe hypotension occurs. The electrocardiogram shows prolonged PR and QT intervals. Thus, nursing assessments for a client who is at risk for serum magnesium excess should include (1) monitoring frequent blood pressure and pulse, (2) assessing the level of consciousness, (3) checking the presence of normal reflexes such as knee jerk, and (4) maintaining careful intake and output records. Magnesium sulfate is considered a high-risk medication by the Institute of Medicine. Review of obstetric accidents with magnesium sulfate has led to 20 more specific recommendations, in addition to the recommendations that apply to all high-risk medications, to promote patient safety (Simpson & Knox, 2004).

In addition to muscle weakness, the client may be confused and thus less aware of the surrounding environment. The nurse must take whatever measures are necessary to protect the client from injury. If the magnesium excess is causing acute problems, the physician may order calcium gluconate or calcium chloride to be given intravenously because calcium is the antidote for magnesium excess. The calcium antidote should be kept in an easily accessible locked kit with the dosage clearly marked on the kit (Simpson, 2006).

Deficient Knowledge Related to Hidden Sources of Magnesium

Clients with chronic renal failure should not be given any medications that contain magnesium. The nurse needs to provide client teaching because several over-the-counter drugs contain magnesium. For example, antacids used should be those that contain aluminum hydroxide gels, not magnesium hydroxide. A popular cathartic, epsom salts, is a compound of magnesium sulfate. Many other laxatives contain magnesium, and those pose a special threat to elderly people with decreased renal function. The dietary restriction of magnesium intake is not a focus for teaching because most foods contain only a trace of this mineral (Table 7–5). For example, people who use alcohol as the primary source of calories may become deficient in magnesium. Deficiencies may result from impaired absorption, such as that associated with a draining intestinal fistula or loss from heavy use of diuretics. Other drugs such as aminoglycosides, cyclosporine, and cisplatin, may also cause hypomagnesemia. Clients with low magnesium levels may also have unexplained hypocalcemia and hypokalemia, which causes complex electrolyte imbalances. Clients with diabetes, especially whose diabetes is not well controlled, may also be having magnesium deficiency.

Possible Nursing Diagnoses Related to Hypomagnesemia

Imbalanced Nutrition: Less than Body Requirements

An assessment for magnesium deficiency is appropriate for clients who have to be fed by artificial means or who are chronically malnourished.

Risk for Injury Related to Alteration in Cardiac Output

The nurse should be on the alert for any change in the rhythm or rate of the pulse because hypomagnesemia is a risk factor for the development of arrhythmias. Originally magnesium was used for clients with digoxin-induced arrhythmias who had low serum magnesium levels. Also, magnesium replacement has been found to have antiarrhythmic effects even in some clients with normal levels, although the mechanisms of this effect are not fully understood (McPhee et al., 2011).

Altered Comfort Related to Neuromuscular Irritability

Early symptoms of a lack of magnesium are related to neuromuscular irritability: The client may have tremors, muscle cramps, and insomnia. The nurse should assess for any involuntary movements or twitching by the client. (See the section on hypocalcemia on how to check for a positive Chvostek's sign and a positive Trousseau's sign.) The client may eventually show symptoms that look very similar to the tetany of hypocalcemia. Often the client may have several deficiencies so the clinical signs and symptoms are not so simple. Laboratory tests have to be performed to identify exactly which electrolyte imbalances coexist. A low calcium or a low potassium that is unresponsive to treatment may be due to a coexisting low magnesium, so interventions may focus on replacements of multiple electrolytes.

Risk for Injury Related to Magnesium Replacements

Magnesium deficits are corrected by the use of magnesium sulfate. If magnesium is being given intravenously, the nurse must assess carefully for the signs and symptoms of magnesium excess discussed in the section on hypermagnesemia. A sliding scale may be used to determine the dosage based on magnesium levels. The intravenous infusion should be stopped if there is a sharp decrease in blood pressure, extreme sedation, or weak reflexes. The importance of assessing for the patellar reflex (knee jerk) has been discussed. Oral placement may cause diarrhea because magnesium has a laxative effect.

MAGNESIUM LOAD TEST WITH 24-HOUR URINE COLLECTION

Sometimes the serum magnesium level may be on the borderline of normal. So this test helps to determine if the body is deficient in magnesium.

Preparation of Patient and Collection of Sample

After a pretest urine sample is collected, the client is given an infusion of 30 mmol/L magnesium sulfate ($MgSO_4$), in 1 L of normal saline, over 8 hours. Urine is collected for 24 hours to measure how much of the drug is excreted (Wu, 2006).

REFERENCE VALUES	
Magnesium deficiency	If less than 18 mmol of the 30 mmol dose is recovered in the 24-hour urine sample, the diagnosis is magnesium deficiency

Questions

1. A home care nurse is visiting an elderly woman who lives alone and who does her own cooking. She considers milk to be "for babies." If she does not wish to drink milk or use it in cooking, which alternative foods would offer the highest calcium intake?
   a. Fresh greens, beans, and whole wheat products
   b. Rice, liver, and chicken
   c. Apples, oranges, and other citrus fruits
   d. Potatoes, shellfish, and cornmeal

2. A nursing diagnosis of "risk for injury related to hypercalcemia" would be most likely for
   a. A client who is beginning dialysis because of chronic renal failure
   b. A baby whose mother has diabetes that is not well controlled
   c. A client whose breast cancer has metastasized to the bones
   d. A client who experiences respiratory alkalosis from hyperventilating

3. A nurse is caring for a client who is receiving normal saline solution intravenously followed by furosemide as a treatment for hypercalcemia. As a next step, the nurse may need to monitor which of the following drugs to further lower the hypercalcemia?
   a. Aluminum hydroxide
   b. Thiazide diuretic
   c. Magnesium sulfate
   d. Zoledronic acid

4. Which nursing action is the most important to prevent complications for clients with a high serum calcium level?
   a. Keeping the pH of the urine alkaline
   b. Checking for signs of tetany
   c. Making sure the client is well hydrated
   d. Checking for tachycardia

5. A lactating mother who drinks only one or two glasses of milk a day will most likely continue to have a normal serum calcium level for which of the following reasons?
   a. Two glasses of milk supply the minimum calcium requirements for lactation
   b. Calcium is also available in most meat products and leafy green vegetables
   c. Lactation causes a decrease in parathyroid hormone
   d. Calcium is being drawn from the reservoir in the bones and teeth

6. Which of the following is a characteristic symptom of a low serum calcium level?
   a. Flank pain
   b. Carpopedal spasms
   c. Bradycardia
   d. Constipation

7. Which of the following clients has little possibility of experiencing symptoms of hypocalcemia?
   a. A premature infant born this morning
   b. The client who had a subtotal thyroidectomy today
   c. The client who has metastatic cancer of the liver
   d. The client who has acute pancreatitis

8. Which of these clients is the most likely to have decreased serum calcium and serum phosphorus levels?
   a. A client who takes a lot of antacids and milk
   b. A client who is in renal failure
   c. A client who eats a low-fat diet and spends little time outdoors
   d. A client who is in a diabetic coma and who is being treated with glucose and insulin

9. A client is undergoing therapy to reduce his serum phosphorus level. Which of the following foods is not high in phosphorus content and would thus be allowed on his diet?
   a. Processed luncheon meat
   b. Skim milk
   c. Soft drinks
   d. Apples

10. In a client with chronic renal failure, aluminum hydroxide may be useful in lowering serum phosphorus levels because the drug
    a. Causes precipitation of insoluble phosphates in the intestine
    b. Increases secretion of phosphorus in the urine
    c. Counteracts the effect of parathyroid hormone
    d. Balances the pH of the serum

11. Which of the following clients is the least likely to have a magnesium deficiency?
    a. A client who has had vomiting and diarrhea for 24 hours
    b. A client who is undergoing hyperalimentation therapy
    c. A client who has a long history of alcohol abuse
    d. A client who has a chronic problem with a draining gastrointestinal fistula

12. An elderly man has had poor nutritional habits over an extended period of time. The home care nurse suspects that magnesium deficiency may be one of his problems. Which of the following symptoms would be least indicative of low serum magnesium?
    a. Leg and foot cramps
    b. Tremors
    c. Irritability
    d. Unusual amount of sleeping

13. A pregnant client is receiving magnesium sulfate ($MgSO_4$) intravenously as treatment for preeclampsia. Which of the following nursing assessments is an indication that she may be experiencing a serum magnesium excess?
    a. Rise in pulse and blood pressure
    b. Exaggerated patellar reflex (knee jerk)

    c. Sedation

    d. Seizure activity

14. An antidote for high serum magnesium levels is the administration of which of the following?

    a. Potassium chloride

    b. Calcium gluconate

    c. Aluminum hydroxide

    d. Calcitonin

References

Beitz, J. M. (2004). Calciphylaxis: An uncommon but potentially deadly form of skin necrosis. *American Journal of Nursing, 104*(2), 36–37.

DeCherney, A. H., Nathan, L., Goodwin, T. M., & Lauter, N. (Eds.). (2007). *Current obstetric & gynecologic diagnosis & treatment* (10th ed.). New York: McGraw-Hill.

Deglin, J. H., Vallerand, A. H., & Sanoski, C. A. (2011). *Davis's drug guide for nurses* (12th ed.). Philadelphia: F. A. Davis.

Hay, W. W., Levin, M. J., Sondheimer, J. M., & Deterding, R. (Eds.). (2011). *Current diagnosis and treatment: Pediatrics* (20th ed.). New York: McGraw-Hill.

Holick, M. F. (2009). Vitamin D status: Measurement, interpretation and clinical application. *Annals of Epidemiology, 19*(2),73–78.

Jackson, R. D., LaCroix, A. Z., Gass, M., Wallace, R. B., Robbins, J., Lewis, C. E., et al. (2006). Calcium plus vitamin D supplementation and the risk of fractures. *New England Journal of Medicine, 354*(7), 669–683.

Katzung, B. G, Masters, S. B., & Trevor, A. J. (Eds.). (2009). *Basic and clinical pharmacology* (11th ed.). New York: McGraw-Hill.

Mangan, P. (2006). Teach your patient about multiple myeloma. *Nursing 2006, 36*(4), 64hn1–64hn4.

McPhee, S. J., Papadakis, M. A., & Rabow, M. W. (Eds.). (2011). *Current medical diagnosis and treatment* (50th ed.). New York: McGraw-Hill.

Plantiga, L. C., Fink, N. E., Melamed, M. L., Briggs, W. A., Powe, N. R., & Jaar, B. G. (2008). Serum phosphate levels and risk of infection in incident dialysis patients. *Clinical Journal of American Society of Nephrology, 3*, 1398–1406.

Quillen, T. F. (2005). About hypercalcemia. *Nursing 2005, 35*(7), 74.

Quillen, T. F. (2006). About primary hyperparathyroidism. *Nursing 2006, 36*(2), 29.

Schmitz C. & Reyes, L. (2009). A case study, calciphylaxis: An exercise in human caring. *MEDSURG Nursing, 18*(4), 239–241.

Simpson, K. R. (2006). Minimizing risk of magnesium sulfate overdose in obstetrics. *MCN: American Journal of Maternal Child Health, 31*(5), 340.

Simpson, K. R. & Knox, G. E. (2004). Obstetrical accidents involving intravenous magnesium sulfate: Recommendations to promote patient safety. *MCN: American Journal of Maternal Child Health, 29*(3), 161–171.

Stephenson, D. W. & Peiris, A. N. (2009). The lack of vitamin D toxicity with megadose of daily ergocalciferol (D2) therapy: A case study report and literature review. *Southern Medical Journal, 102*(7), 765–768.

Thompson, N. (2010). When cancer spreads to the bone. *American Nurse Today, 5*(9), 8–10.

Wu, A. H. (Ed.). (2006). *Tietz clinical guide to laboratory tests* (4th ed.). St. Louis, MO: Saunders Elsevier.

Yantis, M. A. & Velander, R. (2008). How to recognize and respond to refeeding syndrome. *Nursing 2008, 38*(5), 34–39.

Websites

www.cnpp.usda.gov (Information on dietary guidelines from Center for Nutrition Policy and
   Promotion.)
www.iom.edu (Information on vitamin D and calcium requirements.)

Answers

1. a, 2. c, 3. d, 4. c, 5. d, 6. b, 7. c, 8. c, 9. d, 10. a, 11. a, 12. d, 13. c, 14. b

Tests to Measure the Metabolism of Glucose and Other Sugars

- Summary of Glucose Metabolism 181
- Changes in the Diagnosis and Classification of Diabetes Mellitus 182
- Fasting Blood Sugar or Plasma Glucose 183
- Postprandial Blood Sugar or 2-Hour P.C. Glucose 184
- Blood Glucose Monitoring Devices 185
- Oral Glucose Tolerance Test 187
- Hemoglobin A1C 188
- Fructosamine or Glycated Protein 190
- Serum Ketones 196
- Diabetes-Related Autoantibodies: Islet Cell, Glutamic Acid Decarboxylase (GAD) 65 and Insulin 201
- C-Peptide Levels 202
- Lactose Tolerance Test 203
- Serum Test for Galactosemia 204

OBJECTIVES

1. Describe the hormonal control of serum glucose levels.
2. Compare the client preparation, usefulness, and limitations of the various tests of glucose to detect diabetes.
3. Contrast the expected laboratory findings and related assessments in hyperosmolar hyperglycemic nonketotic coma (HHNK) and ketoacidosis.
4. Identify appropriate nursing diagnoses for clients with hyperglycemia of varying severity.
5. Compare and contrast the assessment of hypoglycemia in adults, children, newborns, and the elderly.
6. Determine the priority nursing and medical interventions for various types of hypoglycemia, including reactive hypoglycemia.
7. Identify nursing assessments that would indicate the possibility of a rebound effect from insulin (Somogyi effect).
8. Develop a teaching plan to inform clients about glucose tests performed at home.
9. Analyze the similarities and differences in galactose and lactose intolerances, along with the laboratory tests used to identify each abnormality.

FBS, FPG, OGTT, and A1C—these abbreviations should all be familiar to the nurse because they represent common measurements of glucose in the blood. Clinicians may use several of these tests both to diagnose and to evaluate therapy for diabetes mellitus, as well as for other conditions involving an elevated blood sugar level (hyperglycemia) or a low blood sugar level (hypoglycemia).

Normally, all complex carbohydrates, including sugars and starches, are eventually broken down to glucose. In some metabolic abnormalities, sugars such as lactose and galactose are present in the serum and urine. The tests that may be performed to detect these abnormal sugars are described in the last part of this chapter.

SUMMARY OF GLUCOSE METABOLISM

Although most glucose comes from the dietary intake of carbohydrates, the liver can convert fats and protein into glucose when not enough glucose is available for the cells. The liver also stores extra glucose in the form of glycogen. With an excess of glucose intake, the glucose that is not stored as glycogen is converted into adipose (fat) tissue. Several hormones influence serum glucose levels:

1. *Insulin*, secreted by the beta cells of the pancreas, is essential for the transport of glucose (and potassium) into the cells. A lack of insulin causes an increase in blood glucose levels and a potassium imbalance because glucose and potassium cannot get into the cells.

2. *Glucagon*, secreted by the alpha cells of the pancreas, elevates blood glucose levels by promoting the conversion of glycogen to glucose. The role of glycogen in the treatment of hypoglycemia is explained in the section on hypoglycemia.

3. Other hormones that cause an elevation of blood glucose levels are the *corticosteroids*, *epinephrine*, and *growth hormone*. The hyperglycemic effects of these hormones are discussed under the section on the clinical significance of hyperglycemia.

4. In pregnancy, *human placental lactogen* (HPL) promotes increased blood glucose levels. Other hormones in pregnancy, *progesterone*, *estrogen*, and *prolactin*, are insulin antagonists.

5. *Amylin*, secreted by the beta cells of the pancreas, turns off glucagon, slows down the rate of stomach emptying, and acts on the brain to give a sense of fullness. (Glucagon causes the liver to make glucose from glycogen.) Synthetic amylin came on the market in 2005 as a supplement to insulin, as discussed later.

Table 8–1 summarizes the effect of hormones on glucose metabolism.

For most people, the renal threshold for glucose is about 160–190 mg/dL (i.e., glucose is not spilled into the urine until the blood glucose level is greater than 160–190 mg/dL). For some people, however, the renal threshold may be higher or lower. For example, in elderly people with a high renal threshold, glucose may not be excreted by the kidneys even though the blood glucose is elevated above normal limits. Urine sugar levels need to be compared with blood glucose levels to determine the specific renal threshold for an individual.

Table 8-1 Effects of Hormones on Serum Glucose Levels

Promote Hyperglycemia	Promote Hypoglycemia
Growth hormone	Insulin
Glucocorticoids	Amylin
Epinephrine and norephinephrine	
Glucagon	
Human placental lactogen (HPL)	
Estrogen	
Progesterone	
Thyroxin	

Note: See Chapter 15 for a detailed discussion of the tests for hormones.

CHANGES IN THE DIAGNOSIS AND CLASSIFICATION OF DIABETES MELLITUS

The first type of diabetes, now called type 1 diabetes, is primarily due to pancreatic beta cell destruction, which may be a result of an autoimmune process or may be idiopathic. Uncontrolled type 1 leads to ketoacidosis. The second type of diabetes, now called type 2 diabetes, is more prevalent and is related to some type of insulin resistance with an insulin secretory defect. Both types 1 and 2 may be treated with insulin and the newer types of oral antidiabetic agents. Both types can cause long-term complications if glucose levels are not controlled.

In 2009, another major change occurred when A1C was endorsed as a test to diagnose diabetes, not just to monitor as before. The A1C cannot be used in clients who have rapid cell turnover such as hemolytic anemias or who have had blood transfusions so the fasting plasma glucose (FPG) or oral glucose tolerance test (OGTT) may be needed in some cases. Additionally, the cost may be prohibitive in some parts of the world (Seley, 2009). The American Diabetes Association (ADA) recommends screening for type 2 at 3-year intervals, after age 45. Testing should be done at an earlier age or more frequently if the client has risk factors such as polycystic ovary syndrome (Chapter 15), babies with birthweight over 9 pounds, or others as discussed later. (See www.diabetes.org for a summary of the current recommendations with evidence for each recommendation.)

Type 2 Diabetes in Adults

Major risk factors for type 2 diabetes in adults include advancing age, obesity, and decreased physical activity. Early detection is important to prevent complications from the disease. Diet and exercise are the first step of treatment. If lifestyle modifications are not sufficient, the client may be put on one or more oral antidiabetic agents. A combination of these agents and insulin may give the most effective control.

Type 2 Diabetes in Children

Until recently, diabetes in children was almost always type 1, which formerly was called juvenile-onset diabetes. Type 2 was called adult-onset diabetes. In the past few years, a marked increase in childhood obesity has resulted in many more cases of type 2 in children and adolescents. Severely obese children and adolescents often have impaired glucose tolerance irrespective of their ethnic group. Nurses should be aware that obese children need to be screened for glucose intolerance. A brown, hypersegmented thickening of the skin (acanthosis nigricans) is a warning sign of type 2 diabetes, especially if the client is overweight and/or has a family history of type 2. Children may also have dyslipidemia and polycystic ovary disease.

Type 1.5 or Latent Autoimmune Diabetes in Adults

About 10% of people with diabetes have latent autoimmune diabetes in adults (LADA), which presents in adults as type 2, but has autoantibodies like type 1. Researchers are working on a set of criteria for diagnosis, which includes the following:

1. Presence of autoantibodies in blood
2. Adult age onset
3. No need for insulin in the first 6 months after diagnosis

The client with LADA may be on oral diabetic pills, but research has shown that insulin treatment can preserve beta cell function (Gebel, 2010). Some resources call this slow progressing type 1.

Gestational Diabetes

The exact etiology of gestational diabetes is not known, but it is hypothesized that the combination of genetic and environmental factors contributes to the inability of the pregnant client to produce or utilize insulin. This condition occurs in about 7% of all pregnant women. High-risk factors include marked obesity, a family history of diabetes, and a personal history of gestational diabetes or glycosuria. Gestational diabetes is similar to type 2 diabetes, and the risk for developing gestational diabetes in future pregnancies is at least 60% (DeCherney et al., 2007). The oral glucose tolerance test may be used to assess this condition.

FASTING BLOOD SUGAR OR PLASMA GLUCOSE

In clinical practice, the more general term *blood sugar* is often used interchangeably with the more precise term *plasma glucose*. Hence, one may see an order for a fasting blood sugar (FBS). Whole blood glucose is about 10% lower than plasma values because the red blood cells (RBCs) are not as rich in glucose as in the plasma. Plasma glucose levels are measured in the laboratory, and whole blood samples or plasma equivalent is used for finger sticks.

A fasting plasma glucose (FPG) greater than 126 mg/dL on two occasions indicates diabetes. Borderline results may be followed by a carbohydrate loading test for a definitive diagnosis of diabetes. Although the FPG is the older and most used screening test, the A1C (discussed later) has shown promise as a second screening tool.

Preparation of Client and Collection of Sample

For an FPG test, the client may not eat for at least 8 hours before the test, but water intake may continue. If the client has an intravenous infusion that contains dextrose, the test is not valid. If the client has diabetes and is being treated with insulin, both food and insulin are withheld until the specimen is drawn.

The blood is collected in a tube with an EDTA–fluoride mixture as a glycolytic inhibitor. (Gray-topped vacuum tube is usually used, but check with the laboratory for the specific method.)

REFERENCE VALUES (SERUM VALUES, NOT WHOLE BLOOD VALUES) FOR FPG	
Adult	70–99 mg/dL[a]
Newborn	30–100 mg/dL[b]
Pregnant women	Slightly lower values than in nonpregnant state
Aged	Reference values may be slightly higher with aged, particularly with glucose tests other than FPG; the FPG increases only 1–2 mg per decade

[a]Whole blood glucose levels are 10% lower than plasma levels.

[b]For premature infants, value may be as low as 20–80 mg/dL (Hay et al., 2011). See text for hypoglycemia of newborn.

Prediabetes

An FPG of 100–125 mg/dL is now called "prediabetic" as this is a risk factor for the development of diabetes in the future. The older term "impaired fasting glucose" referred to an FPG above 110 mg/dL. Authorities have estimated that nearly 40% of the adults over 45 are prediabetic. Studies have shown that in the prediabetic clients, development of type 2 diabetes can be slowed by changes in lifestyle that include moderate weight loss (if overweight, as almost all are) and some type of physical exercise most days. Some clients with prediabetes may be prescribed metformin (www.diabetes.org).

POSTPRANDIAL BLOOD SUGAR OR 2-HOUR P.C. GLUCOSE

Purpose of Test and Preparation of Client

Postprandial, or *post cibum* (p.c.), means after a meal. Sometimes the client is given a meal consisting of a standard amount of carbohydrate, or the laboratory draws the blood after a conventional meal. The purpose of the postprandial test is to see how the body responds to the ingestion of carbohydrates in a meal.

The timing of the blood specimen drawing must be accurate. All the factors that affect the glucose tolerance test results may also affect the postprandial blood sugar (PPBS) levels.

> **REFERENCE VALUES FOR PPBS**
>
> Normal is less than 120 mg/dL. A value greater than 120 mg/dL but less than 200 mg/dL may necessitate further study. Levels greater than 200 mg/dL are considered indicative of diabetes. Because the 2-hour value rises about 5 mg/dL for each decade of life, a person 60 years of age has a 2-hour PPBS about 15 mg higher than a person 30 years of age.

BLOOD GLUCOSE MONITORING DEVICES

In the past, most clients with diabetes were monitored by self-testing of urine and occasional blood glucose levels obtained by means of venipuncture by health professionals. (See Chapter 3 on urine tests for glucose.) A "revolution" occurred when self-monitoring of blood glucose became possible with reagent strips and monitors.

Frequent monitoring is needed to maintain tight control of blood glucose levels. Intensive therapy does delay the onset and slow the progression of diabetic retinopathy, nephropathy, and neuropathy.

Preparation of Client and Collection of Sample

A drop of capillary blood is obtained by means of a finger stick, an earlobe stick, or, in the case of an infant, a heel stick. The extremity should be warm to encourage vasodilation. (See Chapter 1 on the procedure for heel and finger sticks.) Monitors use either a light beam (reflectance meter) or an electrical charge (biosensor or biochemical meters) to read the enzymatic change that takes place on the reagent test strip. An older method is a visual comparison of the reagent test strip with a color chart (rainbow method). The accuracy of capillary blood monitoring may be compromised if the client has hypoxia, markedly abnormal hemoglobin, or a glucose level higher than 800 mg/dL. Also, capillary blood monitoring may not be reliable with temperature extremes. Some medications may affect readings, but this varies with the brand of monitors.

> **REFERENCE VALUES FOR FINGER-STICK MONITORING**
>
> | Measurement | Goal |
> |---|---|
> | Whole blood | |
> | Average before meals | 80–120 mg/dL |
> | Average bedtime | 100–140 mg/dL |
> | Plasma | |
> | Average before meals | 90–130 mg/dL |
> | Average bedtime | 110–150 mg/dL |
>
> *Source:* www.diabetes.org, for updates on goals for blood glucose when clients are hospitalized.

For routine monitoring at home, clients may use soap and water rather than alcohol to clean the site. Several different companies make test strips, so it is critical to follow the manufacturer's recommendations for a certain product. General guidelines are as follows:

1. Cover the entire reagent pad with a drop of blood. Newer monitors require less blood. Some tests require only 3 μL—the size of a pin head. Don't let the finger touch the pad because oils from the finger may affect the results.

2. Calibrate the machine to each new batch of strips as instructed by the manufacturer. Test the meter once a week by using a control solution.

3. Use the meter immediately before or after a plasma glucose measurement is performed by the laboratory. A meter value should register within 15% of the lab result. Older monitors reported results only for whole blood, but newer ones may also give the plasma equivalent, which is helpful when comparing to laboratory results.

4. Regular insulin may be given to control the glucose. Sample guidelines are as follows:

   151–200 mg/dL—6 units of regular insulin

   201–250 mg/dL—8 units of regular insulin

   251–300 mg/dL—10 units of regular insulin

   301–400 mg/dL—12 units of regular insulin

5. If the glucose remains 250 mg/dL or more, check urine ketones.

The Annual Consumer Guide in Diabetes Forecast (www.forecast.diabetes.org) lists over 30 different meters, several types of reagent strips, and many brands of equipment for self-sticks. For the visually impaired, there are meters that speak. Glucose meters with built-in timers and digital readouts can be used with memory chips that record each determination so that when they are connected to a microcomputer, a database is available for decision making. A monitor combined with a diabetes manager and personal digital assistant (PDA) fits in the palm of the hand and may be welcomed by those interested in the latest technology. Although glucose photometers or reflectance meters were originally designed for use with capillary blood samples, venous or arterial blood samples may also be used.

Although meters do make blood glucose monitoring easier, clients with diabetes should be confident in just reading the strips. For example, some diabetes camps may encourage the children not to always use a meter so they can "travel light" on a backpacking trip or do a quick check in a variety of other settings in which carrying a monitor may be cumbersome. Newer monitors are very small, so portability is less of an issue. Nurses need to assess if clients are using both the visual strips and the monitors correctly.

The Joint Commission (www.jointcommission.org) requires each nurse who uses a meter to demonstrate competency once a month, so it is important that nurses have a voice in selecting the monitors for a particular setting. Clients, too, need to have a voice in selecting the best monitor for home use. In order to talk to clients, nurses need to be aware of costs of monitors, ease of use, and methods to get accurate readings, as these vary with different types of monitors.

Alternative Site Testing

Clients may draw blood from areas such as the palm, arm, or thigh that have fewer nerve endings than the fingers. Most meters now have instructions for when to use alternative sites. Because readings from alternative sites may lag behind finger-stick readings, clients should still use finger-stick monitoring if they feel they may have a very low glucose level or they need the immediate results for driving or exercise. Studies have shown that the readings from forearm monitors may be 11–13 points higher than those from finger sticks. So a glucose level of 70 mg/dL on the forearm meter might really be 57–59 by finger stick. Any finger-stick reading below 70 mg/dL is considered hypoglycemia and requires treatment (Kordella, 2005). Palm readings may be closer to finger-stick readings (Dale, 2006). People with hypoglycemic unawareness should not use these alternative sites. Manufacturers of alternative-site testing meters provide information on how to compare results to finger sticks and when alternative-site testing is most appropriate.

Continuous Glucose Monitoring Devices

Real-time continuous glucose monitoring (CGM) system uses a fine needle worn in the subcutaneous tissue of the abdomen. This also measures interstitial fluid glucose levels. The monitor is worn on the belt, and results are downloaded to a computer. Insulin pumps also have continuous monitors. One approved test (Dex-Com) uses a sensor on the body to transmit data, wirelessly, to a handheld receiver (Tenderich, 2006). As cost and accuracy (in extreme cases) are issues with these new types of monitors, they cannot yet replace the traditional monitor. Clients who decide to use CGM devices will need encouragement from nurses about the new devices that may help them better manage their diabetes (Ramchandani, Saadon, & Jornsay, 2010). Despite expanded insurance coverage and evidence that (CGM) is effective, widespread adoption has not yet occurred. Body image concerns related to wearing a mechanical device and the complexity of calibrating the monitor are two deterrents (Wolpert, 2010). The reader is encouraged to search the Internet for information on the devices now on the market for noninvasive glucose monitoring.

ORAL GLUCOSE TOLERANCE TEST

The OGTT is no longer recommended for nonpregnant clients as the FPG and A1C are the standards for the diagnosis of diabetes mellitus. All pregnant women may also be tested with the FPG and the A1C to detect diabetes early so treatment can be initiated early to prevent damage to the fetus.

A glucose tolerance test may be done in the second trimester to identify new gestational diabetes. Gestational diabetes mellitus (GDM) is similar to type 2. Women who have GDM have a 50–60% risk of developing diabetes in the future (DeCherney et al., 2007). As many as 18% of pregnant women may be diagnosed with gestational diabetes because the new criterion for diagnosis is one abnormal result rather than the old criterion that requires two abnormal results (Gebel, 2011).

Preparation of Client and Collection of Sample

The client must eat a conventional diet for several days before the OGTT is performed. The test is usually scheduled for early morning after the client has been fasting all night. Water may be consumed.

At the start of the test, blood is drawn for an FPG. The client is then given 75 g of glucose dissolved in water. The glucose drink may be flavored with lemon juice to make it more palatable. Blood samples of glucose are collected at 1- and 2-hour intervals.

The results of all the samples are plotted on a graph to see how long it takes the blood sugar to return to normal.

REFERENCES VALUES FOR OGTT (75 G OF GLUCOSE) IN PREGNANCY

	Pregnancy (upper limits)
FBS	92 mg
Blood sugar in 1 h	180 mg
Blood sugar in 2 h	153 mg

Source: Simpson (2011) and www.labtestsonline.org for updates on the criteria for gestational diabetes testing.

HEMOGLOBIN A1C

With prolonged hyperglycemia, the hemoglobin (Hgb) in RBCs remains saturated with glucose as GHB for the life of the RBC, about 120 days. However, the GHB level is not a simple average of the blood glucose level for 4 months, because RBCs are continually being replaced. The blood glucose levels for the last month count the most, about one-half the total amount. Hence, the test is a weighted average of the glucose level over the last few months. See Table 8–2 for the estimated average based on the A1C.

Table 8–2 Estimated Average Glucose (eAG) Based on A1C

A1C (%)	eAG (mg/dL)
5	97
6	126
7	154
8	183
9	212
10	240
11	269
12	298

Note: www.diabetes.org; the ADA encourages healthcare providers to use the eAG with clients when they are discussing A1C levels.

Beyond 6 months of age, at least 90% of Hgb is Hgb A. The glycosylated part of Hgb is designated A1, or as three subunits—A1A, A1B, and A1C. Hgb A1C is the most abundant of the three and is the test used to monitor clients' control of their glucose levels. In 2009 the ADA endorsed the use of A1C test for diagnosing as well as monitoring. Under the new standard, an A1C of 5.7–6.4% is considered prediabetes and an A1C of 6.5% or higher is diagnostic of diabetes. The advantage of the A1C over a fasting blood glucose is that the A1C provides an overview of the client's blood glucose level for the past 2–3 months (Olahan, 2010), whereas the FBS reflects the results of the blood glucose level only for one particular morning.

A novel use of glycosylated Hgb values was introduced in New York City in 2006. Laboratories are mandated to report these values electronically to the Department of Health. Steinbrook (2006) noted that if confidentiality of clients is maintained, the registry initiative could be a first step toward developing a plan to deal with the diabetes epidemic. Routine A1C testing has also been useful in monitoring blood glucose levels in postsurgical care and discharge planning (Olahan, 2010).

Preparation of Client and Collection of Sample

Usual diet and medications are taken, including insulin or oral antidiabetic agents. (People with diabetes may believe they must fast as they do for other routine tests for blood glucose levels.) A 1-mL specimen of venous blood is collected in a lavender-topped (EDTA) tube. Blood transfusions or hemoglobin anemia make the test invalid.

REFERENCE VALUES FOR HGB A1C

Hgb A1C (measures only one component of Hgb A: A1C)

Reference values for Hgb A1C

4–5.6%	People without diabetes
5.7%	Prediabetes
6.5%	Diabetes
<7%	Optimal for people with diabetes; children may need higher levels to guard against hypoglycemia

Using A1C at Home as Point-of-Care Testing

A prescription was required to buy A1C monitors, but now they can be bought easily over the counter. The test requires a finger stick and three simple steps. Results are ready in 8 minutes. Also, kits can be used to collect a sample on filter paper that is sent to a laboratory.

Possible Nursing Diagnoses Related to Increased A1C

Impaired Home Maintenance Management

An elevated A1C may help motivate clients to reconsider the way they are managing diabetic control. Clients may take more interest and responsibility for their management of diabetes when

(Continued)

> ## Possible Nursing Diagnoses . . . (Continued)
>
> they see their present regimen is resulting in poor control. A high A1C is definitely a risk for diabetic complications, so helping clients understand and use the results of the test is crucial.
>
> The ADA recommends that people with diabetes maintain an A1C no higher than 7%. However, some authorities encourage adults with diabetes to lower the A1C to below 6.5%. Although this may have a benefit in preventing more long-term complications, the client has an increased risk of low blood sugars that must be managed.

FRUCTOSAMINE OR GLYCATED PROTEIN

The fructosamine assay, and the Hgb A1C discussed earlier in the chapter, measure the amount of glucose hooked to another substance. Fructosamine measures the amount of glucose linked to serum proteins, particularly albumin. (Fructosamine refers to the ketoamine linkage between protein and glucose, not to the sugar fructose.) Like the Hgb A1C, this test measures glucose control over a period of time. Because albumin has a half-life of about 3 weeks, the time measured is for the past 3 weeks compared to about 3 months for A1C. Fructosamine assays are particularly useful for clients who are pregnant or have abnormal hemoglobin levels or when control trends are needed sooner. However, low albumin levels will affect results. Fructosamine assays are highly correlated with Hgb A1C results, as shown in the following.

REFERENCE VALUES FOR FRUCTOSAMINE COMPARED TO A1C AND AVERAGE BLOOD GLUCOSE

Level of Control	Fructosamine	A1C	Average Blood Glucose
Excellent	317 μmol/L	7.0%	154 mg/dL
Good	375 μmol/L	8.0%	183 mg/dL
Fair	435 μmol/L	9.0%	212 mg/dL

Note: References are from McPhee, Papadakis, and Rabow (2011).

Elevated Blood Glucose Level (Hyperglycemia)

Clinical Significance

The most common reason for a persistently elevated blood glucose is diabetes mellitus, in which the relative lack of physiologically active insulin results in an increased blood glucose level and can lead to acidosis and a comatose state.

1. In mild diabetic acidosis, the blood glucose level is usually about 300–450 mg/dL.
2. In moderate diabetic acidosis, the blood glucose level is about 450–600 mg/dL.
3. In severe diabetic coma, the blood glucose level is usually greater than 600 mg/dL.

Hyperglycemia from other causes may not be as pronounced as the hyperglycemia in diabetic acidosis. In addition, the test for plasma ketones (discussed in the next section) is positive in diabetic acidosis and not in other types of hyperglycemia. Clients with type 1 diabetes are at much greater risk for diabetic ketoacidosis (DKA) than are clients with type 2 diabetes.

In clinical conditions in which certain hormones are elevated, hyperglycemia may be present.

1. The *glucocorticoids*, for example, tend to raise blood glucose levels because of the breaking down of protein to form new glucose (neoglucogenesis). Clients with Cushing's syndrome or clients taking high doses of cortisone may have higher-than-normal blood glucose levels.
2. Because *epinephrine* increases serum glucose levels, any stress such as shock, burns, or trauma may produce an elevated blood glucose level.
3. *Growth hormone*, secreted by the pituitary gland, produces an elevated blood glucose level by making the cells more resistant to insulin. Tumors or other factors may cause abnormal functioning of the pituitary gland (see Chapter 15).
4. During pregnancy, several hormones tend to cause some hyperglycemia. The placenta secretes human placental lactogen (HPL), also called *human chorionic somatomammotropin* (HCS), which tends to raise the blood glucose level. In addition, the increased levels of *estrogen* and *progesterone* may cause some hyperglycemia.

Hormonal changes in pregnancy may make some women less sensitive to the effects of insulin. See the sections on the OGTT. Transient gestational diabetes develops during the second half of the pregnancy and resolves after delivery, but may lead to diabetes later in life.

Possible Nursing Diagnoses Related to Hyperglycemia

Anxiety Related to Potential Diagnosis of Diabetes

Clients with newly elevated blood glucose levels may be very anxious while further testing is being completed. See the earlier discussion on prediabetes. The possibility of diabetes may be particularly frightening if a client knows someone who has numerous complications of the disease. Assessments may indicate the need for health teaching while the client is undergoing an evaluation for diabetes.

1. Excess glucose in the blood can be deposited in the lenses of the eyes, causing blurred vision. It may be several weeks before the sugar deposits are cleared from the lenses. Thus, eye examinations for fitting glasses should not be performed until the hyperglycemia is controlled.
2. Talking about a specific diabetic diet during testing would be premature. But if the client is overweight, diet counseling may be appropriate if aimed at motivating the client to shed extra pounds.
3. The importance of exercise in helping the body use glucose can be discussed.
4. Because an elevated blood sugar level makes the client more susceptible to infections, good hygiene becomes very important.

(Continued)

Table 8–3 Effect of Elevated Glucose on Serum Osmolality

For an estimate of serum osmolality, the formula is

2(Na + K) + BUN/2.8 + blood glucose/18 = estimate of serum osmolality

Use of formula with normal lab values

2(135 + 4.5) + 15/2.8 + 120/18

279 + 5.36 + 6.67 = 291

Change of values with HHNK

2(146 + 5.0) + 28/2.8 + 300/18

302 + 10 + 16.67 = 329

Note: Reference values for serum osmolality are 282–295 mOsm/kg H_2O, and the values for a calculated one should be within ±9 or 10 mOsm. See Chapter 4 for a discussion of the precise measurement of serum osmolality. Sometimes K is not used in the formula.

Possible Nursing Diagnoses . . . (*Continued*)

Risk for Fluid Volume Deficits and Electrolyte Imbalances

Two of the most important nursing implications for clients with elevated blood sugar levels are (1) to keep them from becoming dehydrated and (2) to assess for electrolyte imbalances. Glucose in high concentrations in the bloodstream functions as an osmotic diuretic because it makes the plasma hypertonic (Table 8–3). Extra water is pulled into the vascular system from the interstitial spaces and even from the cells if the *hyperglycemia* is severe and long lasting. As excess glucose is excreted by the kidneys, so are enormous amounts of water. Thus, the key symptoms of hyperglycemia are thirst (polydipsia) and increased urination (polyuria).

As long as the client can drink large amounts of water, dehydration may not occur, but the continued diuresis causes a loss of potassium and sodium. The loss of these electrolytes leads to some of the specific problems discussed in Chapter 5.

If the hyperglycemia is due to a lack of insulin, the other two cardinal signs of diabetes, polyphagia and weight loss, eventually occur, because the cells are literally starving for glucose.

When dehydration becomes pronounced, the client has characteristic signs and symptoms, such as the loss of skin turgor, flushed warm skin, and soft eyeballs. The soft eyeballs are due to lack of fluid in the interstitial tissue of the eyeball.

Interventions for Hyperosmolar Hyperglycemic Nonketotic Coma. The progression of the foregoing symptoms is called *hyperosmolar hyperglycemic nonketotic coma* (HHNK). A hyperglycemia coma can occur as a result not only of diabetes but also of any pathologic condition that entails a persistently high blood sugar that causes dehydration and electrolyte imbalance. The coma is called *nonketotic* because ketones are not part of the pathologic problem; the serum ketones (see the test for plasma acetone) do not increase. Therapy is geared to reducing the blood sugar level by replacing fluids and perhaps by giving some insulin to help the body use the excess sugar. Because thromboembolic episodes can occur, caused by the increased viscosity of the blood, nurses should institute measures to decrease the chance of venous thrombi. HHNK can be a complication of hyperalimentation therapy if glucose levels are not closely monitored.

Table 8–4 Outstanding Signs and Symptoms of Hyperglycemia and Hypoglycemia

■HYPERGLYCEMIA (most of the symptoms are due to dehydration, occurs gradually)
Frequent urination (positive for sugar)
Thirst, dry mouth, and poor skin turgor
Soft eyeballs
Nausea, vomiting, abdominal pain
Weakness, confusion, blurred vision, headache
Severe dehydration and electrolyte imbalance, flushed face, tachycardia
Possible coma
Urine positive for ketones[a]
Kussmaul's respirations[a]
Acetone breath[a]

■ HYPOGLYCEMIA (many of the symptoms are due to release of epinephrine, also due to lack of glucose for central nervous system, happens quickly)
Diaphoresis (see exceptions for newborns and elderly)
Tachycardia, anxiety, shakiness
Weakness, hunger, nausea, headache
Irritability, confusion, behavioral changes
Tremors or convulsions
Coma
Urine negative for sugar
Low blood sugar

[a]Present only if ketosis and ketoacidosis develop and not present in HHNK. Additionally, the anion gap (Chapter 6) is elevated in ketoacidosis but not in HHNK. See Table 8–5 for laboratory tests in DKA.

Interventions for Diabetic Coma Related to Ketoacidosis. In diabetes, the three levels of glucose intolerance are hyperglycemia, ketosis, and ketoacidosis. Diabetic coma is caused by severe dehydration and by the acidosis resulting from the buildup of ketone bodies. When glucose is not available for the cells because of the lack of insulin, fats and sometimes protein are converted to glucose and used as the source of energy. The incomplete oxidation of fats and proteins leads to the buildup of ketones in the bloodstream (ketosis). Eventually the ketones, which are acid, exhaust the buffering capacity of the blood, and ketoacidosis occurs. The serum bicarbonate level is decreased. Ketoacidosis, as one type of metabolic acidosis, is discussed in Chapter 6 in the section on decreased serum bicarbonate levels. (Note also that the $Paco_2$ level decreases in an attempt to compensate for an overwhelming acidotic state.) Table 8–4 provides a summary of some of the symptoms of hyperglycemia and of hypoglycemia. Table 8–5 shows the laboratory reports used for DKA.

Nursing interventions for ketoacidosis include the careful regulation of intravenous fluid and electrolyte replacements, as for HHNK. Electrolytes must be carefully monitored during the acute stages of diabetic coma. Isotonic saline solution (0.9% NaCl) is usually administered, at a rapid rate, as the first infusion. When the blood glucose falls to 250 or 300 mg/dL, the physician may change the intravenous fluid orders to include dextrose 5% so hypoglycemia will not occur later. Potassium levels are high in the serum because insulin is needed for optimal transportation of potassium into the cells. Potassium also leaves the cell as more hydrogen ions go into it. (See Chapter 5 on the effect of acidosis on the potassium level.) When the acidosis is corrected, hypokalemia may occur if adequate replacement is not given, and hyponatremia may result from the loss of sodium by diuresis. Because dehydration may

(Continued)

Table 8–5 Laboratory Tests Used in Diabetic Ketoacidosis

	Ketoacidosis		
	"Mild"	**"Moderate"**	**"Severe"**
Serum glucose	300–450 mg/dL	450–600 mg/dL	More than 600 mg/dL
Plasma ketones	4+ in undiluted sample	4+ in 1:1 diluted sample	4+ in 1:2 diluted sample
Serum bicarbonate (see Chapter 6)	>15 mEq/L	10–15 mEq/L	<10 mEq/L
pH (see Chapter 6)	>7.3	7.2–7.3	<7.2
BUN (see Chapter 4)	<25 mg/dL	25–40 mg/dL	40–100 mg/dL
Urine glucose (see Chapter 3)	2%	2%	2%
Urine ketones (see Chapter 3)	Small	Moderate	Large

Possible Nursing Diagnoses . . . (*Continued*)

cause a pseudo-elevation of serum sodium levels, osmolality tests of serum and urine (Chapter 4) are useful to assess the magnitude of the dehydration. Additionally, more emphasis is needed to help clients prevent DKA (see Table 8–6).

Administering Insulin. Regular insulin or the rapid-acting insulins are used in treating elevated serum glucose levels that may fluctuate every few hours. The intermediate insulins (NPH and Lente) or 24-hour basal insulins are begun when the severe hyperglycemia in ketoacidosis has been corrected and the client is in a more stabilized condition.

Use of Insulin Drips

In all critically ill clients, hyperglycemia is treated by insulin drips so that a constant tight control can be maintained. However, if the control is too tight, it is associated with a high incidence of hypoglycemia, particularly if patients are not receiving parenteral nutrition. Hospitals need an insulin protocol with suggested glucose targets (Kessler, 2009). The ADA now recommends glucose targets of 140–180 mg/dL for critically ill clients (www.diabetes.org).

A synthetic analogue of human amylin, pramlintide acetate, is used with insulin to help control hyperglycemia by suppressing glucagon release. Because amylin and insulin are both given subcutaneously before meals with the same kind of syringe, nurses and clients must make sure to use the correct dosage of each (Deglin, Vallerand, & Sanoski, 2011).

Deficient Knowledge Related to Management of a Chronic Disease

Education for clients who have just received a diagnosis of diabetes is critical. Many healthcare settings have registered nurses who are certified diabetes educators. However, all nurses in contact with a client with newly diagnosed diabetes can be instrumental in helping the client become proficient in monitoring glucose levels and, if required, insulin injections. In the past few years, there have been significant advances in a number of oral pharmacologic approaches to treatment and more drugs are on the horizon (Capriotti, 2005). Many clients will be on a combination of drugs, so nurses must understand the role of each and the possible

---

Table 8–6 Reasons for Checking Urine Ketones and Follow-Up Care to Prevent DKA

Clients should check for urine ketones:
1. When the blood glucose is 250–350 mg/dL or higher
2. When the urine glucose is 2% or higher
3. During illness—even colds can cause ketone production
4. During emotional stress or times of great anxiety
5. During pregnancy

Actions to take when urine ketones are positive:
1. Check blood glucose and urine ketones every 4 hours to monitor trends (also can check blood ketones on home monitor)
2. Drink plenty of fluids to increase hydration
3. Follow the planned diet if possible or drink fluids with sugar and salt if not able to eat solid foods
4. Continue to take the usual dose of insulin even if not eating
5. Rest and avoid exercise
6. Check with the healthcare provider for concerns about home management

Source: www.diabetes.org, for updates on clinical practice guidelines.

---

side effects. Because the dietary regimen is so important, the nurse can reinforce and expand on the information given by the dietitian. Some clients may be unaware that "sugar-free" foods may have sweeteners such as sorbitol that have as many calories as sucrose or table sugar. Education also needs to focus on possible ways to prevent long-term complications.

Six things to help lower the risk of vascular disease are sometimes grouped under the heading of CHANGE to help clients remember each recommendation:

1. **C**holesterol and lipid control (see Chapter 9)
2. **H**ypertension control
3. **A**ppropriate weight management
4. **N**o smoking
5. **G**lycemic control
6. **E**xercise

The Diabetes Control and Complications Trial Research Group (1993) performed the first important study to demonstrate that intensive therapy effectively delays the onset and slows the progression of three severe complications—diabetic retinopathy, nephropathy, and neuropathy in clients with type 1 diabetes. Since then, further studies such as the United Kingdom Prospective Diabetes Study (UKPDS) have confirmed that complications from both type 1 and type 2 are lessened by controlling glucose levels. In addition to long-term benefits of good control, short-term benefits of intensive insulin treatment in critically ill clients are reduced morbidity and mortality. Nursing research has shown that clients with a myocardial infarction (MI) and hyperglycemia have longer hospital stays (Simpson & Crane, 2005).

Clients with diabetes have an increased frequency of thyroid disease. (See Chapter 15 on thyroid tests.) The ADA has excellent resources, including several monthly publications, for both the general public and professionals who want to be as up-to-date as possible about management of diabetes and related problems. In addition to the tests discussed in this chapter, people with diabetes need to have lipid profiles (Chapter 9) done every 1–2 years, urine microalbumin yearly (Chapter 3), and visual exams, foot inspections, and assessment of blood pressure by a healthcare provider who knows the standards of the ADA. All nurses need to be aware of how they can help clients prevent the complications of diabetes.

SERUM KETONES

When glucose is not available to the cells and the body mobilizes fat as sources of energy, ketone bodies (acetoacetic acid, acetone, and beta-hydroxybutyric acid) are the byproducts. The acidity of these ketone bodies causes the ketoacidosis that results from uncontrolled diabetes mellitus or starvation.

Preparation of Client and Collection of Sample

The laboratory usually needs about 2 mL of blood to complete any form of these tests, and there is no special preparation of the client. The tablets used for urine testing of ketones can also be used to test ketones in serum or blood. For serum testing, the color of the tablet is evaluated 2 minutes after a drop of serum is placed on it. If whole blood is put on the tablet, the clot is removed after 10 minutes, and the tablet is compared with the chart. Except when laboratory facilities are not readily available, such as during a home visit or in a camp, it is better to let the laboratory measure serum ketones under controlled conditions in which serum can be separated from whole blood and properly diluted.

REFERENCE VALUES FOR SERUM KETONES	
Acetoacetate plus acetone levels	0.3–2.0 mg/dL
Serum ketone levels	
Undiluted sample	4+ is considered mild ketoacidosis
1:1 diluted sample	4+ is considered moderate ketoacidosis
1:2 diluted sample	4+ is considered severe ketoacidosis

Note: Some laboratories may simply report abnormal results as small, moderate, or large amounts of ketones.

Blood Ketone Testing at Home

Blood ketone testing monitors are available for home use. Monitoring blood levels of ketones may be particularly useful for a child using an insulin pump. However, insurance companies may not cover the monitor. The ADA recommends using either urine or blood tests for ketones.

Positive Test for Ketones in Serum and Urine

Clinical Significance

The presence of large amounts of ketones in the serum is diagnostic of ketoacidosis. More often, the presence of ketones is assessed by frequent urine testing because ketones are excreted by the kidneys. Urine ketone levels are very important in helping the person with diabetes manage minor illnesses at home (see Table 8–6). (The specific procedure for testing urine for ketones is described in Chapter 3.) As ketones enter the bloodstream, the excess is excreted by the kidneys so that the urine test is positive *before* the buildup in the serum is excessive. However, in severe ketoacidosis, the dehydrated state may cause oliguria, so obtaining urine for testing is difficult. Also, when the acidosis is coming under control with therapy, the serum level is more reflective of the current status of the client because the serum levels begin to drop while the urine level remains high. The serum acetone level is thus more useful as an immediate indicator of the amount of ketones in the bloodstream. When clients have a continuing positive serum acetone level, the nurse may note a fruity odor to their breath similar to the odor of nailpolish remover. The odor is due to the excretion of acetone by the lungs.

Possible Nursing Diagnosis for Clients with Elevated Ketone Levels

Deficient Knowledge Related to Plan of Care at Home

Clients should take care of themselves when sick at home with minor illness, so that they do not develop ketoacidosis. Key points to stress would be

1. How often to check ketones in blood or urine when ill
2. How many extra units of insulin to take based on ketone reading
3. How much fluid to consume to avoid dehydration and how to check for dehydration
4. How often to check the glucose and what diet changes may be necessary
5. When to call healthcare provider, for example, for symptoms such as vomiting or dehydration

See Table 8–6 for a care plan.

Decreased Blood Glucose Level (Hypoglycemia)

Clinical Significance of Hypoglycemia in a Diabetic Client

Hypoglycemia in a diabetic client is caused by (1) too much insulin or, less frequently, by too high a dose of oral antidiabetic agents; (2) too little food; or (3) increased exercise without additional food intake. Less insulin is needed for the utilization of glucose when the body's activity is increased by work or exercise. In stressful events, such as infection or trauma, more insulin is needed to control hyperglycemia. Hence, if bouts of hyperglycemia and hypoglycemia are to be prevented, a client with well-controlled diabetes must have a balance among diet, medication, and exercise, plus a lack of stress.

In pregnant women, hypoglycemia is most likely to occur at two times during the pregnancy. During the first 3 months, because the growing fetus requires additional glucose, the mother may experience some periods of low blood sugar. During labor, the extra exertion may make the woman prone to hypoglycemia. There is wide variation in the change of insulin requirements in pregnant women with type 1 diabetes.

Hypoglycemia is always a potential problem in infants whose mothers have diabetes. During uterine life, the infant's pancreas secretes large amounts of insulin because of the high blood glucose levels in the mother. Glucose crosses the placental barrier, but insulin does not. After birth, the infant's pancreas may continue to secrete large amounts of insulin even though the blood glucose levels are much less than in utero. Usually, glucose levels drop the most an hour or two after birth, reach a plateau in 2–4 hours, and then gradually increase. Infants who are premature or who have a low birth weight are also prone to hypoglycemia caused by a lack of glycogen reserves in the immature liver. After the first few hours of life, glucose levels below 40–45 mg/dL should be considered abnormal (Hay et al., 2011). Current nursing research is investigating whether routine glucose testing should be done on all newborns (Hoops et al., 2010).

Clinical Significance of Hypoglycemia in Nondiabetic Clients

Hypoglycemia in nondiabetic clients is not well understood. Two main groups of hypoglycemia are classified as *fasting* and *postprandial*. Fasting hypoglycemia is likely to suggest serious organic disease. In a few clients, a low blood sugar level can be traced to a tumor of the pancreas, to a lack of cortisone (Addison's disease), to extensive liver disease, or to pituitary hypofunction (see Chapter 15 on growth hormone). Beta cell adenonomas (insulinonmas) continue to secrete insulin even in the presence of severe hypoglycemia; thus, the critical test for diagnosis is an elevated serum insulin level even when the client's glucose level is 40mg/dL or lower (McPhee et al., 2011). Another test that will be elevated is the C-peptide level, as discussed later in the chapter. Self-induced hypoglycemia by medication will not cause elevated C-peptide levels. Alcohol-induced fasting hypoglycemia can cause death if not identified and corrected.

Most cases of hypoglycemia, however, are termed *functional* because their exact cause cannot be attributed to organic abnormality. Sometimes this type of hypoglycemia is termed *reactive* because the hypoglycemia attack may follow a meal high in carbohydrates, particularly one with a large amount of sugar. Sometimes this functional hypoglycemia may be related to anxiety and stress. The diagnosis of "reactive hypoglycemia" usually refers to a blood glucose level of 59 mg/dL or less, which occurs 2–4 hours after ingestion of food

---

Possible Nursing Diagnoses Related to Hypoglycemia

Risk for Injury Related to Lack of Glucose for Normal Cellular Function

For clients who are likely to experience hypoglycemia because of too much insulin, the key nursing implication is to assess for early symptoms of hypoglycemia so that treatment is given quickly. Hypoglycemia occurs rapidly and can lead to coma if it is not treated. (In contrast, the coma of hyperglycemia usually takes much longer to develop as the person becomes progressively more dehydrated and as the ketones build in the bloodstream.)

One of the most outstanding symptoms of hypoglycemia in many adults and children is diaphoresis (excessive sweating). Because infants do not perspire, however, this clinical sign is not useful in the newborn nursery. The diaphoresis, along with tachycardia, dizziness, and tremors, is the result of an increased surge of epinephrine to raise the blood sugar level. Clients taking beta blockers do not exhibit tachycardia or shakiness, two of the classic symptoms of hypoglycemia. However, sweating will still occur. Hypoglycemic unawareness is very common in clients with insulinoma as they adapt to chronic hypoglycemia by increasing the efficiency of transporting glucose to the brain. Other symptoms may not occur (McPhee et al., 2011). If the brain is deprived of glucose for more than a few minutes, the client begins to experience irritability, confusion, and behavioral outbursts. These behavioral changes may resemble an intoxicated state. The onset of hypoglycemia in the elderly may not show the signs and symptoms of increased epinephrine usually seen in the young. As a result, the episodes of confusion or other cerebral dysfunctions may be wrongly attributed to cerebral arteriosclerosis.

Interventions to Raise the Blood Sugar Level. Hospitals have written protocols to follow based on blood glucose levels and whether clients are able to swallow fluids. Treatment for hypoglycemia may be mandated at 60 mg/dL (O'Donnell et al., 2005). More hospitals are now adapting the ADA's 2009 definition of hypoglycemia as a glucose level lower than 70 (McEuen et al., 2010). Clients may be taught to treat themselves when the glucose level is 70 mg/dL and to recheck the glucose level in 15 minutes. Fifteen grams of glucose usually raises the blood glucose by about 50 mg. The strength of over-the-counter glucose tablets is marked in grams per tablet to make it easy for clients to not overindulge. Clients may also take 6 ounces of orange juice (15 g simple carbohydrate) or other sugar-containing beverage or candy to treat mild hypoglycemia. At home, 3 ounces of cake-decorating gel supplies 15 g of simple sugar. Commercial sugar-containing gel or glucose tablets may be less tempting than candy to keep as a reserve. Basic safety requires that a fast-acting sugar must always be readily available when clients are taking insulin. For example, counselors and nurses in diabetes camps are instructed to *always* carry sugar cubes or gel in their pockets because the additional exercise encouraged by an outdoor setting often causes hypoglycemia. Glucose can be given intravenously. In settings where the client is unable to swallow and intravenous access is not possible, glucagon, discussed next, can be used. Honey or cake-decorating gel can be put under the tongue if the client cannot swallow. After the initial sugar to treat the acute hypoglycemia, food with protein and complex carbohydrates should be given if the next meal is more than 30 minutes away.

Assessing and Treating Hypoglycemia in the Newborn. In newborn infants, the symptoms of hypoglycemia are tremors, listlessness, apnea, cyanosis, a shrill cry, changes in muscular tone, and an unstable temperature. When an infant has hypoglycemia, the resultant release of glucagon stimulates the secretion of calcitonin from the thyroid, which may cause a rapid decrease in serum calcium, which causes tetany. (See Chapter 7 for a discussion of hypocalcemia.) Usually, the newborn of a mother with diabetes is fed early with 10–20% glucose by a bottle, by gavage, or by intravenous infusion if necessary. Blood glucose levels are frequently measured (see the procedure for reagent strips discussed earlier in this chapter). Any infant prone to hypoglycemia is usually kept in a special care nursery for close observation.

Assessing for Hypoglycemia Unawareness. Clients who have experienced hypoglycemia are usually aware of the beginning of symptoms and take some orange juice or candy to offset the reaction. For some people, the early symptoms of hypoglycemia may not be obvious, or the hypoglycemia may occur during sleep. For example, with the intermediate-acting insulins (NPH and Lente), the peak action is 8–12 hours after administration and the duration is about 24 hours. Headache and weakness may be the only symptoms, or the client may have nightmares or wake up with damp night clothes and tachycardia. Drinking alcohol raises the risk for hypoglycemia for up to 12 hours. Clients with severe hypoglycemia unawareness who are unable to detect any warning signs may benefit from an awareness program that teaches them to recognize cues. Hypoglycemia unawareness develops when neuropathy results in less release and response of adrenalin. Even though clients may no longer have some of the

(Continued)

Possible Nursing Diagnoses ... (*Continued*)

physical warnings of hypoglycemia, they will still have central nervous system effects such as difficulty concentrating, slowed speech, and lack of coordination.

Deficient Knowledge Related to Use of Glucagon as Treatment of Hypoglycemia

Some physicians may order the hormone glucagon as treatment of an insulin reaction when it is not feasible to give intravenous glucose immediately. For example, this order may be a protocol in nursing homes for clients who have a blood sugar less than 30 or have a cute confusion and delirium from hypoglycemia (Goldstein, 2009). The hormone, available in 1-mg ampules, is injected the same way as insulin, and it should be effective in raising the blood sugar in 5–15 minutes (Katzung, Masters, & Trevor, 2009). Glucagon, secreted by the alpha cells of the pancreas, stimulates the formation of glucose from glycogen stores. So it is not effective for a client who is malnourished and who thus has little stored glycogen. A member of the family needs to be instructed on how to give glucagon when the client has an insulin reaction that does not respond to oral sugar. If glucagon is used, the client needs a feeding of combined simple and complex carbohydrates to replenish the glucose.

Glucagon in School Settings. The ADA launched a campaign "Safe at School" to encourage policies and laws to ensure that all school personnel are educated about diabetic care to identify a diabetic emergency and act appropriately. Glucagon does not harm a child, so one policy is to have some school staff able to give glucagon when a nurse is not available. Hawaii, Kentucky, and Nevada were some of the states that made changes in state laws, first so that school children can get glucagon when they need it (Diabetes Advocate, 2005).

Imbalanced Nutrition: Related to Changes in Activity

The nurse and the diabetic client receiving insulin need to be aware that unusual exercise increases the chance of hypoglycemia. Because active muscular exercise increases the utilization of carbohydrates, the client requires more food intake or less insulin. When a person is in the hospital, the stress of the hospitalization and the lack of normal muscular activity both contribute to increasing the blood sugar level. When the person is discharged, the stress is less and normal muscular activities are resumed. So the insulin requirement may be decreased. Sometimes in pediatric units, children are taken to a park or playground a few times before they are discharged from the hospital so that the insulin maintenance dose matches the food intake and exercise level of the child. This may be very helpful in preventing hypoglycemic attacks after the child is at home.

Deficient Knowledge Related to Insulin Rebound

The Somogyi effect, named after the man who first described the phenomenon, is the occurrence of insulin rebound. After a period of hypoglycemia, several hormones (epinephrine and the glucocorticosteroids) are released to raise serum glucose levels. So repeated episodes of slight hypoglycemia may have the end result of making the client hyperglycemic, which may partially explain why some clients who take insulin have fluctuations of blood sugar levels that are not directly related to food intake. On the basis of this theory, a plan for reducing the insulin dose may bring about a more stable blood sugar level because there is no longer the rebound effect from the periods of slight hypoglycemia.

Unrecognized hypoglycemia most often occurs at night, so the early morning glucose may be higher than normal. However, the *dawn phenomenon*, a term coined in 1984, may also cause a rise in early morning glucose. The dawn phenomenon refers to the surge of growth hormone that may cause blood glucose to rise. To determine if the client needs more or less insulin, 3 am glucose tests are performed for a week. If these nighttime results are elevated, more insulin is needed at bedtime. If the 3 am results are low, less insulin at bedtime prevents insulin rebound.

Imbalanced Nutrition: Related to Functional Hypoglycemia

In contrast to a client who has hypoglycemia caused by an insulin reaction, a client with functional hypoglycemia does not have symptoms that progress to a coma. The light-headedness, sweating, and palpitations may be relieved by the intake of a carbohydrate. For the long-term management of hypoglycemic reactions, the client is usually advised not to eat concentrated sugars at all because they may cause a surge of insulin in the bloodstream. The diet usually is a high-protein, low-carbohydrate diet with frequent feedings. For example, the client should eat cottage cheese and maybe some fruit for a mid-morning snack rather than pastry or a doughnut and coffee. Stimulants such as caffeine should be avoided because the caffeine may cause a sudden rise in blood sugar that stimulates insulin production.

Anxiety Related to Functional Hypoglycemia

The relation of diet, stress, and anxiety to functional hypoglycemia still is not well understood. The nurse needs to evaluate the potential stress in the environment because this may be a contributing factor for the development of hypoglycemic symptoms. Emphasis is placed not on the symptoms but on eradicating the stimulus for the symptoms—be it food indiscretions, anxiety, or an undetected organic abnormality. Measuring blood glucose during a hypoglycemic attack at home may be helpful in documenting the physiologic nature of the symptoms and differentiating them from anxiety symptoms. Psychological support may be more important than dietary manipulation (McPhee et al., 2011).

DIABETES-RELATED AUTOANTIBODIES: ISLET CELL, GLUTAMIC ACID DECARBOXYLASE (GAD) 65 AND INSULIN

Type 1 diabetes, which usually develops before the age of 30 years, involves a destruction of the islet cells in the pancreas. Close relatives of people with diabetes can be screened with a blood test for islet cell autoantibodies (ICA) to see if they are at risk for diabetes. Another type of screening for antibodies that predict susceptibility to type 1 diabetes is the glutamic acid decarboxylase (GAD) 65 antibody test. This test measures antibodies against an enzyme produced primarily by pancreatic islet cells. The presence of this antibody provides early evidence of autoimmune activity and can be useful not only in predicting the type of diabetes, but also in distinguishing type 1 from type 2 diabetes. GAD 65 antibodies may occur years before type 1 diabetes is clinically diagnosed. As GAD test is an easier test to do than ICA test, it is more frequently performed.

Table 8–7 Types of Diabetes

	Presence of Autoantibodies	Progression to Insulin Dependence	Insulin Resistance
Type 1	Yes	Days to weeks	No
Type 1.5	Yes	Months to years	Some
Type 2	No	Over time, if at all	Yes

Note: Identifying LADA can be beneficial as insulin can be started to help preserve beta cell function (Gebel, 2010).

Insulin autoantibodies (IAA) are a third type of diabetes autoantibodies. The test for IAA may be combined with that for ICA for risk prediction (Wu, 2006). People with type 2 do not have diabetes antibodies, so all these tests, and a few others, help make a diagnosis of type 1 diabetes in clients who may be thought to have type 2. The presence of these antibodies may also help diagnose LADA or *slow progressing type 1* or *type 1.5*. See Table 8–7 for types of diabetes.

Preparation of Client and Collection of Sample for GAD 65 Antibodies

Client should not have had radioisotopes in the last 24 hours if radioimmunoassay (RIA) method used. Collect 0.2 to 0.5 mL in red top tube.

REFERENCE VALUES FOR GAD ANTIBODIES

Less than 0.02 nmol/L or less than 1.5 units/mL depending on the method used

Note: Wu (2006) notes GAD 65 antibodies may occur at least 10 years before the onset of type 1 diabetes. These antibodies are probably the effect but not the cause of beta cell destruction (Hay et al., 2011).

C-PEPTIDE LEVELS

C-peptide, pro-insulin, and insulin levels can all be measured in the serum to indicate the activity of the pancreatic beta cells. The serum concentration of C-peptide is proportional to endogenous insulin levels, so this test can be used to document insulin production in the differential diagnosis of hypoglycemia, to classify type 1 diabetes, and to evaluate pancreas transplants. C-peptide levels are also used to determine eligibility for insurance coverage for insulin pumps. The person must produce no more C-peptide than 10% over the lower limit of normal for a particular laboratory measurement. In addition to the C-peptide requirement, clients with either type 1 or type 2 diabetes must meet several other requirements to qualify for Medicare coverage of insulin pumps.

C-peptide levels do not elevate when exogenous insulin is given, so the test can document that hypoglycemia is from an overdose of insulin. Studies are ongoing for other uses of this test. Some research has shown that higher plasma C-peptide in older women without diabetes is related to cognitive impairment (Okereke et al., 2005).

Preparation of Client and Collection of Sample for C-Peptide Levels

The serum should be collected in a fasting state. Two specimens may be drawn: one for the baseline and the second after an intravenous dose of 1 mg glucagon, given to stimulate release of C-peptide. Clients with type 1 will continue to have very low or undetectable levels.

A value above 1.8 ng/mL or above 0.60 nmol/L after glucagon may mean that the client can be managed without insulin (Wu, 2006). Other sources may have different values as they use glucose in the stimulation test.

REFERENCE VALUES	
Baseline	0.78–1.89 ng/mL or 0.26–0.65 nmol/L
Six minutes after glucagon	2.73–5.64 ng/mL or 0.91–1.88 nmol/L

LACTOSE TOLERANCE TEST

Lactase, an enzyme found only in the small intestine, is important for digestion of lactose, a sugar found in milk. Because of genetic and other factors, some people, particularly black and Asian people, may have a deficiency of lactase. Also Jewish people, Hispanics, and Native Americans may have some deficiency. A recent update from the American Academy of Pediatrics, Committee on Nutrition, noted that about 70% of the world's population has primary lactase deficiency. The rate may be as low as 2% in populations who have long had a predominance of dairy foods in the diet, such as Northern European people. In contrast, the rate may be nearly 100% in Asians and American Indians (Heyman, 2006). However, all human ethnic groups are lactase sufficient in the newborn period (Hay et al., 2011). During infancy and childhood, most people may have enough of the enzyme, but the body produces less lactase with age, so lactose intolerance happens later.

A lack of this enzyme leads to an intolerance for milk because the lactose in the milk cannot be converted to galactose and glucose. (One glass [8 oz or 240 mL] of milk contains 12 g of lactose.) The stools are sour and have a low pH, rather than an alkaline pH, because of the presence of undigested milk. The test for lactose tolerance is to give a measured amount of lactose and then test the blood *glucose* level at various intervals. An increase of less than 20 mg of glucose, associated with gastrointestinal symptoms (bloating or diarrhea), is strongly suggestive of lactase deficiency. Most of the hydrogen from the undigested lactose is passed as flatus, but some is absorbed into the bloodstream and expelled in the breath. A breath sample can be analyzed for hydrogen. For the breath test, the fasting client drinks a lactose-loaded beverage (50 g). A rise in breath hydrogen of greater than 20 ppm in 90 minutes is a positive test (McPhee et al., 2011). Certain foods, medications, and smoking should be avoided before the test. The treatment is to remove all sources of dietary lactose until the client is symptom free and then gradually increase lactase until a tolerance level is identified. Several different commercial lactase formulations are available for replacement of the endogenous lactase. Clients need to investigate what is most effective for them. Capsules containing lactase can be taken before or with a meal to help digest dairy products. Additionally, five to seven drops of a liquid preparation of the enzyme can be added to milk 24 hours before consumption. Lactose-reduced milk is a third option. The lactase added to milk makes it sweeter because lactose has already been broken down to glucose and galactose. Soy protein formulas and a lactose-free cow's milk are available for infants.

SERUM TEST FOR GALACTOSEMIA

Galactosemia is an inherited disorder in which galactose cannot be converted to glucose because of a lack of the enzyme galactose-1-phosphate uridyl transferase or two other enzymes. The galactose is wasted in the urine. Once galactose has been detected in the urine, the test for these enzymes verifies that there is a genetic defect in metabolizing galactose. To prevent mental retardation and other complications, a diet containing no galactose should be instituted within the newborn period. If galactose is not eliminated from the diet, cataracts may appear within 1 month and any neurologic defects may be permanent.

Compliance with the diet requires that parents know the galactose content of foods, which includes not only milk but also other foods such as some fruits and vegetables. In severe cases, a galactose-free diet should be followed for life with appropriate calcium supplementation. Prenatal diagnosis is possible if a specific DNA mutation in a family is known. Pregnant women who are carriers of the trait may be advised to maintain a galactose-free diet (Hay et al., 2011).

All parents, especially those who deliver the baby at home, need to be aware of the importance of early detection of the presence of any sugar in the urine or any intolerance to milk. Galactosemia is one of the tests that may be mandated by law for newborns. (See Chapter 18 on genetic screening tests.) Vomiting, liver enlargement, and jaundice are often the earliest signs of the disease. Galactosemia should be considered in any infant with jaundice because of the benefits of early dietary restriction of galactose. The RBC levels of galactose or its metabolites may be used as a monitor to gauge adherence to the diet. This analysis is offered only at specialized laboratories, so monitoring the diet may be achieved simply and with less cost by using whole blood filter paper spot tests.

Questions

1. Blood glucose levels are the least affected by
   a. Growth hormone
   b. Cortisone
   c. Testosterone
   d. Epinephrine

2. In comparing the tests for fasting blood sugar (FBS), postprandial blood sugar (PPBS), and Hgb A1C, which statement is the most accurate?
   a. The client must not take anything by mouth before all three tests are performed
   b. An abnormality of any two of the tests indicates diabetes mellitus
   c. PPBS gives the most accurate assessment of carbohydrate metabolism
   d. The exact timing of drawing of the specimen is most critical for PPBS

3. A nurse working in an ambulatory center should be familiar with the oral glucose tolerance test to assess transient glucose intolerance if the clients are
   a. Newborns
   b. Pregnant women
   c. Women approaching menopause
   d. Elderly men and women

4. Which of the following statements is correct about glucose tests in the elderly client (older than 65 years)?
   a. The curve for a glucose tolerance test for the elderly should return to baseline as soon as the curve for a person younger than 50 years
   b. The renal threshold for glucose is usually decreased in the elderly
   c. The postprandial glucose level in the elderly tends to be higher than postprandial glucose levels for young adults
   d. Normal values for fasting glucose tests tend to border on hypoglycemia in the elderly

5. The plasma ketone level is
   a. Increased in both diabetic coma and hyperosmolar hyperglycemic nonketotic coma (HHNK)
   b. Decreased in both diabetic coma and HHNK
   c. Unchanged in either diabetic coma or HHNK
   d. Increased in diabetic coma and not changed in HHNK

6. A diabetic client is on a sliding-scale insulin coverage for blood glucose greater than 240 mg/dL. Which type of insulin is usually used to control hyperglycemia in acute situations?
   a. Regular insulin
   b. Lente insulin
   c. NPH insulin
   d. Semi-Lente insulin

7. A male client has just received the diagnosis of type 1 diabetes. He asks the nurse what he should do if his blood sugar is always 240 mg/dL before breakfast. The nurse tells him he can find out more information by
   a. Testing his blood sugar at 3 am to see if it is high or low
   b. Restricting fluids because he may be overhydrated
   c. Verifying the reading by performing a urine test for glucose
   d. Keeping a record of his daily caloric intake

8. The risk for injury related to hyperglycemia is the most likely for a client
   a. Born 4 hours ago to a mother with diabetes who is on insulin
   b. Who is in her first trimester of pregnancy and has insulin-dependent diabetes (Lente 20 units)
   c. Whose diabetes has been controlled on NPH 40 units, but who now is undergoing bed rest because of an infected toe
   d. With a possible diagnosis of functional hypoglycemia, who has just eaten two candy bars to "tide him over" until mealtime

9. A characteristic symptom of hypoglycemia in both the adult and the newborn is which of the following?
   a. Diaphoresis
   b. Tremors
   c. Shrill cry
   d. Bradycardia

10. The night nurse discovers a client with newly diagnosed diabetes, wandering about in his room. He says he has a headache. He appears flushed and warm. The nurse knows that he had 55 units of Lente insulin in the morning and 10 units of regular insulin at bedtime to cover a blood glucose of 240 mg/dL. Which action would be the most appropriate for the nurse to perform first?
   a. Get the client back to bed and check to see if he has an order for pain relief for the headache
   b. Call the intern to check the client for possible diabetic acidosis
   c. Obtain a finger stick for a blood glucose and then give the client a glass of orange juice if his blood sugar is low
   d. Assess vital signs, particularly temperature and blood pressure, and wait to see if the client is becoming diaphoretic

11. Glucagon, a hormone from the alpha (α) cells of the pancreas, is sometimes used to do which of the following?
   a. Treat mild cases of diabetes
   b. Counteract the effect of epinephrine
   c. Help promote conversion of glycogen to glucose
   d. Reduce the blood sugar level in newborns

12. A client who has functional or reactive hypoglycemia needs to be taught to avoid a diet that includes
   a. Concentrated sugar
   b. High protein
   c. Low fats
   d. Frequent small feedings

13. A client, age 8, and her parents are in a class for families who have a child with diabetes. Which of the following points should be emphasized to the parents?
   a. Recent research has confirmed that tight glucose control lessens the onset and severity of diabetic retinopathy, nephropathy, and neuropathy
   b. Regular exercise is important, but extra insulin must be given
   c. Urine ketone testing should be performed if the blood glucose level is greater than 400 mg/dL
   d. The hemoglobin A1C is used to assess for glucose control over the past week

14. Which of the following conclusions is incorrect in comparing galactose and lactose intolerances and the tests completed for each?
   a. Both galactose and lactose can be detected in the urine with a test for glucose
   b. Galactose intolerance is a more serious defect than lactose intolerance
   c. A nonmilk diet in the infant eliminates the symptoms of lactose intolerance
   d. The blood glucose level is abnormally elevated in both conditions

References

Capriotti, T. (2005). Type 2 diabetes epidemic increases use of oral anti-diabetic agents. *MEDSURG Nursing, 14*(5), 341–347.

Dale, L. (2006). Make a point about alternate site blood glucose sampling. *Nursing 2006, 36*(2), 52–53.

DeCherney, A. H., Nathan, L., Goodwin, T. M., & Lauter, N. (Eds.). (2007). *Current diagnosis and treatment: Obstetrics & gynecology* (10th ed.). New York: Mc Graw-Hill.

Deglin, J. H., Vallerand, A. H., & Sanoski, C. A. (2011). *Davis's drug guide for nurses* (12th ed.). Philadelphia: F. A. Davis.

Diabetes Advocate. (2005). School safety. *Diabetes Forecast, 58*(9), 79–81.

Gebel, E. (2010). The "other" diabetes. *Diabetes Forecast, 63*(5), 46–48.

Gebel, E. (2011). Blood glucose control is key to having a healthy baby. *Diabetes Forecast, 64*(7), 27.

Goldstein, P. C. (2009). Assessment and treatment of hypoglycemia in elders: Cautions and recommendations. *MEDSURG Nursing, 18*(4), 215–223.

Hay, W. W., Levin, M. J., Sondheimer, J. M., & Deterding, R. (Eds.). (2011). *Current diagnosis and treatment: Pediatrics* (20th ed.). New York: McGraw-Hill.

Heyman, M. B. (2006). Lactose intolerance in infants, children, and adolescents. *Pediatrics, 118*(3), 1279–1286.

Hoops, D., Roberts, P., Van Winkle, E., Trauschke, K., Mauton, N., DeGhelder, S., et al. (2010). Should routine peripheral blood glucose testing be done for all newborns at birth? *American Journal of Maternal Child Nursing, 35*(5), 264–270.

Katzung, B., Masters, S. B., & Trevor, A. J. (Eds.). (2009). *Basic and clinical pharmacology* (11th ed.). New York: McGraw-Hill.

Kessler, C. (2009). Glycemic control in the hospital: How tight should it be? *Nursing, 39*(11), 38–43.

Kordella, T. (2005). Forearm glucose checks may miss lows. *Diabetes Forecast, 58*(7), 33.

McEuen, J. A., Gardner, K. P., Barnachea, D. F., Locke, C. L., Backhaus, B. R., &

Hughes, S. K. (2010). *American Journal of Nursing, 110*(7), 40–46.

McPhee, S. J., Papadakis, M. A., & Rabow, M. W. (Eds.). (2011). *Current medical diagnosis and treatment* (50th ed.). New York: McGraw-Hill.

O'Donnell, M. P., Petersen, J., Hansen-Peters, I., & Nagy, L. (2005). A nursing standards-based system that works! *MEDSURG Nursing, 14*(1), 25–34.

Okereke, O., Hankinson, S. E., Hu, F. B., & Grodstein, F. (2005). Plasma C peptide level and cognitive function among older women without diabetes mellitus. *Archives Internal Medicine, 165*, 1651–1656.

Olahan, K. (2010). Diabetes under control: Improving hospital care for patients with diabetes. *American Journal of Nursing, 110*(6), 65–69.

Ramchandani, N., Saadon, Y., & Jornsay, D. (2010). Diabetes under control: A real-time continuous glucose monitoring. *American Journal of Nursing, 110*(4), 60–63.

Seley, J. J. (2009). Diabetes under control: Diagnosing diabetes. *American Journal of Nursing, 109*(8), 65.

Simpson, R. S. (2011). Diabetes in pregnancy: To screen or not to screen. *MCN: The American Journal of Maternal and Child Nursing, 16*(1), 202.

Simpson, J. P. & Crane, P. B. (2005). The effects of hyperglycemia on patient length of stay following myocardial infarction. *MEDSURG Nursing, 14*(4), 233–239.

Steinbrook, R. (2006). Facing the diabetes epidemic—mandatory reporting of glycosylated hemoglobin values in New York City. *New England Journal of Medicine, 354*(6), 545–548.

Tenderich, A. (2006). The next generation: Continuous glucose monitors. *Diabetes Forecast, 59*(8), 52–55.

Wolpert, H. (2010). Continuous glucose monitoring—coming of age. *The New England Journal of Medicine, 363*, 383–384.

Wu, A. H. (Ed.). (2006). *Tietz clinical guide to laboratory tests* (4th ed.). St. Louis, MO: Saunders Elsevier.

Websites

www.forecast.diabetes.org (Annual consumer guide every January for clients with diabetes.)
www.diabetes.org (Information on practice guidelines for clients with diabetes.)
www.jointcommission.org (Information on use of glucose monitors.)
www.labtestsonline.org (Information on tests for gestational diabetes.)

Answers

1. c, 2. d, 3. b, 4. c, 5. d, 6. a, 7. a, 8. c, 9. b, 10. c, 11. c, 12. a, 13. a, 14. d

Tests to Measure Lipid Metabolism and Other Cardiac Risk Factors

- Serum Cholesterol 210
- Serum Triglycerides 217
- Lipoprotein Electrophoresis and LDL Subclasses 219
- High-Density Lipoprotein Cholesterol 220
- Ratio of Total Cholesterol to HDL 220
- Low-Density Lipoprotein Cholesterol 221
- Homocysteine Levels 222
- Lipoprotein (a) Levels 222
- Apolipoproteins A, B, and E 223
- Lipoprotein-Associated Phospholipase A$_2$ 223
- Possible Risk Factors for Coronary Artery Disease 224

OBJECTIVES

1. Define hyperlipidemia, and discuss factors that seem to contribute to its development.

2. Describe the client preparation necessary for tests of serum cholesterol and serum triglyceride levels.

3. Discuss the controversial aspects of the relation of serum cholesterol and serum triglyceride levels to the development of cardiovascular disease.

4. Plan a diet low in cholesterol and saturated fats.

5. Identify nursing diagnoses that may be useful for clients with elevated serum cholesterol levels.

6. Identify assessments that might indicate a lack of essential fatty acids in the diet.

7. Give examples of how serum triglyceride levels are used as an evaluation tool.

8. Describe research findings on possible risk factors for coronary artery disease.

Hyperlipidemia is a broad term that means high plasma concentrations of cholesterol, triglycerides, or the complex lipoproteins. Lipoproteins transport triglycerides and cholesterol in the plasma.

SERUM CHOLESTEROL

Cholesterol, a natural constituent of the serum, is essential for the production of bile salts, for the manufacture of many of the steroid hormones, and for the composition of cell membranes. Cholesterol is manufactured from saturated fats in the diet. The liver esterifies cholesterol by combining it with a fatty acid. Most of the cholesterol is present in the bloodstream in the esterified form. Cholesterol levels seem to differ greatly depending on variables such as age, diet, geographic location, and genetic influences.

The Third National Cholesterol Education Program updated some of the recommendations from the second panel. Now a complete lipoprotein profile (total, low-density lipoprotein [LDL], high-density lipoprotein [HDL] cholesterol and triglycerides) is the preferred initial screening test. Two other changes were new reference values for (1) optimal LDL cholesterol less than 100 mg/dL and (2) optimal HDL cholesterol greater than 40 mg/dL. The report emphasizes ways to help clients make therapeutic life changes (TLCs) and notes the role of nurses as case managers. In 2004, the NCEP added more therapeutic options for clients at very high and moderately high risk for cardiovascular disease. The overall goal is still an LDL less than 100 mg/dL, but a new optional therapeutic goal of an LDL less than 70 mg/dL was recommended for very high risk clients. Clients with moderately high risk may also benefit from a lower LDL, and drug therapy was recommended for clients with an LDL over 100 mg/dL. See www.nhlbi.nih.gov/guidelines/cholesterol for the latest version.

For clients at low risk, several studies are ongoing to see if the small potential benefit of an LDL under 70 mg/dL is greater than the side effects from medication and justify the high cost of medications, for a large portion of the population. At the present time the average LDL in the United States is about 123 mg/dL (Lee, 2006).

The U.S. Preventive Services Task Force (USPSTF) guidelines recommend that screening for lipid disorders in adult men begins at age 35 and in adult women at age 45 if they also have lipid disorders and are at an increased risk for coronary heart disease. Those with risk factors may need to be tested more often or at a younger age. For example, research supports testing for hyperlipidemia in all overweight children and adolescents (Boyd et al., 2005). Clients on certain types of medications to treat HIV may also develop hyperlipidemia (Capili & Anastasi, 2006).

Preparation of Client and Collection of Sample

The client should consume conventional foods with no dieting for several days. Fasting is not needed unless the cholesterol is part of a lipid profile. Because cholesterol can fluctuate considerably from day to day, at least two samples should be drawn if the first level is 200 mg/dL or greater. If the second level is within 30 mg/dL of the first level, the average of the two can be used. If the first two samples vary by more than 30 mg/dL, a third sample is needed, and the average of the three is used to guide the treatment plan. The two or three samples should be drawn within a period of 1–8 weeks. Because some studies have suggested that volume responses to posture can affect cholesterol, the client should be sitting for at least 5 minutes before the blood is drawn. The venous blood test usually requires 0.5 mL in a tube with no anticoagulant. If plasma is collected (EDTA tube), the blood must clot for 30 minutes before the test can be performed. Finger sticks can be used for initial screening when an automated analyzer is used. Some drugs, such as vitamin E, phenytoin, and steroids, may cause false elevations, whereas other drugs, such as some antibiotics, may cause falsely low readings.

Home Testing for Serum Cholesterol

In 1993, a blood cholesterol test became available for home use by consumers. The test, available without a prescription, required one drop of blood to be placed on a test strip within a cassette. Results took 10–15 minutes. Now, home monitors, approved by the Food and Drug Administration (FDA), are available that give results in 3 minutes not only for total cholesterol but also for HDL and LDL.

REFERENCE VALUES FOR SERUM CHOLESTEROL

Adults, 20 years and older	
Desirable	<200 mg/dL
Borderline high	200–239 mg/dL
High	≥240 mg/dL
Pregnant women	Increases should return to baseline in about 1 month
Newborns	30–70 mg/dL
Children	<170 mg/dL
Aged	Levels >200 mg/dL may not be a concern[a]

[a]See McPhee, Papadakis, & Rabow (2011) for rationale for not screening elderly after age 75.

Skin Test for Cholesterol

The FDA has also approved a skin test for cholesterol called Cholesterol 1,2,3. Skin normally contains cholesterol, and the amount increases when clients have very high blood cholesterol levels. These deposits of cholesterol in the skin may be associated with deposits in vessels such as the carotid and coronary arteries. Thus, this skin test may have value in research and clinical practice in stratifying clients at risk for vascular disease (Sprecher & Pearce, 2006). See Chapter 23 on ultrasound of carotid arteries, which may be done as a follow-up to an abnormal skin test.

The test can be done in a clinic or an office. An adhesive foam pad is placed on the palm of the hand, and drops of an indicator solution are added to a test well in the pad. A handheld spectrophotometer reads the amount of blue color and displays the results on a computer screen.

Increased Serum Cholesterol Levels

Clinical Significance

Three recognized genetic disorders lead to hyperlipidemia: (1) familial hypercholesterolemia, (2) familial combined hyperlipidemia, and (3) familial hypertriglyceridemia. Although these three disorders affect 0.5–1.0% of the population and are the most common genetic diseases, they do not cause most of the high cholesterol levels seen in adults. Familial hypercholesterolemia is an autosomal dominant condition. Screening family members of people who are known carriers is the most cost-effective way for detecting cases in the whole population. As obesity, diabetes, and hypertension are not commonly seen early in familial hyperlipidemia, screening based on family history is important for early detection and intervention.

In some clinical situations, the cause of the increased serum cholesterol level can be identified. For example, liver disease with biliary obstruction, hypothyroidism, and pancreatic dysfunction all cause increased cholesterol levels. Some drugs, such as corticosteroids, may cause an increased cholesterol level, but the clinical significance of this increase is not known. Increased serum cholesterol and triglycerides are also associated with some of the anti-HIV medications. Although cholesterol levels are normally high in pregnancy, they rise even higher in preeclampsia. The cholesterol level also may increase in nephrotic syndromes. Clients with increased serum cholesterol levels need to be tested for hypothyroidism (see Chapter 15).

Recommendations for Follow-Up for Abnormal Lipid Levels

The new guidelines take into account not just the total cholesterol level but also the values for the other parts of the lipid profile discussed later. The clinical significance of the values must be correlated with the number of risk factors the person has for heart disease (see Table 9–1). A point system defines the category of risk for having a myocardial infarction in the next 10 years and helps determine when medication should be prescribed.

Category 1: This highest-risk group needs medication to get the LDL below 70 mg/dL.

Category 2: Clients may begin medication if LDL is above 100 mg/dL.

Category 3: Clients may begin medication if LDL is above 160 mg/dL.

Category 4: Clients with little or no risk factors may not be prescribed medication unless the LDL is above 190 mg/dL.

Although the guidelines suggest when medications should be considered, the healthcare provider must also emphasize the recommended lifestyle changes,

Table 9–1 Major Risk Factors That Modify LDL Goals[a]

Positive Risk Factors

Cigarette smoking

Hypertension or on antihypertensive medications

Low HDL cholesterol (>40 mg/dL)

Family history of premature coronary heart disease (CHD) (<55 in male, <65 in female) in first-degree relatives

Age (men > 45; women > 55)

Negative Risk Factor

HDL (>60 mg/dL) removes one risk factor from the total count

[a]See text for other factors such as diabetes that help determine the category of risk for a myocardial infarction in the next 10 years and the appropriate use of medication for various LDL levels.

Table 9–2 Components of Therapeutic Lifestyle Change (TLC) Diet

Nutrient	Percentage of Total Calories
Total fat	25–35
Saturated fatty acids	<7
Polyunsaturated fatty acids	≤10
Monosaturated fatty acids	≤20
Fiber	20–30 g/day
Carbohydrates	50–60
Protein	15
Cholesterol	<200 mg/day
Total calories	To achieve and maintain desirable weight

which include reducing the intake of saturated fats (<7% of total calories) and lowering dietary cholesterol (<200 mg daily). Eating foods with plant stanols/sterols (2 g daily) and increasing the intake of soluble fiber (10–25 g daily) are other recommendations, as noted in Table 9–2. Achieving and maintaining a healthy weight and sticking to a routine exercise program are other important goals.

Possible Nursing Diagnoses Related to Hyperlipidemia

Deficient Knowledge Related to Alterations in Diet

Once a client has been definitely identified as having hyperlipidemia, the first recommendation is to decrease the amount of fat in the diet and to replace saturated fats with polyunsaturated fats. Vegetable oils tend to be high in polyunsaturated fats, whereas animal fats are high in saturated fats and cholesterol. Meat, egg yolks, and dairy products are the main sources of cholesterol in the U.S. diet (Table 9–3). A fat-controlled diet may have other health benefits. The National Research Council's study on diet, nutrition, and cancer supports a total fat intake not more than 30% of the total calories because of the association between high-fat diets and some types of cancer, which is currently under intense study (McPhee et al., 2011).

The use of soluble fiber, such as oat bran, may be used to implement but not replace the overall dietary plan. Commercial interpretation of the effects of food on cholesterol level may be confusing to both the client and the nurse. Registered dietitians are an excellent resource for evaluating the scientific foundation of many of the claims made about the effects of various foods on serum cholesterol levels. However, dietitians may not always be available, so nurses can have a key role in educating clients. When clients buy prepared foods, they should be aware of not only cholesterol but also the type and amount of fat in the product. The standard American food label notes the amount of cholesterol and the unhealthy saturated as well as the healthier poly- and monounsaturated fat content. Beginning in January 2006, all food labels in the United States also had to contain the amount of trans fat and eight possible allergens. Before this law went into effect, most cookies, crackers, and frozen breakfast products contained a lot of trans fat.

Some cities, such as New York and Philadelphia, and some states, such as California, have mandated that restaurants list trans fat content in their menus.

(Continued)

Table 9-3 Sources of Cholesterol and Saturated Fats in Diet

	Approximate Amount of Cholesterol (mg)	Approximate Amount of Saturated Fat (g)
Liver	370	2.5
Egg, one	275	1.7
Veal	86	4.0
Pork	80	3.2
Hot dog	75	9.9
Lean beef	73	3.7
Chicken		
Light meat	72	1.7
Dark meat	82	2.7
Ice cream, 1 cup	59	8.9
Fish	59	0.3
Lobster	46	0.07
Whole milk, one glass	33	5.1
Cheese, 1 ounce	30	6.0
Butter, 1 tablespoon	31	7.1
Coconut oil	0	11.8
Palm oil	0	6.7
Olive oil	0	1.8
Corn oil	0	1.7
Safflower oil	0	1.2

Note: All meat is 3-ounce servings. Oil is 1 tbsp.

Values have been collected from several sources published by the American Heart Association and others.

Possible Nursing Diagnoses . . . *(Continued)*

This required change in labeling has motivated restaurants and some fast food chains to remove trans fat from their products and substitute healthier vegetable oils. The ones who have made the change make this known to their customers.

Reading labels can also help clients find the type of fat that can lower cholesterol. The use of plant stenols and sterols or phytosterols (2 g daily) can help lower cholesterol levels by 9–20%. These substances derived from soybean oils have been available as margarine spreads since 1999. Several other companies now market or have plans to offer other products that contain these ingredients.

Risk for Noncompliance Related to Need for Long-Term Changes in Dietary Patterns

When a client has a high serum cholesterol level, the nurse's role in diet teaching may be crucial. Rather than emphasizing diet based on restrictions (no eggs, no steak, no ice cream, no butter), it may be better to take a positive approach and emphasize the foods to choose. Thus, the client can be encouraged to choose fish, chicken, lean beef, more vegetables, and fresh

Table 9–4 Drugs Used to Treat Hyperlipidemia (Lipid-Lowering Agents)

Drug	Decrease in ldl Cholesterol (%)	Comments
Cholestyramine	15–30	Can increase triglyceride levels. Alters absorption of other drugs and can cause gastrointestinal (GI) symptoms
Colestipol	15–30	Rash, GI symptoms
Nicotinic acid	15–30	Need to test for hyperuricemia (Chapter 4), hyperglycemia (Chapter 8), and liver enzymes (Chapter 12)
HMG-CoA reductase inhibitors (statins)[a]	20–60	Check liver enzymes and for CK skeletal myopathy (Chapter 12)
Ezetimibe	Varies	Blocks absorption of cholesterol
Fibric acids	5–20	Not used with gallbladder disease Test liver and muscle enzymes (Chapter 12)

[a]Seven statins are now on the market.

Information obtained from Katzung, Masters, and Trevor (2009) and Deglin, Vallerand, & Sanoski (2011). Medications to decrease triglycerides and raise HDL are discussed later in this chapter.

fruits. Clients should also be aware of the food served in "fast food" places, which specialize in selling food that contains high amounts of fats and calories.

Clients at risk for heart disease may be instructed to increase the intake of omega-3 fatty acids by consuming more fish. A supplement of omega-3 fatty acids is discussed in the section on triglycerides. The American Heart Association has excellent material for teaching clients about low-fat diets. Many authorities have suggested that as early as the second year of life, American children should eat the modified low-fat diet described for adults.

Deficient Knowledge Related to Drug Therapy

If dietary changes are not sufficient to lower cholesterol levels, the physician or nurse practitioner may order medications such as those listed in Table 9–4. Cholestyramine is also used to lower an elevated direct bilirubin because it binds bile salts. (See Chapter 11 on direct bilirubin.)

The most popular drugs for treating hyperlipidemia are hydroxymethylglutaryl–coenzyme A (HMG-CoA) reductase inhibitors, which block an enzyme needed for cholesterol production. The HMG-CoA inhibitors, such as lovastatin and the other "statins," improve survival for clients with heart disease and elevated cholesterol levels. Even more encouraging, recent studies have shown that the statins seem to reduce mortality in people with heart disease who do not have elevated cholesterol levels. These findings are important because some people with coronary heart disease do not have abnormal cholesterol levels. The nurse should be aware that researchers are investigating whether statins may also be used to reduce complications of diabetes, slow the progression of osteoporosis, and prevent or slow dementia (Woodruff, 2008). Also see Chapter 10 for the use of statins for elevated C-reactive protein.

Nurses must be aware of the information about the specific drug chosen for the client. With most of the drugs, the serum level of cholesterol may not drop for 1–2 months. The client needs encouragement to continue whatever diet has been prescribed and to report any side effects of the drug.

(Continued)

Possible Nursing Diagnoses . . . (*Continued*)

Imbalanced Nutrition: Less Than Body Requirements

Any plan for diet restriction must be evaluated in relation to the total nutritional needs of the client. A client following a diet very restricted in saturated fats faces the possibility of vitamin E deficiency. If a client does not like skim milk, a calcium deficiency can occur (see Chapter 7). Iron deficiency also may occur with low-cholesterol diets and may be of concern for premenopausal women.

Ineffective Individual Coping Related to the Need to Adopt Healthier Lifestyle

The nursing implications for a client with a high serum cholesterol level are broader than simply teaching about diet and drug therapies because cholesterol seems to be only one of the risk factors for cardiovascular disease. Thus, it is important to identify the other risk factors that may be present, such as lack of exercise, obesity, hypertension, stressful environments, and cigarette smoking. All these risk factors seem to be interrelated, along with other factors such as glucose levels. For example, hypertension may be a critical factor in the development of atherosclerosis because atheromatous plaques do not develop in low-pressure areas of the circulation, although bathed in the same lipid-laden blood, as they do in arteries that have the highest pressures. Obesity and stress both contribute to the development of hypertension. For each 5 lb (2.27 kg) of extra weight, the diastolic pressure rises about 1 mm Hg. It is not enough to tackle just one of the risk factors, because all are part of a still poorly understood pathophysiologic condition.

Hence, a nurse skilled in health teaching and counseling can help clients with a high serum cholesterol level to find ways to achieve a healthier lifestyle. It is essential that clients know both what is known and what is still not known about the role of serum cholesterol and other risk factors in the development of vascular disease. Clients can then make choices about what can be changed in their style of living to reduce some of or all the risk factors.

Altered Health Maintenance Related to Need for Family Follow-Up Care

Although the influence of genetics cannot be controlled by the person, it is important to consider genetic implications in counseling a client with an elevated serum cholesterol level. Because severe hyperlipidemia may sometimes be partly genetically based, the family members of clients with diagnosed hyperlipidemia need to be screened for the same condition. It is usually considered advisable to screen close relatives when a parent or sibling has a coronary event before the age of 55 years if male and before 65 if female.

Children whose parents are known to have blood cholesterol of 240 mg/dL or higher should also be screened (Hay et al., 2011). If familial hyperlipidemia is suspected and a child's lipid levels are normal, rescreening every 3–5 years is recommended. Most authorities believe the prevention of hyperlipidemia, particularly in young people, begins with basic changes in health practices for the entire family. Children with borderline or elevated LDL cholesterol should receive nutritional interventions to help them achieve heart healthy behaviors early in life. A creative approach to dietary change in children can be initiated by pediatric professionals in a variety of disciplines. For example, in familial hyperlipidemia, the maximum dose of the potent statins may be needed as well as a second drug (Table 9–4). Additionally, some lipid specialists prescribe statins to older male teenagers based on their family history, and even young children may also need these drugs (Hay et al., 2011).

Decreased Serum Cholesterol Levels

Clinical Significance

Common conditions that cause low serum cholesterol levels include (1) *hyperthyroidism,* in which the increased metabolism accounts for an increased utilization of fat; (2) *severe liver damage,* after which the liver can no longer manufacture cholesterol; and (3) *malnutrition,* which eventually leads to a deficiency of cholesterol caused by the lack of fats in the diet. Chronic anemia, drug therapy, and acquired immunodeficiency syndrome (AIDS) also cause lowered cholesterol levels. If the low serum cholesterol level is the result of a disease process, treatment is geared toward the particular pathophysiologic condition. The low serum cholesterol level, by itself, is not of specific concern.

If the client is following a diet or taking drugs to reduce cholesterol levels, a gradual lowering of the serum cholesterol levels is an indication of the effectiveness of therapy.

SERUM TRIGLYCERIDES

Triglycerides, like cholesterol and the phospholipids, are lipids that are normally present in the serum. The more precise chemical term for this group of lipids is *triacylglycerols,* but the laboratory test is called serum *triglycerides*. The triglycerides, the most abundant group of lipids, are neutral fat and oils that come from both animal fat and vegetable oils. A heavy meal or alcohol causes a transient increase in serum triglyceride levels. Excess triglycerides, which are useful for energy, are stored in the body as adipose tissue. The triglyceride test is useful in identifying some types of hyperlipidemia and is used as one factor in determining the LDL cholesterol.

Preparation of Client and Collection of Sample

The test should be performed in the fasting state, but the client should consume a conventional diet before the fasting begins. The laboratory needs 2 mL of serum. Because there is much variation in what is considered normal, the client should undergo the test two or three times in a 1- to 8-week period as discussed for serum cholesterol. Certain drugs such as thiazide diuretics, β-adrenergic blockers, protease inhibitors, and corticosteroids may increase the levels of triglycerides.

REFERENCE VALUES FOR TRIGLYCERIDES		
Adult	Normal	<150 mg/dL
	Borderline high	150–190 mg/dL
	High	200–499 mg/dL
	Very high	≥500 mg/dL
Pregnant women	Level rises progressively during pregnancy; note that oral contraceptives also cause an increase	
Newborn	Less than 40 mg at birth but rises to 55–60 mg/dL	
Children (aged 10–14) (aged 15–19)	Boys, 65 mg/dL; girls, 75 mg/dL Men, 80 mg/dL; women, 75 mg/dL	
Aged (older than 65)	130–135 mg/dL	

Note: See Wu (2006) for more details related to age and ethnicity.

Table 9–5 Assessments for Metabolic Syndrome[a]

Clients have metabolic syndrome if three or more of the following are present:

1. Waist measuring at least 40 inches (men) or 35 inches (women)
2. Serum triglycerides at least 150 mg/dL
3. HDL < 40 mg/dL (men) or 50 mg/dL (women)
4. Blood pressure at least 135/80 mm Hg
5. Serum glucose at least 110 mg/dL

[a]This may also be called syndrome X or obesity syndrome.

Increased Serum Triglyceride Levels

Clinical Significance

Many of the clinical conditions that cause an increase in serum cholesterol levels also cause increases in triglyceride levels. Thus, clients with nephrotic syndrome, pancreatic dysfunction, diabetes, toxemia of pregnancy, and hypothyroidism have elevated triglyceride levels. Triglycerides over 500 mg/dL increase the risk for pancreatitis. Fatty meals and alcohol always raise the triglyceride level for a while. The serum triglyceride level peaks about 5 hours after a fatty meal. An increase in serum triglycerides is sometimes associated with certain abnormal patterns of lipid metabolism that are probably genetic in origin. Clients with elevated triglyceride levels often have the metabolic syndrome. See Table 9–5 for the assessments of this syndrome.

Possible Nursing Diagnoses Related to Increased Triglyceride Levels

Deficient Knowledge Related to Diet and Possible Drug Therapy

Clients need the same instructions on diet discussed in the section on cholesterol levels. Often weight reduction and a low-fat diet can lower the serum triglyceride level. Some of the drugs used to lower cholesterol—the statins, nicotinic acid, and fibric acids (Table 9–4)—also reduce triglyceride levels. A fibric acid derivative, fenofibrate primarily inhibits triglyceride synthesis. Fish oils are sometimes used to decrease triglyceride levels that occur with some types of HIV medications (Capili & Anastasi, 2006). A supplement containing omega-3-acid ethyl esters may be prescribed for any client who has triglyceride levels above 500 mg/dL. If levels do not decrease in 2 months, the medication should be discontinued (Deglin et al., 2011).

Risk for Ineffective Coping Related to Unhealthy Lifestyle

The reduction of hyperlipidemia needs to be done in conjunction with other measures to improve the total health of the person. Authorities considered cigarette smoking, hypertension, and LDL cholesterol the three main risk factors for cardiovascular disease. The elevated serum triglyceride level was not as firmly established as cholesterol as a risk factor until a few years ago. Because alcohol causes secondary hyperlipidemia, the possibility of alcohol abuse should be investigated when there are unexplained high levels of triglycerides. Alcohol should be avoided, and a diet plan should be continued even if the client is on medication to reduce triglyceride levels.

Risk for Injury Related to Use of Fat Emulsions

Clients who are deficient in fatty acids can be given fat emulsions intravenously. Because the usual hyperalimentation fluids contain only glucose and amino acids, the fat is given as a separate solution. The fat used for intravenous replacement is composed of soybean oil emulsions and purified egg phosphatides in glycerol and water. This lipid emulsion can be given via a peripheral vein. Maintaining the stability of the emulsion before and during infusion, as well as watching for untoward reactions, is the responsibility of the nurse. As a general rule, treatment should not continue if the serum triglyceride level is above 250 mg/dL during infusion (150 mg/dL in neonates) or if it is greater than 150 mg/dL 6–12 hours after infusion (Hay et al., 2011).

Decreased Serum Triglyceride Levels

Clinical Significance

A decreased triglyceride level is rarely seen as a clinical problem. Some rare genetic defects may cause low serum triglycerides, and severe malnutrition may lead to low levels. Although hypothyroidism may cause an abnormally high triglyceride level, hyperthyroidism does not contribute to a low level. If the low serum triglyceride level is due to an exhaustion of the body's store of essential fatty acids, the client may have sparse hair growth, scaly and dry skin, poor wound healing, and a decrease in blood platelets, which may lead to some bleeding. The nurse should look for these signs when clients are not getting enough fat in their diet.

LIPOPROTEIN ELECTROPHORESIS AND LDL SUBCLASSES

Lipoproteins are complex molecules that contain lipids, such as cholesterol and triglycerides, in combination with various proteins. Researchers have been able to make some broad classifications of these lipoproteins based on the varying density of their molecules: HDL, which weigh the most; LDL; and very low density lipoproteins (VLDL). Electrophoresis can separate these types with an electric current to cause migration of the molecules. The direction of the different protein molecules is based on size and electrical charge. After the lipoproteins have separated into distinct layers, the layers make a distinct pattern that shows the relative distribution of four bands of lipoproteins: (1) chylomicrons (particles representing dietary fat in transport), (2) pre-β lipoproteins (VLDL), (3) β lipoproteins (LDL), and (4) α lipoproteins (HDL).

Certain types of technology such as nuclear magnetic resonance (NMR) spectroscopy can measure many subclasses of VLDL, LDL, and HDL and the size and concentration of the lipid particles. This profile helps identify people at greater risk for cardiac disease, especially those who have normal LDL levels. For example, in pattern A, the majority of LDL particles are large, and in pattern B, the majority of LDL particles are small. Clients with pattern B have a higher risk of heart disease.

Nurse practitioners may order advanced lipid testing and follow up on abnormal results. Medication, in conjunction with any needed weight loss, proper nutrition, and a prescribed exercise regimen, can convert the smaller dense LDL subclass B to the larger LDL subclass A, which reduces the risk of cardiovascular disease (Moredich, Kark, & Keresztes, 2005).

HIGH-DENSITY LIPOPROTEIN CHOLESTEROL

The cholesterol component of HDL (α lipoproteins) is measured as part of a lipid profile. Normally about 20% of cholesterol is HDL cholesterol. Data from the Framingham study, a longitudinal study of the cardiovascular risk for a population in Massachusetts, have supported the theory that low levels of HDL are associated with an increased incidence of CHD.

Preparation of Client and Collection of Sample

The client should fast. Water is allowed. The client should not have had weight changes in the past few weeks. Because many drugs affect the pattern, drugs should be withheld for 24–48 hours, if possible. Radiologic contrast agents interfere with the test. See notes on total cholesterol for timing of repeat samples.

REFERENCE VALUES FOR HDL CHOLESTEROL

Levels below 40 mg/dL are considered a positive risk factor for CHD.

Levels above 60 mg/dL are considered a negative risk factor for CHD.

Note: Wu (2006) reported percentile reference values for various age and ethnic groups.

Possible Nursing Diagnosis Related to Decreased HDL

Altered Health Maintenance

Although low HDLs may be largely due to genetics, some change in lifestyle factors may increase HDL. These lifestyle factors are exercise, weight loss if needed, moderate alcohol (no more than one drink a day for women or one to two for men), smoking abstinence, and avoiding trans fats.

Two groups of medications, the fibrates and niacin (Table 9–4), do raise HDL as well as lower LDL. The statins usually do not increase the HDL level but ezetimibe may. Omega-3 fatty acids, discussed as a treatment for triglyceride levels, may also increase HDL levels (Deglin et al., 2011). Research is continuing to find other treatments that can increase HDL even more.

RATIO OF TOTAL CHOLESTEROL TO HDL

The ratio of total cholesterol to HDL (total divided by HDL) has been used as a predictor of heart attack risk. The desirable ratio is 4.5 or lower. For example, a client with a total cholesterol of 200 and an HDL of 40 would have an undesirable ratio of 5.

LOW-DENSITY LIPOPROTEIN CHOLESTEROL

LDLs carry cholesterol in the plasma. Because this type of LDL cholesterol has been associated with coronary arterial atherosclerosis, it is called "bad" or "*lethal*" cholesterol. HDL cholesterol is the "good" or "*healthy*" cholesterol. The laboratory can determine the amount of LDL by use of the following formula:

LDL cholesterol = Total cholesterol − [HDL cholesterol + (triglycerides/5)]

For example:

$$\text{LDL cholesterol} = 200 - \left(55 + \frac{100}{5}\right)$$

$$200 - 75 = 125$$

The formula is not valid for specimens with chylomicrons present or if triglyceride levels are greater than 400 mg/dL.

Preparation of Client and Collection of Sample

The client should consume a stable diet for at least 2 weeks before lipid profiles are performed. Fasting is required. (See notes on total cholesterol levels, since LDL can be calculated from other blood work. Some laboratories may do a direct test of LDL, so check for the amount of blood needed for the single test.)

REFERENCE VALUES FOR LDL CHOLESTEROL

Adults
Optimal[a]	<100 mg/dL
Near optimal	100–129 mg/dL
Borderline high	130–159 mg/dL
High	160–189 mg/dL
Very high	≥190 mg/dL

[a]An update in 2004 suggested that aiming for less than 70 mg/dL might be appropriate for clients at very high risk for cardiovascular disease. At the present time, in the United States, the average LDL is about 123 mg/dL (Lee, 2006).

Possible Nursing Diagnoses Related to Increased LDL

Altered Health Maintenance

The challenge of achieving an LDL below 70 mg/dL for very high risk clients does usually require at least one or two types of medication. One study predicted approximately 25% of clients with diabetes and cardiovascular disease would require more than two lipid-lowering medications to achieve this goal (Kennedy et al., 2005).

Clients with high LDL cholesterol want to know what else besides diet and drugs may help them decrease the risk of cardiovascular disease. Genetics cannot be changed, but other factors that are related to less of the good HDL cholesterol and more of the bad LDL cholesterol are

(Continued)

Possible Nursing Diagnoses ... (Continued)

obesity and lack of exercise. These factors and smoking are under the control of the person, although making changes does often require professional support. However, being at risk for coronary artery disease can be a strong motivation for clients to evaluate the effect of their total lifestyle on their health. Computer programs are available to help with the assessment of risk factors. Nursing expertise may be one of the most powerful tools in lipid management. Even the use of telephone-delivered intervention by nurses has been shown to improve adherence to a cholesterol-lowering diet (Burke et al., 2005).

HOMOCYSTEINE LEVELS

Although cholesterol, particularly LDL cholesterol, is one predictor of coronary artery disease (CAD), not all clients with CAD have abnormal levels. Another risk factor for atherosclerosis may be homocysteine. Vitamin supplements of folic acid, B_6, and B_{12} may decrease abnormal levels. But Bønaa et al. (2006) and the Heart Outcomes Prevention Evaluation (2006) have not shown that lowering elevated homocysteine levels lowers the risk of major cardiovascular events in clients with vascular disease. Whether lowering levels in clients may *prevent* these events needs further study (McPhee et al., 2011).

Clients with vitamin B_{12} or folic acid deficiencies will most likely have elevated homocysteine levels (See Chapter 2). Certain genetic diseases also cause increased homocysteine in the blood and urine. Homocysteine levels also increase with age, smoking, and the use of some medicines such as methotrexate and phenytoin.

Preparation of Client and Collection of Sample

Fasting EDTA plasma specimen (lavender top) with immediate centrifugation is optimal. Check for specifics with laboratory for other directions. Serial measurements may be done for long-term monitoring of the effect of interventions.

REFERENCE VALUES FOR HOMOCYSTEINE[a]	
Age	**Values in μmol/l**
<30	4.6–8.1
30–59	4.5–7.9 (women); 6.3–11.2 (men)
>59	5.8–11.9

Note: Homocysteine is usually measured as the sum of free homocysteine and homocysteine bound to protein. This "total homocysteine" may be signified by the abbreviation Hcy or Hcys or Homocyst(e)ine.

LIPOPROTEIN (A) LEVELS

Increased levels of lipoprotein (a) [Lp(a)], hair-like projections attached to some LDL particles, are associated with increased risk of premature CAD and strokes. Lp(a) levels, mostly determined by genetic makeup, are higher in African Americans than in Caucasians and higher in women than in men. Other than genetics, factors that increase Lp(a) are uncontrolled diabetes, hypothyroidism, chronic renal failure, and the nephritic syndrome (Wu, 2006).

Preparation of Client and Collection of Specimen

Collect 1 mL of serum from a client who has been fasting for at least 12 hours.

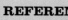

REFERENCE VALUES FOR LP(A) < 75 NMOL/L

Values are from University of California, San Francisco (UCSF). Note that some laboratories report levels in mg/dL and make distinctions based on race and sex.

APOLIPOPROTEINS A, B, AND E

Cholesterol and triglyceride are carried in the bloodstream as lipoproteins. HDL stands for high-density lipoprotein. Connected to these lipoproteins are proteins known as apolipoproteins. These apolipoproteins provide structure for the lipoproteins as well as serve several other functions in the complex metabolism of lipids. Five main types of apolipoproteins (A to E) circulate in the plasma, and each of these has several subtypes. (Confusion may exist between the test for Lp(a) discussed earlier and tests for apolipoprotein A [apo(A)] discussed here.) As a simple summary, apo(A) is the major component of HDL and lower levels of apo(A) are associated with low levels of HDL. Apo(B), measured as subunits, is involved in the binding of LDL particles to LDL receptors. Tests for apo(B) subunits may give more information than routine LDL levels (Wu, 2006). Determining specific subsets of apolipoproteins can help individualize treatment for a client with hyperlipidemia (Agruss & Garrett, 2005). Genetic testing for apo(E) is currently being studied as another risk factor for cardiovascular disease (Foley, 2005).

LIPOPROTEIN-ASSOCIATED PHOSPHOLIPASE A$_2$

Lipoprotein-associated phospholipase A$_2$ (Lp-PLA$_2$) is a cardiovascular-specific inflammatory enzyme that resides mainly in LDL cholesterol. A high level of this enzyme indicates an increased risk of a cardiovascular event or an ischemic stroke even though the LDL cholesterol may be below 130 mg/dL. This risk is independent of other risk factors (Brown, 2006). Lp-PLA$_2$ is also being studied as a predictor of recurrent stroke risk (Elkind et al., 2006). See www.plactest.com for more information on this test.

In addition to lipid levels, other tests that may be predictive of coronary risk are CRP (Chapter 14) and homocysteine levels (Chapter 9). Margolis et al. (2005) found that for women over 50, a WBC count greater than 6,700 may identify high risk for coronary vascular disease. (See Chapter 2 for more information on WBC).

The Lp-PLA$_2$ is not widely available, so a blood sample may be sent to a reference laboratory (www.labtestsonline.org). Statins lower not only cholesterol but also Lp-PLA$_2$ and hs-CRP (See Chapter 14). Braun (2010) discusses the use of Lp-PLA$_2$ to refine the risk status of the client and identify who would benefit from lifestyle changes and lipid-lowering therapies.

INTERPRETATION OF LP-PLA$_2$ RESULTS FOR CARDIOVASCULAR DISEASE	
200 ng/mL or below	Low risk
200–235 ng/mL	Borderline risk
Above 235 ng/mL	High risk

POSSIBLE RISK FACTORS FOR CORONARY ARTERY DISEASE

Although elevated total cholesterol level has long been considered a risk factor for vascular disease, several other possible factors are under investigation such as elevated fasting insulin levels, apolipoprotein A and B levels, the number of small dense LDL particles, and Lp(a) as an altered form of LDL. These tests are not yet recommended for general screening but may be used for clients who have a significant family history for cardiac disease. Apo(A)-1 levels are associated with HDL cholesterol, and apo(B) levels are associated with LDL cholesterol. So a ratio of these two may be calculated (see www.labtestsonline.org). Results must be compared to ethnic- and gender-specific populations to determine the risk percentile. Also, a large number of studies have reported an association between various inflammatory factors and coronary heart disease. Inflammatory factors showing an association are fibrinogen, C-reactive protein, albumin, and leukocyte counts. C-reactive protein is a relatively moderate predictor of coronary heart disease. See Chapter 14 for more on this marker. Other indicators of inflammation such as leukocyte counts (Chapter 2) may be a predictor of cardiovascular events (Margolis et al., 2005). See Table 9–6 for a list of current laboratory tests associated with the development or prediction of cardiovascular disease.

Table 9–6 Examples of Risk Markers for Cardiovascular Disease

Test	**Comments on Test**
Cholesterol	See current screening recommendations See predictive value of skin cholesterol (Sprecher & Pearce, 2006)
HDL	See ways to increase low levels
LDL	Medications often needed to decrease levels below 70 mg/dL
Triglycerides	See effect of diet on levels
LDL subclass B	See section on lipoprotein electrophoresis (Moredich et al., 2005)
Lp(a)	See effect of genetics (Wu, 2006)
Lipoprotein-associated phospholipase A$_2$	See www.plactest.com
Apolipoproteins	Note subsets of A–E and use of each (Agruss & Garrett, 2005; Foley, 2005)
Homocysteine	See effects of B vitamins and folic acid
C-reactive protein	See Chapter 14 for low-, average-, and high-risk CRP levels
WBC	See Chapter 2 on postmenopausal women (Margolis et al., 2005)

See American Heart Association (www.heart.org) for updates on all these markers and www.labtestsonline.org and www.plactest.com for information on PLAC test for lipoprotein-associated phospholipase A$_2$.

Questions

1. Which of the following test results is considered a risk factor for the development of coronary artery disease?
   a. An elevated hemoglobin
   b. A decreased homocysteine level
   c. A decreased lipoprotein (a)
   d. An increased C-reactive protein

2. Which of the following meals contains the least amount of cholesterol?
   a. Steak, baked potato with sour cream, roll and butter, tossed salad with French dressing, and coffee
   b. Lobster, rice, salad with Thousand Island dressing, milk, and apple pie with cheese slice
   c. Chicken, mashed potatoes, green beans, salad with blue cheese dressing, wine, and strawberries with powdered sugar
   d. Liver, rice, peas, cole slaw, tea, and ice cream

3. For clients with hyperlipidemia, the nurse needs to help assess whether the lifestyle contains other high-risk factors for the development of coronary heart disease (CHD). Which of the following has the least impact on development of CHD?
   a. Alcoholic beverages
   b. Cigarette smoking
   c. Hypertension
   d. Obesity

4. A client, 44 years of age, has started drug therapy for a high serum cholesterol level that did not respond to diet and weight control. Which of the following information about hyperlipidemia and drug therapy is appropriate to use to teach him about his disease and drug therapy?
   a. Serum cholesterol levels should drop in a week or two after drugs are begun
   b. Drug therapy eliminates the need for dietary restrictions
   c. Drug therapy always reduces both cholesterol and triglyceride levels
   d. Family members of the client should undergo screening for abnormal lipid levels because they may need treatment

5. Which one of the following lipid-lowering drugs is also used to treat jaundice?
   a. Niacin or nicotinic acid
   b. Cholestyramine
   c. Lovastatin
   d. Gemfibrozil

6. Serum triglyceride levels would be the least useful for
   a. Evaluating the effect of intravenous fat emulsions
   b. Assessing the presence of hyperthyroidism
   c. Evaluating the effectiveness of some drugs used to control hyperlipidemia
   d. Assessing the type of hyperlipidemia that may be present

7. According to data from the Framingham study, which of the following is the type of lipoproteins that may offer some protection against the development of cardiovascular disease?
   a. Chylomicrons
   b. Pre-β (very low density) lipoproteins (VLDL)
   c. β (low-density) lipoproteins (LDL)
   d. α (high-density) lipoproteins (HDL)

8. Which of the following is a factor that tends to increase the level of HDL cholesterol?
   a. Losing weight if obese
   b. Eating meat
   c. Eliminating alcohol from the diet
   d. Lack of exercise

References

Agruss, J. C. & Garrett, K. (2005). New markers for CVD. *Nurse Practitioner, 30*(11), 26–31.

Bønaa, K. H., Njølstad, I., Ueland, P. M., Schirmer, H., Tverdal, A., Steigen, T., et al. (2006). Homocysteine lowering and cardiovascular events after acute myocardial infarction. *New England Journal of Medicine, 354*(15), 1578–1588.

Boyd, G. S., Koenigsberg, J., Falkner, F., Gidding, S., & Hassink, S. (2005). Effect of obesity and high blood pressure on plasma lipid levels in children and adults. *Pediatrics, 116*(2), 442–446.

Braun, L. T. (2010). How inflammatory markers refine CV risk status. *American Nurse Today, 5*(5), 30–31.

Brown, R. A. (2006). Gauging cardiovascular risk with the PLAC test. *Nursing 2006, 8*(1), 9–18.

Burke, L. E., Dunbar-Jacob, J., Orchard, T., & Sereika, S. (2005). Improving adherence to a cholesterol-lowering diet: A behavioral intervention study. *Patient Education and Counseling, 57*(1), 134–142.

Capili, B. & Anastasi, J. (2006). HIV and hyperlipidemia: Current recommendations and treatment. *MEDSURG Nursing, 15*(1), 14–20.

Deglin, J. H., Vallerand, A. H., & Sanoski, C. A. (2011). *Davis's drug guide for nurses* (12th ed.). Philadelphia: F. A. Davis.

Elkind, M. S., Tai, W., Coates, K., Paik, M., & Sacco, R. (2006). High-sensitivity C-reactive protein, lipoprotein associated phospholipase A2 and outcomes after ischemic stroke. *Archives of Internal Medicine, 166*(19), 2073–2080.

Foley, S. M. (2005). Update on risk factors for atherosclerosis: The role of inflammation and apolipoprotein E. *MEDSURG Nursing, 14*(1), 43–50.

Hay, W. W., Levin, M. J., Sondheimer, J. M., & Deterding, R. R. (Eds.). (2011). *Current diagnosis and treatment: Pediatrics* (20th ed.). New York: McGraw-Hill.

Katzung, B., Masters, S. B., & Trevor, A. J. (Eds.). (2009). *Basic and clinical pharmacology* (11th ed.). New York: McGraw-Hill.

Kennedy, A. G., MacLean, S., Littenberg, B., Ades, P., & Pinckney, R. (2005). The challenge of achieving national cholesterol goals in patients with diabetes. *Diabetes Care, 28*, 1029–1034.

Lee, T. H. (2006). High marks for below-average cholesterol. *Harvard Heart Letter, 17*(2), 4–5.

Margolis, K. L., Manson, J., Greenland, P., Rodabough, R., Bray, P., & Safford, M. (2005). Leukocyte count as a predictor of cardiovascular events and mortality in postmenopausal women: The Women's Health Initiative Observational Study. *Archives of Internal Medicine, 165*(5), 500–508.

McPhee, S. J., Papadakis, M. A., & Rabow, M. W. (Eds.). (2011). *Current medical diagnosis and treatment* (50th ed.). New York: McGraw-Hill.

Moredich, C., Kark, D., & Keresztes, P. (2005). Implications of LDL subclass B in patients at cardiovascular risk. *Nurse Practitioner, 30*(7), 16–29.

Sprecher, D. L. & Pearce, G. (2006). Skin cholesterol adds to Framingham risk assessment. *American Heart Journal, 153*(4), 694–696.

Woodruff, D. (2008). Teaching pros and cons of statin therapy. *Nursing 2008, 38*(5), 56.

Wu, A. H. (Ed.). (2006). *Tietz clinical guide to laboratory tests* (4th ed.). St. Louis: Saunders Elsevier.

Websites

www.heart.org (Updates on cardiac markers.)
www.labtestsonline.org (Update on homocysteine, Apo(B), and other lipoproteins.)
www.nhlbi.nih.gov/guidelines/cholesterol (Update on guidelines for cholesterol tests.)
www.plactest.com (Update on lipoprotein-associated phospholipase A_2.)
www.uspreventiveservicestaskforce.org (Updates on screening for lipid disorders in adults.)

Answers

1. d, 2. c, 3. a, 4. d, 5. b, 6. b, 7. d, 8. a

Tests Related to Serum Protein Levels, Tumor Markers, and Cancer Genomics

- Functions of Albumin in the Serum   230
- Functions of Globulins in the Serum   230
- Serum Protein Electrophoresis   231
- Serum Albumin   232
- Pre-albumin or Transthyretin   233
- Alpha-1-Antitrypsin or Alpha-1-Protease Inhibitor   237
- Phenotyping for Protease Inhibitor Genes   237
- Gamma Globulins   239
- Immunoelectrophoresis and Quantification of Serum Proteins: IgG, IgA, IgM, IgD, and IgE, and Free Light Chains   241
- Urine Protein Electrophoresis and Immunoelectrophoresis   243

- Serum Ammonia   243
- Tumor Markers   245
- Alpha-Fetoprotein   246
- Beta-2-Microglobulin   247
- Carcinoembryonic Antigen   248
- CA 125 Antigen   248
- CA 15-3 and CA 27.29   249
- Her-2/neu   249
- CA 19-9   250
- Prostate-Specific Antigen   250
- Free PSA   251
- Bladder Tumor–Associated Antigen Test   251
- NMP22   252
- Tests for Cancer Using Proteomics and Genomics   252
- Genetic Screening for Cancer: BRCA1 and BRCA2   252

OBJECTIVES

1. Identify the serum proteins measured by electrophoresis and immunoelectrophoresis.
2. Illustrate how cellular and humoral immunity are assessed by specific laboratory tests.
3. Identify nursing diagnoses for clients with low serum albumin levels (hypoalbuminemia).
4. Explain the general clinical significance of various aclonal, monoclonal, and polyclonal patterns of immunoglobulins in serum and urine.
5. Identify basic nursing interventions for clients who have an abnormal pattern or deficiency of γ-globulins.
6. Describe how the radioallergosorbent test (RAST) is used in the assessment of allergies.

7. Identify the types of medications and food that must be withheld when a client has an elevated serum ammonia level.

8. Describe the clinical usefulness and limitations of tumor markers and genetic screening.

This chapter focuses on the most common tests used to measure proteins in the serum, including some tumor markers. The difference between serum and plasma proteins is that plasma proteins include those involved in the clotting of the plasma. (Plasma proteins, fibrinogen, and prothrombin are discussed in Chapter 13.)

The two serum proteins measured in the test for total proteins are albumin and globulin. Albumin is a singular type of protein that is either in the serum in sufficient amounts or is not. The tests for globulins are more complex because there are five types of globulins (α-1 and α-2, β-1 and β-2, and γ). In addition, there are many singular types of proteins in each of these main classes.

The exact amounts of albumin and of the five main globulin types are determined with a procedure called *electrophoresis*. If certain of the γ-globulins are shown to be abnormal, a further test, *immunoelectrophoresis*, is performed to separate the five main types of γ-globulins (IgG, IgA, IgM, IgD, and IgE). Electrophoresis uses electric current to separate the six protein fractions, whereas *immunoelectrophoresis* involves, as an added step, the use of antiserum to cause precipitation of the five γ-globulins. Immunofixation uses a similar technique. The proteins identified by these tests are shown in Table 10–1. These tests can be performed not only on serum but also on urine and cerebral spinal fluid.

Table 10–1 Tests of Serum Proteins

Measured As Total Proteins (TP)	Measured with Protein Electrophoresis (PEP)	Measured with Immunoelectrophoresis (IEP) or Quantitative Analysis	
Serum proteins 6.0–8.0 Albumin (3.1–4.3 g/dL) 52–68%			
	α-1 globulins (4.2–7.2%)		
	α-2 globulins (6.8–12%)		
	β-1 globulins (3–10%)		
Globulins[a] 2.6–4.1 g/dL	β-2 globulins (1–9%)	IgG IgA	75% 10–15%
	γ-globulins (13–23%)	IgM IgD	7–10% <1%
		IgE	>1%

[a]Note that many of the α- and β-globulins can be measured by individual tests for α-1-antitrypsin, α-fetoprotein, and so on.

Values are approximate for adults. See text for variations across life span.

FUNCTIONS OF ALBUMIN IN THE SERUM

Albumin, produced only by the liver, is essential in maintaining the oncotic pressure in the vascular system. A lack of albumin in the serum allows fluid to leak out into the interstitial spaces and into the peritoneal cavity. Albumin is also very important in the transportation of many substances in the bloodstream. For example, when the serum albumin level is less than normal, the total serum calcium level decreases. (See Chapter 7 on how albumin affects the interpretation of serum calcium levels.) Many drugs, lipids, hormones, and toxins are bound to albumin while they are circulating in the bloodstream. Once the drug or other substance reaches the liver, it is detached from the albumin and converted to a water-soluble form that can be excreted. (See Chapter 11 for further discussion on the role of albumin in the conjugation process of bilirubin.) Albumin is also one of the buffers that functions to maintain acid–base balance in the bloodstream, as discussed in Chapter 6.

FUNCTIONS OF GLOBULINS IN THE SERUM

As can be seen in Table 10–1, globulins are a very complex and diversified group of serum proteins, for which both the α and β types are synthesized in the liver:

1. *α-1 Globulins* contain various lipoproteins, glycoproteins, antitrypsin, and other proteins such as thyroxine-binding globulin.

2. *α-2 Globulins* contain macroglobulins, haptoglobulins, ceruloplasmin, and hormones such as erythropoietin.

3. *β-1 Globulins* contain hormones, fat-soluble vitamins, transferrin, and plasminogen, in addition to other lipoproteins.

4. *β-2 Globulins* contain most of the various components of the complement system and other proteins.

Unlike the α- and β-globulins, γ-globulins, now called *immunoglobulins*, are not synthesized by the liver. They are made by B lymphocytes in response to a stimulus from an antigen. Classified as five main types that are designated by the letters IgG, IgA, IgM, IgD, and IgE, these five immunoglobulins are changed considerably in different types of immunologic responses. To understand the clinical significance of testing for immunoglobulins, one must recall some facts about the concepts of cellular and humoral immunity.

Immune System

Optimal immunologic defense depends on interactions between cellular and humoral immunity, but much is still to be learned about the interaction between these two systems.

Cellular Immunity

Cellular immunity and delayed hypersensitivity are functions of the T lymphocytes controlled by the thymus. The presence of adequate cellular immunity can be demonstrated by a positive response to various skin tests. Clients with negative tests for all the antigens on a skin test panel have anergy, the inability to mount an immune response. Blood lymphocyte phenotyping (Chapter 2) helps assess the adequacy of T lymphocytes for cell-mediated immunity and for assisting with humoral immunity.

Humoral Immunity

Because the immunoglobulins secreted by the B lymphocytes are found in the bloodstream and in other secretions, such as saliva, tears, and colostrum, this type of immunity is called *humoral*. Humoral immunity is the type directly measured by the assessment of the circulating antibodies in serum and in other body fluids. The *B* stands not for blood but for bursa, because earlier research discovered this type of lymphocyte in the bursae of chickens. In humans, the B lymphocytes are thought to be matured in the lymphoid tissue at various locations. The B lymphocytes produce the IgM class of antibodies as a first response to a potential infection. As the response proceeds, the B lymphocytes can be switched to produce other isotypes such as IgG, IgA, or IgE (see the section on immunoglobulins).

The complement system contains several proteins that are classified by the letter C and a number (e.g., C2, C4). The complement system enhances the antibody–antigen reaction of the humoral system. The tests involving the complement system are discussed in Chapter 14.

SERUM PROTEIN ELECTROPHORESIS

In serum protein electrophoresis (SPEP), the laboratory uses an electric current to separate normal human serum into six distinct protein fractions, through a migration of protein molecules. Various protein molecules, after separating out in a gel mixture or on a coated film, are fixed on a sheet of paper. Albumin, the largest component, has the greatest mobility, so it moves the farthest away from the point of the electrical circuit. The α-globulins line up next, and then the β-globulins. Because the γ-globulins migrate the least from the electrical point, this group makes the last large, distinct band on the paper. Once the six protein fractions have been separated on the strip of paper, the sheet is stained to identify the pattern.

This pictorial representation of the amounts of each protein type is useful as a screening device because changes in the patterns can be seen and further testing carried out if deemed necessary by the clinician. For example, protein electrophoresis is a screening test for multiple myeloma. The pathologist is usually the one to compare the pattern with known abnormal patterns seen in various disease states. The strip of paper, or electrophorectogram, can be put into a machine that quantifies the serum protein fractions and reports the amount in percentages. This report in percentages can be read by the nurse, who can compare the numbers with reference values for each type of protein fraction.

Preparation of Client and Collection of Sample

The client should be fasting but can have water. One milliliter of whole blood is ample for total protein (TP) and SPEP. Fresh samples are ideal, but older samples can be used.

REFERENCE VALUES FOR SPEP

Essentially the same for all people. Variations noted for electrophoresis results are as follows:

Total serum protein	6.0–8.0 g/dL
Serum albumin	3.1–4.3 g/dL
Serum globulins	2.6–4.1 g/dL

Electrophoresis (reported as a percentage of total protein):

Adult	Albumin	52–68%	
	Globulins		
	α-1	4.2–7.2%	
	α-2	6.8–12.0%	
	β-1	3–10%	(Some laboratories
	β-2	1–9%	report β together
	γ	13–23%	as 9.3–15.0%)

Newborn	See details about γ-globulins in text
Pregnant women	Albumin falls quickly the first few months and then more slowly during rest of pregnancy
	Overall decrease is about 1 g/dL with a return to normal within 8 weeks postpartum
Children	Tend to have slightly lower amounts of albumin until 4 years of age or later; types and amounts of γ-globulins depend on age (see text)
Aged	The γ-globulins, or at least the immunologic response, decreases with age; albumin levels gradually decrease

See Hay et al. (2011) for details on newborn and pediatric values.

SERUM ALBUMIN

Increased Serum Albumin Level

Clinical Significance

No pathologic conditions cause the liver to produce extra amounts of albumin. So an increased value of albumin on a laboratory report is a reflection of dehydration. (Recall that many tests can be falsely elevated by dehydration.) The inclusion of excess amounts of protein in the diet does not raise the serum albumin level, because protein is first broken down into amino acids and then used for various purposes, including storage as adipose (fat) tissue.

Decreased Serum Albumin Level

Clinical Significance

Because albumin is totally synthesized by the liver, liver dysfunction is a common reason for a decreased serum albumin level (hypoalbuminemia). Reduced albumin levels are not seen in acute liver failure because it takes several weeks of lack of production before the albumin level decreases. The most common reason for a lowered level is chronic liver dysfunction caused by cirrhosis. Clients with acquired immunodeficiency syndrome (AIDS) have hypoalbuminemia. A loss of albumin in the

Table 10–2 Conditions That Change Serum Albumin Levels

Increased Levels

Dehydration

Decreased Levels
Cirrhosis
AIDS
Nephrotic syndrome
Preeclampsia
Burns
Severe malnutrition

Note: See text for further explanation of the pathophysiology of these conditions.

urine caused by renal dysfunction (nephrotic syndrome) can also cause a decrease in albumin in the serum. Although a decrease of about 1 g/100 mL is normal in pregnancy, there is even more of a decrease with preeclampsia. (Albuminuria, or albumin in the urine, is a sign of both renal disease and eclampsia. See Chapter 3.) Severe burns, with related damage to capillaries and blood vessels, result in a large loss of serum proteins, including albumin. The increased capillary permeability caused by the burn damage may cause a continual leak of serum proteins out of the vascular system. Also, the long-term depression of protein synthesis after a burn may last for a couple of months. See Table 10–2 on conditions that change the albumin level.

If there is inadequate intake of protein, the body begins to break down muscles (catabolism) to obtain enough amino acids for the continuing synthesis of serum albumin. Thus, albumin levels do not decrease in fasting states or in malnutrition until the condition is severe. Protein requirements may be greatly increased during stress, infection, or injury. The client is in a negative nitrogen balance when the catabolic process is greater than the anabolic process. (See Chapter 4 on the test for urinary urea nitrogen for calculating negative nitrogen balance.)

PRE-ALBUMIN OR TRANSTHYRETIN

Pre-albumin, also known as thyroxin-binding pre-albumin or transthyretin, has a half-life of less than 2 days. Because of its short half-life, pre-albumin is a sensitive indicator of recent changes in catabolism (Mulden, 2009). This test is used for nutritional assessment. Other tests such as transferrin, an iron-supporting protein (half-life of 7 days), and retional-binding protein (half-life of 12 hours) may be used to assess malnutrition, but pre-albumin is more common (DiMaria-Ghalili & Amella, 2005).

Preparation of Client and Collection of Sample

Serum samples without hemolysis or lipidemia are preferred. Sometimes a CRP (Chapter 14) is ordered to rule out inflammation because inflammation lowers the pre-albumin level (Wu, 2006). Renal failure causes an increase, as do some medications such as corticosteroids.

REFERENCE VALUES FOR PRE-ALBUMIN (FASTING)	
Cord blood	8.1–18.7 mg/dL
Newborns	4–19 mg/dL
Adults	12–50 mg/dL

Clinical Significance

Low levels of pre-albumin signify the need for a comprehensive nutritional evaluation including a nutritional history, weight, anthropometric measurements, and calorie counts. The Joint Commission (www.jointcommission.org) states that clients must have a nutritional assessment within 24 hours of admission to a hospital. In addition to physical assessment, pre-albumin values are the gold standard to determine risks and to gauge the effect of therapy. A pre-albumin level of less than 5 mg/dL requires aggressive nutritional support. The target is to increase pre-albumin by 2 mg per day or to achieve normal level by 8 days. Thus, clients may have pre-albumin levels drawn twice a week (Kuszajewski & Clontz, 2005). Clients with end-stage renal disease exhibit increased levels of pre-albumin because of lack of excretion by the kidneys. Low serum pre-albumin levels in renal clients are associated with increased mortality.

Possible Nursing Diagnoses Related to Hypoalbuminemia

Impaired Skin Integrity Related to Development of Edema

Because albumin is responsible for the oncotic pressure in the vascular system, a reduction in serum albumin causes edema. Edema occurs when the albumin level decreases to 2.0–2.5 g/dL. Without adequate albumin in the bloodstream, fluid leaks out into the interstitial spaces and into the peritoneal cavity. Unlike the edema caused by too much volume in the vascular space, this type of edema is not found primarily in dependent areas. For example, clients with an increased volume caused by congestive heart failure have edema in the feet if they are sitting up or in the sacral area if in bed. In contrast, clients with edema caused by a lack of albumin may also have puffy eyelids or hands and a swollen abdomen caused by leakage of fluid into the peritoneal cavity. (A client with cirrhosis who has hypoalbuminemia is also likely to have portal hypertension that intensifies the collection of fluid in the peritoneal cavity.) In addition to weighing these clients and checking their ankles and sacral area for edema, the nurse should also measure the abdominal girth to check the progression of edema. Besides causing edema, the lack of protein also escalates the risk of decubitis ulcers because cellular nutrition is inadequate. Skin breakdown is always a potential problem. These clients need superb skin care. A transjugular intrahepatic portosystemic stent (TIPS) as a shunt may be performed to manage refractory ascites (Lee & Grap, 2008).

Assisting with Interventions to Decrease Edema. A collection of fluid in the peritoneal cavity may make it impossible for the client to breathe comfortably in a reclining position. Sometimes

Table 10–3 Requirements of Protein Across Life Span

Age	Protein (g/kg)
0–6 months	2.2
6–12 months	2.0
1–3 years	1.8
4–6 years	1.5
7–10 years	1.2
11–14 years	1.0
15–18 years Girls Boys	 0.84 0.85
19 and older	0.8[a]

[a]A 70-kg man would need (70 × 0.8) = 56 g of protein each day, and a 50-kg woman would need only (50 × 0.8) = 40 g.

Note: Many adults in the United States consume much more protein than is required.

a paracentesis must be performed to take the pressure off the diaphragm. (See Chapter 25 for a description of paracentesis.) The disadvantage of a paracentesis is that proteins are lost in the peritoneal fluid. Diuretics, along with some restrictions of fluids and sodium, may be ordered because an increased amount of aldosterone may also be contributing to the formation of edema. (See Chapter 5 for a discussion of hypernatremia.)

Imbalanced Nutrition Related to Protein Requirement

The primary treatment of edema caused by a lack of serum albumin is to increase the albumin level. If the liver can still synthesize albumin, a diet with adequate protein is appropriate for long-term therapy. The recommended daily allowance for protein for various ages is shown in Table 10–3.

Often the clients who need the protein the most can tolerate it the least because their livers are unable to handle the ammonia that results from protein breakdown. (See the test for serum ammonia at the end of this chapter.) If protein is well tolerated, however, eggs, cheese, fish, and meat are excellent sources, along with a correct mixture of nuts, grains, and vegetables. Dried milk is economical and can be added to many foods and beverages. Commercially made protein supplements can be used. If the client is also deficient in minerals and vitamins, these liquid diets may ensure a higher level of many necessary nutrients. The client must have plenty of calories from carbohydrates, so that protein is not used as an energy source. See Table 10–4 for a comparison of the protein content in various foods.

Risk of Injury Related to Intravenous Albumin Replacement

For a client who needs albumin replacement immediately, albumin can be given intravenously. Albumin is also used as a plasma expander. Some albumin, which is collected from human donors, is obtained from placental blood, which is important because the infusion of

(Continued)

Table 10–4 Foods High in Protein

Food Item	Protein (G)
■ **COMPLETE PROTEINS**	
1 egg	7.0
1 oz (28 g) meat or fish	7.0–8.0
1 oz (28 g) cheese	6.0–7.0
8 oz (240 mL) milk	8.5
1 tbsp dried milk	1.6
■ **INCOMPLETE PROTEINS**[a]	
1 tbsp peanut butter	4.0
2 slices wheat bread	4.0
1 cup nuts	7.0–8.0
3 oz lentils	7.0
1/4 cup garbanzo beans	10.0

[a]Consult a nutrition text on how incomplete vegetable proteins can be balanced to supply all needed amino acids.

Note: Estimates are from various food labels and nutritional pamphlets.

Possible Nursing Diagnoses . . . (*Continued*)

some albumins causes an increase in alkaline phosphatase level. (See Chapter 12 for this enzyme test.) Albumin does not need to be refrigerated as does whole blood. It does not have any preservatives added, so it must be used soon after it is opened.

Albumin comes in a 5% and a 25% concentration. Except in shock, the intravenous infusion must be given slowly because of the danger of circulatory overload. Vital signs must be monitored.

As the oncotic pressure returns to normal, edematous fluid is pulled back into the vascular system. The mobilization of edema from the tissues causes increased urine output. The albumin remains in the bloodstream for several days, but with a severe albumin deficiency, the client may need repeated infusions over time.

Risk for Injury Related to Drug Toxicity

Some drugs are highly bound to protein (mostly albumin) while they circulate in the bloodstream so that only a small portion of the drug is unbound and thus active. Therefore, if a client has low levels of serum albumin, toxicity might occur when drugs that are known to be highly protein bound are given in the usual dosage. However, as long as the drugs are cleared by the kidneys, this theoretical problem does not occur (Katzung, Masters, & Trevor, 2009).

Risk for Infection Related to Associated Lymphopenia

Protein malnutrition in the hospitalized elderly may greatly increase the risk for infection. Severe protein malnutrition inhibits lymphocyte and antibody synthesis. Thus, a client who has a decreased serum albumin level may have a low lymphocyte count. In fact, lowered albumin levels and a lowered lymphocyte level ((1,500 mm³) are two markers of malnutrition that are used in research on nutrition. Poor nutrition may also lead to impaired neutrophil functioning. Nursing interventions should be geared to protect the client from infection, as discussed in Chapter 2 (lymphocytes and neutrophils) and Chapter 16 (culture and sensitivity tests), and to promote a healthful diet.

ALPHA-1-ANTITRYPSIN OR ALPHA-1-PROTEASE INHIBITOR

α-1-Antitrypsin (AAT) is an example of a special α-globulin that can be measured. A decrease or near-absence of AAT can be a factor in chronic obstructive pulmonary disease (COPD). AAT deficiency, also known as *α-1-antiprotease inhibitor deficiency*, results from an autosomal recessive genetic mutation. Alpha-1-antitrypsin deficiency (A1AD) has the highest incidence in Scandinavia and is at least as common as cystic fibrosis in Caucasians. However, other ethnic groups may also have the gene, and current data suggest that less than 10% of people living with A1AD have been properly diagnosed (www.alpha1.org). AAT is an important protein for inhibiting the damaging effects of a proteolytic enzyme, neutrophil elactase, released by phagocytes in the lungs in response to irritation or infections. Thus, people with A1AD develop chronic bronchitis and "hereditary" emphysema. Smokers develop the disease earlier than do nonsmokers who may not be diagnosed until midlife.

A1AD may also cause jaundice and severe liver disease, particularly in young children, and an increased rate of cirrhosis and liver cancer in adulthood. Much rarer are dermatological manifestations that include panniculitis, characterized by necrotizing lesions and inflammation of the skin.

Screening tests are recommended for clients suspected to have AAT deficiency such as those with early onset of emphysema, neonates with hepatitis or jaundice, adults with unexplained liver disease or panniculitis, or those with a family history of these conditions.

Early detection is needed so clients can avoid factors that could damage the lungs or liver. Avoidance of smoke and air pollution is critical. Prompt treatment of respiratory infections, use of pneumococcal vaccine, influenza shots, and hepatitis A and B vaccines may be recommended. See Chapter 14 on hepatitis vaccines and ways to prevent hepatitis C.

Preparation of Client and Collection of Sample

Serum is used and can be stored for later use. Most serum samples are usually refrigerated. Hyperlipemic samples are rejected.

REFERENCE VALUES FOR AAT	
Newborn	142–270 mg/dL
Adult with MM phenotype	78–200 mg/dL
Aged	115–200 mg/dL

PHENOTYPING FOR PROTEASE INHIBITOR GENES

Several different variants of AAT deficiency or alpha-1 disease exist, so phenotyping is done after low levels are discovered by the screening test. Because A1AD is an inherited disorder, relatives of the client should be offered phenotyping and genetic counseling. The normal type of the protease inhibitor (pi) gene is called the M variant. Some common abnormal variants are the S and Z variants. The null pi gene produces no AAT. A phenotype of these abnormal variants can predict the risk for developing emphysema and help with treatment decisions about the replacement therapy of AAT. In addition to clarifying the diagnosis, phenotyping is indispensable for identifying carriers of the disease. AAT deficiency can also be assessed by amniocentesis (Chapter 28).

REFERENCE VALUES FOR AAT IN DIFFERENT PHENOTYPES OF THE PROTEASE INHIBITOR GENE

pi MM	Level within normal reference ranges (see earlier section)
pi MZ, SS, or M null	80% of normal
pi SZ	35–45% of normal
pi ZZ or pi Z null	10–20% of normal
pi null (rare)	Undetectable

Reference Values from Wu (2006). See *www.alpha1.org* for other values.

Possible Nursing Diagnoses Related to Decreased Alpha-1-Antitrypsin

Risk for Ineffective Health Maintenance Related to Development of Chronic Lung Disease

People with a moderate deficiency of AAT whose environment is healthful may live a normal life span, but those who smoke or live in a polluted environment may develop lung disease and die at an early age. Lung transplantation is an option for some clients. Hence, clients need information on how to protect themselves from air pollutants. Referrals to stop-smoking programs may be needed. In addition to helping clients prevent further damage to their lungs, nurses can help clients with AAT deficiency identify how to manage the consequences of their disease, such as dyspnea. (See Chapter 24 on testing for FEV_1 and the use of bronchodilators).

In the late 1980s, human alpha-1-proteinase inhibitor became available as replacement therapy for clients with severe AAT deficiencies. At present, the replacement is given intravenously every few weeks. Studies are ongoing about the long-term effects of replacement therapy. Investigations are under way for delivery of recombinant AAT via a high-efficiency nebulizer. The Alpha-1 Association (www.alpha1.org) has current information on treatment options and information on local chapters and support groups.

Risk for Impaired Health Management Related to Liver Dysfunction

Some clients with AAT deficiency may develop cirrhosis. Treatment is supportive, as discussed in the section on low albumin levels. The American Liver Foundation has information on this condition. Liver transplantation has been successful for children who have AAT deficiency (Hay et al., 2011).

GAMMA GLOBULINS

Changes in Patterns

Clinical Significance

There may be an increase either of various types (polyclonal) or of only one type (monoclonal) or there may be an absence (aclonal) of γ-globulins. The use of the term *clonal* refers to the origin of the globulins from a particular *clone* of plasma cells.

Polyclonal Patterns

This pattern is a reflection of an overproduction of almost all the immunoglobulins in response to antigens. Several different clones of plasma cells produce increased amounts of various immunoglobulins. The result is general hypergammaglobulinemia, a characteristic response to infections (the inflammatory response). Autoimmune diseases and some liver diseases also cause a generalized increase.

Monoclonal Patterns or M Protein

In this pattern, only one type of γ-globulin is increased. Patterns of this sort may be diagnostic because they involve a spike of a single globulin, which can be closely examined by means of immunoassay to detect paraproteins or abnormal variants of an immunoglobulin. Monoclonal patterns are found in a number of situations:

1. Most clients with multiple myeloma have a peak of a paraprotein or abnormal globulin. (The discussion on immunoelectrophoresis explores paraproteins.) The diagnostic criteria for multiple myeloma include a 10% involvement of plasma cells in the bone marrow (Chapter 25) plus one or more of the following: M spike or band in serum, M spike or band in urine as discussed later, and/or osteolytic lesions on skeletal radiographs (Mangan, 2005).

2. Sometimes the elderly have a monoclonal pattern that appears to be more the result of the aging process than of a specific disease, but some clients who show a monoclonal pattern may eventually have multiple myeloma. In fact, those with monoclonal gammopathy of undetermined significance (MGUS) do have a rate of progression to multiple myeloma or a related malignancy of about 1% a year. Thus, a client who has MGUS will be followed up for long term as the progression rate does not decrease with time (Kyle et al., 2006).

3. Macroglobulinemia, an increase in IgM, is characterized by an increase in only one type of immunoglobulin.

4. Malignant lymphomas and amyloidosis may cause an increase in only one type of immunoglobulin.

Aclonal Patterns

In aclonal patterns, or hypogammopathies, some of the γ-globulins are absent or markedly decreased.

1. The lack of γ-globulins may be congenital. Infants with an aclonal pattern may appear to have a normal pattern at birth because of the presence of immunoglobulins from the mother. But then frequent and severe infections begin to occur when the passive immunity from the mother no longer exists.

2. Acquired hypogammaglobulinemia is most often seen with chronic lympho-cytic leukemia, malignant lymphomas, or other diseases that affect the bone marrow.

3. Drugs, such as corticosteroids and cytotoxic drugs used for treatment of malig-nant tumors, may reduce γ-globulin levels or at least make the γ-globulins inef-fective.

4. Radiation therapy and toxins in the environment can produce an acquired lack of γ-globulins.

Possible Nursing Diagnoses Related to Abnormal Gamma Globulins

High Risk for Infection Related to Ineffective Immune Response

A person with either fewer γ-globulins or abnormal γ-globulins is susceptible to diseases caused by opportunistic pathogens. Bacterial pneumonia is often the cause of death. The client must be protected from others who have upper respiratory infections. Sometimes it may be necessary to initiate reverse isolation to protect the client, particularly infants who have a severe immunodeficiency disorder. With older clients, meticulous handwashing is most important, because reverse isolation, with its extra cost, still does not protect people from the bacteria on their own skin or from the bacteria in food. An effort should be made to keep the environment relatively free of pathogens. Because the main defense against invading organisms is intact skin and mucous membranes, the nurse must promote good skin care. Proper nutrition with adequate protein is important for the production of immu-noglobulins and lymphocytes. (See the discussion on albumin for ways to ensure adequate protein intake.)

Risk for Injury Related to Infusions of Gamma Globulins

γ-Globulin may be administered to increase immunoglobulin levels temporarily. Immune serum globulin may prevent serious infection if circulatory levels of IgG (discussed next) are kept at about 200 mg/dL. However, immune globulin may not prevent chronic infections of the secretory tissues, such as those of the respiratory tract. The γ-globulin may be needed every 3–4 weeks. Although immune globulin is generally safe, it can cause allergic reac-tions, increased viscosity of the blood, or renal failure. Premedication with diphenhydramine, acetaminophen, or methylprednisolone may be used to reduce the risk of allergic reaction (Rosenthal, 2006). After an infusion is completed, the client should be kept well hydrated and urine output should be monitored.

Deficient Knowledge Related to Technical Aspects of Therapy

In addition to the replacement of normal γ-globulins, there may also be an attempt to remove abnormal proteins from the bloodstream by pheresis. Pheresis is the process by which a spe-cific plasma constituent is separated from other blood constituents and removed from the client's plasma. If the client has an excessive amount of abnormal IgM (see the discussion on macroglobulinemia), this protein can be filtered out of the blood by the pheresis machine. Another therapeutic alternative is bone marrow transplantation (Hay et al., 2011).

IMMUNOELECTROPHORESIS AND QUANTIFICATION OF SERUM PROTEINS: IgG, IgA, IgM, IgD AND IgE, AND FREE LIGHT CHAINS

Immunoglobulins are defined as proteins of animal origin that are endowed with known antibody activity. Although there are only five main groups of immuno-globulins (IgG, IgA, IgM, IgD, and IgE), 40 or more fractions can be differentiated by researchers. This discussion is limited to general knowledge about the five main types of immunoglobulins.

Preparation of Client and Collection of Sample

A fresh sample is the sample of choice, but aged serum or plasma can be used. Depending on the technique, only 1 mL of blood may be needed. Any blood transfusions or blood component therapy within the past 6 weeks, as well as any immunizations or vaccines within the past 6 months, should be recorded on the laboratory requisition.

REFERENCE VALUES FOR IMMUNOGLOBULINS		
Adult	IgG	639–1,349 mg/dL (usually about 75% of total)
	IgA	70–312 mg/dL (10–15%)
	IgM	56–352 mg/dL (7–10%)
	IgD	0.5–3.0 mg/dL (<1%)
	IgE	0.01–0.04 mg/dL (<1%)
Newborn	IgG	640–1,250 mg/dL
	IgA	0–11 mg/dL
	IgM	5–30 mg/dL
	IgD	—
	IgE	—
Children	Depends on age; by 6 months to 1 year of age, levels begin to gradually increase; adult values may be reached by late teens	
Pregnant women	Evidently IgE falls somewhat during pregnancy, but the others show no significant change	
Aged	Even healthy older people may show abnormal patterns with increase in paraproteins; in response to a challenge, such as an infection, immunoglobulin production is likely to be reduced or be a less vigorous response	

Changes in Immunoglobulins

IgG

This immunoglobulin, which makes up about three-fourths of the total immuno-globulins, is the only one that crosses the placenta. Hence, infants have a high level, which shows a decrease until about 6 months to 1 year, when the infant begins production of IgG.

IgG protects against viruses, bacteria, and toxins. It is more for a secondary response. Thus, specific IgG antibodies against infections such as hepatitis or rubella indicate past exposure and probable immunity (see Chapter 14). In the newborn, IgG levels indicate passive immunity. A lack of IgG causes severe immunodeficiency. Injections of immune serum globulin contain primarily IgG.

IgA

The second most common immunoglobulin in the bloodstream, IgA is also present in other fluids and in surface secretions, such as saliva, tears, and colostrum. These immunoglobulins are thought to be the first line of defense against organisms invading the respiratory, gastrointestinal, and urinary tracts. The infant begins producing IgA after a few months. Deficiencies of IgA may be combined with other deficiencies or may occur alone.

IgM

Present in the bloodstream in slightly lower levels than IgA, IgM does not cross the placenta, but the infant begins synthesizing IgM sooner than IgA. IgM is the most important component in a primary immune response. IgM antibodies are indicators of an active infection. IgM activates the complement system, its level remaining high as long as the antigen is present. The antibodies to blood group antigens are in the group of IgM immunoglobulins. (See Chapter 14 for discussion of IgM antibodies for hepatitis and rubella.)

Because IgM has a high molecular weight, abnormal increases are called *macroglobulinemia*. These immunoglobulins tend to make the blood highly viscous. Normal viscosity of blood is 1.4–1.8 compared with the viscosity of water. The increase in macroglobulins also makes the client very sensitive to cold. As discussed earlier, pheresis therapy may be used to remove abnormal immunoglobulins.

IgD

This immunoglobulin is present in the bloodstream in very small amounts and may increase in IgD myeloma or with some central nervous system tumors.

IgE

IgE, which is present in the bloodstream in very small amounts, increases in allergic states and in the event of parasitic infestation. Evidently, IgE is responsible for severe hypersensitivity reactions. A measurement of specific IgE antibodies in the serum helps establish the diagnosis of allergic disease by identifying which allergens are causing clinical symptoms such as hay fever, asthma, or skin rashes. An allergen-specific IgE antibody test is sometimes called the radioallergosorbent test (RAST).

Free Light Chains

Immunoglobulins produced by the plasma cells include the heavy chains—G, A, M, D, and E, discussed earlier—and the light chains called kappa (κ) and lamda (λ). Most of these light chains are attached to the heavy chains, but some unattached light chains are found in healthy people. Certain diseases such as different types of myelomas cause an increase in the free light chains in the serum, urine, and cerebral spinal fluid.

URINE PROTEIN ELECTROPHORESIS AND IMMUNOELECTROPHORESIS

The techniques of electrophoresis and immunoelectrophoresis (IEP) of urine are similar to those of serum testing. If an abnormal amount of protein is detected in the urine, these tests can identify exactly which kinds of proteins are being excreted. (See Chapter 3 for the screening technique for proteinuria.) Normally, a 24-hour urine has a protein content of about 40–150 mg, with no more than 10 mg in a random specimen. The dipstick used for screening registers 1+ when there are about 30 mg in the specimen; less than 30 mg causes a trace showing.

The dipstick method of screening for proteinuria tests for albumin, so a dipstick for protein is not reliable as a screening test for proteins other than albumin. The laboratory uses other methods to screen for abnormal proteins, such as Bence Jones protein, which may occur with multiple myeloma. Bence Jones protein in the urine is now called light-chain disease. Light chains are the polypeptide chains that compose immunoglobulins.

REFERENCE VALUES FOR URINE PROTEIN ELECTROPHORESIS

Three main types of pathologic patterns may be identified by separating the protein fractions in urine.

1. There may be a marked increase in the albumin fraction and some increase in α- and β-globulins. This signifies increased glomerular permeability such as that seen in some renal diseases and in eclampsia.

2. There may be a marked increase in α- and β-globulins with a decrease in albumin, most likely signifying tubular damage.

3. There may be various abnormal proteins or paraproteins, such as those found in multiple myeloma or in other disorders of the γ-globulins. This finding is considered a prerenal pattern. Just as in the serum, quantitative assay and, if needed, immunofixation electrophoresis can be used to identify exactly which globulins are present.

SERUM AMMONIA

The liver normally converts ammonia (NH_3), a byproduct of protein metabolism, into urea, which is excreted by the kidneys. When the liver is unable to convert ammonia to urea, toxic levels of ammonia accumulate in the bloodstream. In severe liver failure, the blood urea nitrogen (BUN) decreases as the ammonia level increases. (See Chapter 4 on the use of the BUN as a test for renal function.)

Preparation of Client and Collection of Sample

Some laboratories may require a fasting state; water is allowed. One milliliter of either venous or arterial blood can be used. The blood is put into a heparinized tube (green-topped vacuum tube) and packed in ice for transport to the laboratory. The specimen is stable for about 20 minutes. If the client is on antibiotics (such as neomycin) for treatment of hepatic coma, record this fact on the laboratory slip.

REFERENCE VALUES FOR SERUM AMMONIA	
Adult	35–65 µg/dL
Newborn	90–150 µg/dL
Children	45–80 µg/dL

Note: Values may vary considerably from laboratory to laboratory.

Increased Ammonia Level

Clinical Significance

Increased ammonia levels, which occur in liver dysfunction, may be due either to blood not circulating through the liver well or to actual hepatic failure. Clients with cirrhosis who have portacaval shunts performed to relieve portal hypertension may have increased ammonia levels after the operation because blood is shunted away from the liver. Reye's syndrome, which sometimes occurs with viral infections, leads to elevated ammonia levels. The number of reported cases of Reye's syndrome has decreased in the past few years, perhaps because salicylates are no longer given to young children who have viral infections (Hay et al., 2011). (See www.reyessyndrome.org for more information on the detection and treatment of Reye's syndrome.)

Possible Nursing Diagnoses Related to Increased Ammonia Levels

Risk for Injury Related to Disturbed Sensory Perception

Although high levels of ammonia occur in hepatic coma (hepatic encephalopathy), the ammonia is not the only factor that causes the neurologic symptoms. Because of a lack of relationship between the plasma levels of ammonia and the clinical degree of hepatic encephalopathy, routine use of serum ammonia levels for monitoring severity is no longer done (Wu, 2006). Most likely, many toxins in hepatic failure cause the symptoms of disorientation and tremors seen in hepatic encephalopathy. Increased intracranial pressure may accompany severe liver failure, and a bioartificial liver may help bring down serum ammonia levels and other toxins until a transplant is possible. The client should be checked for a certain kind of tremor of the hand called liver flap or asterixis (which can also be caused by high levels of uremia or other central nervous system toxins). Ask the client to extend his or her arms out in front of the body, spread the fingers, and hold the hands in a dorsiflexed position. Clients who have a high level of ammonia in their blood and in whom hepatic encephalopathy is developing cannot hold their palms up in a steady manner. The hands flap. Asking the client to write his or her name or to draw a star is another way to assess the neurologic dysfunction. The nurse may often be the first one to notice subtle changes in the client's ability to perform simple tasks that require coordination and mental alertness. The lack of mental alertness and coordination may progress to a coma unless treatment is begun. Renal failure (see Chapter 4) is often associated with liver failure. The development of hepatorenal syndrome carries a poor prognosis unless a liver transplant is feasible (McPhee, Papadakis, & Rabow, 2011).

Imbalanced Nutrition Related to Need to Reduce Sources of Ammonia from Protein Breakdown

Because an increased serum ammonia level indicates an inability of the liver to handle the breakdown of protein, the client should have limited protein intake until the ammonia level returns to normal. An enteral amino acid formula may be used to prevent muscle breakdown. If the patient in hepatic failure has gastrointestinal bleeding, the progression to hepatic coma accelerates because ammonia is produced when the blood proteins in the intestine are digested. Gastric lavage may be needed to get as much of the blood out of the gastrointestinal tract as possible. Because intestinal bacteria produce ammonia by breaking down protein, the amount of bacteria may be reduced with administration of neomycin, a nonsystemic antibiotic, which may be given orally or by means of enemas.

When the ammonia level returns to normal, protein is cautiously put back into the diet in increasing amounts. The diet may be limited to no more than 0.6 g of animal protein per kilogram of body weight. (See Table 10–4 for a list of the protein content of foods.) As the protein level in the diet is increased, the nurse must watch carefully for any signs of hepatic encephalopathy. Lactulose, an ammonia detoxicant, may be given orally or rectally to help reduce ammonia levels. Because lactulose inhibits the diffusion of ammonia from the gut to the bloodstream, the drug is used to both treat and prevent hepatic encephalopathy. The dose should be adjusted until the client has 2–3 soft bowel movements daily (Deglin, Vallerand, & Sanoski, 2011). Oral lactulose may be continued as long-term treatment.

Risk for Injury Related to Use of Sedatives and Diuretics

In addition to the amount of protein in the diet, other factors that contribute to the development of hepatic coma include hypokalemia and the use of sedatives and opioids. The body is less able to handle ammonia when the potassium level is low or when alkalosis is present. Thus, diuretic therapy (which often causes potassium loss) may be contraindicated when the client has an increased ammonia level. In addition, the failing liver is unable to detoxify many drugs, including sedatives and opioids. When a client has an increased ammonia level, all previous medication orders need to be reevaluated to see if they are still appropriate in respect to the change in the client's condition.

TUMOR MARKERS

Tumor markers are substances associated with malignant growths. (See Table 10–5.) An example already discussed was the paraprotein found in the serum or urine of clients with multiple myeloma. Hormones, such as human chorionic gonadotropin (HCG) (Chapter 15), are sometimes tumor markers. The appearance of fetal proteins such as carcinoembyronic antigen (CEA) or α-fetoprotein (AFP) in some types of malignant tumors in adults gives support to the theory that cancer somehow arises from very primitive cells. The oncofetal antigens discussed later in this chapter have been used to assess some tumors. Other tumor antigens or proteins are designated simply by numbers such as CA 125, CA 15-3, or CA 19-9. A more tissue specific antigen, such as prostate-specific antigen (PSA), is also a tumor marker. Researchers are continuing to refine the specificity and sensitivity of these tests so they can be even more useful as screening tests and for evaluating treatment outcomes.

Table 10–5 Examples of Tumor Markers

Type of Tumor Marker	Examples of Malignancies
Specific proteins	
Beta-2-microglobulin	Multiple myeloma
HER-2/neu	Breast cancer
Immunoglobulins	Multiple myeloma[a]
Prostate-specific antigen (PSA)	Prostate cancer
Bladder tumor antigen	Bladder cancer
NMP22	Monitor bladder cancer
Tissue polypeptide antigen (TPA)	Many types of cancer
Oncofetal antigens	
α-fetoprotein[b]	Liver and testicular cancer
CEA	Colon, stomach, and other cancers
	Metastatic breast cancer
Glycoproteins	
CA 125	Ovarian cancer
CA 15-3 and CA 27.29	Breast, lung, and ovarian cancer
CA 19-9	Pancreas and biliary tract cancer
Hormones	
Human chorionic gonadotropin (HCG)	Trophoblastic tumors (Chapter 18)
	Testicular cancer
Calcitonin	Medullary cancer of thyroid (Chapter 15)
Catecholamines	Pheochromocytomas (Chapter 15)
Thyroglobulin	Some forms of thyroid cancer (Chapter 15)
Estrogen receptors	Breast cancer (Chapter 15)
Progesterone receptors	Breast cancer (Chapter 15)
Chromogranin A	Neuroendocrine tumors (Chapter 15)
Enzymes	
Acid phosphatase or prostatic acid phosphatase (PAP)	Prostate cancer (Chapter 12)
ALP (SGPT)	Bone metastasis (Chapter 12)
LDH	Non-Hodgkin's lymphoma, testicular cancer, and other cancers (Chapter 12)

[a]All tumor markers discussed in this chapter unless another site specified.

[b]See Chapter 18 for another use of α-fetoprotein.

Note: For more details on tumor markers, see *www.labtestsonline.org* and *www.cancer.org*.

ALPHA-FETOPROTEIN

Normally this globulin, formed only in the yolk sac and liver of the fetus, disappears from the bloodstream after birth, except for trace amounts. The test for AFP is performed on amniotic fluid to detect specific congenital defects (see Chapter 28) and on the serum of pregnant women and other adults to detect pathologic conditions.

The serum AFP, recommended since 1985, has the distinction of being the first maternal serum test to screen for a genetic defect in the fetus. In the fetus, if the neural tube fails to close properly, enormous amounts of fetal protein leak into the amniotic fluid throughout the pregnancy. In the pregnant woman, levels greater than the usual reference values for a particular gestational age may indicate a neural tube defect in the fetus. The AFP is also used with two other tests, estriol and HCG, to assess for Down syndrome. (See Chapter 18 for the discussion of these three tests.)

In a nonpregnant woman, a markedly increased AFP level is associated with primary carcinoma (hepatoma) of the liver and some types of testicular cancer. Metastatic cancer of the liver does not cause such a rise. Very small amounts of AFP are present in some nonmalignant liver diseases in children and adults. Clients with cirrhosis and those who are carriers of hepatitis B or C (Chapter 14) are at greater risk for liver cancer. These clients may have periodic screens with AFP and ultrasound (Chapter 23) to detect tumors that may still be amenable to treatment (McPhee et al., 2011).

Preparation of Client and Collection of Sample

There is no special preparation of the client for a serum sample. The laboratory needs 1 mL of clotted blood.

REFERENCE VALUES FOR AFP	
Men and nonpregnant women	<12.8 IU/mL
Pregnant women	Serum levels increase during pregnancy (see Chapter 18)

BETA-2-MICROGLOBULIN

Beta-2-microglobulin (B2M) is a light chain protein found on cell wells, especially lymphocytes. Multiple myelomas, chronic lymphocytic leukemia, and some lymphomas cause an increase in B2M. As elevated levels of B2M correlate with more aggressive tumors, the test is used to predict prognosis after treatments (Mangan, 2005). Hepatitis and chronic inflammations such as Crohn's disease also cause elevations.

In addition to being a tumor marker to predict prognosis after treatment for certain malignancies, B2M can also be used to evaluate renal function because the protein is excreted by the glomeruli and partially reabsorbed into the bloodstream by the tubules. Glomerular damage causes an increase in B2M in the blood level and a decrease in the urine, while tubular disease causes low blood levels and high urine levels. Also, blood levels of B2M become high when a kidney transplant is failing.

Preparation of Client and Collection of Sample

An overnight fast is preferred. Serum is used. Requests other than for predicting the prognosis in multiple myeloma may require special approval.

REFERENCE VALUES FOR BETA-2-MICROGLOBULIN	
Neonates	0.30 mg/dL
Adult	0.19 mg/dL
Aged	0.21–0.24 mg/dL
References are from Wu (2006).	

CARCINOEMBRYONIC ANTIGEN

Carcinoembryonic antigen (CEA), a glycoprotein that circulates at a high level during fetal life, is detectable in only tiny amounts in the blood of healthy adults. CEA is elevated in malignant tumors, such as colonic cancer and metastatic breast disease. Most clients with colonic cancer have elevated CEA levels. Although CEA may be used as part of a diagnostic evaluation for cancer of the colon, it is most useful as a marker to determine the effectiveness of treatment. For example, CEA levels usually return to normal about 6 weeks after a malignant tumor of the colon is surgically removed. CEA is helpful but not conclusive and is thus of little value in a diagnostic evaluation for cancer of the colon because (1) not all people with cancer of the colon show elevated CEA levels and (2) several conditions other than colonic cancer may cause elevated CEA levels. Other conditions that cause elevated CEA levels are heavy cigarette smoking, cirrhosis, ulcerative colitis, diverticulitis, rectal polyps, peptic ulcer disease, pancreatitis, and many malignant tumors.

Preparation of Client and Collection of Sample

Venous blood is collected in a lavender-topped tube. The specimen must be sent on ice.

REFERENCE VALUE FOR CEA

0–3.4 ng/mL

Note: Smokers may have values as high as 5.0 ng/mL or even higher.

CA 125 ANTIGEN

Like other tests discussed in this section, CA 125 is a tumor marker. CA 125 antigen is not specific enough to be used to screen healthy clients for ovarian cancer. Research has not supported the use of this test as a general screening test for women because of so many false-positive results (Lockwood-Rayermann et al., 2009). Women at high risk for this disease because of a history of ovarian cancer in the family may undergo the test and intra-abdominal or transvaginal ultrasonography on a routine basis. Additionally, women who have unexplained symptoms of bloating and pelvic or abdominal pain may also be evaluated with these tests. The test is used to follow clients once they have been diagnosed as having ovarian cancer. As many as 90% of clients with persistent CA 125 elevations after surgical intervention do have residual tumor.

For asymptomatic women, CA 125 is not very sensitive ((50% abnormal for stage I ovarian cancer) or specific as it may be elevated in a number of other conditions. The addition of transvaginal ultrasound (Chapter 23) improves the predictive value somewhat, but this is still not an effective way to screen all women. The ultrasound will differentiate between cysts and tumors but not between benign and malignant tumors. The use of color Doppler imaging (Chapter 23) may enhance the specificity of ultrasound. Once an ovarian mass is detected, the use of CA 125 levels determines the next step, but unfortunately it is elevated in only 50% of women with early cancer (McPhee et al., 2011). Nurses should be aware of current research in this area and the variety of resources available from ovarian cancer advocacy groups. Researchers are looking at the MUC16 gene that encodes the CA 125 molecule. An understanding of MUC16 may be helpful to develop new assays and improve the sensitivity and specificity of CA 125 (McLemore & Aouizerat, 2005).

Nurses need to help educate women about ovarian cancer as research has shown a low awareness of the symptoms of ovarian cancer and the risk factors for the disease (Lockwood-Rayermann et al., 2009).

Preparation of Client and Collection of Sample

One milliliter of serum is needed in a serum separator tube (SST).

REFERENCE VALUE FOR CA 125

<35 U/mL

CA 15-3 AND CA 27.29

CA 15-3 is a breast cancer–associated antigen. Higher serum levels are often found in clients with breast cancer metastasis, especially at multiple sites or to bone. Both CA 15-3 and CA 27.29, another test that measures the same breast tumor antigen, are used as markers for recurrent breast cancer as they begin to rise before clinical evidence of a relapse.

REFERENCE VALUE FOR CA 15-3

0–30 U/mL

REFERENCE VALUE FOR CA 27.29

0–38 U/mL

HER-2/neu

Human epidermal growth factor receptor 2 (HER-2/neu), a protein expressed in normal epithelial cells, is overexpressed in certain types of tumors. This factor can be measured in breast tissue and in the serum (Wu, 2006). Estrogen and progesterone receptors may also be measured in the breast tissue sample (Chapter 15) as all three tests help with treatment decisions. Breast cancers that display overexpression of HER-2/neu may be given a monoclonal antibody, trastuzumab, to inhibit the expression of the growth factor (Deglin et al., 2011). Serum levels, if elevated, may be used to check if the level drops with therapy.

CA 19-9

CA 19-9 is a tumor antigen used to help evaluate the outcome of therapy for malignancies of the pancreas or biliary tract. Like most other tumor markers, the test is not sensitive enough for early detection (McPhee et al., 2011), but it may be used to follow colon cancer when the CEA is not elevated.

REFERENCE VALUE FOR CA 19-9

0–37 U/mL

PROSTATE-SPECIFIC ANTIGEN

Unlike the other tumor markers, PSA, introduced in 1987, is relatively specific for both benign and malignant prostate epithelium. For men with symptoms, the PSA and the digital rectal examination are commonly used for diagnostic purposes and as follow-up assessment after therapy. PSA testing is now recommended with and without the digital rectal exam. But the current focus is on informed decision making, and not just informed consent, so that the client understands both the benefits and the risks of being tested. Controversy exists over whether early diagnosis is useful because early treatment may have no added benefit for some very slow growing tumors, and evidence is lacking on what is the best treatment for early-stage disease. Another concern is the rate of false-positive results that lead to unnecessary follow-up tests with the associated anxiety and cost. Transrectal ultrasound (Chapter 23) may be used as a follow-up but is not recommended for first-line screening.

Research by Concato et al. (2006) suggested that widespread screening with PSA is not effective in reducing mortality. However, many physicians do support the use of PSA in men above 50 (Barry, 2006). Men age 50 or above, who have at least a 10-year life expectancy, may be offered a yearly digital rectal exam (DRE) and a PSA. African-American men and those having a first-degree relative with prostate cancer before age 65 may be offered the test, beginning at age 45 or even at 40 (Ficorelli & Weeks, 2006). In 2009, two studies for PSA screening found only a slight benefit and possible harm, so wide-scale testing remains controversial (McPhee et al., 2011).

Treatment of localized prostate cancer may include prostatectomy, radiation, insertion of radioactive seeds, hormone therapy, or watchful waiting in older men. "Watchful waiting" may now be called active surveillance. The Prostate Cancer Foundation (www.pcf.org) offers the latest diagnostic and treatment options.

Preparation of Client and Collection of Sample

Collect serum in red-topped tube. Fasting specimen is preferred. May be elevated after rectal exams. Finasteride or other drugs or herbs such as saw palmetto that are used to treat an enlarged prostate may affect PSA levels.

REFERENCE VALUES FOR PSA

Men[a]

	40–49	<2.5 mg/dL
	50–59	<3.5 mg/dL
	60–69	<4.5 mg/dL
	70–79	<6.5 mg/dL
	After prostatectomy	0–0.5 mg/dL
Women[b]		0–0.5 mg/dL

[a]Age-specific values need to be validated in larger populations and in various ethnic groups (McPhee et al., 2011).

[b]Small amounts of PSA may arrive from other tissues such as breast tissue. PSA may be elevated in breast cancer.

FREE PSA

Elevated levels of PSA do not always signify cancer because benign prostate hyperplasia and other conditions may cause an elevation. Measuring the free amount of PSA may help determine a likely benign condition. Studies have shown that PSA exists in a form bound by α-1-antichymotrypsin and in an unbound or free state.

The free PSA tends to be lower in men with prostate cancer than in those with benign disease, so an elevated PSA with a low amount of free PSA is more likely to signify a malignancy than an elevated PSA with a high free PSA. Use of the free PSA may reduce unnecessary biopsies for clients who have a modest rise in the total PSA and whose prostate appears palpably benign.

REFERENCE VALUE FOR FREE PSA

Expressed as a percentage of the total amount.

Clinical Significance of Low Free PSA

A biopsy may be recommended for a client who has a total PSA between 4.0 and 10.0 ng/mL and a free PSA of 25% or less. McPhee et al. (2011) found that using 25% as a cutoff detected 95% of cancers while avoiding 20% of unnecessary biopsies in clients whose prostate glands were palpably benign.

BLADDER TUMOR–ASSOCIATED ANTIGEN TEST

In the past, clients with bladder cancer had repeat cystoscopies (Chapter 27) and/or urine cytology because reoccurrence is very common. Now a urine test that uses monoclonal antibodies can detect the presence of a bladder tumor–associated antigen (BTA). The test should not be used for screening or for diagnosis but may be useful for individuals who need surveillance for biopsy-confirmed bladder cancer. The test requires five drops of urine and results are ready in 5 minutes. In addition to use in a clinic, the test may also be prescribed for home use. (This is the first tumor marker cleared for home use.)

NMP22

Like the BTA discussed earlier, NMP22 is a tumor marker found in the urine of clients with bladder cancer and is used to monitor recurrences. It is not widely used at the present time.

Possible Nursing Diagnosis Related to Elevation of Tumor Markers

Risk for Ineffective Coping Related to Severity of Malignant Condition and Possible Need for More Treatment

Persistent or rising levels of a tumor marker indicate that the tumor is still active and prognosis is thus less favorable than if the levels remain normal. Additional treatments may be needed, and the client and family may need help in coping with the less-than-favorable news from the physician. Nurses often help clients deal with unpleasant news and can be very effective in helping clients use their coping skills.

TESTS FOR CANCER USING PROTEOMICS AND GENOMICS

The American Cancer Society (www.cancer.org) has updates on many types of tests for cancer. *Proteomics* looks at the pattern of many proteins in the blood rather than the single proteins discussed earlier. Patterns of proteins in ovarian cancer, as discussed earlier, and rectal cancer (Chapter 13) are current examples of research in this area. *Genomics* looks at patterns of changes in the DNA of cancer cells. Tests may use samples from blood, stool, or urine.

GENETIC SCREENING FOR CANCER: BRCA1 AND BRCA2

The mapping of the human genome has led to rapid advances in identifying many genes that make a person *susceptible* to a specific disease. This is different than genes that are definite causes such as those discussed in Chapter 18. This predisposition to a disease is not 100% because other factors, most of which are not known, must be present to have the disease develop. For example, mutation of BRCA1 or BRCA2 makes a person more susceptible to breast and ovarian cancer. Carriers of a BRCA1 mutation are thought to have a 50–85% lifetime risk for breast cancer and a 20–40% lifetime risk for ovarian cancer. A mutation of BRCA2 carries about the same risk for breast cancer and a 10–20% risk for ovarian cancer. Another breast cancer gene, CHK2, is located on chromosome 22. Those who have a mutation are also at risk of breast cancer, but the BRCA mutations are the ones linked to a significant risk. The U.S. Preventive Services Task Force (2005) recommends against routine testing for genetic risk of breast or ovarian cancer in the general population. This was the first time the Task Force addressed the issues of DNA-based genetic testing. Women who have a family history should be referred for genetic counseling and evaluation for BRCA testing. See Chapter 20 for information on mammograms and MRI (Chapter 21) for high-risk clients.

Genetic Screening Hereditary Non-polyposis Colon Cancer

Hereditary Non-polyposis Colon Cancer (HNPCC) accounts for 5–10% of all colorectal cancers. Causative genes are transmitted through an autosomal dominant pattern. In addition, women are more susceptible to uterine and ovarian cancer. Nurses need to be aware that potetial carriers of HNPCC will seek genetic testing only if they are aware of the risk (Razmus, Jackson, & Wilson, 2008). Clients who do have the HNPCC gene may have a colonoscopy every 1–2 years beginning at age 25 or 5 years younger than a family member who had the cancer (McPhee et al., 2011).

As these tests and others become more readily available, nurses must be aware of the psychological, medical, ethical, and legal implications of tests that may predict cancer.

Nurses are involved in obtaining family histories to track cases of cancer, giving psychosocial support to clients undergoing genetic screening for cancer, and maintaining records that ensure privacy. See Chapter 18 for more discussion on other types of genetic screening and the role of the nurse in keeping up-to-date on this relatively new area of nursing. The reader is encouraged to search the current literature for more on the impact of genomics on nursing practice.

Questions

1. A young woman is caring for her sister who has advanced ovarian cancer. She asks the home care nurse the name of the test being used to monitor her sister's response to treatment. The nurse explains that the test is
   a. CA 15-3
   b. PSA
   c. CEA
   d. CA 125

2. Which of the following is the only clinical condition that creates an elevated serum albumin level?
   a. Early liver dysfunction
   b. Increased protein intake over a long period
   c. Dehydration
   d. Kwashiorkor

3. A nursing diagnosis of altered nutrition related to hypoalbuminemia would be most likely for
   a. A client who is in her last trimester of pregnancy and is expecting twins
   b. A client, aged 6, who has severe asthma
   c. A client who has advanced cirrhosis
   d. A client, aged 17, who has been on a very restricted diet (only juices) for the past 8 days

4. Which of the following is the most important clinical manifestation of a lowered serum albumin level?
   a. Decreased susceptibility to infection
   b. Edema
   c. Loss of weight
   d. Tendency to bleed

5. A client is receiving a 25% solution of albumin intravenously because his serum albumin level was 2 g/dL. Which of the following nursing actions is appropriate?
   a. Infuse the solution as quickly as possible
   b. Observe the client frequently for possible circulatory overload
   c. Tell the client that he will probably have decreased urination over the next several hours
   d. Keep the albumin refrigerated until 30 minutes before it is hung

6. For a client who can tolerate oral feedings, the most efficient and economical way to increase protein is to do which of the following?
   a. Use commercially prepared protein mixtures or powders
   b. Add extra tablespoons of powdered milk to foods and beverages
   c. Increase meat consumption
   d. Reduce carbohydrate intake so the person can eat more protein

7. Which of the following is the principal nursing diagnosis for a client who is deficient in α-1-antitrypsin?
   a. Risk for injury related to smoking
   b. Knowledge deficit related to dietary changes
   c. Altered cardiac output related to fluid volume excess
   d. Impaired skin integrity related to edema

8. Which of these clients is the least likely to have low levels of immunoglobulins? A client who is
   a. A premature infant born yesterday
   b. 6 months pregnant and has diabetes
   c. Undergoing corticosteroid therapy and is malnourished
   d. Eighty-five years of age and has been admitted because of a malignant tumor

9. Which of the following is the single most important nursing diagnosis in caring for any client with an abnormal γ-globulin pattern?
   a. Fluid volume deficit
   b. Fluid volume excess
   c. High risk for infection
   d. Impaired skin integrity

10. Which immunoglobulin crosses the placenta and provides immunity for the newborn for several months?
    a. IgG
    b. IgA
    c. IgM
    d. IgD

11. The radioallergosorbent test (RAST) is useful for which of the following?
    a. To measure all types of immunoglobulins in the serum
    b. To differentiate between cellular and humoral immunity
    c. To measure the quantity of antigen-specific IgE antibodies in the serum that increase in immediate allergic reactions
    d. To discriminate the globulins of high molecular weight macroglobulin from other globulins

12. A client with cirrhosis has an ammonia level greater than 100 µg/100 mL. He states he wants "something to eat." Which breakfast would be appropriate for the client this morning?
   a. Eggs, toast, jelly, and coffee
   b. Grapefruit juice, cereal, and a glass of milk
   c. Orange juice and sliced banana
   d. Pancakes, syrup, butter, and coffee

13. In a nonpregnant state, what might the continuing presence of large amounts of α-fetoprotein in the serum indicate?
   a. Infertility
   b. Lack of adult proteins
   c. Congenital enzyme defect
   d. Malignant tumor of liver

References

Barry, M. (2006). The PSA conundrum. *Archives of Internal Medicine, 166*, 7–8.

Concato, J., Wells, C. K., Horwitz, R. I., Penson, D., Fincke, G., Berlowitz, D. R., et al. (2006). The effectiveness of screening for prostate cancer. *Archives of Internal Medicine, 166*, 38–43.

Deglin, J. H., Vallerand, A. H., & Sanoski, C. A. (2011). *Davis's drug guide for nurses* (12th ed.). Philadelphia: F. A. Davis.

DiMaria-Ghalili, R. A. & Amella, E. (2005). Nutrition in older adults. *American Journal of Nursing, 105*(3), 40–51.

Ficorelli, C. T. & Weeks, B. (2006). Facing up to prostate cancer. *Nursing 2006, 36*(5), 66–68.

Hay, W. W., Levin, M. J., Sondheimer, J. M., & Deterding, R. (Eds.). (2011). *Current diagnosis and treatmen: Pediatrics* (20th ed.). New York: McGraw-Hill.

Katzung, B., Masters, S. B. & Trevor, A. J. (Ed.). (2009). *Basic and clinical pharmacology* (11th ed.). New York: McGraw-Hill.

Kuszajewski, M. L. & Clontz, A. S. (2005). Prealbumin is best for nutritional monitoring. *Nursing 2005, 35*(3), 70–71.

Kyle, R. A., Therneau, T. M., Rajkumar, S. V., Larson, D. R., Plevak, M. F., Offord, J. R., et al. (2006). Prevalence of monoclonal gammopathy of undetermined significance. *New England Journal of Medicine, 354*, 1362–1369.

Lee, L. & Grap, M. J. (2008). Care and management of the patient with ascites. *MEDSURG Nursing, 17*(6), 376–381.

Lockwood-Rayermann, S., Donovan, H. S., Rambo, D., & Kuo, C. J. (2009). Women's awareness of ovarian cancer risks and symptoms. *American Journal of Nursing, 109*(9), 36–45.

Mangan, P. (2005). Recognizing multiple myelomas. *Nurse Practitioner, 30*(3), 14–27.

McLemore, M. R. & Aouizerat, B. (2005). Introducing the MUC16 gene: Implications for prevention and early detection in epithelial ovarian cancer. *Biological Research in Nursing, 6*(4), 262–267.

McPhee, S. J., Papadakis, M. A., & Rabow, C. A. (Eds.). (2011). *Current medical diagnosis and treatment* (50th ed.). New York: McGraw-Hill.

Mulden C. (2009). Prealbumin testing for early malnutrition detection. *American Nurse Today, 4*(9), 44.

Razmus, I., Jackson, J., & Wilson, D. (2008). Hereditary non-polyposis colon cancer: Change the name to protect the innocent. *MEDSURG Nursing, 17*(6), 400–404.

Rosenthal, K. (2006). Administering immune globulin. *Nursing 2006, 36*(3), 20–21.

U.S. Preventive Services Task Force. (2005). Genetic risk assessment and BRCA mutation testing for breast and ovarian cancer susceptibility: Recommendation statement. *Archives of Internal Medicine, 143*, 355–361.

Wu, A. H. (Ed.). (2006). *Tietz clinical guide to laboratory tests* (4th ed.). St. Louis, MO: Saunders Elsevier.

Websites

www.alpha1.org (Alpha-1 Association for updates on alpha-1-antitrypsin deficiency.)
www.cancer.org (American Cancer Society for updates on tumor markers.)
www.jointcommission.org (Joint Commission for Standards for nutritional support.)
www.labtestonline.org (Information on tumor markers.)
www.pcf.org (Prostate Cancer Foundation offers latest updates on diagnostic and treatment options.)
www.reyessyndrome.org (Information on Reye's syndrome and the danger of salicylates for treating fever in those under age 19.)

Answers

1. d, 2. c, 3. c, 4. b, 5. b, 6. b, 7. a, 8. b, 9. c, 10. a, 11. c, 12. c, 13. d

Tests to Measure the Metabolism of Bilirubin

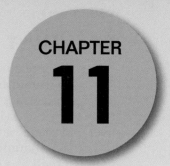

- Pathway of Normal Bilirubin Excretion   258
- Total Bilirubin   259
- Unconjugated (Indirect) Bilirubin   261
- Conjugated (Direct) Bilirubin   262
- Urine Bilirubin   263
- Urine Urobilinogen   264
- Fecal Urobilinogen   265
- Bilirubin in Amniotic Fluid   269
- Transcutaneous Bilirubinometer   269

OBJECTIVES

1. Diagram the normal pathway for bilirubin excretion, and explain the five laboratory tests used as assessment tools.
2. Distinguish between prehepatic, intraheptic, and posthepatic jaundice in regard to causation, symptoms, and changes in laboratory values.
3. Compare and contrast the nursing diagnoses appropriate for elevated unconjugated and conjugated serum bilirubin levels in infants and adults.
4. Describe the role of the nurse in assisting with medical interventions for newborns with markedly elevated serum unconjugated bilirubins (BU).
5. Describe the nurse's role in assisting with medical interventions for clients with elevated serum conjugated bilirubin (BC).
6. Discuss the psychological impact of jaundice on the client and on significant others.
7. Explain the clinical significance of measuring the bilirubin content in amniotic fluid.
8. Describe the usefulness of the transcutaneous bilirubinometer in the care of the newborn.

This chapter begins with a discussion about the normal pathway of bilirubin excretion and differences between the two types of bilirubin, conjugated (BC) and unconjugated (BU). The clinical symptom of any elevated bilirubin is jaundice, but the nursing implications are somewhat different depending on whether the jaundice is prehepatic, posthepatic, or hepatic in origin. This chapter ends with a discussion about general nursing diagnoses for any client with an elevated bilirubin (jaundice), along with more specific implications that depend on the origin of the jaundice.

PATHWAY OF NORMAL BILIRUBIN EXCRETION

When the reticuloendothelial system breaks down old or nonuseful red blood cells (RBCs), bilirubin is one of the waste products. This "free" bilirubin, which is not water soluble, is a lipid-soluble waste product that needs to be made water soluble to be excreted. So it is carried by albumin to the liver, where it is conjugated by the liver and made water soluble. Only water-soluble BC can be excreted in the urine.

The liver handles bilirubin in a way similar to other poorly water soluble compounds, such as steroids, drugs, and toxins. In general, such substances are carried by the plasma proteins (see Chapter 10) to the liver, where they are detached from the protein and converted to a form that can be excreted.

The enzyme glucuronyl transferase is necessary for the transformation, or conjugation, of bilirubin. Either a lack of glucuronyl transferase or the presence of drugs that interfere with this enzyme renders the liver unable to conjugate bilirubin.

Urine, however, is not the most important pathway of excretion for BC, almost all of which is excreted as one of the components of bile salts. In fact, bilirubin, a vivid pigment, gives bile the characteristic bright greenish-yellow color. When the bile salts reach the intestine via the common bile duct, the bilirubin is acted on by bacteria to form chemical compounds called *urobilinogens*. Technically, the breakdown of BC in the intestine produces several other compounds, but the end product that is measured in both urine and feces is labeled *urobilinogen*. These breakdown products give feces their dark color; hence, an absence of bilirubin in the intestine causes clay-colored stools. Most of the urobilinogen is excreted in the feces, but some is reabsorbed and goes through the liver again, and still another small amount is excreted in the urine. Thus, tests for fecal and urine urobilinogens can detect abnormalities in bilirubin excretion.

Because the bilirubin is chemically different after it goes through the conjugation process in the liver, laboratory tests of the serum can differentiate between the bilirubin that is free (prehepatic) and the bilirubin that is conjugated (posthepatic). If the laboratory reports the test results as "direct" or "indirect" bilirubin, these older terms refer to the way the two types react to certain dyes (sometimes referred to as the van den Bergh reaction):

1. The conjugated water-soluble (posthepatic) bilirubin reacts *directly* when dyes are added to the blood specimen.
2. The non-water-soluble, free (prehepatic) bilirubin does not react to the reagents used for the test until alcohol is added to the solution; hence, their measurement is *indirect*.

A newer method of bilirubin measurement can also measure fractions of the serum bilirubin, and the results are listed as *BU* for unconjugated bilirubin and *BC* for conjugated bilirubin. Another less common term is *delta bilirubin,* which refers to a fraction of conjugated bilirubin associated with cholestasis. Delta bilirubin remains elevated longer than other conjugated bilirubin (Wu, 2006). Table 11–1 can be used as a quick summary of how each of the bilirubin tests is related to the normal pathway of bilirubin excretion. Table 11–2 summarizes how each of the five tests of bilirubin is changed in the three types of jaundice (prehepatic, hepatic, and posthepatic).

Table 11-1 Relation of Normal Bilirubin Excretion to the Five Tests Used to Measure Bilirubin Metabolism

Red blood cell breakdown by reticuloendothelial system

↓

Unconjugated bilirubin in bloodstream carried by albumin

→*Test 1*
Serum bilirubin indirect (prehepatic or free) 0.1–1.0 mg/dL

↓

Liver conjugates bilirubin and makes it water soluble

→*Test 2*
Serum bilirubin direct (posthepatic or conjugated) 0.0–0.4 mg/dL

↓

Conjugated bilirubin excreted in bile salts to intestine

↓

Bacteria in intestine break down bilirubin to urobilinogens

Test 4
Urine urobilinogen: Small amount of urobilinogen is absorbed into bloodstream and goes to urine or back to the liver to be excreted again

Test 3
Fecal urobilinogen: Most of the urobilinogens are excreted in feces—40–280 mg/day

Test 5
No bilirubin is normally in urine. It can be detected with Icotest tablets in pathologic conditions.

Note: Total bilirubin measures both unconjugated (BU) and conjugated (BC) bilirubin. See Wu (2006) for a discussion on some of the problems with including delta bilirubin and some unconjugated bilirubin as direct bilirubin.

TOTAL BILIRUBIN

Preparation of Client and Collection of Sample

Most laboratories require the client to fast for 8 hours before the test because a large intake of fat interferes with the chemical testing. The test requires 1 mL of serum. The specimen should be protected from bright light because bilirubin is broken down by exposure to sunlight or to high-intensity artificial light. The test should not be performed for 24 hours after a dye has been used for radiographic studies. For neonatal use, blood is drawn from a heel stick by means of a capillary pipette (see Chapter 1). This "micro" bilirubin measures only totals and is appropriate for the first 10 days of life.

Table 11-2 Changes in Serum Urine and Feces in Three Types of Jaundice

	Unconjugated Serum Bilirubin	Conjugated Serum Bilirubin	Urine Bilirubin	Urine Urobilinogen	Fecal Urobilinogen
Reference values	Average 0.5 mg/dL	Average 0.1 mg/dL	None	0.4–1.0 mg/day	40–280 mg/day
Prehepatic jaundice (hemolytic)	Elevated usually not more than 5 mg in adults—may be > 20 mg in newborns	Normal	None	Up to 10 mg	Up to 1,400 mg
Hepatic jaundice	Elevated—may be 15–20 mg in severe liver failure	Elevations depend on amount of stasis of bile	Elevated if obstruction present	Normal or increased (see text)	Normal or little decrease (see text)
Posthepatic jaundice (obstruction)	Normal in beginning	Elevated—may be 30–40 mg if obstruction complete	Elevated—urine dark and foamy	Slight decrease or normal	Absent—clay-colored stools

Note: See McPhee, Papadakis, & Rabow (2011) for discussions on causes of jaundice.

REFERENCE VALUES FOR SERUM BILIRUBIN

Most laboratories report only the figures for the total and the direct. The indirect is calculated by subtracting the direct from the total. Measurement of direct bilirubin is usually not needed if the total bilirubin is less than 1.2 mg/dL.

Adults and children past newborn stage
BU, or indirect bilirubin	0.1–1.0 mg/dL Mean 0.5 mg	This is the prehepatic, free, or unconjugated bilirubin
BC, or direct bilirubin	0.0–0.4 mg/dL Mean 0.1 mg	Posthepatic, conjugated, or esterified bilirubin (water soluble)
Total bilirubin	0.1–1.0 mg/dL	Includes both types of bilirubin

Newborn		See text for explanation of physiologic jaundice in newborns Examples used here reflect *total* bilirubins; check with individual laboratory for newer methods that use a layered technology for neonatal bilirubin
Term infant	First 24 hours	<6 mg
	Up to 48 hours	<8 mg
	2–5 days	<12 mg
Premature infant	First 24 hours	<8 mg
	Up to 48 hours	<12 mg
	2–5 days	<16 mg
Pregnant women		Bilirubin levels usually remain in normal ranges, but some normal pregnancies may have increased bilirubins

See www.bilitool.org for treatment guidelines for newborn based on bilirubin levels and age in hours.

UNCONJUGATED (INDIRECT) BILIRUBIN
Increased Level of BU
Clinical Significance

An increase in the BU can be caused in two different ways. First, the breakdown of RBCs can increase, causing an excess of free bilirubin in the bloodstream. Many conditions cause an increased destruction (hemolysis) of RBCs:

1. Sickle cell disease
2. Autoimmune disease
3. Hemorrhage into a body cavity when the RBCs are broken down
4. Drug toxicity
5. Any physical or physiologic stress (a slight increase)
6. A transfusion reaction caused by incompatible blood (see Chapter 14 on transfusion reactions)
7. Rh or ABO incompatibility in an infant

The BU of a newborn with Rh incompatibility (erythroblastosis fetalis) is often greater than 20 mg. Usually, the BU in an adult does not rise much above 5 mg because of hemolysis. The BU is about 6 mg with sickle cell disease.

Second, the BU can be elevated when the ability of the liver to conjugate the free bilirubin that circulates in the bloodstream is decreased. Liver dysfunction causes high elevations of BU in both adults and newborns. In severe liver disease, the BU may be greater than 20 mg. Although the most common reason for severe liver dysfunction in adults is cirrhosis, hepatitis may also make the liver less capable of conjugating bilirubin. Some infants are born with a deficiency in the enzyme glucuronyl transferase (Crigler–Najjar syndrome), which is necessary for the conjugation of bilirubin in the liver. This syndrome is rare but may be very severe (Hay et al., 2011). On the other hand, a relatively common, benign type of familial hyperbilirubinemia (Gilbert's syndrome) is associated with a mild decrease in enzymatic activity. Bilirubin levels increase with fasting or illness, but no treatment is needed for the fluctuating bilirubin levels (McPhee et al., 2011). Drugs, viral diseases, and other toxins may injure the liver or interfere with enzymatic actions, so that the liver cannot conjugate bilirubin efficiently.

Jaundice in the Newborn

An increase in the total bilirubin is a physiologic occurrence in the newborn that is due both to increased hemolysis and to slower conjugation by the liver. The infant is born with a large number of fetal RBCs that have a short life span. So the hemolysis that occurs after birth is a normal adaptation to the new environment. Because the newborn's liver has inadequate glucuronyl transferase, the liver takes longer to conjugate and to remove bilirubin from the bloodstream. The synthesis of the enzyme occurs a few days after birth in a full-term infant and a little longer after birth in a premature infant. Because of these events, many newborns have some physiologic jaundice that begins *after* 24 hours and begins to decline by the fifth day. For infants born before 37 weeks, 80% will have jaundice. For those born at 37 weeks or later, 60% will have jaundice (Brethauer & Corey, 2010).

Differentiating physiologic jaundice from any other kind is important. If the BU is elevated the first day, or if it does not begin to drop after 3–5 days, the jaundice may be pathologic rather than physiologic. For example, an infant with Rh incompatibility has a high BU immediately after birth. (See Chapter 14 for other tests for Rh babies.) Lowered serum albumin levels, hypoxia, cold, stress, drugs, and other metabolic factors may also cause abnormal increases in BU by interfering with the transportation or conjugation of bilirubin (DeCherney et al., 2007).

In a few instances, breast-feeding may intensify physiologic jaundice because an enzyme present in some women's milk inhibits the action of glucuronyl transferase. However, breast-feeding should continue and be done frequently, every 2–3 hours even though feeding a sleepy baby is challenging. The peak for jaundice usually occurs before 3 weeks (Hay et al., 2011).

Guidelines of the American Academy of Pediatrics for the prevention and treatment of elevated hyperbilirubinemia in the newborn stress the following: (1) promote breast-feeding, (2) perform a systematic assessment for hyperbilirubinemia that includes a total serum bilirubin (TSB) or transcutaneous monitoring, (3) provide early and focused follow-up based on the risk assessment, and (4) use phototherapy or exchange transfusions, when indicated, to prevent possible kernicterus. (Complete treatment guidelines are available at www.bilitool.org.)

Acute bilirubin encephalopathy can occur with very high levels of bilirubin. If this toxicity causes permanent damage, the condition is called kernicterus (kern = kernel, icterus = yellow). Kernicterus is largely preventable, but sometimes parents do not understand what to do (Simpson, 2007).

For infants born near term, the development of kernicterus rarely occurs unless the TSB is above 25 mg/dL, and in most reported cases it has occurred at levels above 30 mg/dL (McDonagh & Maisels, 2006). Some evidence exists that the free bilirubin is better than TSB in discriminating risks for newborns with very high bilirubin levels (Wennberg et al., 2006). Hankø (2006), commenting on the use of free or unbound bilirubin to assess newborn, notes that the concept that only free bilirubin crosses the blood–brain barrier is a theory and not an established fact. More research is warranted to determine which type of test actually measures the bilirubin that causes brain damage. In 2000 an organization of parents on infants with kernicterus was formed. See www.pickonline.org for more information on kernicterus.

CONJUGATED (DIRECT) BILIRUBIN

Increased Level of BC

Clinical Significance

Normally the amount of BC circulating in the bloodstream is very small because the larger portion of this type of bilirubin is excreted in the bile salts into the intestine. Thus, a marked increase in this type of bilirubin is a sign of obstruction in the normal flow of bile. Jaundice caused by an elevation in BC, or direct bilirubin, is called *obstructive jaundice*. The obstruction may be in the collecting channels in the liver, in the hepatic ducts, or in the common bile duct. For example, a gallstone lodged in the common bile duct prevents the normal excretion of bile salts (which contain the BC) into the intestine. The BC is absorbed into the bloodstream in much larger amounts than normal. In complete biliary obstruction, the BC may be as high as 30–40 mg. Another example of an obstruction is cancer of the head of the pancreas, of which jaundice is often the first symptom. Newborns with a congenital malformation in the biliary tree (biliary atresia) also have high BCs.

Sometimes the BC may be elevated even though biliary obstruction is not apparent. Some drugs, notably estrogen and some of the phenothiazines such as chlorpromazine, may cause stasis of bile in the liver (intrahepatic cholestasis). The bile tends to be viscous, and the small bile ducts in the liver become dilated. The BC is elevated because of this partial obstruction to the normal outflow of bile. A similar condition of stasis occurs in what is called the *benign jaundice* of pregnancy. The rise in bilirubin is an occasional occurrence in pregnancy, and the bilirubin returns to normal after delivery. Inflammation of the liver, as in hepatitis, or scarring, as in cirrhosis, may also cause partial obstruction to the flow of bile out of the liver and thereby cause an elevation of the BC.

Combination of Conjugated and Unconjugated Elevations

Although the previous discussion attempts to clarify the distinction between elevations of BC and of BU, clinical situations often entail elevations of both. Any clinical condition, any drug, or any toxic condition that causes obstruction to the flow of bile may eventually cause an increase in BU as well, because stasis of bile in the collecting ducts eventually impairs normal functioning of the liver. Intrahepatic disease, such as cirrhosis or hepatitis, and drug toxicity may cause elevations in both BC and BU. Urine bilirubin and urine urobilinogen may give additional information about the nature of the jaundice. Table 11–2 summarizes the usual findings in jaundice that is prehepatic (hemolytic), intrahepatic (liver dysfunction), or posthepatic (obstruction).

For clinical jaundice, tests other than those for bilirubin and urobilinogen may be needed. For example, alkaline phosphatase and (-glutamyl transferase (GGT) are enzymes normally excreted in the bile and are elevated in the serum with biliary obstruction. The transaminases aspartate transaminase (AST) and alanine transaminase (ALT) are released into the serum when liver cells are damaged. (See Chapter 12 on using these enzymes in detecting liver and biliary disease.) For cholestatic jaundice, ultrasonography (Chapter 23) may help detect gallstones. Transhepatic cholangiography (Chapter 20) and endoscopic cholangiography (Chapter 27) are two other diagnostic approaches to obstructive jaundice.

URINE BILIRUBIN

Because only the water-soluble conjugated (direct) bilirubin can cross the glomerular filter, it is the only type of bilirubin ever found in the urine. Normally, even this type of bilirubin is not in the urine in detectable amounts because it has been converted to urobilinogen in the intestine. Bilirubin becomes apparent in the urine when there is an obstruction to the normal pathway of BC. This test is, therefore, used to detect obstructive jaundice, and it is sometimes said incorrectly to be a test for "bile" in the urine. Because the test is likely to be positive for bilirubin before the client has signs of clinical hepatitis, it may be a screening procedure performed on populations that were known to be exposed to hepatitis. It may also be useful to screen blood donors, food handlers, and other possible carriers of the disease when controlling the spread of subclinical cases of hepatitis is imperative.

Preparation of Client and Collection of Sample

A few milliliters of freshly voided urine are needed. The urine must be fresh because oxidation affects the results, and exposure to strong lights also changes the chemical composition of the bilirubin.

Sometimes the nurse or the client may test urine for bilirubin by using either a tablet or a dipstick. For the Icotest, five drops of urine are placed on a special test mat. A tablet is then placed on the mat and two drops of water are added. If the mat turns blue or purple within 30 seconds, the test is positive for bilirubin. With the dipstick method, the positive reaction is a tan-to-purple color. The dipstick method is two to four times less sensitive than the tablet method. Drugs that change the color of the urine may mask the color change on the tablet or strip of paper. (See Chapter 3 for a list of drugs that cause color changes in urine, as well as for a dipstick method to check for ascorbic acid, because this may interfere with the bilirubin tests.)

REFERENCE VALUE FOR URINE BILIRUBIN

All groups   Normally, bilirubin is present in such small quantities in the urine that it is not detected with routine screening procedures

---

Possible Nursing Implication Related to Bilirubin in the Urine (Bilirubinuria)

Large amounts of bilirubin make urine a dark orange color, and they also make urine foam when it is shaken (shake test). Urine does not foam or become dark if it contains only urobilinogen. Because the nurse or the client may be the first to notice that the urine color is abnormal, the color of urine and stools should always be a priority assessment when an obstruction of the common bile duct is suspected. (The stools become clay colored when complete obstruction occurs.)

URINE UROBILINOGEN

Urobilinogen is formed in the intestine from the BC normally present in bile salts. Most of the urobilinogen is excreted in the feces, but a small amount that finds its way into the bloodstream either goes through the liver again or is excreted in the urine. This test may be used to detect hemolytic jaundice or early liver dysfunction.

An increase in urine urobilinogen follows hemolysis, with the increase in fecal urobilinogen even more pronounced than that in urinary urobilinogen. Because some of the urobilinogen in the feces is picked up by the portal circulation and carried to the liver again and because urinary urobilinogen excretion is increased when the liver cannot excrete the recycled urobilinogen, urinary urobilinogen can also be used to detect early liver dysfunction. The inability of the liver to handle urobilinogen occurs before bilirubin excretion is affected.

In obstructive jaundice, the lack of bilirubin excreted into the intestine causes a decrease in the amount of urobilinogen in the urine, which is not important to measure because it is very small even in normal health. The amount of urinary urobilinogen also decreases when there is a lack of intestinal flora to convert bilirubin to urobilinogen; this effect, however, is more of academic interest than of clinical usefulness.

Preparation of Client and Collection of Sample

The common procedure is to collect a 2-hour urine sample in the afternoon, because the excretion of urobilinogen is at a maximum from mid-afternoon to evening when food is being digested. The urine should be protected from light and taken to the laboratory immediately after collection. Strongly acid urine may make the results inaccurate, so if a client is taking drugs, such as high doses of salicylates, record this fact on the laboratory slip.

The nurse can also check for urobilinogen by using a dipstick, which shows 0.1–1.0 Ehrlich units as normal. For amounts from 2 to more than 12 Ehrlich units, the color goes from dark yellow to orange when read after 45 seconds.

REFERENCE VALUE FOR URINE UROBILINOGEN
All groups   0.3–1.0 Ehrlich units in a 2-hour sample (1–3 pm)

FECAL UROBILINOGEN

The amount of urobilinogen in the feces depends on the amount of BC excreted in the bile salts into the intestine and the presence of bacteria in the intestine. A lack of urobilinogen causes the stools to be clay colored. A lack of bacteria to break down the bilirubin may reduce the urobilinogen in the intestine, and thus the feces become lighter in color. For example, this lighter color may occur with antibiotic use.

The fecal urobilinogen is increased when there is an increased breakdown of RBCs (hemolytic jaundice) because much more bilirubin is conjugated by the liver and excreted into the intestine.

Possible Nursing Diagnoses Related to Hyperbilirubinemia

Deficient Knowledge Related to Clinical Signs of Jaundice

Although serum tests are used to monitor the exact level of the bilirubin from day to day, the nurse or client should also record color changes on a daily basis. Because clients may be the best judges of day-to-day changes in their own skin color, this source of data should never be overlooked, and clients should be instructed on changes that are important to note. An excess of serum bilirubin, either the BU or the BC, gives a yellowish coloration to the sclera of the eyes,

(Continued)

Possible Nursing Diagnoses . . . *(Continued)*

skin, and mucous membranes. The symptoms of jaundice begin to appear when the total bilirubin is about 2–4 mg in adults or older children. In infants, jaundice may not be apparent until the total bilirubin is about 5–7 mg. Often the yellow is noted first in the sclera of fair-skinned clients. In dark-skinned clients, the inner canthus of the eye may show more change. In dark-skinned or Asian clients, the yellowish tinge also becomes apparent in the mucous membranes of the hard palate. The palms and plantar surfaces of the feet are other areas to assess for jaundice in people of color. Blanching the skin of newborns by pressing on the sternum makes the jaundice of the skin more apparent. With proper lighting, one can see jaundice on the abdomen nearly as easily as in the sclera. Observations for jaundice should be carried out in natural daylight, if possible.

In a community health setting or clinic, the nurse may be the first to notice the beginning of jaundice. In high-risk populations composed of abusers of alcohol or other drugs, inspections of the eyes and skin are especially important to detect liver damage.

Differences in BU and BC. Nurses must also know whether the BU or BC is elevated, because the nursing implications vary for each type of elevation. Some of the implications, such as changes in body image or ways to assess for jaundice, are the same for both types. However, the danger to the central nervous system (CNS), itching, discomfort, and bleeding are problems associated more with one type than with the other.

Anxiety of Parents Related to Risk for Central Nervous System Damage in the Newborn

In older children and adults, an increase in BU is not in itself dangerous or uncomfortable for the client. After infancy, the blood–brain barrier prevents the BU from affecting the CNS. A high BU in newborns, however, is of grave concern.

A nurse may be able to alleviate some anxiety with a brief explanation of a specific protocol for jaundice in the newborn and the importance of frequent laboratory testing. Parents may prefer not to see the heel sticks performed to obtain blood. Anxiety may also be lessened by helping the mother be successful with breast-feeding, because an adequate milk supply will be useful in reducing the level of breast milk jaundice.

Risk for Ineffective Health Maintenance of Newborns

As discussed earlier in the section on jaundice in the newborn, current guidelines recommend that all infants be examined again for hyperbilirubinemia in the first few days after birth. Very early discharges, poor communication with parents, and a fragmented healthcare system are barriers to having all infants get appropriate follow-ups. Also, a delay in treatment may occur if nurses do not have standing orders to obtain a bilirubin level on any infant they assess to be jaundiced, on a home visit. Nurses need to be involved so that their organization can do timely follow-ups and treatment plans for all newborns.

Risk for Injury Related to Treatments to Decrease Indirect Bilirubin in Newborns

Researchers are exploring the use of protoporphyrins to decrease bilirubin production (Hay et al., 2011), but the two standard treatments to decrease the indirect bilirubin in newborns are exchange transfusions and phototherapy.

Exchange Transfusions. These are used primarily for severe cases of blood-type incompatibility. (See Chapter 14 for safety needs with transfusions.) In recent years, phototherapy has been so successful that exchange blood transfusions are not widely used (McDonagh & Maisels, 2006).

Phototherapy. High-intensity light is used to help break down the BU to a nontoxic substance. Phototherapy converts bilirubin to derivatives that apparently can be excreted in the bile and urine without being conjugated by the liver. It is important that the baby's eyes be protected under the lights. It is also crucial to monitor the temperature to prevent hypo- or hyperthermia. Extra fluids should be given to prevent dehydration. Sometimes phototherapy can be easily and safely provided by using a small blanket embedded with a fiberoptic bili-light. The blanket, wrapped around the baby to touch as much skin as possible, eliminates the need for goggles. Also, the baby can be held and more easily fed so that the risk of dehydration and hyperthermia is less than with the traditional bili-lights. Fiberoptic blankets are most often used as adjuncts, but prove inadequate as the sole therapy for term infants (Hay et al., 2011).

Because the BU itself is not a danger to older children or adults, little effort is made to decrease the level itself. Theoretically, sitting in the sun would be beneficial to a child who has a high BU, but it is more important to correct the pathophysiologic process causing the elevation.

One research study found that new mothers may be confused by caregivers who tell them that sunlight exposure is another treatment for hyperbilirubinemia as it is not a recommended procedure (Brethauer & Carey, 2010).

Pain Related to Pruritus

It is presumed that the severe itching (pruritus) that often accompanies an elevated BC is due to something toxic in the "bile salts" deposited in the skin. Keeping the environment cool is useful because perspiration may accentuate the pruritus. Soothing baths and lotions may give some relief. Aveeno, a colloidal oatmeal bath for irritated skin, contains no soaps or synthetics that can harm the skin. The bath soothes and cleanses naturally because of its unique adsorption action. Oatmeal baths or cornstarch baths can be used for infants as well as adults who have pruritus. Children may need to be restrained from scratching. Excess bilirubin levels may also irritate connective tissue in the sclera. Clients may have photophobia and thus a need to avoid bright lights.

Although there is no direct evidence that the pruritus is directly attributed to bile salts, the use of medications that bind bile salts may relieve the itching. Cholestyramine is a resin that is taken orally to bind bile salts in the intestine and prevent their reabsorption (Katzung, Masters, & Trevor, 2009). This treatment may be helpful when the obstruction is not complete. To prevent constipation, a person taking cholestyramine needs a large intake of fluids and a diet high in fiber. Because the drug may bind with other drugs, it should be given at least 1 hour before or 4 hours after administering other drugs. Pruritis should decrease in 1–2 weeks (Deglin, Vallerand, & Sanoski, 2011). Supplements of fat-soluble vitamins may be needed if the client is undergoing long-term therapy with the drug. (Cholestyramine is also used as a drug to lower cholesterol levels [see Chapter 9].)

Risk for Injury Related to Bleeding Caused by Hypoprothrombinemia

For fats and fat-soluble vitamins to be emulsified and absorbed from the intestine, there must be adequate bile salts. For this reason, a client with an elevated BC may have a tendency

(Continued)

Possible Nursing Diagnoses . . . *(Continued)*

to bleed. Without bile salts, fat-soluble vitamins, including vitamin K, are not absorbed from the small intestine. If vitamin K is not absorbed into the bloodstream, the liver cannot make enough prothrombin and other factors needed for normal blood clotting. Clients with obstructive jaundice thus often have increased prothrombin times. Clients with elevated prothrombin times caused by obstructive jaundice are given parenteral injections of vitamin K. Parenteral vitamin K can reach the liver because the bile salts are not needed to get the vitamin from the intestine into the bloodstream. Specific methods to prevent bleeding when the client has an increased prothrombin time are discussed in Chapter 13 on clotting tests.

Risk for Pain Related to Obstructive Jaundice

Although jaundice caused by an elevation of BU is painless, pain, other than that associated with pruritus, may or may not be associated with jaundice caused by an elevation of the BC. Because obstruction of the biliary tree by a pancreatic tumor may be painless for quite a while, the first indications of biliary obstruction could be jaundice and a tendency to bleed. However, jaundice caused by a gallstone in the common bile duct tends to cause severe abdominal pain in the right upper quadrant. In such a case, the client may need opioids to relieve the pain. Characteristically, the pain tends to radiate to the right shoulder, and it may be intensified by an attempt to eat fatty foods.

Imbalanced Nutrition: Related to Inability to Tolerate Fats and Other Nutrients

Clients with an elevated BC usually have marked intolerance to fatty foods. Their nutritional status must be carefully assessed so that their caloric needs are met. If indicated, an operation is performed to relieve the obstruction. Before the operation, the client may need intravenous feedings to maintain hydration and caloric intake. Fat-soluble vitamins can be added to intravenous fluids. Even with only a partial or clearing obstruction, the client may have little appetite for food, so the nurse must plan meals carefully. (As a rule, an increase in the BU does not seriously interfere with appetite unless the liver is involved, and then anorexia can be profound.)

Hepatitis, which causes cholestasis and elevations of both BU and BC, is accompanied by anorexia. Even if foods are not desired, the client should be encouraged to drink fruit juices. These provide some calories and help flush the water-soluble BC into the urine. As the client's appetite returns, food is needed to supply adequate calories and protein for liver regeneration. Protein in the diet is encouraged only if serum ammonia levels are normal (see Chapter 10). Otherwise, hepatic coma can result from too much protein. Fats can be allowed as tolerated.

Disturbed Body Image

A concentration on the physical aspects of care for clients with an elevated bilirubin must not overshadow their psychological needs. Nurses need to be aware that jaundice is a definite change in the body image of the person. Jaundice may be very upsetting not only to clients but also to their families. Some clients are afraid to look in a mirror, and others may prefer not to have any visitors. If these clients must come to a clinic, they may not want others to stare at them. (In addition, other clients may be afraid that the jaundice is contagious.) Soft, subdued lights make the jaundice less apparent while treatments are begun to reduce the bilirubin level.

Clients' reactions, of course, can also be unexpected. A young man was once admitted to the hospital with severe jaundice caused by cirrhosis. Blue dye for a lymphogram (Chapter 20) turned the man's sclera and skin from yellow to green. One might jump to the conclusion that the client would not want anyone to see him and that he would be upset by the parade of nursing students, residents, and interns who came to examine the "green man." On the contrary, the client enjoyed all the extra attention from being unique and seemed a little disappointed when his color began to return to normal. So, as with all generalizations about nursing implications, nurses must choose which ones are applicable for a certain client in a certain setting. Nurses should also recognize that a change in body image caused by a specific external source (such as the dye) may be quite a different experience from the change due to a longer-term and less specific internal source such as jaundice caused by an inoperable tumor.

BILIRUBIN IN AMNIOTIC FLUID

It is not known for sure how bilirubin reaches the amniotic fluid; some of it may diffuse across the skin. The bilirubin in the amniotic fluid is the unconjugated, non-water-soluble type and cannot be excreted in the urine of the fetus. The bilirubin content of amniotic fluid is often high during early pregnancy, but it should fall progressively after midpregnancy. (See Chapter 28 for a discussion on the procedure for amniocentesis.) The importance of measuring bilirubin content of amniotic fluid is to determine whether the normal downward progression of bilirubin concentration in the last half of pregnancy is continuing. If the bilirubin content is not dropping or if it begins to rise for the fetus of an Rh-negative mother, medical interventions may be necessary to save the fetus. Laboratories may use either light or chemical methods to determine the amount of bilirubin in the amniotic fluid. (See Chapter 14 for Rh antibody titers and the Coombs' test, which are used to determine the need for amniocentesis.)

A new alternative to serial amniocentesis is the use of ultrasound to determine the peak velocity of systolic blood flow in the middle cerebral artery (MCV) of the fetus. High flow in this area correlates well with the severity of fetal anemia (DeCherney et al., 2007). Research suggests that this noninvasive monitoring should be used to monitor the mother who is Rh negative and may have antibodies against the RBCs of the fetus (Sau et al., 2009).

TRANSCUTANEOUS BILIRUBINOMETER

A transcutaneous bilirubinometer is a handheld device that contains a fiberoptic probe to measure the color intensity of the skin. The probe is placed on the neonate's forehead, and a button is pressed to activate the meter. An audible click and a flash of light are emitted. Measurements of how the light travels through and reflects off the skin are converted to a digital display. The digital readings correlate with total serum bilirubin levels. Each institution must establish its own criteria for correlating the readings with approximate serum bilirubin levels and for determining a protocol for when follow-up serum bilirubin levels are indicated. For example, if the digital reading is less than a certain number, the infant may be spared the discomfort of having blood drawn. The use of this transcutaneous method as adjunctive screening can enhance client care by reducing the number of blood draws (Wu, 2006).

Questions

1. When the body is using the normal pathway of bilirubin excretion, which laboratory test is negative?
   a. Serum bilirubin level (indirect portion)
   b. Fecal urobilinogen
   c. Urine urobilinogen
   d. Urine bilirubin

2. Which of the following terms is a synonym for indirect bilirubin?
   a. Conjugated bilirubin
   b. Water-soluble bilirubin
   c. Posthepatic bilirubin
   d. Free bilirubin

3. The laboratory slip on a client's chart shows a total bilirubin of 3.0 mg and a direct bilirubin of 0.3 mg. Which of the following is the indirect bilirubin?
   a. Unknown at the present time
   b. 3.3 mg/dL
   c. 2.7 mg/dL
   d. 3.9 mg/dL

4. A client has been admitted with a diagnosis of complete obstructive jaundice related to a gallstone in the common bile duct. The nurse would expect to observe for
   a. Dark stools and dark orange urine with a high specific gravity
   b. Clay-colored stools and pale yellow urine with a low specific gravity
   c. Clay-colored stools and dark orange urine that foams when shaken
   d. Dark stools and pale yellow urine that foams when shaken

5. In an infant, clinical jaundice becomes apparent when the total bilirubin level is about which of the following levels?
   a. 3–5 mg/dL
   b. 5–7 mg/dL
   c. 7–9 mg/dL
   d. More than 9 mg/dL

6. In an adult, clinical jaundice becomes apparent when the serum bilirubin (total) is about which of the following levels?
   a. 2–4 mg/dL
   b. 5–7 mg/dL
   c. 7–9 mg/dL
   d. More than 9 mg/dL

7. An elevation of the direct or conjugated bilirubin would be an expected finding for
   a. A client, aged 31, who has anemia caused by a lack of iron in her diet
   b. A infant, 2 days old, breast-feeding and slightly jaundiced
   c. A client, aged 7, who has been admitted to the pediatric unit in a sickle cell crisis
   d. A client, aged 42, who has cholestatic jaundice related to drug therapy

8. An elevation of the indirect or unconjugated bilirubin would be an expected finding for
   a. A client who has gallstones in the common bile duct
   b. A client who is undergoing an operation (Whipple procedure) for cancer of the head of the pancreas
   c. A client who has a malformation in the biliary tree (biliary atresia)
   d. A client, aged 7, who had a transfusion reaction caused by incompatible blood

9. An infant has been diagnosed with breast-feeding jaundice. Which of the following points is appropriate to include in a teaching plan for the parents of this baby?
   a. Breast-feeding should not be continued
   b. Phototherapy is usually begun if bilirubin levels are greater than 12 mg/dL
   c. Inadequate milk intake may intensify the jaundice
   d. Phototherapy always requires the baby to stay in the hospital

10. A possible nursing diagnosis for an adult client with an elevated indirect or unconjugated bilirubin is
    a. Alteration in self-concept related to changes in body image
    b. Risk for bleeding related to hypoprothrombinemia
    c. Altered nutrition related to intolerance for fats
    d. Risk for injury related to central nervous system damage

11. The most common method used to treat high levels of bilirubin in the newborn is
    a. Complete elimination of breast milk to reduce the factors that interfere with glucuronyl transferase in the liver
    b. Exchange transfusions to remove toxic products from the bloodstream
    c. Phototherapy with high-intensity lights to help break down the bilirubin
    d. Drug therapy with phenobarbital to promote the hepatic clearance of bilirubin

12. A home care nurse is visiting a client, who is recovering from hepatitis. The nurse knows that the drug cholestyramine is proving effective if the client states that
    a. Constipation is no longer a problem
    b. Itching is less
    c. Appetite is better
    d. Bright lights no longer hurt her eyes

References

Brethauer, M. & Carey. L. (2010). Neonatal jaundice. *Maternal Child Nursing, 25*(1), 9–14.

DeCherney, A. H., Nathan, L., Goodwin, T. M., & Lauter, N. (Eds.). (2007). *Current diagnosis & treatment: Obstetrics & gynecology* (10th ed.). New York: McGraw-Hill.

Deglin, J. H., Vallerand, A. H., & Sanoski, C. A. (2011). *Davis's drug guide for nurses* (12th ed.). Philadelphia: F. A. Davis.

Hankø, E. (2006). Unbound bilirubin and risk assessment in the jaundiced newborn: Possibilities and limitations. *Pediatrics, 117*(2), 526–527.

Hay, W. W., Levin, M. J., Sondheimer, J. M., & Deterding, R. (Eds.). (2011). *Current diagnosis and treatment: Pediatrics* (20th ed.). New York: McGraw-Hill.

Katzung, B., Masters, S. B., & Trevor, A. J. (Eds.). (2009). *Basic and clinical pharmacology* (11th ed.). New York: Lange Medical Books/McGraw-Hill.

McDonagh, A. F. & Maisels, M. (2006). Bilirubin unbound: Déjà vu all over again? *Pediatrics, 117*(2), 523–525.

McPhee, S. J., Papadakis, M. A., & Rabow, M. W. (Eds.). (2011). *Current medical diagnosis and treatment* (50th ed.). New York: McGraw-Hill.

Sau, A., El-Matary, A., Newton, L., & Wichramarachchi, D. C. (2009). Management of red cell alloimmunized pregnancies using conventional methods with that of middle cerebral artery peak systolic velocity. *Acta Obstetricia et Gynecologia Scandinavica 2009, 88*(4), 476–478.

Simpson, K. (2007). Kernicterus prevention. *MCN: The American Journal of Maternal Child Nursing, 32*(2), 132.

Wennberg, R. P., Ahlfors, C., Bhutani, V., Johnson, L., & Shapiro, S. (2006). Toward understanding kernicterus: A challenge to improve the management of jaundiced newborns. *Pediatrics, 117*(2), 474–485.

Wu, A. H. (Ed.). (2006). *Tietz clinical guide to laboratory tests* (4th ed.). St. Louis, MO: Saunders Elsevier.

Websites

www.bilitool.org (Guidelines from American Academy of Pediatrics for treatment of increased bilirubin in newborn based on age in hours.)

www.pickonline.org (Official site for parents of infants and children with kernicterus has useful information for clients.)

Answers

1. d, 2. d, 3. c, 4. c, 5. b, 6. a, 7. d, 8. d, 9. c, 10. a, 11. c, 12. b

Tests to Measure Enzymes and Cardiac Markers

- Alkaline Phosphatase   274
- γ-Glutamyl Transferase or γ-Glutamyl Transpeptidase   278
- Carbohydrate-Deficient Transferrin   279
- Acid Phosphatase or Prostatic Acid Phosphatase (PAP)   279
- Alanine Aminotransferase or Serum Glutamic-Pyruvic Transaminase   279
- Aspartate Aminotransferase or Serum Glutamic-Oxaloacetic Transaminase   281
- Creatine Kinase or Creatine Phosphokinase   282
- Lactic Dehydrogenase   285
- Troponins As Cardiac Markers   286
- Cardiac Analyzers As Point of Care   287
- B-Natriuretic Peptide   288
- Serum Aldolase   289
- Serum Amylase   290
- Urinary Amylase   293
- Serum Lipase   294

OBJECTIVES

1. Identify factors, other than pathologic processes, that tend to cause elevations in most of the serum enzyme tests.
2. Explain the usual clinical significance of an elevated serum alkaline phosphatase (ALP) level and compare with the γ-glutamyl transferase (GGT) level.
3. Compare and contrast the use of the serum acid phosphatase level with the use of the prostate-specific antigen (PSA) test.
4. Describe possible nursing diagnoses when a client has marked elevations of the transaminases, alanine aminotransferase (ALT) (formerly serum glutamic-pyruvic transaminase [SGPT]), and aspartate aminotransferase (AST) (formerly serum glutamic-oxaloacetic transaminase [SGOT]).
5. Discriminate between the cardiac markers—creatine kinase (CK) and the troponins—in relation to the onset, peak, and duration of elevation after a myocardial infarction.
6. Explain why measurements of isoenzymes of CK are more valuable than measurement of the total amounts of the enzyme.
7. Identify the most important nursing diagnosis for a client with cardiac disease who has increased levels of B-natriuretic peptide.

8. Plan an appropriate activity schedule for a client who has an elevated CK level or serum aldolase level caused by a muscular disorder.

9. Explain how serum amylase and lipase and urinary amylase are used as assessment tools for pancreatitis.

10. Identify the nursing diagnoses for clients who have marked elevations of serum amylase and lipase levels.

This chapter covers the most common enzymes measured in the serum. As an additional assessment, only one of the enzymes, amylase, is measured in the urine. Almost all cells contain the principal enzymes, although some types of tissue contain larger concentrations of particular enzymes. So when tissue cells are damaged, the enzymes leak into the serum.

Although the enzymes are not tissue specific, various types of tissue have isoenzymes with different chemical and physical properties. Isoenzymes of a particular enzyme all control the same specific metabolic function even though their molecular forms vary slightly from one to another.

Enzymes are often named for the reaction that they catalyze. For example, lipase is an enzyme used for the reaction of a lipid or fat, and transaminases transfer amino groups in energy production. Enzymes are easy to recognize because their names almost always end in -ase. However, because many of the serum enzyme tests are known by initials rather than by names, there is no way to know that CPK is an enzyme test unless one sees it written out as *creatine phosphokinase*, and more recently *CPK* has become just *CK* for *creatine kinase*.

Table 12–1 summarizes the most important enzyme elevations for several common pathologic conditions. With a quick glance at the table, the reader sees that none of the enzyme tests is totally specific and that many are changed by several pathologic conditions. Also, various nonpathologic factors, such as vigorous exercise, cause elevated serum enzymes. Treatments such as intramuscular injections and the administration of opiates cause serum elevations of some enzymes. Improper handling of the specimens also brings about elevations caused by hemolysis.

ALKALINE PHOSPHATASE

Two types of phosphatases are measured in the bloodstream: alkaline and acid. These two types of phosphatases are so termed because their activity is best measured in a pH of about either 10 (alkaline) or 5 (acid).

ALP is found in the tissues of the liver, bone, intestine, kidneys, and placenta. Its three isoenzymes can be identified by electrophoresis:

1. Band I: Liver, vascular endothelium, and lung
2. Band II: Bone, kidney, and placenta
3. Band III: Intestinal mucosa

However, unlike the other isoenzymes, the isoenzymes of ALP are not commonly used in clinical evaluations of pathologic conditions.

Except in pregnancy, most of the serum ALP is made up of liver and bone isoenzymes. Because ALP is increased with new bone formation (osteoblastic

Table 12–1 Enzyme Elevations in Common Pathologic Conditions

Serum Enzymes	Eclampsia	Cancer of Prostate	Biliary Obstruction	Bone Metastasis	Malignant Tumor of Liver	Hepatitis	Cirrhosis	Myocardial Infarction	Infectious Mononucleosis	Hemolytic Disease	Pulmonary Infarction	Muscular Necrosis or Inflammation	Pancreatitis	Brain Tissue Injury
1. Alkaline phosphatase	↑	↑	(↑)	(↑)	(↑)	↑	↑						↑	
2. Acid phosphatase	↑	(↑)								(↑)				
3. GGT			(↑)	↑	(↑)	↑	↑							
4. ALT (SGPT)	↑	↑	↑	↑	↑	(↑)	↑	↑	(↑)		↑	↑	↑	
5. AST (SGOT)	↑		↑	↑	↑	(↑)	↑	(↑)	(↑)	↑	↑	↑	↑	
6. CK (total)								(↑)				(↑)		↑
CK-I (BB)														↑
CK-II (MB)								(↑)						
CK-III (MM)												(↑)		↑
7. LDH Total	↑	↑		↑	↑			↑[a]	↑	(↑)		↑	↑	
LDH_1								↑		↑				
LDH_2										↑	↑			
LDH_3											(↑)		↑	
LDH_4					↑	↑			↑				↑	
LDH_5			↑		↑	↑	↑		↑					
8. Aldolase		↑						↑			↑	(↑)		
9. Amylase			↑										(↑)	
10. Lipase			↑										(↑)	

[a] See discussion on troponins as a newer cardiac marker.

↑ Clinically significant elevation. Note that any tissue injury causes *slight* increase in many of these enzymes.

(↑) Used as principal diagnostic tool. See text for elaborations.

activity), children have higher levels than adults, and because the placenta is a rich source of ALP, a high level of this enzyme is also normal in pregnancy. The ALP from liver tissue is normally excreted into the bile, so biliary obstruction causes an increase in ALP. The ingestion of a fatty meal also causes a temporary increase in serum ALP.

Preparation of Client and Collection of Sample

The client should be fasting, because a fatty meal may cause an elevation. If the client is taking oral contraceptives, phenothiazines, morphine, or phenytoin, record use of the drug on the laboratory slip, because elevations in the enzyme level may be related to the drug. The laboratory needs 1 mL of serum. Some methods require immediate refrigeration of the sample.

REFERENCE VALUES FOR ALP	
Adult	Men 45–115 U/L Women 30–100 U/L
Pregnant women	Levels increase because of production by placenta; levels return to normal about 3–6 weeks after delivery
Infant and children	1.0–2.0 times adult levels[a]
Aged	Values tend to increase after the age of 50 years

[a]See Hay et al. (2011) and Wu (2006) for more details.

Increased ALP Level

Clinical Significance

A markedly increased ALP level in a nonpregnant woman is a general warning of bone or liver abnormality. If there is question whether bone or liver is the origin, other enzyme tests more specific for hepatobiliary disease may be done (see discussion on GGT).

In Paget's disease, in which there is considerable bone destruction and bone rebuilding, the ALP level is higher than normal. Cancer metastatic to the bone also often causes an elevated ALP if the body attempts to continue to form new bone. If bone is only being broken down (osteolytic process), ALP is not elevated. However, most types of osteolytic processes are accompanied by some osteoblastic activity. A healing fracture causes a modest rise in the ALP level. Conditions such as hyperparathyroidism and vitamin D or calcium deficiencies cause an increased amount of ALP, even though bone growth may be abnormal.

Liver dysfunction is the other main reason for increased ALP levels. The elevation may be either due to actual liver tissue damage or, because ALP is excreted in the bile, due to an obstruction of bile flow. Morphine sulfate and other opioids may cause some spasm of the sphincter of Oddi and thus elevate the ALP level. Conditions that cause obstructive jaundice, such as a stone in the common bile duct or cancer of the head of the pancreas, cause a markedly elevated ALP.

Certain drugs, such as the estrogens and phenothiazines, may cause a stasis of bile (cholestatic effect), thus elevating the ALP in the serum. Anticonvulsants and other drugs may induce a synthesis of increased amounts of ALP and other liver enzymes. The elevation of the ALP may be the first indication of an adverse reaction to a drug and indicates that the drug should be stopped.

In eclampsia, the ALP levels are increased above the normally high levels of pregnancy, probably because of a liver dysfunction.

Possible Nursing Diagnoses Related to Increased ALP Level

Risk of Injury Related to Pathologic Fractures

One of the most common uses of the ALP test is to screen for the possibility of bone metastasis in clients with malignant tumors. The possibility of bone metastasis is an indication that the client may be prone to pathologic fractures and thus should be handled very carefully and protected from injury. Remember that the metastatic destruction of bone causes an increase in ALP only if osteoblastic activity is occurring along with bone destruction. So not all bone metastases cause elevated ALP levels. In metastatic disease, any elevated ALP is usually followed with a bone scan (see Chapter 22) to determine the exact points of bone destruction.

Ineffective Health Maintenance Related to Development of Obstructive Jaundice

If the elevated ALP is due to any type of obstruction in the common bile duct, specific nursing implications are related to the presence of obstructive jaundice. (The problems associated with obstructive jaundice are discussed in Chapter 11 in the section on conjugated bilirubin levels.)

Deficient Knowledge Related to Need to Change Therapeutic Regime

If the client is taking drugs that can cause cholestasis, such as estrogens or phenothiazines, an increase in the ALP level may be an indication that the client should not continue taking the drug. A client taking oral contraceptives that contain estrogen needs information about other forms of birth control.

Decreased ALP Level

Clinical Significance

In a child who has not yet reached puberty, a decrease in ALP indicates a lack of normal bone formation. This condition may be caused by pathologic conditions, such as hypothyroidism, celiac disease, cystic fibrosis, or chronic nephritis. A decreased ALP may also be caused by a genetic defect. Dentists may observe that these children have premature bone loss. Very low levels of ALP are seen in scurvy. Adults with a lack of bone formation caused by malnutrition or excessive vitamin D intake may have lowered ALP levels.

> ## Possible Nursing Diagnosis Related to Decreased ALP Level
>
> ### Imbalanced Nutrition: Less Than Body Requirements
> The exact nursing implications depend on the reason for a lack of normal bone formation. Usually, a dietary plan is needed to ensure an adequate intake of protein, vitamins, and minerals for optimal bone growth.

γ-GLUTAMYL TRANSFERASE OR γ-GLUTAMYL TRANSPEPTIDASE

Gamma-glutamyl transferase (GGT), an enzyme useful in amino acid transport, is found chiefly in the liver, kidneys, prostate, and spleen. When ALP is elevated, the GGT may be used to assess whether the increase is due to liver and biliary involvement, because the GGT is more specific for the hepatobiliary system, whereas the ALP can be elevated in bone or liver disease. The GGT is also raised by alcohol and hepatotoxic drugs and thus is useful to monitor drug toxicity and alcohol abuse.

Preparation of Client and Collection of Sample

Some laboratories may require fasting for 8 hours, with water allowed. Serum is collected in a red-topped tube.

REFERENCE VALUES FOR GGT	
Adult	
Men	7–71 U/L
Women	5–39 U/L
Children	Varies by age[a]

[a]See Hay et al. (2011)—levels vary with the methods used.

Clinical Significance

Elevated GGT levels are found in liver disease, including liver metastasis, and in biliary obstruction. The GGT may also be used to monitor the course of hepatitis; a return to normal shows an excellent prognosis.

Because liver damage from alcohol causes immediate increase in the GGT, this enzyme has been the test of choice in investigating alcohol abuse. The use of CDT, discussed next, improves the sensitivity of detecting excessive alcohol consumption (Hietala et al., 2006).

Possible Nursing Diagnoses for Elevated GGT

Elevation of GGT is related to liver damage or biliary stasis. For diagnoses related to liver damage, see the discussion on ALT (SGPT) in this chapter. For diagnoses related to biliary stasis, see the discussion on obstructive jaundice in Chapter 11. If the GGT and the CDT are elevated, the client may need referral for alcohol abuse counseling (see Chapter 17).

CARBOHYDRATE-DEFICIENT TRANSFERRIN

Carbohydrate-deficient transferrin (CDT) is useful as a marker for excessive alcohol consumption and a sign of possible alcohol dependency. CDT is a collective term referring to isoforms of transferrin that are elevated when alcohol interferes with the normal production of transferrin. As these isoforms have a half-life of about 14 days, they will disappear with abstinence. Several different assay methods are used, and so reference values will vary. CDT levels are markedly affected by various factors including the factors that alter iron homeostasis. The combined use of CDT with GGT (discussed earlier) and the mean corpuscular volume (MCV) of erythrocytes (Chapter 2) increases the sensitivity of the assessment for alcohol dependence. CDT is also used to assess congenital disorders of glycosylation, a group of autosomal recessive disorders that have several phenotypes (Hay et al., 2011). See Chapter 18 on nursing diagnoses for genetic defects.

ACID PHOSPHATASE OR PROSTATIC ACID PHOSPHATASE (PAP)

Acid phosphatase is found in high concentrations in the prostate gland, erythrocytes, and platelets. Because this enzyme is excreted in the seminal fluid, a test for acid phosphatase is sometimes performed on vaginal secretions as supportive evidence for alleged rape (McPhee, Papadakis, & Rabow, 2011). The test has also been a tumor marker for prostatic cancer, but the current marker is prostate-specific antigen (PSA), which is discussed in Chapter 10.

ALANINE AMINOTRANSFERASE OR SERUM GLUTAMIC-PYRUVIC TRANSAMINASE

Formerly known as serum glutamic-pyruvic transaminase (SGPT), alanine aminotransferase (ALT) is found in the largest concentration in liver tissue, but it is also present in kidney, heart, and skeletal muscle tissue. Like the other aminotransferase or transaminase (AST or SGOT), ALT is increased in various types of tissue damage, and so it is not very specific. ALT may be used if there is a specific need to evaluate the possibility of liver tissue necrosis or liver damage from drugs. ALT has been useful in screening blood donors to reduce the incidence of non-A, non-B hepatitis (now known as hepatitis C). (See Chapter 14 for more specific tests for hepatitis C.)

Preparation of Client and Collection of Specimen

The client does not need to fast. The laboratory needs 1 mL of blood. Many medications and herbs may cause false elevations of liver enzymes (Wu, 2006; Deglin, Vallerand, & Sanoski, 2011).

REFERENCE VALUES FOR ALT OR SGPT	
Adult	Men 10–55 U/L
	Women 7–30 U/L
Aged	Very slight increase

Note: Newborns have higher levels.

Elevated ALT or SGPT

Clinical Significance

In severe hepatitis, the ALT is often greater than 1,000 IU and may rise to 4,000 IU. In chronic hepatitis and cirrhosis, the levels are not so markedly elevated. Infectious mononucleosis, which often involves the liver, causes a substantial rise in ALT. (See Chapter 14 for tests for infectious mononucleosis.) Shock, Reye's syndrome, congestive heart failure, and preeclampsia all cause an increased ALT because of some liver tissue damage. (See Chapter 18 on preeclampsia.) Hydatidiform moles also cause elevations of the ALT. (Chapter 15 discusses the diagnosis of hydatidiform moles by hormone assay.)

Possible Nursing Diagnoses Related to Increased ALT Levels

Risk for Impaired Liver Function

Nurses and clients must be aware of medications that need to be monitored by ALT. Liver injury from medications is defined as an ALT of more than three times the upper limit of normal range, but increases far above this level may not lead to permanent liver damage because the liver has a great capacity to heal from injury once the medication is stopped. However, the appearance of jaundice suggests a much more serious problem with possible fatal outcome (Navarro & Senior, 2006).

Because a markedly elevated ALT especially with jaundice may be indicative of severe liver tissue damage, nurses must carefully assess for any signs of liver insufficiency, which could progress to a hepatic coma. (See Chapter 10 for the test of ammonia levels as a sign of liver dysfunction and for details of the symptoms that may be present. Chapter 11 discusses the special needs of the patient with jaundice.)

Imbalanced Nutrition: Less Than Body Requirements

The basic ingredients for the encouragement of liver tissue regeneration are the promotion of rest, the avoidance of drugs toxic to the liver, and the provision of a nutritious diet. Liver disease often causes anorexia, so meeting nutritional needs is challenging.

> **Activity Intolerance Related to Fatigue**
>
> Nurses may have to teach clients how to conserve energy. For clients at home, someone should be available to see that they do indeed rest. Rest is not a luxury here; it is often the basic therapy. Enzyme levels, tested over a period of weeks, may be used to gauge the amount of activity allowed. Boredom and depression can occur because of a long convalescent period with prolonged restrictions on usual activities.

ASPARTATE AMINOTRANFERASE OR SERUM GLUTAMIC-OXALOACETIC TRANSAMINASE

Formerly called serum glutamic-oxaloacetic transaminase (SGOT), aspartate aminotranferase (AST) is found predominantly in heart, liver, and muscle tissue, although all tissues contain some of the enzyme. Because the transaminases or aminotransferases are very important to energy transformation, the highest amounts of them are found in high-energy cells such as the heart, liver, and skeletal muscle. As discussed in the previous section, the highest concentration of ALT or SGPT is in the liver, and it is used primarily to detect liver necrosis. AST can also be used to detect liver necrosis, because both transaminases rise before there are any signs of jaundice. Neither the ALT nor the AST is used to evaluate skeletal muscle necrosis because two other enzymes (CK and aldolase) are more specific for muscle tissue necrosis.

Preparation of Client and Collection of Sample

The client is prepared and the specimen collected in the same way and under the same conditions as for the other aminotransferase, ALT. Various drugs may interfere with the test.

REFERENCE VALUES FOR AST OR SGOT	
Adult	Men 10–40 U/L Women 9–25 U/L
Newborn	Values are 2–3 times higher
Aged	Slight increase

Increased AST or SGOT Level

Clinical Significance

In hepatitis, the AST may reach levels greater than 500 U/L, and it is elevated in the bloodstream even before jaundice appears. The return to normal may take weeks to months after hepatitis. Other types of liver involvement, such as that with shock, trauma, or cirrhosis, may cause lesser elevations of the AST. Reye's syndrome and pulmonary infarction are other causes of an elevated AST. GGT also helps identify liver involvement.

Possible Nursing Diagnoses Related to Elevated AST or SGOT

Because the AST can be elevated from many different causes, nursing care must be based on the underlying pathophysiologic condition. If the AST level is due to hepatic damage, the nursing diagnoses for ALT elevations would be useful as general guidelines.

Decrease in ALT and AST

Clinical Significance

Because the levels of transaminases or aminotransferases are normally very low, a decrease is unlikely. In *rare* instances, both are decreased or nonexistent because the liver can no longer make the enzymes. Uremia sometimes causes a pseudodecrease, as can chronic dialysis and ketoacidosis. Also, some medications may cause a decrease (Wu, 2006).

CREATINE KINASE OR CREATINE PHOSPHOKINASE

Creatine phosphokinase, or CK as it is now called, is very important in energy utilization and is involved in the reaction that changes creatine to creatinine. Because almost all circulating CK comes normally from muscular tissue, muscular activity and intramuscular injections are two common ways that CK values are elevated. CK can be measured as one total enzyme in the serum, or it can be separated into three different isoenzymes. The three types of CK isoenzymes are as follows:

1. CK-I (BB): produced primarily by brain tissue and smooth muscle
2. CK-II (MB): produced primarily by heart tissue
3. CK-III (MM): produced primarily by muscle tissue

The isoenzymes of CK are particularly useful in detecting myocardial infarction and progressive muscular diseases that cause muscle necrosis as well as drugs that cause muscle damage.

Preparation of Client and Collection of Sample

The timing of the drawing for the CK is crucial because the enzyme may disappear from the bloodstream in less than 24 hours after a myocardial infarction. If possible, intramuscular injections should be delayed until the sample is drawn.

REFERENCE VALUES FOR CK			
Adult			
Women	Total: 40–150 U/L[a]		
Men	Total: 60–400 U/L[a]		
Isoenzymes	CK-I	(BB)	Brain 0–1%
	CK-II	(MB)	Heart 3% or 0–7.5 ng/mL
	CK-III	(MM)	Muscle 95–100%
Pregnant women	Levels are reduced in first half of pregnancy but rise in second half of pregnancy. Slight increase during labor and delivery; surgical procedures, such as an episiotomy, cause more increase		
Newborns	Higher values, which may be very high because of birth trauma		

[a]Intramuscular injections and exercise may elevate the total CK.

Increased Serum CK

Clinical Significance of Elevation of CK-II

CK, the first enzyme to be elevated after a myocardial infarction, begins to rise in 3–6 hours and may peak in the first 24 hours (Table 12–2). In some clients, the CK returns to normal within 16 hours after the chest pain.

If the CK total is above normal, measurement of CK-II or CK-MB is needed. (Laboratories may perform a CK-MB only if the total CK is above normal.) When the CK-MB is reported in U/L, the laboratory may note the following:

- If less than 10 U/L, a myocardial infarction is improbable.
- If 10–12 U/L, the finding is inconclusive.
- If greater than 12 U/L, a myocardial infarction is probable.

See the discussion on troponins for more current cardiac markers. The CK is more useful than the troponins to detect a reoccurrence infarction as troponins remain in the bloodstream for 5 days or longer after the initial infarction.

Table 12–2 Time Frame for Changes in Serum Enzyme Levels and Cardiac Markers After an Acute Myocardial Infarction

	Appears in serum (H)	**Peaks (H)**	**Duration (days)**
CK (isoenzyme II-B)	3–6	18–24	3 or less
Troponins[a]	2–6	14–48	5–7

[a]See text for more details on variations for troponin T and troponin I.

Note: These time frames are general approximations based on several references. Not all clients fall exactly into these patterns.

Possible Nursing Diagnoses Related to Changed Levels of CK

Altered Cardiac Output Related to Extension of Myocardial Infarction

A sudden increase in the CK after a day or two should be reported to the physician immediately and the client assessed for the possibility of an extension of the infarction. If the client undergoes thrombolytic therapy, a high peak of CK followed by a dramatic drop is indicative of reperfusion.

Deficient Knowledge Related to Diagnostic Procedures for Muscle Necrosis

If the elevated CK is related to muscle necrosis, the client may need to undergo a battery of tests to identify the exact problem. Women who are found to be carriers of the sex-linked gene for muscular dystrophy may need to be referred for genetic counseling if they want to bear children (see Chapter 18). The enzyme aldolase is another test for muscular inflammatory diseases. Some general nursing implications for clients with myositis are covered in the section on aldolase later in this chapter.

Clinical Significance of Elevation of CK-III

CK-III (MM) elevations are never diagnostic of a specific muscular disease, but high levels are an indication for further specific testing of muscular function. In the early stages of muscular dystrophy, CK is as high as 3,000 IU/L. As the disease progresses, the CK levels drop, and by the time the client is bedridden, they may be normal. Healthy female carriers of X-linked Duchenne muscular dystrophy have raised levels of CK. Once these women are pregnant, however, the lowering of the CK in the first half of pregnancy may mask the elevation.

Total CK, which is mostly CK-III, is used as a screening test for some drug reactions (Katzung, Masters, & Trevor, 2009). For example, neuroleptics or psychotropic drugs that are dopamine antagonists can cause a neuroleptic malignant syndrome that causes fever, muscle rigidity, and possible death. In susceptible individuals, certain anesthetics and muscle relaxants can cause malignant hyperthermia with severe muscle contractions. The CK will be over five times normal in rhabdomyolysis, a pathologic syndrome associated with disintegration of skeletal muscle. Rhabdo means "rodlike," and rhabdomyo refers to striated muscle. Darkened reddish urine, due to myoglobin, is a cardinal sign. Rhabdomyolysis can be caused by many factors that can damage muscles including drugs such as the hepatic hydroxymethylglutaryl coenzyme A (HMG-CoA) reductase inhibitors (the statins). Graham et al. (2004) found the risk for rhabdomyolysis is low unless the statin is combined with fibrate therapy. (See Chapter 9 for more information on these medications). Combining vigorous exercise, drugs, and extreme heat increases the risk of rhabdomyolysis or "rhabdo."

Clinical Significance of Elevation of CK-I

The isoenzyme CK-I (BB) may be elevated in the case of extreme shock, brain tumors, or severe cerebral accidents, but it is rarely used.

LACTIC DEHYDROGENASE

Lactic dehydrogenase (LDH) is an enzyme that helps remove a water molecule from lactic acid. LDH is found in large amounts in the heart, liver, muscles, and erythrocytes. It is also present in other organs such as the kidneys, pancreas, spleen, brain, and lungs. Like the enzyme CK, LDH can be separated into various isoenzymes:

1. LDH_1 is primarily from the heart and erythrocytes.
2. LDH_2 comes mostly from the reticuloendothelial system.
3. LDH_3 is from the lungs and other tissue.
4. LDH_4 comes from the placenta, kidneys, and pancreas.
5. LDH_5 is largely from the liver and striated muscle.

Preparation of Client and Collection of Sample

The sample must be handled carefully because any hemolysis of the RBCs falsely elevates the results. Even if the hemolysis is not enough to turn the serum pink, there is still an increased LDH.

REFERENCE VALUES FOR LDH

Adults	45–90 U/L (reference ranges dependent on the method used)	
Pregnant women	Normal in pregnancy but increases slightly during labor and delivery, as with other vigorous exercise	
Newborns	First week of life: 160–450 U/L	
Children	60–170 U/L (decreases with age)	
Aged	55–102 U/L	
Isoenzymes	LDH_1 (erythrocytes, heart tissue)	17–27%
	LDH_2 (reticuloendothelial tissue, kidney)	23–28%
	LDH_3 (lungs, lymph nodes, spleen, and various other tissues)	18–28%
	LDH_4 (kidneys, placenta, liver tissue)	5–15%
	LDH_5 (liver tissue, skeletal tissue, kidney)	5–15%

Note: See Hay et al. (2011) and Wu (2006) for more age-related values.

Increased Serum LDH

Clinical Significance

Although LDH isoenzymes are no longer used to diagnose myocardial infarctions (as discussed in the section on troponins as cardiac markers), they may still be useful in the differential diagnosis of certain other diseases, as noted in the following:

1. Hemolytic and macrocytic anemias tend to cause elevations in LDH_1 and LDH_2.
2. In pulmonary infarction, LDH_3 is elevated.

3. Leukemia and malignant tumors, in general, cause large increases in LDH$_3$. LDH is a tumor marker for non-Hodgkin's lymphoma, testicular cancer, and metastatic melanoma. (See Chapter 10 for more information on tumor markers).

4. Liver damage increases the last two isoenzymes, LDH$_4$ and LDH$_5$. Because these two isoenzymes make up only a small portion (10%) of the total LDH, such an increase may not change the total drastically.

5. Shock and trauma may cause an elevation of all the isoenzymes, as do cardiac operations. If a heart–lung machine is used, the LDH is four to six times the normal reference values.

6. In pregnancy, placental disturbances such as abruptio placentae affect an elevation in the isoenzymes.

7. Hepatitis and pancreatitis cause elevations in the total.

8. More than 90% of clients with *Pneumocystis carinii* pneumonia (PCP), now called *Pneumocystis jiroveci,* have elevations of LDH.

TROPONINS AS CARDIAC MARKERS

Troponin, a regulatory protein found in striated muscles, occurs in three forms: I, T, and C. These troponins function together in the contractile apparatus for striated muscle in skeletal muscles and in the myocardium. C troponin is identical from both sources, while I and T troponins have different isoforms for skeletal and cardiac origin. Sensitive assay tests, using antibodies, have been developed to measure serum levels of cardiac troponin I (cTnI) and cardiac troponin T (cTnT). Increased amounts of troponins are released into the bloodstream when an infarction causes damage to the myocardium. After a myocardial infarction, troponin I begins to increase in about 4–6 hours, peaks in 14–18 hours, and remains elevated for 5–7 days. Troponin T begins to increase in 3–4 hours and remains elevated for 10–14 days. A large trial of troponin I, troponin T, and other markers determined that a sensitive assay for troponin improves early diagnosis regardless of the time of onset of chest pain (Keller et al., 2009).

Recommendations on the use of troponins as cardiac markers should take into consideration the following:

1. Current practice is to obtain troponins on admission, at 6–9 hours, and if the clinical picture suggests an myocardial infarction such as symptoms of ischemia, new pathologic Q waves on ECG (Chapter 24) or imaging, evidence of a new loss of viable myocardium, or new regional wall abnormality (Brown, 2009), and then repeat troponins in 12–24 hours. Check the protocol for your specific hospital as well.

2. All current cardiac markers detect myocardial necrosis only, not ischemia, so clients may still have dangerous arrhythmias.

3. No tests of a single cardiac marker are 100% sensitive and specific for the diagnosis of a myocardial infarction in all patients. Clinical pathways help determine alternative testing for unusual cases.

4. Because cardiac troponins remain elevated for at least 5–7 days, a suspected reinfarction should be evaluated with CK-MB (McPhee et al., 2011).

Preparation of Client and Collection of Sample

Client does not need to be fasting. Specimens may be drawn in a gel tube to obtain serum. Check for interferences related to the type of testing.

REFERENCE VALUES FOR TROPONINS[a]

Troponin I	>1.5 ng/mL consistent with myocardial infarction
Troponin T	>0.1–0.2 ng/mL consistent with myocardial infarction

[a]Check with the laboratory at your institution as references are method dependent.

CARDIAC ANALYZERS AS POINT OF CARE

The need for quickly diagnosing clients who present with chest pain has led to the development of several point-of-care cardiac analyzers. For example, as noted in the reference table for troponins, a portable handheld device as a bedside assay can provide information on the troponin T level within a few minutes. Portable cardiac analyzers can also test for troponin I as well as CK-MB. These tests provide a reliable determination of several cardiac markers from a single whole blood sample. Comparison of the various point-of-care tests is available at www.medcompare.com.

Possible Nursing Diagnosis Related to Increased Cardiac Enzymes or Other Markers

Altered Cardiac Output Related to Extension of Infarction or Other Complications

When the presence of an infarction is open to question, it is prudent to continue to treat the client as having a possible myocardial infarction until the condition is definitely ruled out. The key nursing actions are to promote physical and mental relaxation and to watch the vital signs carefully. The use of a cardiac monitor does not take the place of the nurse. The nurse must be able to recognize that the client is having a potentially dangerous arrhythmia so that early treatment can be initiated. The nurse can also detect distended neck veins, crackles, or slight dyspnea as signals of fluid overload. Even a slight change in vital signs may indicate impending cardiogenic shock. This very careful watching of the client is essential any time there is a question of myocardial infarction. (See Chapter 24 for more information on monitoring.) Once a client is diagnosed with an acute myocardial infarction, evidence-based guidelines from the American Heart Association (www.heart.org) and American College of Cardiology (www.acc.org) can be followed. Lackey (2006) outlined the role of the nurse in following these guidelines in caring for the client and in preventing future infarctions.

B-NATRIURETIC PEPTIDE

Human natriuretic peptides have been isolated in several forms, including atrial-type natriuretic peptide (ANP) and brain-type natriuretic peptide. B-Natriuretic peptide (BNP), found in the ventricles of the heart, increases in the serum when ventricular filling pressures are high. The serum levels of BNP increase before the client has symptoms, so it is a way to detect early congestive heart failure (CHF) as well as distinguish cases in which symptoms are not related to CHF. The Food and Drug Administration (FDA) approved BNP in 2001. BNP had high sensitivity and specificity for detecting abnormal ventricle function. BNP has become very important in improving the detection of heart failure when the clinical signs and symptoms are not obvious. The test must be carefully interpreted because pulmonary hypertension and some cardiac diseases may also cause an increase in the BNP level (Wu, 2006).

Preparation of Client and Collection of Sample

Collect one tube of EDTA whole blood. Plasma may also be used.

REFERENCE VALUES FOR BNP

<100 pg/mL

Note: Women and the elderly have higher values. Age- and gender-specific ranges are listed by specific manufacturers.

NT-proBNP

NT-proBNP is a precursor protein (pro-BNP) and an inactive N-terminal fragment. This N-terminal fragment has a longer half-life than BNP; thus, it may be a better marker than BNP in some situations such as mild cardiac failure (Dakin, 2008). This test is also available as point of care (see www.medcompare.com).

Nesiritide is a human B-type natriuretic peptide used to treat clients with acute decompensated heart failure (Deglin, Vallerand, & Sanoski, 2011). Since the synthetic BNP will falsely elevate the BNP test, a test that measures precursor protein, proBNP, needs to be ordered. Nesiritide is usually not used for acute heart failure if clients respond well to diuretics and nitrates as safety of the medication is being researched (McPhee et al., 2011). A standard reference range is not available for proBNP.

Clinical Significance of BNP Levels

BNP levels increase with the severity of heart failure. Mild heart failure may have levels above 100 pg/mL, moderate failure may have levels from 200 to 400 pg/mL, and severe failure from 400 to over 1,000 pg/mL. As noted earlier, BNP may be elevated in some other lung and heart conditions. So the test cannot be used alone to diagnose heart failure as levels between 101 and 400 pg/mL could be related to other conditions. After heart failure is diagnosed and treatments begun, the BNP may be used to monitor the effects of therapy. Although low BNP levels indicate a low probability of heart failure, a complete cardiopulmonary assessment should be done to rule out heart failure.

SERUM ALDOLASE

Like most of the other enzymes discussed in this chapter, aldolase is present in most cells. Its highest concentrations are found in skeletal muscles, heart, and liver tissue. Because damage to muscular tissue causes marked elevations of aldolase, it is a diagnostic test for some types of muscle damage. (CK, discussed earlier, is a more common test for muscular damage.)

Preparation of Client and Collection of Sample

Fasting is not necessary. Aldolase is in erythrocytes, so the specimen must not be hemolyzed. The laboratory needs 2 mL of fresh serum.

REFERENCE VALUES FOR ALDOLASE	
Adults	0–7 U/L
Children	Two times adult level
Newborns	Up to four times adult level

Increased Serum Aldolase Level

Clinical Significance

Muscular disorders that cause inflammation of the muscles (myositis) cause an elevation of aldolase (McPhee et al., 2011). In the event of muscular wasting caused by a muscular disease of the central nervous system, such as myasthenia gravis or multiple sclerosis, the aldolase level is not elevated. In progressive muscular dystrophy, the level may be 10–15 times normal in the early stages of the disease, but the level subsides as muscle wasting continues. In some types of acute myositis, the levels of aldolase return to normal when corticosteroid treatment is effective.

Possible Nursing Diagnoses Related to Increased Aldolase Serum Level (or CK-MM)

Self-Care Deficit Related to Muscle Fatigue

The key nursing implication for a client with a skeletal muscular problem is to help the client be as independent as possible while conserving muscle strength. If the muscular disorder is due to an acute condition, the client is comforted to know that the lack of muscle strength

(Continued)

> ## Possible Nursing Diagnoses . . . (Continued)
>
> is temporary. Return of muscle strength occurs after the enzymes return to normal. Nursing care during the acute phase may center on preventing any complications from disuse of muscles.
>
> ### Risk for Ineffective Coping Related to Problems of Chronic Muscular Disease
>
> If the muscular disorder is a chronic problem, such as muscular dystrophy, the client is faced with learning how to cope with a progressively debilitating disease. Because each case of muscle disease differs from all others, the nursing care plan must be individualized to the severity of the disease and to its effects on the client. The home care nurse may be very involved in helping clients adapt to a crippling disease by suggesting ways to be independent in doing personal care and housekeeping while using limited energy wisely. The nurse needs to emphasize to clients that a schedule that allows frequent and short rest periods is much better than one with a long rest period. Clients may be able to do much more if they are not hurrying to accomplish several activities in a limited time. In addition to emphasizing a planned exercise and rest schedule, the nurse may also need to teach about the expected effects of the prescribed medications and the necessity for follow-up diagnostic tests.

SERUM AMYLASE

Amylase, an enzyme that helps with the digestion of starch, is found in high concentrations in the salivary glands and in the pancreas, each of which contains a different isoenzyme. These two isoenzymes can be separated to rule out nonpancreatic sources. Clients with bulimia nervosa often have enlarged salivary glands and elevated serum amylase levels (Hay et al., 2011). An amylase test may be used to see if induced vomiting is still occurring during treatment.

Amylase may be measured in both serum and urine. The serum amylase may be done as a stat procedure in clients with acute abdominal pain to differentiate pancreatitis from other acute abdominal problems that necessitate surgical intervention. Both lipase and amylase are used for diagnosing pancreatitis as well as ultrasound (Chapter 23), Cat scan (CT) (Chapter 21), and endoscopy (Chapter 26).

Preparation of Client and Collection of Sample

About 60% of the total amylase is from the salivary gland. If healthcare workers talk over an uncovered urine or blood sample, this can falsely elevate total amylase levels. Drugs that cause spasm of the sphincter of Oddi, such as the opiates, may cause an elevation in serum amylase. The increase is at a maximum 5 hours after drug administration. So, if possible, the stat amylase should be drawn before the use of opiate drugs. Thiazide diuretics and diagnostic dyes may cause false elevations.

The client does not need to be fasting. Hemolysis does not affect the results of this test. The laboratory needs 0.5 mL of serum.

REFERENCE VALUES FOR AMYLASE	
Adults	53–123 U/L
Pregnant women	Pregnancy causes moderate increases; women taking oral contraceptives have slightly increased amylase levels
Children	Levels increase to adult levels by age 1 (Wu, 2006)
Aged	May have higher values

Test of Drainage Fluid

Clients who have pancreatic surgery, such as a Whipple procedure, will have drains placed around the surgical site. Before the drains are removed, a test for amylase in the drainage fluid can be performed to identify if there is any leakage.

Increased Serum Amylase Level

Clinical Significance

Pancreatitis is the most common reason for marked elevations in serum amylase, which begins to increase about 3–6 hours after an attack of this disease. (See Table 12–3 for a comparison with serum lipase, the other pancreatic enzyme.) The severity of the disease is not always directly related to the levels of the enzyme. In fact, about 10% of patients with fatal pancreatitis have normal serum amylase levels. High levels in alcoholism, pregnancy, and diabetic ketoacidosis are of salivary rather than pancreatic origin. Renal failure may also cause abnormal elevations not related to pancreatic disease. Certain tumors, such as pheochromocytomas, myelomas, and bronchial cell carcinomas, are associated with high amylase levels

In adults, the two most common reasons for pancreatitis are gallstones (45% of cases) and alcohol abuse (35% of cases) (Pool, 2008). Some cases of presumed "idiopathic" pancreatitis are caused by gallstones too small to be discovered by ultrasound (Chapter 23) but can be identified in the microscopic exam of bile obtained by endoscopy of the bile ducts (see Chapter 27 on ERCP). Evidently, the obstruction of the pancreatic ducts or pancreatic ischemia triggers an acute inflammatory response, and autodigestion of the pancreas begins. Oral contraceptives, hyperlipidemia, and hyperthyroidism are less common reasons for such response. Ruptured ectopic pregnancies, perforated ulcers, and other acute abdominal conditions may cause some elevation of the serum amylase level due to trauma to the pancreas. In children, pancreatitis is rare and often of an unknown cause. Sometimes it appears to have a hereditary base (Hay et al., 2011). Obesity and the beginning of puberty have been related to the incidence of pancreatitis in girls.

Table 12–3			
	Begins Elevation[a]	**Peaks**[a]	**Duration**[a]
Serum amylase	3–6 hours	20–30 hours	2–3 days
Urine amylase	6–10 hours after serum levels	Varies	1–2 wk
Serum lipase	Increases after amylase	Varies	Up to 14 days longer than amylase

[a]Time frames are *general* approximations based on several references.

Possible Nursing Diagnoses Related to Increased Serum Amylase Level

Risk for Deficient Fluid Volume

Among clients with massive hemorrhagic necrosis, the mortality may be as high as 50–80%. If the pancreatitis is not hemorrhagic, the prognosis is much better, but fluid loss can still lead to shock. Thus, one key nursing implication for a client with an elevated serum amylase level is to observe for any change in vital signs that may indicate hypovolemia from the loss of pancreatic fluids or blood. The Hct (Chapter 2) needs to be checked periodically. Optimal hydration can be maintained by the use of intravenous fluids.

Pain Related to an Acute Inflammatory Process

Clients with pancreatitis usually have severe abdominal pain. Comfort measures and pain relief are important. Despins, Kivlahan, and Cox (2005) noted that although opiates such as morphine and fentanyl may increase common duct pressure, they are very effective pain relievers and are usually given by patient-controlled analgesia (PCA). Once pain is resolved, a clear liquid diet is begun, but if pain resumes, an amylase level may be drawn a couple of hours after the resumption of pain.

Imbalanced Nutrition: Related to Measures to Decrease Pancreatic Stimulation

Stimulation of the pancreas needs to be minimized as much as possible. The client must take nothing by mouth and continue to receive intravenous fluids. Total parenteral nutrition may be needed. Bowel sounds may be hypoactive or absent if the inflammation is severe. Current practice is to not use NG tubes unless vomiting is severe or ileus is present (Brenner & Krenzer, 2010).

Risk for Infection

Clients may develop an infection of the necrotic tissue in the pancreas. (See Chapter 2 on white blood cell [WBC] differentials to assess infections.) The temperature should be assessed every 4 hours. Antibiotics are usually reserved for severe pancreatitis with necrosis of more than 30% as demonstrated on a CT scan (Whitcomb, 2006).

Risk for Injury Related to Possible Hypocalcemia, Hypokalemia, Hyperglycemia, and Jaundice

When a client has pancreatitis, laboratory tests and diagnostic procedures often influence nursing care:

1. *Calcium levels:* Serum calcium may be lowered because calcium is deposited in the pancreas because of fat necrosis. The hypocalcemia may be severe enough to cause tetany. (See Chapter 7 for possible nursing diagnoses for clients with a decreased serum calcium level.) Levels lower than 7 mg/dL when albumin levels are normal are associated with an unfavorable prognosis (McPhee et al., 2011).
2. *Potassium levels:* Hypokalemia may result from a lack of intake and a loss of body fluids. (See Chapter 5 for the implications of a lowered potassium level.)

3. *Glucose levels:* Hyperglycemia may be brought about because the damaged pancreatic cells may not be able to produce sufficient insulin. (See Chapter 8 for serum glucose levels.)

4. *Bilirubin levels:* Conjugated bilirubin may increase if the pancreatic inflammation is due to obstruction of the common bile duct. (See Chapter 11 for the implications when the client has obstructive jaundice.)

5. *Triglyceride levels:* Triglyceride levels may be high, particularly if alcohol was a triggering event (see Chapter 9).

6. *Blood urea nitrogen (BUN) and creatinine levels:* Impaired renal function may occur (see Chapter 4).

7. *Other criteria*: Other criteria used to assess the severity of acute pancreatitis include arterial oxygen saturation (Chapter 6) and LDH and AST levels (Chapter 12).

8. *Assessing for chronic complications:* Once the client is over the acute stage of pancreatitis, the most common complications are abscess formation in the pancreas or pseudocysts, which are collections of fluids in sacs outside the pancreas. Gallium scans (Chapter 22) may be used to detect abscesses, whereas sonograms (Chapter 23) may show the presence of the pseudocysts.

Deficient Knowledge Related to Measures to Prevent Recurrent Attacks

Clients who have had an elevated serum amylase level benefit from discharge planning that focuses on the ways that recurrent attacks can be reduced. Alcohol in all forms should be avoided. If alcohol abuse was the precipitating factor, the client may need to seek professional help to deal with a chronic problem. If gallstones are present and a cholecystectomy is to be performed later, dietary fat restriction may be needed.

URINARY AMYLASE

Amylase, the enzyme elevated in the serum in acute pancreatitis, can also be measured in the urine. The amylase may be elevated in the urine for as long as 2 weeks after an acute episode of pancreatitis. Monitoring amylase levels in urine may be useful after the acute peak in the serum has diminished. (See Table 12–3 for a comparison of the time frames for serum and urine amylases.) A continued elevation of urine amylase suggests formation of a pseudocyst (Wu, 2006).

Preparation of Client and Collection of Sample

Usually the test is completed on a collection of urine for a 2-hour period, but sometimes a 24-hour specimen is used. (See Chapter 3 for tips on collecting 24-hour urine specimens.) Send a blood sample with the urine specimen.

REFERENCE VALUE FOR URINARY AMYLASE

4–400 U/L

SERUM LIPASE

Lipase is a pancreatic enzyme that breaks down fat into glycerol and fatty acids. In acute pancreatitis (see Table 12–3), lipase rises later in the serum than does amylase. So lipase may be used as a secondary test for pancreatitis when the diagnosis is questionable. Other types of pancreatic disease, such as carcinoma or traumatic injury, cause some release of the enzyme into the serum. (See the discussion of amylase for nursing diagnoses related to acute pancreatitis.)

Preparation of Client and Collection of Sample

The precautions are the same as those for amylase, except there is no concern about contamination from saliva. The laboratory needs 1 mL of serum.

REFERENCE VALUE FOR LIPASE	
All groups	3–19 U/dL

Questions

1. A markedly elevated alkaline phosphatase level is a general warning of either
   a. Increased bone formation or obstruction to bile flow
   b. Myocardial infarction *or* angina
   c. Cancer of the prostate *or* of the liver
   d. Increased bone destruction *or* liver dysfunction

2. Intravenous administration of albumin solutions may cause an elevated serum alkaline phosphatase level for which of the following reasons?
   a. Albumin obtained from placentas is rich in this enzyme
   b. Alkaline phosphatase is transported by albumin
   c. Oncotic pressure is increased in the serum
   d. The method used to purify albumin causes the release of the enzyme

3. A client has a history of alcohol abuse but is now in a rehabilitation program. Which of the following tests is used to assess for hepatic injury caused by alcohol abuse?
   a. ALP
   b. LDH
   c. Amylase
   d. GGT

4. When a client has a marked elevation of the ALT (formerly SGPT) and AST (formerly SGOT), a priority nursing diagnosis is
   a. Activity intolerance
   b. Fluid volume deficit

    c. Fluid volume overload

    d. Impaired gas exchange

5. In myocardial damage, which of the following enzymes is most useful for detecting an extension of 2 days after the initial infarction?

    a. CK

    b. AST (SGOT)

    c. BNP

    d. Troponin T

6. Troponins are very useful in diagnosing

    a. Myocardial infarction

    b. Pancreatitis

    c. Hepatitis

    d. Smooth muscle injury

7. A 50-year-old businessman has been admitted to the observation unit with severe chest pain. His CK and troponins were normal at admission. He wants to make several business calls. He has asked where he can find a phone. Which nursing action is appropriate?

    a. Allow him to go to a phone via wheelchair, because his first tests are normal

    b. Tell him he has most likely had a heart attack, so he must stay on complete bed rest

    c. Make sure that he understands the need for further assessment of ECG readings, serial levels, and a medical exam to rule out a possible myocardial infarction

    d. Tell him that phone calls are not allowed and continue to observe him for arrhythmias, hypotension, or distended neck veins

8. A 44-year-old mother has two teenaged girls. She has increased CK and aldolase levels caused by a still-undiagnosed muscular disease. Which advice by a home health nurse would be the most appropriate?

    a. "Schedule most of your activities for the morning when you have the most strength."

    b. "Ask your teenagers to take care of your personal needs such as baths and shampoos."

    c. "Why not hire someone to do all your housework?"

    d. "Try to alternate each small activity with a short period of rest."

9. A 35-year-old man has been admitted with recurring pancreatitis. Both his serum and urine levels of amylase are markedly increased. The nurse should be alert for any signs of which of the following?

    a. Hypocalcemia

    b. Hypoglycemia

    c. Hypernatremia

    d. Hyperkalemia

10. A client's amylase levels have returned to normal, and he is being discharged. When he returns to the clinic next week, it would be *most important* to reemphasize a diet plan that includes which of the following?

    a. Decreased intake of starches and other carbohydrates

    b. Total restriction of alcoholic beverages

    c. Foods high in fat-soluble vitamins

    d. Frequent small feedings with an emphasis on high-calorie foods

References

Brenner, Z. R. & Krenzer, M. E. (2010). Understanding acute pancreatitis. *Nursing 2010, 40*(1), 32–37.

Brown, R. (2009). Detecting AMI with cardiac biomarkers. *Nursing 2009, 39*(10), 63.

Dakin, C. L. (2008). New approaches to heart failure. *American Journal of Nursing, 108*(3), 68–71.

Deglin, J. H., Vallerand, A. H., & Sanoski, C. A. (2011). *Davis's drug guide for nurses* (12th ed.). Philadelphia: F.A. Davis.

Despins, L. A., Kivlahan, C., & Cox, K. R. (2005). Acute pancreatitis. *American Journal of Nursing, 105*(11), 54–57.

Graham, D. J., Staffa, J. A., Shatin, D., Andrade, S. E., Schech, S. D., Grenade, L., et al. (2004). Incidence of hospitalized rhabdomyolysis in patients treated with lipid-lowering drugs. *Journal of the American Medical Association, 292*(21), 2585–2590.

Hay, W. W., Levin, M. J., Sondheimer, J. M., & Deterding, R. (Eds.). (2011). *Current diagnosis and treatment: Pediatrics* (20th ed.). New York: McGraw-Hill.

Hietala, J., Kolvisto, H., Anttila, P., & Niemela, O. (2006). Comparison of the combined marker GGT-CDT and the conventional laboratory markers of alcohol abuse in heavy drinkers, moderate drinkers and abstainers. *Alcohol and Alcoholism, 41*(5), 528–533.

Katzung, B. G., Masters, S. B., & Trevor, A. J. (2009). *Basic and clinical pharmacology* (11th ed.). New York: Mc Graw-Hill.

Keller T., Zeller, T., Peetz, D., Tzikas, S., Roth, A., Czyz, E., et al. (2009). Sensitive troponin 1 assay in early diagnosis of acute myocardial infarction. *The New England Journal of Medicine, 361*(9), 868–877.

Lackey, S. A. (2006). Suppressing the scourge of AMI. *Nursing 2006, 36*(5), 37–42.

McPhee, S. J., Papadakis, M. A., & Rabow, C. A. (Eds.). (2011). *Current medical diagnosis and treatment* (50th ed.). New York: McGraw-Hill.

Navarro, V. J. & Senior, J. R. (2006). Drug-related hepatotoxicity. *New England Journal of Medicine, 354*(7), 731–739.

Pool, D. (2008). Prevailing over acute pancreatitis. *American Nurse Today, 3*(3), 10–12.

Shatzer, M. & Saul, L. (2003). Using a BNP test to identify heart failure. *Nursing 2003, 33*(1), 68.

Whitcomb, D. C. (2006). Acute pancreatitis. *New England Journal of Medicine, 354*(20), 2142–2150.

Wu, A. H. (Ed.). (2006). *Tietz clinical guide to laboratory tests* (4th ed.). St. Louis, MO: Saunders Elsevier.

Websites

www.acc.org (American College of Cardiology guidelines for treatment of myocardial infarction.)
www.heart.org (Information on myocardial infarctions and heart failure.)
www.medcompare.com (Information on various types of point of care cardiac analyzers.)

Answers

1. a, 2. a, 3. d, 4. a, 5. a, 6. a, 7. c, 8. d, 9. a, 10. b

Coagulation Tests and Tests to Detect Occult Blood

- Coagulation Process   298
- Prothrombin Time   300
- Partial Thromboplastin Time (Activated) (aPTT)   310
- Antiphospholipid Antibodies: Lupus Anticoagulants and Anticardiolipin Antibodies   313
- Activated Clotting Time   313
- Tests for Low-Molecular-Weight Heparin   314
- Direct Thrombin Inhibitors Monitored by PTT   314
- Heparin Antifactor Xa Assay (Anti-Xa)   314
- Hemophilia Tests: Factors VIII and IX   315
- Screening for von Willebrand Disease   315
- Platelet Count and Mean Platelet Volume   317
- Clot Retraction Test   320
- Aspirin Resistance Tests   320
- Clopidogrel Resistance Tests   320
- Fibrinogen   321
- D-Dimer Screen: ELISA and Latex Agglutination Slide Test   322
- Thrombin Time: Fibrinogen Screen, Thrombin Clotting Time with Reptilase   323
- Plasminogen Assay   323
- Proteins C and S Anticoagulant System   324
- Factor V Leiden   324
- Prothrombin G 20210A Mutations   325
- Occult Blood Testing in Various Specimens   326
- Screening Tests to Detect Colorectal Cancer   326

OBJECTIVES

1. Describe the four main stages of the coagulation process, and the difference between the intrinsic and extrinsic systems of clotting as a basis for laboratory tests.

2. Describe clinical situations in which vitamin K is useful for returning the prothrombin time (PT or Pro Time) to normal.

3. Identify important nursing diagnoses for a client who has a bleeding tendency caused by a lack of clotting factors.

4. Devise a teaching plan for a client who is discharged to undergo long-term coumarin therapy.

5. Compare and contrast the two most common coagulation tests, PT and partial thromboplastin time (PTT).

6. Describe possible nursing interventions when a client has an abnormally decreased PT or PTT or other signs of hypercoagulability.

7. Explain the screening tests and confirmatory tests for classic hemophilia (hemophilia A).

8. Identify possible nursing diagnoses for clients with increased and decreased platelet counts.

9. Identify the changes in fibrinogen levels, along with the changes in other laboratory tests, that are clues that disseminated intravascular coagulation (DIC) or consumption coagulopathy may be occurring.

10. Describe the important facts a nurse should know about tests used to detect occult blood in the feces or other specimens.

The delicate balance of the coagulation process makes it possible for a healthy person to experience neither hemorrhage nor thrombus formation. Tests such as the PT, PTT, and platelet counts are routine tests for the clotting ability of the blood. Tests of individual factors are needed to detect specific diseases, such as hemophilia A (test for factor VIII). Other tests, such as fibrinogen assays, help in the assessment of severe coagulation problems, such as DIC.

Besides the common tests for clotting ability, this chapter includes information on guaiac and other tests used to detect hidden or occult blood. Occult blood tests are used not only to detect bleeding tendencies but also to screen for rectal cancer.

Coagulation tests are of use to the nurse in three primary ways. First, these tests may alert the nurse to the possibility that the client is vulnerable because of an increased bleeding tendency. Second, some of these tests may indicate that the client is vulnerable because of an increased risk of thrombus formation. Third, three of these tests are specifically used to monitor the effects of anticoagulant drugs.

COAGULATION PROCESS

Twelve factors are involved in the clotting process. Remembering all the factors is not necessary, but knowing which test measures which factors is useful. A list of the 12 factors, along with the tests that show the deficiencies and the relation of vitamin K, is presented in Table 13–1. Vitamin K was named K because it is the "koagulation" factor. If the liver cannot obtain vitamin K, four coagulation factors cannot be manufactured: factors II, VII, IX, and X. Note that the table contains 13 numbers, because one factor (VI) was found to be part of another factor. The factors were numbered, instead of named, in the order of their discovery, so there could be a universal understanding of which factor was being discussed.

Table 13–1 illustrates that both the PT and the PTT are used to test several factors but not always the same ones. Although the PTT is a broader screening test, certain deficiencies can be assessed by using both the PT and the PTT. Also the laboratory can add one factor at a time to see which factor is missing.

The coagulation process can be initiated in two ways. With the *extrinsic system,* the clotting is triggered by the release of tissue thromboplastin. With the *intrinsic system,* the coagulation process requires only the factors that are present in the plasma.

Regardless of how the process is initiated, the coagulation process occurs in four stages. Stage I involves the release of platelet factors that begin the clotting process.

Table 13–1 Coagulation Factors Tested by Specific Tests and Relation to Vitamin K

Name of Factor	Test of Deficiency	Vitamin K Needed for Production By Liver
I (fibrinogen)	Fibrinogen level[a] PT, PTT	
II (prothrombin)	PT, PTT	Yes
III (thromboplastin)		
IV (calcium)		
V (labile or proaccelerin)	PT, PTT	
VI (unassigned at present time)		
VII (stable factor or proconvertin)	PT	Yes
VIII (antihemophilic globulin)	PTT	
IX (partial thromboplastin component [PTC], Christmas factor)	PTT	Yes
X (Stuart–Prower factor)	PT, PTT	Yes
XI (plasma thromboplastin antecedent)	PTT	
XII (Hageman factor)	PTT	
XIII (fibrin-stabilizing factor)		

[a]Specific assays can be performed to test for each factor. See Wu (2006).

Stage II is the generation of thromboplastin as calcium and other factors interact. Stage III is the conversion of prothrombin to thrombin, and Stage IV is the formation of fibrin from fibrinogen. Some sources list three stages of coagulation because Stages I and II are combined as Stage I. Table 13–2 outlines the stages of clotting.

Table 13–2 Stages of Clotting and Common Laboratory Tests

Time of Stage	Stage	Factors Involved[a]	Tests for Stage
	I	Platelets initiate clotting	Platelets, clot retraction
Takes 3–5 minutes	II	Thromboplastin (factor III) is generated by reaction of factors VIII, IX, X, XI, and XII. Factor IV, CA^{2+} also needed	PTT very sensitive
Takes 8–16 minutes	III	Factor II (prothrombin) is converted to thrombin. Accelerator factors V, VII, and X are involved.	PT very sensitive
Almost instantly	IV	Factor I (fibrinogen) is converted to fibrin. Factor XIII, the fibrin-stabilizing factor, is needed.	Fibrinogen levels

[a]Moderate reductions in multiple factors prolong PT and PTT, but this synergistic action usually imposes little clinical risk of hemorrhage.

Some references combine Stages I and II so that

Stage I: Formation of thromboplastin or activation of factor X

Stage II: Prothrombin to thrombin

Stage III: Fibrinogen to fibrin

The importance of calcium in the clotting process should be noted. Usually, a lack of calcium is not a problem because of the tremendous reservoir of calcium in the bones and teeth (see Chapter 7 on calcium). About 90% of all clotting defects occur in Stage II, the thromboplastin generation stage. Thus, the PTT is a useful screening tool for many bleeding disorders.

After the factors are used in the coagulation process, fibrin inhibitors, such as antiplasmin, protein C, and antithrombin III, inactivate excess amounts of certain clotting factors so that clotting does not occur inappropriately. Pathologic defects or decreases in these factors may be responsible for thrombotic episodes, so these fibrin inhibitors may sometimes be measured to help determine a coagulation problem. Inactive plasminogen is converted to plasmin by a tissue plasmin activating factor (TPA). Plasmin is useful as a fibrinolytic agent. TPA derived from human cells and synthesized by recombinant DNA technology is used to dissolve clots.

PROTHROMBIN TIME

Prothrombin, or factor II, is a plasma protein produced by the liver. The confusing thing about the test is that although it is called *prothrombin time,* it does not measure just prothrombin but also several other factors (see Table 13–1). The point to remember is that a change in all, or any, of these factors causes an abnormal PT. Just like prothrombin, these other factors are manufactured in the liver, and most of the factors require vitamin K for their manufacture.

The PT is the specific, and the only, laboratory test used to measure the effectiveness of the coumarin type of anticoagulant drugs, such as warfarin sodium. Although heparin, a different type of anticoagulant, in large doses may change the PT, two other tests are used to monitor heparin therapy. These are the PTT and the activated clotting time (ACT), both of which are discussed later in this chapter. Although the abbreviations PT and PTT are very similar and thus often confusing to the novice, the tests are very different and used for two very different anticoagulants (Table 13–3).

Use of International Normalized Ratio

The International Normalized Ratio (INR), first used in European laboratories and now common in North America, adjusts for the variability in the type of tissue thromboplastin used for the PT. In the 1980s, the World Health Organization developed a plan to standardize the PT by comparing various commercial preparations of rabbit brain thromboplastin with the more sensitive human brain tissue thromboplastin. This comparison of the thromboplastin from the animal source to the purer human source gives the International Sensitivity Index (ISI). The ISI, obtained from the manufacturers of the thromboplastin reagents, is used with the PT ratio to obtain the INR. The laboratory uses a table like Table 13–4 to match the PT ratio with the ISI for the reagent used. For example, if the control is 12 seconds and a patient has a PT of 24 seconds, the PT ratio is 2.0. If the reagent used is 1.6, the corresponding INR is 3.0, based on Table 13–4. However,

Table 13–3 Comparisons of PT and PTT

	PT	**PTT (Activated)**
Drugs monitored	Warfarin sodium	Heparin
Reference values (control)	60–140% activity 12–15 seconds	Not reported in percentage 25–37 seconds
Desirable therapeutic levels	INR usually 2.0–3.0[a]	1.5–2.3 times control
Time of drug to affect laboratory test	Oral warfarin takes several *days* to achieve therapeutic level.	Intravenous heparin acts immediately Subcutaneous heparin takes several hours.
Usual timing of laboratory test	On daily basis until stabilized, then once every 4–6 wk for long-term control	Once a day if continuous intravenous infusion or more often if unstable
Measures used to return laboratory test to normal	1. Reduction of dosage 2. Fresh frozen plasma concentrate 3. Vitamin K_1 parenterally	1. Reduction of dosage 2. Fresh frozen plasma concentrate 3. Protamine sulfate parenterally
Time of reversibility	1. Varies with dosage reduction 2. Immediate with transfusion 3. Several hours for vitamin K	1. Varies with dosage reduction 2. Immediate with transfusion 3. Immediate with protamine

[a]See text on INR—some conditions require slightly higher INR.

Many drugs may affect test results. See Katzung, Masters, and Trevor (2009) and Deglin, Vallerand, and Sanoski (2011).

if the ISI were 1.8, the INR would be 3.5. Laboratories report both the PT ratio and the INR for decision making about anticoagulation. Recommendations for monitoring oral anticoagulant therapy are usually an INR of 2.0–3.0 for most clients, except those with mechanical heart valves, who require a higher INR of 2.5–3.5 (Turka, 2005). Clients usually reach an INR of 2.0–3.0 in 3–5 days after oral anticoagulation is begun. A lower INR (1.3–1.9) may be the goal if the client is on low-dose warfarin to prevent thrombosis from a central venous catheter (Hadawoy, 2004).

Measurement in Seconds

The INR is not used to monitor clients with liver disease. In liver disease, other clotting factors are decreased, so the INR does not detect or adjust to these changes. Thus for liver disease, seconds should be used to determine the severity of the bleeding disorder.

Preparation of Client and Collection of Sample

Many drugs can affect the PT (see Table 13–3). Record on the laboratory slip any heparin dosage because the PT may be affected at the peak of heparin activity. Venous blood (1.8 mL) is collected in plastic tubes with sodium citrate (blue top). For point-of-care testing, a portable laser photodetector measures the PT in 2 minutes. Only a finger stick is needed.

Table 13–4 Table for Conversion of Prothrombin Time Ratio to International Normalized Ratio

Prothrombin Time Ratio	International Sensitivity Index (ISI)																				
	1.0	1.1	1.2	1.3	1.4	1.5	1.6	1.7	1.8	1.9	2.0	2.1	2.2	2.3	2.4	2.5	2.6	2.7	2.8	2.9	3.0
1.0	1.0	1.0	1.0	1.0	1.0	1.0	1.0	1.0	1.0	1.0	1.0	1.0	1.0	1.0	1.0	1.0	1.0	1.0	1.0	1.0	1.0
1.1	1.1	1.1	1.1	1.1	1.1	1.2	1.2	1.2	1.2	1.2	1.2	1.2	1.2	1.2	1.3	1.3	1.3	1.3	1.3	1.3	1.3
1.2	1.2	1.2	1.2	1.3	1.3	1.3	1.3	1.4	1.4	1.4	1.4	1.5	1.5	1.5	1.5	1.6	1.6	1.6	1.7	1.7	1.7
1.3	1.3	1.3	1.4	1.4	1.4	1.5	1.5	1.6	1.6	1.6	1.7	1.7	1.8	1.8	1.9	1.9	2.0	2.0	2.1	2.1	2.2
1.4	1.4	1.4	1.5	1.5	1.6	1.7	1.7	1.8	1.8	1.9	2.0	2.0	2.1	2.2	2.2	2.3	2.4	2.5	2.6	2.7	2.7
1.5	1.5	1.6	1.6	1.7	1.8	1.8	1.9	2.0	2.1	2.2	2.3	2.3	2.4	2.5	2.6	2.8	2.9	3.0	3.1	3.2	3.4
1.6	1.6	1.7	1.8	1.8	1.9	2.0	2.1	2.2	2.3	2.4	2.6	2.7	2.8	2.9	3.1	3.2	3.4	3.6	3.7	3.9	4.1
1.7	1.7	1.8	1.9	2.0	2.1	2.2	2.3	2.5	2.6	2.7	2.9	3.0	3.2	3.4	3.6	3.8	4.0	4.2	4.4	4.7	4.9
1.8	1.8	1.9	2.0	2.1	2.3	2.4	2.6	2.7	2.9	3.1	3.2	3.4	3.6	3.9	4.1	4.3	4.6	4.9	5.2	5.5	5.8
1.9	1.9	2.0	2.2	2.3	2.5	2.6	2.8	3.0	3.2	3.4	3.6	3.8	4.1	4.4	4.7	5.0	5.3	5.7	6.0		
2.0	2.0	2.1	2.3	2.5	2.6	2.8	3.0	3.2	3.5	3.7	4.0	4.3	4.6	4.9	5.3	5.7					
2.1	2.1	2.3	2.4	2.6	2.8	3.0	3.3	3.5	3.8	4.1	4.4	4.7	5.1	5.5	5.9						
2.2	2.2	2.4	2.6	2.8	3.0	3.3	3.5	3.8	4.1	4.5	4.8	5.2	5.7								
2.3	2.3	2.5	2.7	3.0	3.2	3.5	3.8	4.1	4.5	4.9	5.3	5.7									
2.4	2.4	2.6	2.9	3.1	3.4	3.7	4.1	4.4	4.8	5.3	5.8										
2.5	2.5	2.7	3.0	3.3	3.6	4.0	4.3	4.7	5.2	5.7											
2.6	2.6	2.9	3.1	3.5	3.8	4.2	4.6	5.1	5.6												
2.7	2.7	3.0	3.3	3.6	4.0	4.4	4.9	5.4	6.0												
2.8	2.8	3.1	3.4	3.8	4.2	4.7	5.2	5.8													
2.9	2.9	3.2	3.6	4.0	4.4	4.9	5.5														
3.0	3.0	3.3	3.7	4.2	4.7	5.2	5.8														
3.1	3.1	3.5	3.9	4.4	4.9	5.5															
3.2	3.2	3.6	4.0	4.5	5.1	5.7															
3.3	3.3	3.7	4.2	4.7	5.3	6.0															
3.4	3.4	3.8	4.3	4.9	5.5																
3.5	3.5	4.0	4.5	5.1	5.8																
3.6	3.6	4.1	4.7	5.3	6.0																
3.7	3.7	4.2	4.8	5.5																	
3.8	3.8	4.3	5.0	5.7																	
3.9	3.9	4.5	5.1	5.9																	
4.0	4.0	4.6	5.3																		
4.1	4.1	4.7	5.4																		
4.2	4.2	4.8	5.6																		
4.3	4.3	5.0	5.8																		
4.4	4.4	5.1	5.9																		
4.5	4.5	5.2																			
4.6	4.6	5.4																			
4.7	4.7	5.5																			

Note: See text for prothrombin time ratio determination. The ISI is supplied by the manufacturer.

302

REFERENCE VALUES FOR PT	
Adult	Control 11.2–13.2 seconds (± 2 seconds). INR around 1.0*
Newborn	Some clotting factors are lower than in adults, so reference values may be about 12–21 seconds. Premature infants may have even higher reference values in seconds.
Pregnant women	In late pregnancy, some clotting factors are increased, so reference values may be slightly decreased for time in seconds.

*See text for explanation of INR, which is used to monitor anticoagulants.

Testing Prothrombin Times at Home

Since the late 1980s, portable PT monitors have been used by hospital laboratory personnel to accurately measure PT in seconds, a PT ratio, and an INR. Capillary blood from a finger stick is placed into a cartridge inserted in the monitor, a procedure similar to testing glucose levels. Because the monitor is easy to use, studies were begun to see if clients could do the monitoring at home. Clients were able to use the home monitors to get results similar to laboratory results. The Food and Drug Administration (FDA) approved the monitor for home use in 1997. Self-testing requires that individuals feel comfortable taking on this responsibility and that they understand the meaning of the results and when to call their health care provider (Pence & McErlane, 2005).

Increased PT (Increase in Time) or Hypoprothrombinemia

Clinical Significance

A client may have an increased PT because the liver is unable to make prothrombin and the other factors measured with the PT test. An increased PT is characteristic of advanced cirrhosis of the liver because a large amount of scar tissue takes the place of functioning liver cells, and these nonfunctioning liver cells can no longer make prothrombin. PT is a valuable tool in assessing the amount of liver damage in a client with liver disease. Unlike other situations in which the PT is increased, vitamin K injections usually do not help much with advanced liver disease. The inability of the liver to respond to vitamin K, as evidenced by little change in the PT after vitamin K injection, demonstrates that the liver is so damaged that it cannot produce more prothrombin and other factors, even with abundant vitamin K.

Another clinical reason for an increased PT is the inability of the body to absorb vitamin K from the gastrointestinal (GI) tract. Because vitamin K is a fat-soluble vitamin, absorption depends on the presence of bile salts. With an obstruction of the common bile duct, bile salts cannot be released into the duodenum. So a client who has obstructive jaundice, which is caused by an obstruction in the common bile duct, has an increased PT because the liver cannot get vitamin K.

Much rarer is a true deficiency of vitamin K in the body, because humans do not depend much on dietary sources for vitamin K. This vitamin is manufactured by the bacteria that normally reside in the intestinal tract. So if a client is undergoing long-term antibiotic therapy that depletes the normal bacteria in the GI tract, he or she may have an increased PT caused by a deficiency of vitamin K. Unlike a client with a failing liver, a client with a vitamin K deficiency or malabsorption problem has an increased PT that can be returned to normal by the administration of vitamin K. When the vitamin is given parenterally, it is absorbed into the bloodstream and bypasses the digestive step that requires bile salts. (See Chapter 11 for more discussion on obstructive jaundice and hypoprothrombinemia in relation to the test of direct bilirubin.)

A newborn's PT is slightly prolonged because infants do not have the same quantity of some of the clotting factors as adults. Newborns also do not have a store of vitamin K, and they have not yet acquired the normal intestinal bacteria to produce the vitamin. Newborns of mothers who are deficient in vitamin K are thus susceptible to a disease called *hemorrhagic disease of the newborn*. A dose of vitamin K, given prophylactically to all newborns, guards against the possibility of hemorrhage in the first few days. Vitamin K prophylaxis in newborns has been the standard of care since 1961 (DeCherney et al., 2007).

Another hemorrhagic situation with an increased PT is in the complex bleeding disorder called *DIC*. This clinical situation is discussed in detail at the end of this chapter, as are fibrinogen levels.

Effect of Warfarin on PT. Coumarin-type drugs cause a decrease in the production of prothrombin and of other factors because these drugs interfere with the use of vitamin K by the liver. Because the coumarin-type drugs work in this indirect way, by depressing liver function, the change in the PT does not occur for a day or longer. It usually takes several days for the PT to reach the desired INR. Vitamin K, taken orally or parenterally, reverses the effects of these drugs, returning the PT to normal within several hours. A PT in the normal range may be dangerous for a client who needs to undergo anticoagulation in the first place. (Refer to Table 13–3 for a summary of information about coumarin drugs and PT monitoring with the INR.)

Use of Vitamin K for Elevated INR

Research supports maintaining the same warfarin dosage in asymptomatic clients with an INR no higher than 3.3. If the INR is above the therapeutic range but below 5, the client may skip the next dose and the dosage may be reduced (Turner, 2006). The website of the American College of Chest Physicians (www.chestnet.org) has detailed guidelines for the treatment of elevated INR that may include small doses of vitamin K for an INR between 5 and 9 and high doses for an INR over 9. Administering too high a dose of vitamin K must be avoided because this may make the client resistant to the oral anticoagulant for up to a week. Serious bleeding or immediate reversal of the anticoagulation may be treated with intravenous infusion of concentrated clotting factors or fresh frozen plasma as noted in Table 13–3.

Genetic Tests to Determine Warfarin Dosage

Determining the correct dosage of warfarin can be difficult as clients metabolize the drug differently. Most clients need about 5 mg a day, but lower doses may be needed for those who have changes in the CYP2C9 or the VKORCI genes (McPhee, Papadakis, & Rabow, 2011). However, these tests are expensive and slow to perform.

The warfarin label recommends but does not require genetic testing for newly prescribed clients. See www.labtestsonline.org for updates on these tests.

A New Type of Oral Anticoagulant

A new type of oral anticoagulant, dabigatron, may be as effective as warfarin and can be given in fixed dosages. This anticoagulant does not require laboratory monitoring (Schulman et al., 2009).

Possible Nursing Diagnoses Related to Increased PT

Risk for Bleeding Related to Hypoprothrombinemia

A nurse caring for a client with an increased PT needs a clear understanding of whether this client is likely to be vulnerable to bleeding for a long time or if this abnormal PT is of short duration. For example, if the client has an increased PT as a result of obstructive jaundice, vitamin K brings the PT back to normal within a few hours or at most within a day or so. In this case, one should not need to burden the client and family with a long list of all the possible ways to protect the client from bleeding. However, a client who is being discharged to take a coumarin-type drug needs to know that a PT that represents 20–50% normal clotting activity makes a client vulnerable to bleeding. These clients and their families need detailed instructions on how to treat bleeding episodes. Vitamin K is one antidote for coumarin overdosage (frozen plasma is the other), but many physicians do not want clients to carry this drug if they are close to a medical facility. (See the earlier discussion on the usual treatment for an elevated INR.) Clients with severe liver disease may also be functioning with an increased PT that is of a chronic nature. They need to be taught how to protect themselves from bleeding. As mentioned earlier, vitamin K probably does not help this PT very much. Clients with liver disease are very likely eventually to have severe bleeding episodes.

Assessing and Preventing Bleeding Episodes. Nurses must always be looking for symptoms that could indicate a client might be bleeding because a bleeding episode is the possible consequence in any client with an increased PT. Nurses must also be aware of the ways to prevent bleeding. They must use their own judgment about which parts of the following assessment and interventions are needed for an individual client. The degree of client involvement in protecting him- or herself from bleeding depends on the level of illness and the setting of home or hospital. Nurses must assess the client's level of understanding, readiness for information about the condition or treatment, and willingness and ability to participate in health care.

When caring for a client who has a bleeding tendency because of an abnormal PT and other factors, nurses need to be aware of all the subtle clues that can be a symptom of bleeding. As the professionals who probably spend the most time with the client, nurses have the opportunity and responsibility to detect these subtle changes before a bleeding episode becomes a catastrophe. A complete assessment and prevention of bleeding includes the following:

1. Headaches or changes in neurologic status could indicate bleeding into the cranium. A headache is of particular concern for a client who has sustained a head injury.
2. Clients with an increased PT must be protected from falls. Sports or other activities that could lead to head blows are risky.

(Continued)

Possible Nursing Diagnoses . . . *(Continued)*

3. Clients who shave should do so with an electric razor to prevent bleeding from accidental cuts.
4. Epistaxis (nose bleeding) and gum bleeding may occur. So too-vigorous tooth brushing, hard coughing, or blowing the nose may trigger bleeding. Nose bleeding in these clients can be a serious matter.
5. Nurses must be particularly careful when suctioning a client who has a bleeding tendency.
6. Vomiting or coughing blood can be quite serious. The physician should be notified immediately, even if the vomitus contains only a small amount of blood. Often the small amount of blood that is vomited first is only the first indication. Fresh blood looks like blood. Older blood, which has been acted on by the gastric juices, has a characteristic dark brown color called *coffee-ground*.
7. In a client with a nasogastric (NG) tube, the drainage may be coffee-ground color rather than the yellowish to pale green of normal stomach contents. Not all coffee-ground drainage from NG tubes means the client is experiencing a large amount of bleeding. Sometimes simply the presence of the NG tube causes enough irritation to produce minimal and clinically insignificant bleeding. Yet for a client with an increased PT, any bleeding may be serious.

   Tests can be performed to detect occult bleeding in gastric secretions. Yet, obviously, if there is frank blood, a guaiac test is a waste of time and effort. The nurse must also be very careful about irrigation of an NG tube for a client with bleeding tendencies. Iced saline lavage may be used to control gastric bleeding. Antacids and histamine-2 blockers such as cimetidine may be ordered to decrease gastric hyperacidity. (See the section on guaiac and other tests at the end of this chapter.)
8. A client with severe liver disease may also have esophageal varices (varicosities) that can be the source of massive bleeding. A client with suspected varices may have dietary restrictions so that only soft foods are served.
9. Abdominal or flank pain may indicate slow internal bleeding. Internal bleeding can be very subtle in the beginning, with few symptoms, because the bleeding usually is slow. A client may describe a backache that cannot be relieved with back rubs, a change of position, or the administration of a mild analgesic. No one may consider a possible connection to the anticoagulant the client is receiving until the client faints when he or she tries to get out of bed. Then it is discovered that the client has been slowly bleeding into the retroperitoneal area.

   Internal bleeding can cause pain because of the increasing pressure as blood collects. If the bleeding is into the GI tract, however, there is probably no associated pain because the blood does not cause undue pressure, and if the client has an ulcer, the blood acts as a buffer. The blood eventually passes into the stool, making the stool a dark color.

   Clients with a bleeding tendency should periodically test the stools for occult blood. Hematocrits (Hcts) are useful to assess the exact amount of blood loss (see Chapter 2). The tests for occult blood, described at the end of this chapter, are simple enough that clients can be taught to conduct a test at home if the situation warrants doing so. If the bleeding is fairly copious and high enough in the GI tract to be in contact with the digestive juices, the stools take on a dark black color that is described as "tarry." Straining at stool may cause bleeding, especially if the client has hemorrhoids, so the nurse needs to help the client find ways to avoid constipation.

10. Dark or smokey-looking urine may indicate blood in the urine. Hematuria is often the first indication of overdosage with anticoagulants. Sometimes the blood is bright red if it is fresh. Clients who have catheters may bleed because of irritation caused by the catheter. Nurses should make sure the catheter is securely anchored with tape so it does not slide up and down the meatus.

11. Women with bleeding tendencies caused by an abnormal PT probably have heavy menses, and they should be aware of this possibility.

12. Pain in or immobility of a joint can indicate bleeding into the joint. Nurses must consider all precautions necessary to protect the client from falls and trauma. When active children are clients, doing so may be a real challenge to the parents and to the nurse. Specific points about bleeding caused by classic hemophilia (hemophilia A) are discussed with the test for factor VIII.

13. Measuring blood pressure and pulse are two other ways to detect bleeding. A slight but steady increase in pulse may be a subtle sign of bleeding, long before the blood pressure decreases.

14. It is wise to have a policy of avoiding intramuscular injections, if at all possible, for clients with bleeding tendencies. If an intramuscular injection must be given, choose the smallest-gauge needle possible and apply pressure for 10 minutes after the injection.

When laboratory personnel come to draw blood, a nurse needs to remind them of the potential bleeding problem. The finger-stick method to obtain blood should be used whenever possible if the bleeding tendency is severe (see Chapter 1 for the finger-stick procedure). Some hospitals put a sign on the client's door to alert all personnel to the bleeding tendency. The nurse can be inventive in particular settings to make sure everyone caring for the client knows about the bleeding tendency. See Chapter 25 on invasive procedures.

Special Needs for a Client Receiving Surgical Care. If a client with an increased PT must undergo an invasive procedure or operation, it is imperative that the PT be medically corrected before the procedure. To get the PT back to a safe level, vitamin K injections may be ordered. For example, clients who have undergone valve replacements are usually receiving long-term anticoagulation therapy to prevent thrombus formation about the valve. If the client needs an emergency appendectomy, the conversion to a normal PT is done in conjunction with heparin replacement for anticoagulation. When anticoagulant therapy is necessary during a surgical procedure, the client's drug is switched to heparin because this short-term anticoagulant can be more easily controlled (see PTT) and quickly reversed with protamine. Whole blood or fresh frozen plasma should always be available for a client with an abnormal PT who must undergo an operation. A type and a cross match are performed as part of the preoperative preparation (see Chapter 14 on type and cross match).

Impaired Home Management Related to Need for Frequent PT

Dosages of a long-term anticoagulant must be adjusted frequently until the PT reaches the desired INR for the client. The PT may be drawn daily during the adjustment phase. Once the client knows the maintenance dose, the PT can be measured about once a month or as little as every 6 weeks. On discharge, clients need written instructions about the anticoagulant and the time for the next PT. In the past, clients would be kept in the hospital until dosages were

(Continued)

Table 13–5 Examples of Foods Containing Vitamin K*

Asparagus

Avocado

Broccoli

Brussels sprouts

Cabbage

Cauliflower

Chickpeas

Greens such as endive, lettuce, spinach, collards, and chard

Egg yolk

Herbal and green teas

Kale

Sauerkraut

Soy products

Turnips

Yogurt

*Compiled from various patient instruction sheets. The intake of these foods should be consistent.

Possible Nursing Diagnoses . . . (*Continued*)

stabilized. Because hospital stays are short now, a steady anticoagulation state may not be reached before discharge, so the problem of home management of the anticoagulant is intensified. Clients may also do home monitoring.

Deficient Knowledge Related to Long-Term Anticoagulation and Other Medications

When a client is taking coumarin-type drugs, a wide variety of other drugs may interact with them to cause changes in the PT, either to increase or to decrease the PT. Aspirin, other salicylates, and acetaminophen potentiate the effect of warfarin, thus increasing the PT time. Often the client is not aware that many pain medications, such as cold remedies, contain aspirin. In fact, more than 500 aspirin-containing compounds are available. Certainly the client needs to be instructed not to take any medication without consulting the physician who is prescribing the anticoagulant. Sometimes physicians will prescribe aspirin concurrently with a coumarin-type drug to avoid higher doses. A free booklet titled "Your Guide to Coumadin/Warfarin Therapy" is available at www.ahrq.gov/consumer/btpills.htm. This booklet is also featured on www.mybloodthinner.org.

Deficient Knowledge Related to Amount of Vitamin K and Other Nutrients in the Diet

Clients on warfarin should strive for a steady intake of vitamin K so that the INR does not fluctuate. (See Table 13–5 for examples of foods containing vitamin K that clients may have in moderation.) If obtaining a constant INR is problematic, the client should be referred to a dietician for a detailed list of foods to avoid, foods known to be very high in vitamin K, such as some types of tea, mangos, papayas, and tart cherries.

Not only does vitamin K activate clotting factors, but it also plays an essential role in building and maintaining bones. Long-term use of warfarin has been associated with osteoporosis in some elderly men (Gage et al., 2006). Although more research is needed to confirm these findings, researchers suggest that clients on long-term warfarin should maintain adequate intake of vitamin D and calcium (see Chapter 7), exercise regularly, and take precautionary measures to avoid falls.

Deficient Knowledge Related to Effects of Anticoagulation During Pregnancy

Women undergoing anticoagulation therapy need information on birth control and the risks of anticoagulation in pregnancy. Oral anticoagulants may cause nasal hypoplasia, neurologic deficits, and other malformations known as the fetal warfarin syndrome (Katzung et al., 2009). Women who need anticoagulants during pregnancy usually take maintenance doses of low-molecular-weight (LMW) heparin, and transition to warfarin in the postpartum state (DeCherney, 2007).

Decreased Prothrombin Time

Clinical Significance

Sometimes clients may have a PT of 8 or 9 seconds, compared with a control of 11 or 12 seconds. It may reflect a pathologic condition, such as thrombophlebitis or a malignant tumor. The reduced PT, however, is not of clinical significance as a diagnostic tool.

Possible Nursing Diagnosis Related to Decreased PT Time

Risk for Injury Related to Formation of Venous Thrombi

A decreased PT may indicate hypercoagulability of the blood. Hypercoagulability of the blood, venous stasis, and injury to the venous wall are the three conditions that contribute to the formation of venous thrombi. (Note that the condition associated with arterial thrombosis is atherosclerosis. See Chapter 9 on lipid metabolism.) It is thought that at least two of the three conditions (Virchow's triad) must be present to have thrombosis formation in the veins. Venous thrombi are found most often in the deep veins of the legs or in the pelvic veins.

When a client has known hypercoagulability of the blood, the primary goal of the nurse is to decrease the possibility of venous thrombus formation by such measures as leg exercises, adequate hydration, and no venous constrictions, such as crossing the legs. (See the discussion in the section on PTT on the effectiveness of low doses of heparin to prevent deep venous thrombosis [DVT].)

PARTIAL THROMBOPLASTIN TIME (ACTIVATED) (APTT)

The PTT, a nonspecific test, can demonstrate a lack of any of the various clotting factors, except factor VII (stable factor), that function in the intrinsic clotting system (see Table 13–1). Because some clotting tests, such as PT, bypass the intrinsic clotting system, they are not useful to screen for general plasma deficiencies. The PTT, on the contrary, is useful in detecting the presence of many types of bleeding disorders caused by defective or deficient circulating factors that compose the intrinsic system. If the PTT is abnormal, further tests are needed to pinpoint exactly which factor is defective or deficient.

PTT is also used to monitor heparin therapy because heparin, a short-acting anticoagulant that circulates in the plasma, increases the PTT. Table 13–3 summarizes the use of the PTT for monitoring heparin. Newer drugs, such as the direct thrombin inhibitors (i.e., lepirudin, desirudin, orgatroban) will also be monitored with the PTT (Deglin et al., 2011).

Preparation of Client and Collection of Sample

Venous blood is collected (1.8 or 4.5 mL) in tubes containing sodium citrate (blue vacuum tube). If the client is undergoing anticoagulation therapy, record the time, dosage, and route of administration of the heparin.

REFERENCE VALUES FOR PTT*	
Adult	22.1–34.1 seconds for activated PTT
Pregnant women	May be normally decreased by a few seconds.
	Also may be decreased with oral contraceptives.
Newborn	Range is increased above adult level for about 3 mo.

*Labs now all do activated PTT so the symbol may be aPTT or just PTT.

Increased PTT

Clinical Significance

An increased PTT, when the client is not taking heparin, signifies a bleeding disorder. Further tests must be performed to determine which factor is deficient. Also, the client may have abnormal factors such as the lupus anticoagulant factor as discussed later.

A relatively common hereditary disorder is lack of factor VIII (antihemophilic globulin), which results in the classic hemophilia, or hemophilia A. An inherited deficiency in factor IX (plasma thromboplastin component or Christmas factor) results in the condition known as *Christmas disease,* or hemophilia B. Often the client's history gives clues that the increased PTT is due to a familial condition (see the tests for factors VIII and IX). Specific assays for different factors in the plasma definitively establish the diagnosis.

Acquired deficiencies may be more subtle and difficult to connect to any specific cause. The PTT becomes elevated in a complex bleeding disorder in which the clotting factors are used up at an abnormal rate. This disorder, DIC, is discussed in detail at the end of this chapter, along with fibrinogen levels. Autologous blood transfusions may cause an elevated PTT.

If the client is taking heparin, an increase in the PTT is the result of the effects of the circulating anticoagulant in the plasma. Usually the PTT is kept about 1.5–2.5 times the control value. So if the control is 36 seconds, a report greater than 90 seconds indicates more-than-adequate anticoagulation for the moment the blood is drawn. A report of less than 53 seconds indicates inadequate anticoagulation for the moment the blood is drawn. The PTT is an indirect measure of the functional activity of heparin. A test that directly measures the activity of heparin and is not affected by the factors that affect the PTT is the heparin anti-Xa (activated factor X) assay discussed later.

Effect of Lupus Anticoagulant. The lupus anticoagulant produces a prolonged PTT by binding to the phospholipid used in the test. Because this is a laboratory artifact, the increased PTT is a false increase. In fact, lupus anticoagulant may be suspected in clients when the PTT is markedly elevated, but the client has no signs of bleeding (McPhee et al., 2011). The lupus anticoagulant and anticardiolipin antibodies are types of antiphospholipids associated with an increased risk for arterial or venous thrombosis, thrombocytopenia, and spontaneous abortions. (See the section on antiphospholipid antibodies).

Possible Nursing Diagnoses Related to Elevated PTT

Risk for Injury Related to Bleeding

An abnormal PTT necessitates postponement of an operation unless it is an emergency. If the PTT is being used as a routine check before an operation such as a tonsillectomy, the test must be completed early enough so that the reports are on the chart before the client goes to the operating room. Easy bruisability does not always mean a bleeding disorder, but any evidence of past bleeding difficulties needs to be assessed medically before operative or other invasive procedures, such as an arteriogram, are performed. (See Chapter 25 for the risk of bleeding with invasive procedures.)

Anxiety Related to Bleeding Disorder

If the PTT is elevated, several tests may be needed to evaluate the client's clotting ability. Nurses may be helpful in allowing the client and the family to express their concerns and anxieties about an unknown medical diagnosis. Any client with an elevated PTT has an increased tendency to bleed, and thus client teaching for preventing bleeding, discussed earlier, is appropriate. Stress may activate the bleeding process, so biofeedback and imagery may be useful tools to decrease the client's stress.

Risk for Injury Related to Heparin Therapy

The introduction of weight-based heparin protocols has made achieving therapeutic goals easier and faster but the process is still complex (Ridge & Antonacci, 2008).In recent years,

(Continued)

Possible Nursing Diagnoses . . . (*Continued*)

hospitals have developed protocols for intravenous heparin to allow nurses to adjust the heparin dosage based on the current PTT value. The nurse may stop the infusion for a specified time or change the drip rate to more or fewer units per hour. The protocols also specify the times to repeat the PTT and other tests such as platelet counts.

Platelet counts are essential because some clients develop heparin-induced thrombocytopenia (HIT) a few days after therapy is begun. Mild HIT (Type I), a nonimmune response, usually occurs up to 3 days after initiation of therapy. Watchful waiting may be the plan. The much more rare but very serious type of HIT (Type II) occurs in 4–14 days after the start of heparin. The decrease in platelet count (usually over 50%) may lead to bleeding but a greater danger is thrombosis (white clot syndrome) due to the activation of platelets by the immune response. The presence of antibodies to heparin helps distinguish the immune-mediated type from the nonimmune. These antibodies to heparin may cross-react with LMW heparin. Therefore, these clients must be prescribed other types of anticoagulants. (See the section on direct thrombin inhibitors). Serotonin is released from activated platelets, so a serotonin release assay (SRA) may also help diagnose HIT Type II. Although HIT is rare when heparin is used to flush lines, researchers are investigating if reducing the client's exposure to heparin flushes will reduce the occurrence of HIT Type II (Rosenthal, 2006). If HIT develops, all types of heparin are discontinued (McPhee et al., 2011).

Checking for Drug Interferences. Drugs that interfere with the action of heparin are not as numerous as those that interfere with the coumarin-type drugs, but some drugs do affect the PTT. The potential interaction of these drugs may be important if the drugs are added or deleted during the time the client is undergoing heparin therapy. Because drugs containing aspirin increase the bleeding time, they should be avoided when the client is taking heparin. Platelet aggregation is the main defense against bleeding, and aspirin decreases the adhesiveness of platelets, potentiating the bleeding tendency from any type of anticoagulation.

Deficient Knowledge Related to Possible Need for Long-Term Anticoagulation

If long-term use of anticoagulants is necessary to prevent other thromboembolic episodes, the usual pattern is to begin with a coumarin-type drug after a few days of heparin therapy and continue both types of anticoagulants until the PT is within the desired range. For example, long-term anticoagulation might be needed for a client who has had a pulmonary embolus. During this switch from heparin to long-term oral anticoagulants, both the PT and the PTT need to be monitored, and clients need the instructions about coumarin described earlier. (Also see the section on tests for LMW heparin.)

Decreased PTT

Clinical Significance

A PTT lower than the control sample is not diagnostically significant, but it may be a clue reflecting hypercoagulability. (See the discussion of PT for nursing interventions to help prevent venous thrombus formation.) Some degree of hypercoagulability is normal in pregnancy.

ANTIPHOSPHOLIPID ANTIBODIES: LUPUS ANTICOAGULANTS AND ANTICARDIOLIPIN ANTIBODIES

As discussed earlier, the presence of an antibody called lupus anticoagulant makes the PTT falsely elevated. The antibody was named the lupus anticoagulant because it was first discovered in clients with lupus. Now researchers have discovered that the antibody may also be found in various conditions. Lupus anticoagulant is a misnomer because this antibody can cause clotting, not anticoagulation (Gigler & Oertel, 2010). Because of the teratogenic effects of warfarin, pregnant women who have antiphospholipid antibody syndrome (APLAS) are usually prescribed baby aspirin and subcutaneous heparin (McPhee et al., 2011).

Clients who have increased lupus anticoagulants may also have anticardiolipin antibodies. These two major categories of antiphospholipid antibodies are found increased in clients having primary antiphospholipid syndrome (APS) and sometimes secondary to having other autoimmune disorders such as systemic lupus erythematosus (SLE). Antiphospholipid antibodies are present in 20% of women with recurrent miscarriages and 30% of clients with SLE (Pullen, Cannon, & Rushing, 2004). In addition to repeated miscarriages, three other signs of APS are recurrent clotting problems (usually venous), a lace-like rash (livedo reticularis) due to sluggish blood flow, and thrombocytopenia. Wound healing may be impaired. A client with medium to high titers of antiphospholipid antibodies who develops a clot will be prescribed long-term anticoagulant therapy. A client who has antiphospholipid syndrome but has no clotting or skin changes may begin life-long low-dose aspirin (Sarvis, 2005).

ACTIVATED CLOTTING TIME

Although the PTT is more precise to monitor heparin therapy, the ACT also can be used. The ACT, measured at the bedside, is commonly used during cardiovascular operations and in intensive care units (Wu, 2006).

Preparation of Client and Collection of Sample

The test is performed at bedside by a technologist or other clinician. Whole blood is drawn into special tubes that contain an activator such as siliceous earth (tubes and syringes should be warmed to 37°C). Time to clot is observed immediately. If the client is receiving a continuous heparin drip, the venous sample is obtained from the arm without the intravenous catheter.

REFERENCE VALUES FOR ACT

70–120 seconds (depends on type of activator used)

Desirable range for anticoagulation may be 150–190 seconds

TESTS FOR LOW-MOLECULAR-WEIGHT HEPARIN

The introduction of low-molecular-weight (LMW) heparin, enoxaparin, made it much easier to care for clients with thromboembolism in the hospital and at home. Administration of LMW heparin is less time consuming and does not require as much laboratory monitoring as conventional heparin (unfractionated heparin [UFH]). The PTT is never needed, and only rarely is the anti-Xa assay needed. However, periodic monitoring of a complete blood count (Chapter 2), platelet count, and stool for occult blood is routine. Two other LMW heparins, dalteparin and tinzaparin, have similar recommendations, but these drugs may elevate levels of the liver enzymes AST and ALT (Deglin et al., 2011).

DIRECT THROMBIN INHIBITORS MONITORED BY PTT

Lepirudin and argatroban are direct thrombin inhibitors that are not derived from heparin, so there is no cross-reaction with heparin antibodies. They may be used to remedy HIT. Both are given by intravenous infusion and are monitored by the PTT much like heparin, as discussed earlier (Deglin et al., 2011).

Lepirudin is similar to naturally occurring hirudin. Thus, some clients develop anti-hirudin antibodies that may increase the anticoagulation effect; therefore, the PTT must be closely monitored (Devlin, 2009).

HEPARIN ANTIFACTOR XA ASSAY (ANTI-XA)

The heparin anti-Xa assay is based on the ability of heparin to inhibit the activity of Xa. The client's plasma is added to a known amount of Xa and antithrombin. If heparin or LMW heparin is present in the client's sample, the medication binds to antithrombin and inhibits Xa. Thus anti-Xa assay directly measures the functional activity of heparin. (The PTT discussed earlier is an indirect measurement of the functional activity of heparin.) Also, anti-Xa is not affected by concurrent therapy with warfarin as is the PTT, nor is the test affected by clotting disorders as the PTT may be. (See the discussion on lupus anticoagulants.) The disadvantages of anti-Xa compared to PTT are expense and low availability.

Two different anti-Xa assays are used—one for UFH, the type of heparin used for continuous intravenous drips, and one for LMW heparin. Routine monitoring is not required for LMW heparin but may be needed for some conditions such as renal failure, pregnancy, or morbid obesity. Continuous heparin infusions always require monitoring and each institution has a policy for the timing of the samples.

Preparation of Client and Collection of Sample

Whole blood is collected in a light blue citrate tube. The optimal amount is 2.7 mL, but as little as 1.8 mL will suffice. Timing should be 4–6 hours after the third subcutaneous injection, depending on the type of LMW heparin. For continuous heparin infusions, the first sample should be collected 6 hours after initiation of therapy. The timing of further samples depends on how often the dosage needs to be adjusted. The two types of assay are calibrated differently, so the correct type of assay must be specified on the laboratory requisition. Date and time of last dose is needed for LMW heparin and dosage per hour for continuous infusion. Any dosage adjustments should also be documented.

REFERENCE VALUES FOR HEPARIN ANTI-XA ASSAY

Therapeutic range for unfractionated heparin	0.30–0.70 units/mL*
Therapeutic range for LMW heparin	q 12 hr dosing 1.00–2.00 units/mL
	q 24 hr dosing 0.50–1.00 units/mL

*Target range may vary depending on condition being treated; for example, range may be less when heparin is used for a cardiac protocol rather than to treat deep vein thrombosis.

These values are from Kaiser Permanente Hospital, San Francisco, CA.

HEMOPHILIA TESTS: FACTORS VIII AND IX

The two main types of hemophilia are called A (*classic hemophilia*) and B (*Christmas disease*). Classic hemophilia has affected several royal families in Europe. Christmas disease was named for the family who was studied with the genetic defect of factor IX. The specific diagnosis of classic hemophilia is made by means of assay of factor VIII and of Christmas disease by means of assay of factor IX. The cause of more than 80% of all hemophilias is a deficiency of factor VIII. Because the PTT is prolonged in hemophilia, it is a screening test for bleeding disorders. The client has a normal PT and platelet counts.

Preparation of Client and Collection of Sample

Venous blood (4.5 mL) is collected in plastic tubes with sodium citrate (blue vacuum tube).

REFERENCE VALUES FOR FACTORS VIII AND IX

Factor VIII (antihemophilic globulin)	50–200%
Factor IX (plasma thromboplastic cofactor)	60–140%

SCREENING FOR VON WILLEBRAND DISEASE

Although not as well known as the hemophilias, von Willebrand disease (vWD) is the most common inherited bleeding disorder. It is not sex linked, so men and women are equally affected, but women have more severe problems because of menses and childbirth. There are several types of this disease, but all show a decrease in quantity or diminished activity of the von Willebrand factor (vWF). The vWF, a plasma protein, carries factor VIII and is a cofactor for platelet adhesion.

Clients may have easy bruising, frequent nosebleeds, heavy menstrual periods, and excessive bleeding from injuries or surgical procedures. Symptoms may be mild to severe. Screening tests such as the PT and PTT do not detect the disorder. Clients with a familial history or who have abnormal bleeding need to have specialized tests for vWF antigen, vWF activity (ristocetin cofactor), factor VIII, and vWF multimers to analyze the vWF molecule structure. In 2010, the American Academy of Nurse Practitioners (www.aanp.org) launched a program to help consumers and health care providers become aware of vWD signs and symptoms and treatment options.

Possible Nursing Diagnoses Related to Deficiency in Coagulation Factors

Impaired Home Maintenance Management

The general nursing implications for a client with bleeding tendencies are discussed in the section on PT. Because factor replacement therapy can be provided, many bleeding episodes can be prevented or treated before damage occurs to joints or to other vital areas. Older children and their parents are taught to mix the factor concentrate and to administer the intravenous infusion. The slogan of the Prevention Program of the National Hemophilia Foundation is "Do the Five." The five are as follows:

1. Get an annual comprehensive checkup at a hemophilia treatment center.
2. Get vaccinated for hepatitis A and B.
3. Treat bleeds early and adequately.
4. Exercise to protect joints and maintain a healthy weight.
5. Get tested regularly for blood-borne infections.

Anxiety Related to Transmitting a Genetic Disease

See Chapter 18 for a discussion of genetic counseling. Both hemophilia A and B are inherited as X-linked recessive traits. Females who receive the defective gene do not have the disease because they also have another "healthy" X chromosome. On the contrary, any male who receives the defective X shows symptoms because he does not have a healthy X chromosome to balance the effect. Hemophilia may be mild, moderate, or severe, depending on how much of the factor is produced. Hemophilia can also result from spontaneous mutations, since some affected males do not demonstrate the disease in the family tree.

Anxiety Related to Safety of Factor Transfusions

The contamination of pooled factors with the human immunodeficiency virus (HIV) was possible until 1985, when viral inactive clotting factor concentrates were introduced. (See Chapter 14 on the current status of testing for HIV.) More than 7,000 people with hemophilia were infected with HIV, and some clients may fear that such a catastrophe could occur again if the blood supply is contaminated. Cost and availability help determine whether clients have plasma-derived or recombinant factor VIII or factor IX as replacement therapy.

Anxiety Related to Development of Factor Inhibitors

Some clients who receive factor infusions develop antibodies against the factor. These antibodies may lead to treatment failure and the need to use much more expensive specialty products. These factor inhibitors are measured by an assay that measures the amount in Bethesda Units (BU). Parents and the client, if old enough, need to know the type of inhibitor the child has and whether the titers are low or high (greater than 5 BU). Close communication with the health team is imperative in planning an inhibitor treatment regimen. The National Hemophilia Foundation (www.hemophilia.org/inhibitors) has useful information on factor replacements and the problem of inhibitors.

PLATELET COUNT AND MEAN PLATELET VOLUME

Sometimes platelets are considered as a third type of blood cell in the plasma (see Chapter 2 for RBCs and white blood cells [WBCs]). Actually, platelets are not intact cells but only fragments of cytoplasm that function in blood coagulation. As platelets adhere to the wall of an injured vessel, they clump together (or aggregate) and release a substance that begins coagulation. Platelets are formed by the bone marrow and removed by the spleen when they are old or damaged.

Preparation of Client and Collection of Sample

The laboratory uses 0.5 mL of blood. EDTA is used as the anticoagulant (lavender-topped tube). If platelets clump with EDTA, a blue-topped tube may be used. The count is usually performed with a machine, but if the count is low, it is confirmed by means of microscopic examination. Smears can also be performed to estimate the number of platelets.

REFERENCE VALUES FOR PLATELETS AND MPV[a]

Adults have 150,000–450,000/mm³

Women have a greatly decreased platelet count for the first few days of menses.

Platelets are increased after labor and delivery.

Newborns have lower values.

[a]Mean platelet volume (MPV) can be measured. Reference values are 6.4–11.0 μm³. Larger platelets apparently have better hemostatic function.

Increased Platelet Count (Thrombocytosis)

Clinical Significance

Malignant tumors, especially advanced or metastatic lesions, may cause an elevated platelet count, or thrombocytosis. Many clients with an "unexpected" high platelet count are found to have a malignant neoplasm. Clients with polycythemia vera often have high platelet counts. (Polycythemia vera is discussed in Chapter 2 in the section on RBCs.) Another reason for an increased platelet count is the splenectomy, which causes a temporary increase in the platelet count.

Possible Nursing Diagnoses Related to Increased Platelet Counts

Risk for Injury Related to Thromboembolic Episodes

A logical assumption is that an increased amount of platelets tends to make the blood more coagulable. As discussed in the section on decreased PT and hypercoagulability, dehydration could be dangerous for a client with a high platelet count. Venous stasis may be of particular concern. Depending on the reason for the thrombocytosis, thrombus formation may or may not be a possibility. For example, the increased platelet count after a splenectomy does not seem to cause any problems.

Essential thrombocytosis may be treated with drugs such as hydroxyurea or anagrelide (Agrylin), to keep the platelet count below 500,000 mm³. Low-dose aspirin may reduce the risk of thrombosis (McPhee et al., 2011).

Risk for Injury Related to Bleeding

Surprisingly, an increased number of platelets does not always mean an increased tendency to clot. In fact, it may mean an increased tendency to bleed. This paradox can be partially explained by the fact that sometimes the increased numbers of platelets are abnormal ones that cannot function properly in the coagulation process. Thus, a client with thrombocytosis may need to be watched for bleeding tendencies. (See the detailed assessment guide in the section on PT.)

Low Platelet Count (Thrombocytopenia)

Clinical Significance

If the cause of the low platelet count, or thrombocytopenia, is unknown, the condition is called *idiopathic* (unknown cause) thrombocytopenic purpura (ITP). *Purpura* refers to bruising. As more has been learned about ITP, some sources, such as the Immune Thrombocytopenic Association, consider that at times the *I* is to denote immune thrombocytopenia purpura. Platelet-associated antibodies of both the IgG and the IgM type (Chapter 14) can be measured in clients with the immune type of thrombocytopenia. Acute thrombocytopenia, the most common cause of childhood bleeding, usually has spontaneous remission, but about 20% become chronic due to an immune process (Hay et al., 2011). Chronic idiopathic thrombocytopenia in adults, an autoimmune disease, is more difficult to treat. Immune thrombocytopenic purpura may be primary or secondary. The diagnosis remains one of exclusion of other causes. Low platelet counts may occur after viral infections and are common with acquired immunodeficiency syndrome (AIDS). Thrombocytopenia is also common in clients with systemic lupus erythematosus. A low count can be associated with some types of anemias or other hemolytic disorders. Entities that depress bone marrow function, such as chemotherapeutic drugs or radiation, also depress the platelet count. An overactive spleen (hypersplenism) or an enlarged spleen (splenomegaly) destroys platelets at too fast a rate. Severe thrombocytopenia often follows any type of extracorporeal bypass or autotransfusion. Because heparin can cause thrombocytopenia, platelet counts must be monitored while a client is taking heparin. The LMW heparins have less effect on platelets than does conventional heparin (Deglin et al., 2011). Low platelet counts occur with disseminated intravascular coagulation (DIC) and with preeclampsia (See Chapter 18).

Possible Nursing Diagnoses Related to Thrombocytopenia

Risk for Injury Related to Bleeding

When a client has a low platelet count, the most important nursing concern is protecting the client from bruising and bleeding. Petechiae are the most common manifestations of thrombocytopenia because the many microscopic injuries that occur continuously in the capillaries are not immediately sealed off because of the lack of platelets. Invasive procedures may be withheld if platelet counts are as low as 50,000/mm^3. The risk of spontaneous hemorrhage is about 50% if the level drops to 20,000/mm^3. Some activities may need to be curtailed until the platelet count returns to normal. Flossing of the gums and hard-bristled toothbrushes may cause bleeding. Clients should not have rectal exams or suppositories. In the case of an active child, protection from trauma requires a great deal of ingenuity on the part of the nurse and the parents. Symptoms that indicate bleeding are described in detail in the section on nursing implications for an increased PT. Clients may be embarrassed by the bruises on their arms and legs, and so they appreciate clothing that conceals the bruises from curious onlookers.

Risk for Injury Related to Clotting

In some conditions, a low platelet count actually leads to clotting rather than the expected bleeding because of the pathophysiology. (See the earlier discussion on why heparin antibodies cause clotting.) Thrombotic thrombocytopenic purpura (TTP), a rare condition probably caused by damage to endothelial cells, results in a low platelet count and widespread thrombi (Burruss & Holz, 2005). Thus, protecting the client with thrombocytopenia includes assessment of symptoms of thrombosis as well as bleeding.

Risk for Infection

If the thrombocytopenia is a result of general bone marrow depression, the implications about leukopenia (low WBC) and anemia (low RBC) must also be considered. (Related nursing diagnoses are discussed in Chapter 2.) Adult clients, and sometimes children, with a low platelet count may undergo corticosteroid therapy, which is given to raise the platelet count to normal. The risk for infection is due to the use of the cortisone-type drugs. (See Chapter 15 on cortisone therapy and other nursing diagnoses.)

In adults, sometimes the removal of the spleen is necessary to return the platelet count to normal. If such an operation is scheduled, the nurse can help prepare the client for the surgical experience. The risk associated with splenectomy is small, but clients do have a lifelong increased risk of bacterial sepsis (Bromberg, 2006).

Risk for Injury Related to Platelet Transfusions or Drugs

If thrombocytopenia results from a malignant tumor or from treatment with chemotherapeutic drugs, platelet transfusions may be given. One unit of platelet concentrate increases the platelet

(Continued)

> ### Possible Nursing Diagnoses . . . *(Continued)*
>
> count by at least 5,000. Clients with counts less than 10,000/mm³ require platelet transfusions, whereas those with more may receive transfusions only if hemorrhage begins (Weaver & McDonald, 2006). Because patients may become sensitized to the platelet concentrates, transfusions are reserved for those who are at great risk. Three of the most important problems in platelet transfusions are allergic reactions, hypervolemia, and bacterial sepsis.
>
> Oprelvekin, a thrombopoietic growth factor, was approved by the FDA in 1998, and also called interleukin-II. This colony-stimulating factor increases platelets after chemotherapy. Clients may be taught to do their own subcutaneous injections, of oprelvekin. They must also know about possible unwanted effects, such as fluid retention, that can occur with the beginning of therapy. Platelet counts are monitored, and therapy is discontinued when the count is over 50,000 (Deglin et al., 2011).
>
> Two newer medications to treat ITP in adults are romiplastin and eltrombopag. These thrombopoietin receptor agonists are only used when clients have not responded to other treatments (McPhee et al., 2011).

CLOT RETRACTION TEST

Platelets have an important role in clot formation and in making the clot firm by causing retraction. If platelets are lacking or defective, the clot does not shrink or retract but stays soft and watery. Also, if fibrinolysins are present in the serum, no clot retraction takes place. (Fibrinolysis is discussed in the section on decreased levels of fibrinogen.)

REFERENCE VALUE FOR CLOT RETRACTION
50–100% in 2 hr

ASPIRIN RESISTANCE TESTS

Tests for aspirin resistance usually evaluate platelet function after the client is on aspirin. Several tests for aspirin resistance have been developed, but these tests are more useful for clinical research than routine screening. (See www.labtestsonline.org for more information on these tests.)

CLOPIDOGREL RESISTANCE TESTS

The FDA has mandated that the manufacturers of clopidogrel include a black box warning indicating that some clients may not respond well to the medication due to their genetic makeup. Clients who are carriers of loss-of-function CYP2C19 alleles may not convert or metabolize clopidogrel to its active form. This genetic variation is found in approximately 2% whites, 4% blacks, and 14% Asians (Deglin et al., 2011). However, some studies suggest that this genetic variant may not modify the efficacy and safety of clopidogrel (Pare et. al, 2010).

FIBRINOGEN

Fibrinogen (factor I) is a plasma protein manufactured by the liver. Vitamin K is *not* necessary for the formation of this factor, as it is for many of the others manufactured by the liver (see Table 13–1). The sole purpose of fibrinogen seems to be the formation of fibrin as the end product (Stage IV) of blood coagulation (see Table 13–2).

Preparation of Client and Collection of Sample

Venous blood (4.5 mL of plasma) is collected in a tube with sodium citrate (blue-topped tube).

REFERENCE VALUES FOR FIBRINOGEN	
Adult	175–400 mg/dL Women tend to have slightly higher levels.
Pregnant women	Values may be as high as 600 mg/dL.

Decreased Levels of Fibrinogen

Clinical Significance

Low fibrinogen levels can result from rare genetic disorders or from severe liver disease, either of which might first be detected with the PTT.

More commonly, however, the decrease of fibrinogen is due to DIC. DIC is a pathologic overstimulation of the coagulation process. Not a primary disorder, DIC is secondary to other severe illnesses. The theory is that widespread tissue injury somehow triggers the clotting mechanism so that a pathologic formation of small thrombi occurs in the microcirculation. Paradoxically, the client begins to bleed because the clotting factors are eventually depleted. Besides the low fibrinogen level, the PT is increased, the PTT is increased, and the platelet count is lowered. Thrombocytopenia is a cardinal diagnostic finding. Because the placenta is a rich source of tissue thromboplastin, abnormalities such as abruptio placentae and fetal death can trigger massive clotting problems. Pregnant women have a reduced activity of the fibrinolytic system. The increase of clotting factors and the decrease in fibrolysis protect against severe hemorrhage, but these changes can also contribute to coagulation problems in pregnancy (DeCherney et al., 2007). Other clients most likely to experience this abnormal clotting process are those with toxemia of pregnancy, metastatic cancer, shock, sepsis, or burns. Respiratory distress syndrome, malaria, snake bite, and extracorporeal bypass also may contribute to DIC.

If the PT, PTT, platelet count, and fibrinogen levels are positive for DIC, additional tests to check for fibrinolysis and fibrin degradation products may be ordered. (See the following section for values for these tests.)

Possible Nursing Diagnoses Related to Decreased Fibrinogen Levels

Risk for Injury Related to Bleeding and Clotting in the Microcirculation

Because a low fibrinogen level is often part of a complex pathologic situation, clients most likely to experience DIC are usually those who are already in an intensive care unit with a primary illness.

(See the tests for FDP and D-dimer.) Shock is often present. In the obstetric area, women with toxemia or with any abnormality of the placenta should be observed for DIC. The nurse giving direct care may be first to notice signs of bleeding, such as bruise marks or the appearance of blood in drainage tubes or on dressings. (Refer to the section on PT to review the ways a nurse can make objective assessments for occult or hidden bleeding.) If thrombi have developed in the microcirculation, the client may have unexplained pain or symptoms of poor circulation to specific areas, such as cyanosis of the fingers or toes (Dressler, 2004).

Assisting with Medical Interventions. Whole blood or blood components may be given intravenously to replace the clotting factors. Nurses must understand the correct rate of flow for the particular blood component used as well as the complications that may occur. (See Chapter 14 for tests used to screen blood products.) Not only is bleeding occurring, but also thrombus formation may be taking place. So heparin may be part of the therapy for this complex situation if there is a large thrombus (DeCherney et al., 2007; McPhee et al., 2011).

D-DIMER SCREEN: ELISA AND LATEX AGGLUTINATION SLIDE TEST

D-Dimer refers to the degradation products of cross-linked fibrin. This byproduct of clot lysis may be measured by enzyme-linked immunosorbent assay (ELISA) or a slide test. ELISA is time consuming and expensive but may be needed to confirm a screening test. A rapid screening test is the latex agglutination slide test. Sensitivity and negative predictive values were similar for both types of tests when used to evaluate for venous thrombosis in an emergency unit. The D-dimer slide test also has proved useful for screening for abruptio placentae. The D-dimer test is now the initial diagnostic step for clients with suspected DVT or pulmonary embolus (PE). The use of D-dimer with a formal scoring system to assess for thromboembolism may rule out this pathology and make imaging tests unnecessary.

The use of D-dimer to rule out deep vein thrombosis (DVT) is usually performed only on outpatients in an emergency department because results are likely to be elevated in an inpatient population due to stasis, chronic illness, or surgery. However, D-dimer may be used for inpatients to rule out pulmonary emboli or disseminated intravascular coagulation (DIC). The D-dimer should only be ordered when there is a clinical suspicion of PE because an elevated D-dimer is a nonspecific finding that sometimes occurs in healthy people. A negative test essentially rules out thrombosis, but a positive test does not confirm a diagnosis of thrombosis and so further testing may be needed (Andrews & Habashi, 2010.

Preparation of Client and Collection of Sample

The blood sample is collected in a blue-topped tube, 1.8 mL in a 2-mL tube or 4.5 mL in a 5-mL tube. If D-dimer is being used to diagnose DIC, other related tests such as PT, PTT, platelet count, and fibrinogen level are also done.

REFERENCE VALUE FOR D-DIMER SCREEN	
If used to assess for venous thromboembolism (VTE)	<500 ng/mL
If used to assess for DIC	<1000 ng/mL

Note: Some healthy people and many inpatients may have elevated D-dimer levels, even though no clotting has occurred. Pregnancy causes a slight increase.

THROMBIN TIME: FIBRINOGEN SCREEN, THROMBIN CLOTTING TIME WITH REPTILASE

The thrombin time measures the time it takes blood to clot when thrombin is added to the sample. If a clot does not form immediately, a fibrinogen deficiency is present. Heparin therapy also keeps the blood sample from clotting. A reagent called *reptilase* (derived from snake venom) has an action similar to thrombin as it clots fibrinogen. However, reptilase is not inhibited by heparin, so it can be substituted for the conventional thrombin time test when the client is receiving heparin. In addition to assessing for some bleeding disorders, the thrombin time is also used to monitor clients receiving fibrinolytic therapy.

Preparation of Client and Collection of Sample

Whole blood, 4.5 mL, is collected in a plastic tube with sodium citrate (blue top). For the reptilase test, a special tube is obtained from the hematology laboratory.

REFERENCE VALUES FOR THROMBIN TIME AND REPTILASE TIME	
Thrombin time	14–16 seconds or within 5 seconds of control
Reptilase time	18–22

PLASMINOGEN ASSAY

Plasminogen is the inactive precursor of plasmin, an enzyme that has the ability to dissolve clots. The amount of this substance is useful information when the client is taking thrombolytic agents. The test also may be used to evaluate a client who has DIC. A decrease in plasminogen activity may be associated with the tendency for thrombosis.

Preparation of Client and Collection of Sample

Venous blood is collected in a special tube with a plasmin inhibitor.

REFERENCE VALUES FOR PLASMINOGEN ACTIVITY AND ANTIGEN	
Functional	80–130%
Antigen	8.4–14.0 mg/dL

PROTEINS C AND S ANTICOAGULANT SYSTEM

Protein S is a naturally occurring anticoagulant, and protein C is necessary for its action. Congenital or acquired decreases or a defect in either of these proteins increases the risk for vascular thrombosis. Thrombotic episodes often occur in high-risk situations such as pregnancy, a surgical procedure, or trauma. Tests for the protein C and protein S antigens and a functional assay of each are conducted.

Preparation of Client and Collection of Sample

The coumarin drugs alter the results, so blood is drawn before administration of oral anticoagulants or after a stable therapeutic level is established. Whole blood, 4.5 mL, is collected in a blue-topped vacuum tube. This procedure may require approval from the laboratory. The turnabout time for results may be 2–4 weeks.

REFERENCE VALUES FOR PROTEINS C AND S	
Protein C (immunoassay for antigen and functional clotting assay)	70–140%
Protein S (immunoassay for antigen and functional clotting assay)	70–140%

FACTOR V LEIDEN

Factor V, a protein that helps form the fibrin in the clotting cascade (see Table 13–2), is "turned off" by an activated protein C once enough fibrin is made. In some people, particularly European Caucasians, a gene mutation causes an abnormal version of factor V called the Leiden factor. The name "Leiden" refers to the Dutch city where a family with this gene mutation was studied in the 1990s (Gigler & Oertel, 2010). This factor V Leiden resists the action of protein C, so the person is prone to thrombosis if there are additional risk factors for clotting. No more than 10% of people with this abnormality and other mutations that cause clotting will ever experience a thrombosis. So screening family members for these genetic clotting disorders has been controversial (Crawford, 2005). Clients who have the mutated gene from both parents are at greater risk. The laboratory will initially test for activated protein C (APC) resistance, and if this is positive, a genetic test for factor V Leiden will be done. See www.labtestsonline.org for more details.

PROTHROMBIN G 20210A MUTATIONS

Normally prothrombin factor II is converted into thrombin, which helps to form a blood clot to prevent hemorrhaging. The mutation in the gene that makes prothrombin is called G20210A or factor II mutation. Clients with this mutated gene tend to make larger quantities of prothrombin, which can lead to excessive clot formation. Thus, the PT 20210 mutation, more common in Caucasians, must be diagnosed by genetic testing.

Possible Nursing Diagnosis Related to Tests for Hypercoagulability (Inherited Thrombophilla)

Risk for Injury Related to Clotting

About half of the people in the United States who die from arterial or venous thrombosis have an inherited or acquired defect that predisposes them to clotting. At least 15 blood-coagulation proteins and platelet defects have been identified as causes of hypercoagulability (Mulroy & DeJong, 2003). See Table 13–6 for some of the more common tests to detect a risk for clotting. If clients have one of these factors, they need to be taught ways to reduce their risk. For example, preventive measures when flying long distances include leg exercises, adequate hydration, and, perhaps, compression stockings to decrease the possibility of DVT. In a hospital setting, the nurse takes the responsibility of measures to decrease DVT, as is done with all immobile clients. (See nursing assessments under the section on a decrease in PT time.) As noted earlier, genetic screening of family members is controversial because many people with some of the known risk factors never have a difficulty with hypercoagulability. At this time, experts do not recommend screening for the general population (www.labtestsonline.org).

Table 13-6 Common Tests for Hypercoagulable States

Antiphospholipid syndrome (lupus anticoagulant and anticardiolipin antibodies)

Antithrombin defects

Elevated factor VIII

Factor V Leiden present

Heparin-induced thrombocytopenia (antibodies to heparin)

Plasminogen assay for defective plasminogen

Protein C defects

Protein S defects

von Willebrand disease (vWD)*

---

*Most common hereditary blood coagulation disorder. See text.

OCCULT BLOOD TESTING IN VARIOUS SPECIMENS

Occult (hidden) blood can be detected by simple tests that cause color changes in the presence of blood. Although all tests for blood in stool, urine, or other secretions are sometimes called *guaiac tests*, not all of them use the chemical guaiac. Some tests, Hematest (Ames) being the common one, use another chemical, orthotolidine. Although tests such as Hematest and Hemostix (Ames) can be used to detect occult blood in urine, a microscopic examination is needed to detect intact erythrocytes. (See Chapter 3 on tests for hematuria.) The various tests for occult blood can also be performed on emesis, but note that a histamine-2 blocker may make the test falsely positive and a low pH falsely negative. Gastroccult (SmithKline Diagnostics) is specifically designed to test for occult blood and the pH of gastric secretions. Nurses may use Gastroccult for on-the-spot assessment of occult blood in emesis or nasogastric (NG) drainage. Only a drop of gastric juices is needed. Some hospitals have eliminated the use of gastric occult blood analysis for lack of evidence that the test is significant for client care decisions (Dierdorf, 2002).

SCREENING TESTS TO DETECT COLORECTAL CANCER

The U.S. Preventive Services Task Force (2008) recommends several screening methods for colorectal cancer including home fecal occult blood testing (FOBT), sigmoidoscopy, or colonoscopy (Chapter 27). One method of FOBT screening uses the guaiac-based test FOBTg (guaiac) with 2 stool specimens collected for 3 days at home by the client. More recently, FOBTi (immunoassay), which uses an immunochemical method to detect intact protein from human hemoglobin, has also been approved as a screening test (Greenwald, 2005). FOBTi does not require any dietary restrictions and requires only 2 stool samples, but it is more expensive than FOBTg. A third screening test uses an entire stool specimen for DNA analysis for changes that may indicate cancer or precancerous growth. The tests for fecal DNA for 22 gene mutations is not yet practical for general population screening due to the cost and necessity of mailing stool specimens (McPhee et al., 2011).

Some type of FOBT should be done annually after age 50 years (Ransohoff & Sandler, 2002). Although clinical trials have demonstrated a reduction in mortality from colorectal cancer when yearly screening is done, many clients over 50 years do not take advantage of this basic screening. Also, FOBT may be done on only one sample, which is not considered adequate (Nadel et al., 2005). Nurses are involved in research to find why nearly half of the Americans over age 50 years are not being screened. Greenwald (2006) found that some clients preferred using toilet paper rather than wooden sticks to smear samples.

Preparation of Client and Collection of Sample for FOBT (guaiac)

The client may be instructed to avoid meat, raw fruits, and vegetables and to eat a high-fiber diet for 1–3 days before a screening test of the feces. Meat, especially red meat, may cause a false-positive result, and a high-fiber diet increases the chances of finding occult blood if a lesion is present in the GI tract. Some places may restrict a client's diet or medication only after an initial screening test is positive. Three specimens are recommended. Stool specimens do not have to be tested immediately but must be protected from sunlight.

Nurses should be aware of influences on these tests. Vitamin C (>250 mg) may produce false-negative results, whereas iron pills may give false-positive results. Turnips and horseradish, which contain peroxidase, may also cause a false-positive result. Aspirin and anti-inflammatory drugs, which tend to cause slight GI bleeding, may make the test positive, but this effect is usually small. Check if the client should withhold any drugs before the test. Long-distance runners may have occult blood in the feces after a vigorous run.

The client can collect stool at home with a commercially prepared filter paper in a protective cover. The written instructions tell the client to collect a small specimen of stool on an applicator and smear the stool on part A of the paper. A second specimen from a different part of the stool is put on part B of the paper. After three samples are collected and brought to the clinic or laboratory, two drops of a commercially prepared developing solution are placed on each smear, and the color change is noted after 30 seconds.

Preparation of Patient and Collection of Sample for FOBTi (immunoassay)

There are no diet restrictions and one sample is collected for 2 days.

REFERENCE VALUES FOR FECAL OCCULT BLOOD (FOB)

Blue indicates the presence of blood. A second test may be completed to confirm a positive report.

Possible Nursing Diagnosis Related to Occult Blood

Deficient Knowledge Related to Health Maintenance by Checking for Occult Blood

Nurses may be involved in instructing clients on how to test stools for blood as a screening measure at home. Nurses can educate the public about the importance of the resources available in their communities. The tests discussed previously can be bought without prescriptions and are advertised in publications for the general public. As discussed in Chapter 1, screening for occult blood in the feces is one of only a few tests that are generally recommended routinely for even apparently healthy people older than 50 years of age. The community health nurse or the family nurse practitioner can offer this screening test to clients. (See Chapter 27 for information on colonoscopy, which may be needed as a follow-up to the screening test for occult blood in the feces.)

Questions

1. The case manager is scanning the laboratory reports that were just sent to the unit. A PT reported as an INR of 2.5 would be evidence of an appropriate therapeutic outcome for
   a. A client who is undergoing warfarin therapy
   b. A client who is undergoing heparin therapy
   c. A client who is scheduled for a liver biopsy
   d. A client who had an injection of vitamin K_1 yesterday

2. A prophylactic injection of vitamin K_1 is given to newborns because the
   a. PT of newborns is increased in seconds
   b. Fibrinogen level of newborns is decreased
   c. Platelet count may be lowered in some instances
   d. Intestinal bacteria may destroy the vitamin K

3. Vitamin K injections are the least likely to return the PT to normal for which client?
   a. A client who is suffering from malnutrition
   b. A client who has liver dysfunction
   c. A client who is undergoing long-term warfarin therapy
   d. A client who has obstructive jaundice caused by a pancreatic tumor

4. A client with cirrhosis has had two episodes of gastrointestinal bleeding but seems stabilized now. His PT is 20 seconds (control, 13 seconds), and his platelet count is 100,000/mm^3 (reference value, 150,000–350,000/mm^3). He eats a conventional diet but has little appetite. The most important instruction for the nurse to give the client when he goes home is to
   a. Maintain a balanced diet with emphasis on foods containing vitamin K
   b. Check his pulse regularly and report a rate greater than 100 beats per minute
   c. Always drink a glass of milk when he takes aspirin
   d. Report any dark-colored or black stools to his physician immediately

5. A client is being discharged to undergo long-term warfarin therapy. When the nurse formulates a discharge teaching plan, the least important topic to include is the necessity of
   a. Carrying identification that she is undergoing long-term anticoagulant therapy
   b. Having periodic INRs drawn
   c. Not taking nonprescription drugs that contain aspirin
   d. Assessing the amount of potassium (K^+) in her diet

6. A client has a PTT of 100 seconds (control, 35 seconds). She is receiving an intravenous heparin drip at a rate of 700 U/hr. Which action by the nurse is most appropriate after the physician is notified of the laboratory result?
   a. Prepare an injection of vitamin K for emergency use by the physician
   b. Increase the heparin rate, as ordered, because this will decrease the PTT
   c. Encourage walking to increase circulation
   d. Keep the client on bed rest and assess the client often for any symptoms of bleeding

7. A 66-year-old postoperative client had deep venous thrombosis (DVT) after a previous operation. His PTT is slightly lower than the normal control value. He takes a "minidose" of heparin as a preventive measure. Thus, the nursing action that has the highest priority is to
   a. Assess frequently for bleeding
   b. Encourage as much walking as possible

   c. Ascertain if protamine, the antidote for heparin, is readily available

   d. Monitor fluids to prevent circulatory overload

8. If a client has a low platelet count, the initial physical assessment is most likely to reveal
   a. Large hematomas on abdomen and back
   b. Delayed capillary filling when the skin is blanched
   c. Evidence of gastrointestinal bleeding, such as a positive test for blood in the feces
   d. Petechiae on the legs

9. Which of the following nursing actions is the most appropriate for a teenager who reports a headache and is asking if she may take an over-the-counter medication for pain? Her platelet count today is 20,000/mm³ (reference value, 150,000–350,000/mm³).
   a. Allow her to take her usual over-the-counter medication for headache because it is usually very effective
   b. Offer her fluids to decrease the viscosity of her blood
   c. Obtain an order for aspirin for her headache
   d. Assess her for any changes in level of consciousness (LOC)

10. A teenager has a platelet count of 10,000/mm,³ caused by idiopathic thrombocytopenia. An elderly man has a platelet count of 780,000/mm,³ caused by a malignant tumor (reference value, 150,000–350,000/mm³). Because of these laboratory reports, both of these clients should be assessed for
   a. Bone marrow depression and polycythemia
   b. Thrombus formation in lower extremities
   c. Bleeding episodes from minor trauma
   d. Infection of mucous membranes

11. Which of the following changes in laboratory tests are most indicative of the complex bleeding disorder that is called disseminated intravascular coagulation (DIC), or consumption coagulopathy?
   a. Increased PT, increased PTT, and increased platelet count
   b. Decreased PT, decreased PTT, and decreased fibrinogen levels
   c. Increased PT, decreased platelet count, and increased fibrinogen levels
   d. Increased PTT, decreased platelet count, and decreased fibrinogen levels

12. A client is scheduled for a liver biopsy tomorrow. He has a tentative diagnosis of cirrhosis caused by alcohol abuse. Which two of these laboratory tests are used in assessing adequate liver function before the invasive procedure of a liver biopsy?
   a. PTT and fibrinogen levels
   b. PT and platelet counts
   c. Fibrinogen levels and platelet counts
   d. PT and antihemophilic factor (factor VIII)

13. A 32-year-old woman delivered a premature infant yesterday. Because of massive blood loss, she received three units of blood. Today she is having only slight vaginal bleeding. The laboratory data to best substantiate the need for continued close observation of vital signs would be
   a. PT, 11 seconds (control, 12 seconds)
   b. Fibrinogen, 0.10 g/dL (reference value, 0.15–0.60 g/dL)
   c. PTT, 37 seconds (control, 35 seconds)
   d. Platelet count, 400,000/mm³ (reference value, 150,000–350,000/mm³)

14. Two days ago, a 58-year-old man underwent a complex abdominal operation for cancer of the colon. He has a nasogastric tube, which is draining greenish secretions. He can walk

with help. Today's laboratory reports show a PT of 9 seconds (control, 12 seconds), a PTT of 30 seconds (control, 34 seconds), and a platelet count of 350,000/mm³ (reference value, 150,000–350,000/mm³). Based on this laboratory data, a priority nursing action is to
   a. Encourage the client to walk
   b. Check the nasogastric secretions for occult (hidden) bleeding
   c. Check stools for occult (hidden) bleeding
   d. Monitor for infection or other signs of bone marrow depression

15. Which of the following statements is accurate about testing for occult blood in the feces?
   a. Red meat may cause false-negative results in the feces
   b. The test is useful as a screening test for cancer of the colon
   c. The stool specimen must be tested within 2–4 hours after collection
   d. Blue indicates a negative reaction for the presence of blood

References

Andrews, P., & Habashi, N. M. (2010). Detecting, managing and preventing pulmonary embolism. *American Nurse Today, 5*(9), 21–25.

Bromberg, M. E. (2006). Immune thrombocytopenia purpura—The changing therapeutic landscape. *New England Journal of Medicine, 355*(16), 1643–1645.

Burruss, N., & Holz, S. (2005). Managing the risks of thrombocytopenia. *Nursing 2005, 35*(6), 32hnl–32hn5.

Crawford, S. (2005). Factoring the risks of factor V Leiden. *Nursing 2005, 35*(3), 26.

DeCherney, A. H., Nathan, L., Goodwin, T. M., & Lauter, N. (2007). *Current diagnosis and treatment obstetrics & gynecology* (10th ed.). New York: McGraw-Hill.

Deglin, J. H., Vallerand, A. H., & Sanoski, C. A. (2011). *Davis's drug guide for nurses* (12th ed.). Philadelphia: F. A. Davis.

Devlin, M. M. (2009). Lepirudin: Test your drug IQ. Careful dosing is key with this anticoagulant. *Nursing 2009, 39*(6), 56cc6.

Dierdorf, B. (2002). Is gastric occult blood analysis affecting patient care delivery? *MEDSURG Nursing, 22*(1), 30–32.

Dressler, D. K. (2004). Coping with a coagulation crisis. *Nursing 2004, 34*(5), 58–62.

Gage, B. F., Birman-Deych, A., Radford, M., Nilasena, D., & Binder, E. (2006). Risk of osteoporotic fracture in elderly patients taking warfarin. *Archives of Internal Medicine, 166,* 241–246.

Greenwald, B. (2005). A comparison of three stool tests for colorectal cancer screening. *MEDSURG Nursing, 14*(5), 292–300.

Gigler, C. R., & Oertel, L.B (2010). Understanding hypercoagulopathies. *Nursing 2010, 40*(8), 53–56.

Greenwald, B. (2006). A pilot study evaluating two alternate methods of stool collection for the fecal occult blood test (2006). *MEDSURG Nursing, 15*(2), 89–94.

Hadaway, L. (2004). Keep catheters clear with low dose heparin, *Nursing 2004, 34*(10), 73.

Hay, W. W., Levin, M. J., Sondheimer, J. M., & Deterding, R. (Eds.). (2011). *Current diagnosis and treatment: Pediatrics* (20th ed.). New York: McGraw-Hill.

Katzung, B., Masters, S., & Trevor, A. (Ed.). (2009). *Basic and clinical pharmacology* (11th ed.). New York: McGraw-Hill.

McPhee, S. J., Papadakis, M. A., & Rabow, M. W. (Eds.). (2011). *Current medical diagnosis and treatment* (50th ed.). New York: McGraw-Hill.

Mulroy, J. F., & DeJong, M. (2003). Syndromes of hypercoagulability. *American Journal of Nursing, 103*(5), 64KK–64SS.

Nadel, M. R., Shapiro, J., Klabunde, C., Seeff, L., Uhler, R., Smith, R., et al. (2005). A national survey of primary care physicians' methods for screening for occult blood. *Annals of Internal Medicine, 142*(2), 86–94.

Paré, G., Mehta, S. R., Yusuf, S., Anand, S. S., Connolly, S. J., Hirsh, J., et al. (2010).

Effects of CYP2C19 genotype on outcomes of clopidogrel treatment. *The New England Journal of Medicine, 363*(18), 1704–1714.

Pence, C., & McErlane, K. (2005). Anticoagulation self-monitoring. *American Journal of Nursing, 105*(10), 62–65.

Pullen, R. L., Cannon, J., & Rushing, J. (2004). Managing antiphospholipid syndrome. *Nursing 2004, 34*(3), 32hn1–32hn4.

Ransohoff, D. F., & Sandler, R. S. (2002). Screening for colorectal cancer. *New England Journal of Medicine, 346*(1), 40–44.

Ridge, R. A., & Antonacci, L. M. (2008). Shining a spotlight on anticoagulation safety. *Nursing 2008,38*(8), 22–23.

Rosenthal, K. (2006). Breaking the link between IV therapy and HIT. *Nursing 2006, 36*(5), 22.

Sarvis, C. M. (2005). Antiphospholipid antibody syndrome: When wounds won't heal. *Nursing 2005,* 35(9), 24.

Schulman, S., Kearon, C., Kakkar, A.K., Mismetti, P. Schellong, S. Eriksson, H., et al. (2009). Dabigatran versus warfarin in the treatment of acute venous thromboembolism. *The New England Journal of Medicine, 361*(24), 2342–2352.

Turka, J. (2005). Understanding international normalized ratio (INR). *Nursing 2005, 35*(8), 18–19.

Turner, L. (2006). Keeping warfarin therapy in balance. *Nursing 2006, 36*(11), 43–44.

U.S. Preventive Services Task Force. (2008). Screening for colorectal cancer: U.S. Preventive Services Task Force recommendations statement. *Annals of Internal Medicine, 149*(9), 1–44.

Weaver, R., & McDonald, M. (2006). What you need to know about transfusing platelets. *Nursing 2006, 36*(6), 26–27.

Wu, A. H. (Ed.). (2006). *Tietz clinical guide to laboratory tests* (4th ed.). St. Louis, MO: Saunders Elsevier.

Websites

www.aanp.org (Toolkit for von Willebrand Disease.)

www.ahrq.gov/consumer/btpills.htm (Information on oral anticoagulants or blood thinners.)

www.chestnet.org (American College of Chest Physicians for evidence-based guidelines for antithrombotic and thrombolytic therapy.)

www.hemophilia.org (National Hemophilia Foundation for information on factor products and factor inhibitors.)

www.labtestsonline.org (Update on genetic testing for warfarin dosing, aspirin resistance, Factor V Leiden, and prothrombin G20210A.)

www.mybloodthinner.org (Information on warfarin for clients and health professionals.)

Answers

1. a, 2. a, 3. b, 4. d, 5. d, 6. d, 7. b, 8. d, 9. d, 10. c, 11. d, 12. b, 13. b, 14. a, 15. b

Serologic Tests: Immunohematology Microbiology and Immunology

- Common Techniques in Serologic Testing — 333
- Screening Blood for Transfusions — 335
- ABO Grouping — 336
- Rh Factor — 339
- Rh Antibody Titer Test — 340
- Direct Antiglobulin (Coombs' Test) or RBC Antibody Screen — 341
- Antibody Screening Test (Indirect Coombs') — 341
- Microbiologic Serologic Tests — 342
- Hepatitis B Surface and E Antigens and Antibodies Against Hepatitis B Antigens and the Delta Agent — 343
- Hepatitis A Tests: Anti-HAV, IgG, and IgM — 346
- Tests for Hepatitis C Virus — 347
- HIV Testing — 349
- Rapid Tests for HIV as Point of Care — 351
- Home Tests for HIV — 351
- CD4 Counts — 352
- Viral Load Tests — 352
- Human T-Cell Lymphotropic Virus Types I and II — 353
- West Nile Virus Test — 353
- Serologic Tests for Syphilis — 354
- Infectious Mononucleosis (Epstein–Barr Virus [EBV]) — 355
- Streptococcal Infections — 356
- Rubella — 357
- Parvovirus B19 (Erythema Infectiosum or Fifth Disease) — 358
- Toxoplasmosis — 359
- Amebiasis — 360
- Serologic Tests for Lyme Disease — 360
- Serologic Tests for Helicobacter pylori — 361
- Herpesvirus Family — 361
- Cytomegalovirus Titers — 362
- Varicella-Zoster Antibody Titer — 362
- Hantavirus — 363
- Fungal Antibodies: Histoplasmosis and Coccidioidomycosis — 363
- Fungal Antigens — 364
- Immunologic Tests — 364
- C-Reactive Protein Routine and High Sensitivity (Cardiac CRP) — 365
- Antinuclear Antibodies — 366
- Other Tests for Systemic Lupus Erythematosus — 367
- Rheumatoid Factor — 367
- Thyroid Autoantibodies — 368

OBJECTIVES

1. Explain the basic techniques for serologic tests for blood bank, microbiologic, and immunologic procedures.
2. Describe the role of the nurse in the prevention and assessment of transfusion reactions due to ABO incompatibility.

3. Explain the rationale for the administration of Rh immunoglobulins.

4. Identify the most important nursing diagnoses when a client has a positive report for hepatitis B surface antigen (HBsAg) or for hepatitis C.

5. Describe the usefulness of the test for antibodies against human immunodeficiency virus (HIV) and compare with viral load tests.

6. Describe what a client should be taught about the various serologic tests for syphilis (STS).

7. Describe the clinical usefulness of serologic tests for common bacterial, viral, and fungal diseases.

8. Describe the information that should be given to a woman of childbearing age who has a negative titer of rubella antibodies.

9. Explain why positive serologic tests or skin tests may not be indicative of an active infection.

10. Describe how C3 and C4, two components of the complement system, are altered by antigen–antibody reactions.

11. Describe how humoral antibodies, such as rheumatoid factor (RF) and antinuclear antibodies (ANAs), are useful in assessing autoimmune disease.

The category of serologic tests is broad. It includes blood bank procedures (immunohematology), identification of antibodies against infectious diseases (microbiology), and studies of immune diseases (immunology). The basic principle underlying serologic tests is that a reaction between an antibody and an antigen results in a recordable event. In some tests, the client's blood sample is mixed with an antigen to see if there are antibodies in the serum. In other tests, antibodies may be added to the blood sample to see if the antigen exists.

The first part of this chapter describes the techniques used in blood banking procedures. The ABO blood types demonstrate in a dramatic way the antigen–antibody basis for tests. Many other tests are done to make blood transfusions as safe as possible.

The second part of this chapter discusses the common serologic tests used in microbiology. (Specific microbiologic tests, such as cultures and microscopic examinations, are described in Chapter 16.)

The last part of this chapter contains a discussion on the common serologic tests used to assess immunologic diseases, such as systemic lupus erythematosus (SLE).

COMMON TECHNIQUES IN SEROLOGIC TESTING

Serologic testing is based on the fact that antigen–antibody reaction causes an observable event. From a nursing point of view, the exact testing technique is not of primary interest. Nonetheless, to understand the description of the test, nurses do need to be familiar with the general meaning of these techniques:

1. Agglutinations and titer levels
2. Immunofluorescence antibody test (IFA)
3. Radioimmunoassay (RIA)
4. Enzyme immunoassay (EIA) and enzyme-linked immunosorbent assay (ELISA)
5. Immunoglobulins G and M

Table 14–1 Titer Dilution Chart for ASO

1:60	Positive
1:85	Positive
1:120	Positive
1:170	Positive
1:240	Negative

ASO, anti-streptolysin-O antibodies.

An antibody titer is reported as the last dilution that causes an antigen–antibody reaction, or agglutination. Thus, in this example, the laboratory report would read "ASO titer 1:170." See text for further explanation.

Agglutination and Titer Levels

Agglutination, or clumping, which often occurs when antibodies attach to an antigen, is the most basic type of serologic testing. The Coombs' test is an example of an observable clumping of cells in the blood sample when there is a certain ratio of antibodies to antigens.

The serum is diluted with normal saline solution in graduated amounts. For many serologic tests, rather than reporting only agglutination (positive) or no agglutination (negative), the laboratory represents the results as a *titer*, which is the last dilution at which a reaction occurred. For example, the laboratory uses the standard dilutions in Table 14–1 to test for antibodies against streptolysin-O (ASO) that is produced by group A β-hemolytic streptococci. In the example in the table, the last dilution to cause a reaction was 1:170, which would be the titer reported. In essence, this finding means that the client's serum contained enough antibodies still to cause a reaction with the antigenic material when the serum was diluted 1:170.

One titer does not give as much information as do two titers separated by a time interval, because a *rise* in titer is more significant than any one high number. So, to catch a rise or fall, the timing of titers is very important. A fourfold increase in titer between an acute and a convalescent sample is usually necessary to confirm the presence of an infection. The time interval between acute and convalescent phases depends on the organism causing the disease.

Immunofluorescence Antibody Tests

The IFA test can be direct or indirect. In the direct method, an antibody labeled with a fluorescent dye (fluorescein) is mixed with a sample of blood from the client. If an antigen is present, the antigen–antibody complex can be seen under a microscope with an ultraviolet light source. With the indirect method, the known antigen is mixed with the serum and any antigen–antibody complex is then mixed with fluorescein-labeled anti-immunoglobulin antibodies.

Immunoassays with Radioactive Material and Enzymes (RIA, EIA, and ELISA)

As noted in Chapter 1, RIA is one way to detect very small particles in a blood sample. A newer way uses EIA or ELISA to detect specific proteins or antigens. For examples, see tests for HIV and other diseases.

Immunoglobulin G and M Identification

The specific identification of immunoglobulins supplements the information gained from serologic testing. IgM antibodies are indicative of an acute infection, and IgG antibodies are indicative of past exposure and probable immunity. (For examples, see the discussion on tests for rubella and hepatitis.)

SCREENING BLOOD FOR TRANSFUSIONS

Several routine laboratory tests are performed on a unit of donor blood (see Table 14–2). Nurses need to be up to date about these tests because clients are concerned about the safety of blood.

Blood banks take precautions to ensure that donor blood is as safe as possible to administer to a client and also that it is safe for the person to donate blood. For example, the donor must weigh at least 110 lb (50 kg) and have a hemoglobin (Hgb) level of 13.5 g for men and 12.5 g for women. (See Chapter 2 on the measurement of Hgb levels.) The donor must have a temperature no higher than 98.6°F (37°C), a heart rate of 50–100 beats per minute with no irregularities, and a blood pressure between 160/90 and 100/50 mm Hg. The blood bank physician may modify these guidelines depending on the individual situation. Overall, the donor must be in generally good health with no upper respiratory infections or allergies. Blood donations are not taken from people who have ever had hepatitis, malaria, jaundice, or a history of IV drug use. Pregnancy or a blood transfusion excludes donors for 6 months. Travel to other countries may exclude donors. Dental operations or tooth extraction in the 72 hours before the donation excludes a donor. (See Chapter 16 on how even minimal dental work can cause transient bacteria in the bloodstream [bacteremia].) Vaccines and some immunizations are other reasons for deferral.

Table 14–2 Routine Tests on Donor Blood

1. ABO and Rh typing

2. General antigen and antibody screening

3. Hepatitis B virus (HBV)—HBsAg (surface antigen) and anti-HBc (core antibody)

4. Hepatitis C virus (HCV)—anti-HCV (antibodies) and NAT (nucleic acid test for virus)

5. Human immunodeficiency virus (HIV)—anti-HIV-1 and anti-HIV-2 (antibodies) and NAT for virus[a]

6. Serologic test for syphilis

7. Human T-cell lymphotropic virus type I or II (HTLV-I/II)—anti-HTLV-I and anti-HTLV-II (antibodies)

8. Alanine transaminase (ALT) (see Chapter 12)

9. Cytomegalovirus (CMV) if requested[b]

10. West Nile virus

11. Serologic test for antibodies for a parasite, *Trypanosoma cruzi*, that causes Chagas disease.[c]

[a]Before use of NAT, the HIV p24 antigen was used (see text).

[b]Blood that has leukocytes removed (leukoreduction) will not need this test as CMV and some other viruses are transferred in the leukocytes.

[c]Once just a threat in Mexico, Central and South America, but now threatens blood supplies in the United States. Many blood banks are now performing this test. (See www.labtestsonline.org)

Typing and Crossmatching of Blood

To type and crossmatch (T&C) blood, the laboratory needs at least 15–30 minutes to make sure that the donor unit of blood is compatible with the blood of the recipient. The client's blood type and Rh factor are determined so that a matching unit of blood can be taken from the blood bank. It is never safe to assume that any unit of A-positive blood can be given to any client with A-positive blood. So the cross match mixes a small sample of the two bloods to see if any clumping occurs. The full range of tests for a T&C is discussed later.

Typing and Screening

If there is only a faint possibility that blood will be needed, the physician may order typing and screening (T&S) rather than crossmatching. In a screening, the client's blood is tested, so that if blood is needed, the actual crossmatching can be performed in a few minutes. The advantage of screening is that it does not tie up a unit of blood when the need is slight. For example, if two units of blood are typed and crossmatched for a surgical client, those two units of blood cannot be used for another client until the operation is over and the blood is released for re-crossmatching for another client.

Typing for Packed Cells

A unit of packed RBCs contains only about one-fourth the amount of plasma as a unit of blood. T&C is as necessary for packed cells as it is for whole blood. Packed cells are now much more commonly used for blood transfusions than is whole blood. In this discussion, *blood transfusion* refers to either whole blood or packed cells.

Preparation of Client

There is no special preparation of a client for T&C or for T&S. For either procedure, the laboratory needs whole blood collected in a lavender-topped (EDTA) tube. Dextran, a plasma expander, should not be started before a T&C because it interferes with crossmatching.

ABO GROUPING

All humans have one of four blood types—A, B, AB, and O—which are genetically determined. Even though type A has subgroups, one generally speaks of only four types, the frequency of which is shown in Table 14–3, along with a description of the antigens and antibodies in each type. Each of these blood types may be Rh positive or Rh negative, so this gives eight major blood types. Other antigens also do exist, so crossmatching of the donor red cells with some plasma from the prospective recipient is necessary to rule out incompatibility.

Understanding the concept of the universal donor and recipient may help the nurse visualize, in a simple way, the importance of antibody–antigen response in immunologic testing. Type O blood is theoretically the universal donor because none of the principal antigens occur on the RBCs of people with type O blood. Type O blood does have antibodies against A and B, but in one unit of donor blood, the donor antibodies become so diluted in the plasma of the recipient that the antibodies are of minimal importance. In fact, in an emergency situation such as a

Table 14–3 ABO Blood Typing		
Estimated Percentage of Population	**Type**	**Description**
46	O	No A or B antigens on RBCs. Antibodies against A and B antigens[a] (universal donor)
41	A	Antigen A on RBCs. Antibodies against B antigens
9	B	Antigen B on RBCs. Antibodies against A antigens
4	AB	Antigens A and B on RBCs. No antibodies against A or B antigens (universal recipient)

[a]From birth, the person has the antibodies, even with no exposure to the antigens. In contrast, a person with Rh-negative blood does not have antibodies against the Rh factor until exposed to the factor.

disaster, health care personnel ask the blood bank to send O-negative packed cells so they are ready even before victims arrive at the hospital (McPhee, Papadakis, & Rabow, 2011). A person with AB blood has both A and B antigens on the RBCs, so the plasma contains no antibodies against A or B antigens. Thus, people with AB blood are sometimes called universal recipients. It is interesting to note that a person born with one type of ABO antigens has the antibodies against the other antigens, even though the person has never had contact with the other types of blood. In contrast, a person with Rh-negative blood does not have antibodies against the Rh factor until there is sensitization. (The Rh factor, which, like ABO types, is genetically determined, is discussed later in this chapter.)

Clients must *never* be given a type of blood that contains foreign A or B antigens. For example, a client with type A blood who is given a unit of type B blood would undergo a severe hemolytic reaction. The antibodies against the B antigen, which are present in the A client, attack the RBCs of the type B donor blood. The hemolysis of the RBCs causes the release, directly into the bloodstream, of free hemoglobin, which can be damaging to the renal tubules. The end result of a transfusion of incompatible blood may be renal failure and death.

Possible Nursing Diagnosis Related to Blood Transfusion

Risk for Injury Related to Complications of Blood Transfusion

Client identification must follow institutional policy which usually mandates that the blood tag, blood bag, and client identification be checked by two licensed professionals, at least one of whom is an RN. Verification includes name, medical record number, transfusion number, ABO and Rh factor type, expiration date, and volume of blood. After the unit of blood is hung, the nurse's responsibility is to see that the blood is given correctly. (See Chapter 13 for a discussion of platelet transfusion and Chapter 2 for leukocyte replacement.)

Assessing for Complications. The nurse must also be aware of the signs and symptoms of an adverse reaction to a blood transfusion. The most severe hemolytic reaction is due to donor–recipient ABO incompatibilities. Rh and other factors may also cause some hemolysis,

(Continued)

Possible Nursing Diagnoses . . . (Continued)

but usually the reaction is not as pronounced as with ABO incompatibility. (See the next section on laboratory tests done after a hemolytic transfusion reaction.) Checking of vital signs before and during the blood transfusion is the basic nursing action. When possible, the addition of pulse oximetry may be helpful to detect very early respiratory distress. See the discussion on transfusion-related acute lung injury (TRALI). Also, running the blood slowly for the first 15 minutes minimizes the severity of a reaction, should it occur. The nurse should also be alert for other transfusion reactions, such as allergic reactions, febrile reactions, circulatory overload, and air embolism. Febrile reactions were more common before leukocytes were removed from blood transfusions (leukoreduction or leukodepletion). Removal of leukocytes from the blood is more expensive and causes loss of some RBCs. To combat febrile or mild allergic reactions, clients may be given acetaminophen and diphenhydramine about 30 minutes before the transfusion.

If a client begins to exhibit symptoms such as fever, chills, and low back pain, it is essential that the nurse not let the transfusion continue. Normal saline solution can be infused to keep the intravenous line patent when the unit of blood is discontinued.

The unfinished unit of blood must be sent back to the laboratory with a specimen of the client's blood for the laboratory to try to determine what caused the reaction. The client's blood and the donor's blood are re-crossmatched to see if they are truly incompatible.

Because one of the dreaded complications of an incompatible blood transfusion is renal failure, the laboratory may want a urine specimen to check for the presence of Hgb in the urine. Intake and output should be meticulously recorded, and all urine should be saved for laboratory examination for at least 24 hours.

The laboratory checks for free Hgb in the plasma and, if needed, indirect bilirubin and haptoglobin, the presence of which helps confirm hemolysis. (See Chapter 11 for an explanation of why unconjugated bilirubin is elevated with hemolysis.) Haptoglobin is a serum glycoprotein, the role of which is to bind free Hgb released from destroyed RBCs. Evidently, haptoglobin is diminished in severe hemolysis because it cannot be replaced quickly enough. Reference values for haptoglobin vary considerably, depending on the methods of evaluation used. A 2-minute slide test is available.

Assessing for and Preventing Bacterial Contamination. In addition to the tests for hemolysis, the laboratory may also perform a blood culture from the donor bag of blood. (See Chapter 16 on culture reports from blood specimens.) Blood at room temperature becomes an attractive culture medium for bacteria. Nursing actions to prevent sepsis from blood transfusions include the aseptic technique for starting the transfusion, hanging the blood within 30 minutes after it is taken from the blood bank, and ensuring that the entire unit is transfused within 2–4 hours.

Assessing for Lung Injury After a Transfusion. TRALI presents as acute hypoxemia and non-cardiac pulmonary edema during transfusion or up to 6 hours after a transfusion of blood or blood components. The syndrome, mild to fatal, is more common in clients who are very ill and who have been exposed to multiple blood products. Research is ongoing to see if leukocyte antibodies or other active substances incite or exacerbate lung injury (McAdams-Jones, 2009; Toy et al., 2005). Male plasma donors have less anti-leukocyte antibodies than female donors (McPhee et al., 2011). Use of pulse oximetry detects very early respiratory distress. The nurse must stop the transfusion, summon medical assistance, and give maintenance oxygen when TRALI occurs. Diuretics are not indicated for this type of pulmonary edema (Knippen, 2006).

Table 14–4 Rh Factor		
Estimated Percentage of Population	**Type**	**Description**
85–90	Rh+	Rh antigen on RBCs. No antibodies against Rh factor
10–15	Rh–	No Rh antigen on RBCs. Develops antibodies against Rh factor if sensitized by transfusion of Rh-positive blood. Also, the pregnant woman can be sensitized by an Rh-positive fetus.

RH FACTOR

The Rh factor is named after the rhesus monkey used in the original research on this factor. Actually, several different Rh factors have been identified, but usually only the main factor is clinically significant. The Rh factor, like the ABO types, is genetically determined.

There are two different nomenclatures for the Rh factors. In the Weiner system, the main Rh factor is RhO. In the Fisher–Rose system, the main Rh factor is *D*. In the literature, RhO or *D* is often called the *Rh factor*. In this discussion, the term *Rh factor* specifies the main factor involved when one speaks of Rh-positive or Rh-negative blood. Table 14–4 provides a description of Rh positive and Rh negative.

Normally, a person with Rh-negative blood does not have any antibodies against the Rh factor. An Rh-negative male can become sensitized (i.e., antibodies develop against the Rh factor) by transfusion with Rh-positive blood. In an Rh-negative female, antibodies can develop against the Rh factor, not only through blood transfusions with Rh-positive factors but also through a pregnancy in which the fetus is Rh positive. Once an Rh-negative person has antibodies against the Rh factor, another transfusion with Rh-positive blood, or another pregnancy with an Rh-positive fetus, can have serious consequences.

Rh Factor in Blood Transfusions

To keep antibodies against the Rh factor from developing in a person with Rh-negative blood, the Rh-negative person is given only Rh-negative blood. Hence, Rh typing is one of the components of crossmatching. The administration of Rh-positive blood to an Rh-negative person who has antibodies against the Rh factor (i.e., who is sensitized) causes a hemolytic reaction because the person's antibodies attack the RBCs that contain the Rh factor. The severity of this hemolytic reaction is usually not as great as it is in ABO incompatibility, but it is nevertheless to be avoided. (See the nursing implications for when a client has any kind of transfusion reaction.)

Rh Factor in Pregnancy

An Rh-negative mother and an Rh-positive father can produce either an Rh-negative or an Rh-positive baby, depending on the gene passed from the father. Laboratory tests can be performed to determine if the Rh-positive father has either two positive genes for Rh or one positive and one negative. (Note that an Rh-positive mother can carry an Rh-negative fetus without any Rh-related problems.)

A problem occurs when an Rh-negative mother is carrying an Rh-positive child. Hemolytic disease of the newborn, formerly called *erythroblastosis fetalis*, occurs when an Rh-negative mother produces antibodies against the Rh-positive RBCs of her fetus. With the first pregnancy, the fetus is usually not affected because the mother has not had time to build antibodies against the Rh factor. However, at the time of the infant's separation from the placenta (a full-term birth or an abortion), some of the RBCs from the fetus enter the mother's general circulation and trigger the production of antibodies against the Rh factor. Subsequent pregnancies with another Rh-positive fetus may present problems because the woman's serum is now sensitized against Rh-positive antigens.

Possible Nursing Diagnosis Related to the Rh Factor

Deficient Knowledge Related to the Use of Rh Immunoglobulins

About 13% of all Rh-negative mothers become sensitized (i.e., antibodies develop against the Rh factor) by their first pregnancy with an Rh-positive fetus. If the woman is not immunized by the administration of Rh immunoglobulins, each subsequent pregnancy with an Rh-positive fetus incurs a further 13% risk of starting antibody production. The use of Rh immunoglobulins is based on the principle of passive immunity. Because the mother has been given antibodies against the Rh factor, her body is not stimulated to begin active production of antibodies against the Rh factor.

Nurses who work with women in the childbearing years should have a good understanding of the Rh factor so that they can help these women understand the possible implications in relation to pregnancy. The laws of some states make it mandatory that any woman whose blood is typed must be told the results of the Rh factor.

RH ANTIBODY TITER TEST

The Rh antibody titer test is used to monitor the course of an Rh-negative woman who is carrying an Rh-positive fetus. If the mother is in a second pregnancy and did not receive Rh0 (D) immunoglobulin (RhoGAM) after a first pregnancy or abortion, the rise of the titer helps determine the need for medical intervention, such as exchange transfusions or an early delivery.

Preparation of Client and Collection of Sample

The laboratory needs 10 mL of blood. This test may also be performed on a sample of cord blood.

REFERENCE VALUES FOR RH TITER

A normal Rh antibody titer is negative. A rising titer may indicate the need for immediate medical intervention to prevent serious damage to the fetus or newborn. (See Chapter 28 on amniocentesis for titers of 1:16 or greater.)

DIRECT ANTIGLOBULIN (COOMBS' TEST) OR RBC ANTIBODY SCREEN

In certain types of sensitization, such as to the Rh factor, the erythrocytes become coated with antibodies or immunoglobulins. The Coombs' test is used as a screening test to detect whether immunoglobulins have become attached to the RBCs.

The test is referred to as a direct antiglobulin test (as opposed to the indirect or antibody screening test discussed next), because the RBCs are tested without any intervening manipulations. A sample of the client's blood is mixed with Coombs' serum, which is a rabbit serum that has antibodies against human globulins. If the client's RBCs are coated with immunoglobulins, agglutination occurs. The Coombs' test is performed for the following reasons:

1. To screen blood for crossmatching. If a client's erythrocytes have been exposed to incompatible blood, the erythrocytes are coated with an antibody or globulin complex.
2. To check for hemolytic transfusion reactions.
3. To assess for hemolytic disease of the newborn. In hemolytic disease of the newborn, the antibodies from a sensitized Rh-negative mother cross the placenta and coat the fetal red cells. (See Chapter 28 on amniocentesis.)

Other factors may also cause the client's RBCs to be coated with immunoglobulins. For example, many drugs, as well as autoimmune diseases that cause hemolytic anemia, may cause a positive Coombs' reaction. If necessary, further testing can be completed to identify the specific immunoglobulins present. (See Chapter 10 on immunoglobulin testing.)

Preparation of Client and Collection of Sample

In the newborn, the blood sample is taken directly from the umbilical cord. In children and adults, a venous sample is used. This test is routine for one aspect of T&C, which requires 10 mL.

REFERENCE VALUES FOR COOMBS' TEST

The Coombs' test should be negative. A positive test indicates that some type of globulin is coating the RBCs.

ANTIBODY SCREENING TEST (INDIRECT COOMBS')

An antibody screen is used to detect Rh antibodies in maternal serum. This test used to be called the *indirect* Coombs' test because the serum is subjected to several different conditions to detect various antibodies. If there is a positive result from the antibody screening, the laboratory performs more tests to identify the specific antibodies. This test is also performed as part of a cross match.

Preparation of Client and Collection of Sample

Red-topped or lavender-topped (EDTA) tube.

REFERENCE VALUE FOR ANTIBODY SCREEN

The antibody screening test should be negative.

MICROBIOLOGIC SEROLOGIC TESTS

The tests in this section are used for various types of diseases with infectious agents. Table 14–5 provides an overview.

Table 14–5 Common Serologic Tests Used in Microbiology

Test	Organism	Remarks
VDRL RPR TTPA	*Treponema pallidum*, which causes syphilis.	Confirming tests are performed if screening tests are positive.
HBsAg	Hepatitis B virus (formerly called serum hepatitis)	Can also measure antibodies against HBsAg and other antigens
Anti-HAV	Hepatitis A virus (formerly called infectious hepatitis)	See Table 14–6 for all tests for hepatitis.
Anti-HCV	Hepatitis C virus	Useful in blood screening
HIV antibodies and antigen	Virus associated with AIDS	See text and current literature for update.
Cold agglutinins	Eaton agent of pleuropneumonia-like organism (PPLO) may cause atypical pneumonia.	Positive in some cases, not all
HSV	Herpes simplex virus	Not used routinely. See Chapter 16 for other tests.
CMV	Cytomegalovirus	Problematic in pregnancy and for immunosuppressed clients
EBV Monospot	Epstein–Barr virus of infectious mononucleosis	Also see WBC with differential in Chapter 2.
ASO Anti-DNase-B Streptozyme test	Group A β-hemolytic streptococci	Measures antibodies *after* an acute infection with streptococci. Not useful during initial infectious stage.
Rubella titer	Rubella virus (3-day measles)	Even a low antibody titer probably indicates immunity.
TPM or Toxo	*Toxoplasma gondii*, a protozoan that causes toxoplasmosis	Most tests are indirect measurements of the protozoan.
Hemaglutination for amebiasis	*Entamoeba histolytica* (causes amebic dysentery and hepatic abscess)	Stool cultures also performed (see Chapter 16)
Fungus antibody tests	Histoplasmosis Coccidiosis	Cultures also performed (see Chapter 16)

Note: A TORCH screen includes toxoplasmosis, others such as syphilis or hepatitis, rubella, cytomegalovirus, and herpes.

Serologic Tests for Hepatitis

The several different forms of viral hepatitis are designated as hepatitis A (formerly called *infectious hepatitis*), hepatitis B (formerly called *serum hepatitis*), and hepatitis C (formerly called *non-A, non-B hepatitis*). Hepatitis D, caused by the delta virus, appears as a coinfection with hepatitis B. Hepatitis E, a type of enteric hepatitis, is most common in countries with poor sanitation. Before the onset of clinical symptoms, which usually resolve in 2–4 weeks, hepatitis E virus (HEV)-RNA can be detected in the stool. Serum antibodies to HEV can be identified in both the acute phase (IgM) and months to years afterward (IgG). In most cases, hepatitis E is self-limiting but has a high mortality rate of nearly 20% in pregnant women (DeCherney et al., 2007). The occurrence of hepatitis E is very low in the United States, so testing for anti-HEV is not included in routine panels (Wilson, 2005). Another viral agent, designated hepatitis G virus (HGV), has been found in some blood donors, intravenous drug users, hemodialysis clients, and clients with hemophilia. At the present time, HGV does not appear to cause significant liver disease or alter the course of clients with chronic B or C hepatitis (McPhee et al., 2011). Table 14–6 describes a wide array of tests used to detect hepatitis.

HEPATITIS B SURFACE AND E ANTIGENS AND ANTIBODIES AGAINST HEPATITIS B ANTIGENS AND THE DELTA AGENT

The virus that causes hepatitis B was discovered in 1965 in an Australian man. It was originally named the *Australian antigen*, and early laboratory tests were called HAA, for hepatitis Australian antigen. The commonly used test now is called *hepatitis B surface antigen* (HBsAg). Because a typical virus has many different antigens, a surface antigen is but one component of the hepatitis B virus (HBV). In addition to measurement of HBV antigens and antibodies to those antigens, the direct measurement of HBV-DNA can be done with molecular biological techniques (Wu, 2006).

The detection of HBsAg in a client's serum means that the client either is ill with the disease or is a carrier. In either case, the person is a possible source of infection for other people. Most people do not carry the virus after the disease is over, but 5–15% do become carriers. Hepatitis B is spread primarily by blood and body secretions. Because the incubation period is 50–180 days, a client who gets hepatitis B from a blood transfusion may not show symptoms for as long as 6 months. Thus, no one who has undergone a blood transfusion is permitted to donate blood for 6 months. Tests of HBsAg have become very useful in screening blood donors, many of whom are not aware they are carriers.

In addition to testing for the presence of HBsAg, the laboratory can also test for antibodies against the hepatitis B antigens. A person who has antibodies against HBsAg is presumed to be immune to hepatitis B. Table 14–6 summarizes information about the usefulness of three different antibody tests, including antibodies to the delta agent, a defective RNA virus that seems to infect only people who already have HBV infection.

Table 14–6 Tests Used to Diagnose Hepatitis A, Hepatitis B, and Hepatitis C

Name of Test	Explanation
Anti-hepatitis A virus (anti-HAV) IgM IgG	Measures antibodies to the hepatitis A virus. Antibodies of IgM type indicate *current* infection, whereas IgG antibodies represent past infection and probable immunity. Used to diagnose or rule out hepatitis A in a suspected case of hepatitis.
Hepatitis B surface antigen (HBsAg)	Measures surface antigen of hepatitis B virus. Indicates infection with hepatitis B and carrier state if it persists. Used to screen potential blood donors and to diagnose or rule out hepatitis B in suspected cases of hepatitis.
Hepatitis B virus DNA	Primarily used to assess effectiveness of therapy and to monitor liver transplants for viral load.
Hepatitis B e antigen (HBeAg)	Measures the e antigen of the hepatitis B virus. Correlates well with high titers of the virus, so used to evaluate infectiousness, particularly in chronic states.
Anti-HBsAg	Measures antibodies to hepatitis B surface antigen. Demonstrates immunity to hepatitis B virus, except for a few unusual subtypes. Used to demonstrate if vaccine is needed for a person at risk for hepatitis B.
Anti-HBcAg IgM IgG	Measures antibodies to the core antigen of hepatitis B. Appears in the serum earlier than anti-HBsAg, so may be used to diagnose hepatitis B in the "window" or convalescent state. IgM indicates *current* infection. IgG indicates past infection and probably immunity. Also can demonstrate if vaccine is needed for a person in the high-risk group.
Anti-HBeAg	Measures antibodies to the e antigen of hepatitis B virus. Appears late in infection and may be an index of infectivity. May be too weak to be detected.
Antibody to delta antigen (anti-delta) (delta antibody)	Suggests recent infection or carrier for a defective virus active only in the presence of hepatitis B.
Hepatitis C antibodies (anti-HCV)	Measures antibodies to the hepatitis C virus, which was formerly known as one type of non-A, non-B hepatitis.
HCV antigens	See text for discussion on RIBA and HCV-RNA assays.

Note: See section on serologic tests for hepatitis information, especially hepatitis E and G.

Preparation of Client and Collection of Sample

The laboratory uses venous blood to test for hepatitis B. The exact amount needed depends on the test used.

REFERENCE VALUES FOR HEPATITIS B TESTS

A positive HBsAg test indicates either active hepatitis or a carrier state. In either case, the client's body fluids and blood may be a source of infection.

A negative HBsAg with positive anti-HBsAg and anti-HBcAg occurs with natural immunity.

A negative HBsAg with positive anti-HBsAg occurs after successful vaccination.

Negative antigen and antibody tests for HBsAg indicate the client is susceptible to hepatitis B.

Possible Nursing Diagnoses Related to Positive Test for Hepatitis B

Deficient Knowledge Related to Spread of Infection

Clients who are carriers of HBV must be informed of their risk to others through blood or contact with body secretions such as semen. Printed information on safer sexual practices should be made available. Information about safer sex has become readily available since the AIDS epidemic began. Although universal precautions, now called standard precautions, are expected practice in all clinical settings and dental offices, clients should be told to notify health care workers about the positive test for hepatitis B if these workers will be handling the client's blood.

Of particular concern is the spread of hepatitis B to newborns, which usually occurs on entry into the birth canal. The use of hepatitis B immune globulin (HBIG), which gives immediate passive immunity, and hepatitis B vaccine, which promotes active immunity, is usually effective in protecting the babies of mothers who are carriers of HBV.

Hepatitis B, which can lead to liver cancer, is very prevalent in Asians and Pacific Islanders. A campaign to reach these ethnic groups and eliminate HBV has been launched in San Francisco by public health officials and Asian community leaders. The goal is to make HBV screening a basic part of health care among Asians (www.sfhepbfree.org).

Deficient Knowledge Related to Prevention of Disease

γ-Globulin may lessen the severity of hepatitis, but only a vaccine totally prevents the disease. The first vaccine for hepatitis B, made from pooled donors, was marketed in 1981. Now the vaccine is produced by DNA recombinant technology. After completion of three injections, antibody titers may be performed to validate the effectiveness of the vaccine. The vaccine was first used for groups at high risk, such as homosexuals, abusers of intravenous drugs and their sexual partners, and health care workers who might be contaminated with blood. One of the most effective provisions of the 1992 regulations on protecting health care workers from blood-borne pathogens was the requirement that free HBV vaccines be made available to all health care employees who are at risk for exposure to hepatitis B.

Immunization of all newborns is recommended because the estimated cost of universal use of the vaccine is less than 5% lifetime risk of infection. A comprehensive prevention and treatment plan endorsed by the Centers for Disease Control and Prevention includes screening all pregnant women for HBV. Infants of affected mothers can then be given HBIG at birth, as well as the recommended vaccine given at birth, 1 month, and 6 months. Children not vaccinated as infants should be given the complete series by age 12 years. Several states have laws requiring screening in pregnancy. Adolescents should receive the hepatitis B vaccine before they become sexually active. Pregnant woman can also be given the vaccine. Stringer, Ratcliffe, and Gross (2006) found that re-offering the vaccine was a successful intervention in a population of pregnant adolescents who had less-than-optimal prenatal visits. In some states, immunization with the three-dose series may be a legal requirement to enter middle school or even earlier (e.g., kindergarten). Nurses working in perinatal and pediatric settings need to know current recommendations because they can help educate clients about these prevention strategies.

(Continued)

Possible Nursing Diagnoses ... *(Continued)*

Activity Intolerance Related to Extreme Fatigue

See the sections on hepatitis A and on bilirubin levels (Chapter 11) and ALT levels (Chapter 12) for more information on other nursing diagnoses for clients with hepatitis. Hepatitis B tends to be more severe than hepatitis A. About 90% of clients with acute hepatitis B have complete recovery and lifelong immunity. Those clients who do develop chronic hepatitis may be treated with interferon or other antivirals to achieve sustained suppression of HBV replication (McPhee et al., 2011). Initially treatment may cause fatigue, but later the client should be able to resume most activities.

HEPATITIS A TESTS: ANTI-HAV, IgG, AND IgM

Hepatitis A is spread primarily by the oral–fecal route. It is often spread by food handlers or by means of sexual contact. The incubation period is about 15–45 days, which is much shorter than the 50–180 days for hepatitis B. There is no evidence of progression to chronic liver disease. Clinical features cannot be used to differentiate hepatitis A from other types of hepatitis. As noted in Table 14–6, there are two tests for hepatitis A and many more for hepatitis B, as well as several for hepatitis C.

Preparation of Client and Collection of Sample

The laboratory needs 2 mL of serum in a serum separator tube (SST).

REFERENCE VALUES FOR HEPATITIS A

A positive test for hepatitis A antibodies of the IgM type is strong evidence of acute infection with the virus. Antibodies of the IgG type are indicative of past exposure to hepatitis A. About 40–50% of adults have IgG antibodies against hepatitis A.

Possible Nursing Diagnoses Related to Positive Hepatitis A Test

Deficient Knowledge Related to Prevention of Disease

If the test indicates acute infection, the most important nursing implication is to initiate enteric precautions so that feces-to-mouth transmission of the virus does not occur. The person should not be allowed to handle or prepare any food for others. The disease can also be transmitted by means of sexual contact. In a hospital, a patient with poor hygiene may need a private room. Vaccines for hepatitis A are available and are recommended for people who plan to travel in areas where HAV is common. Immunization of children and adolescents is recommended in areas that have a high incidence of hepatitis A, as determined by local or state public health departments. In the past, immune globulin was administered to clients exposed to someone with hepatitis A. Now post-exposure prophylaxis has been updated to include use of the vaccine in healthy people between the ages of 1 and 40 years.

Risk for Injury Related to Immune Globulin

Immune globulin as post-exposure prophylaxis continues to be recommended for clients who are not candidates for the vaccine, such as the very young, the elderly, and those who are immunocompromised or have chronic liver failure disease (Dentinger, 2009). Immune globulin, which can be given up to 2 weeks after exposure, does not prevent the disease, but it may lessen the severity. The immune serum globulin against hepatitis A comes from human sources. The product information sheet gives the recommended dosages based on weight. Note that anaphylactic reactions, although very rare, can occur.

Activity Intolerance Related to Extreme Fatigue

There is no drug to cure hepatitis; the mainstays of treatment are rest and a diet that promotes liver regeneration. (For other nursing diagnoses, see bilirubin levels [Chapter 11] and ALT levels [Chapter 12], which are used to monitor the progress of the client.) Older clients tend to have more severe symptoms. For young children, the disease may be totally asymptomatic and thus can be easily spread in a day care setting.

TESTS FOR HEPATITIS C VIRUS

In the late 1980s, researchers cloned a protein associated with the hepatitis C virus (HCV). This protein was used to develop a test to detect antibodies to HCV (anti-HCV) in the blood. This was the first time a viral genome was used to develop a serologic assay without actually first isolating the agent. Studies revealed that the predominant virus for non-A, non-B transfusion hepatitis was this C virus, which could be detected with the antibody test. This anti-HCV is not a protective antibody, so its presence signifies a carrier state, not immunity. By May 1990, the U.S. Food and Drug Administration (FDA) approved the use of test kits to detect anti-HCV, and the test became part of the routine screen of donor blood (see Table 14–2). The risk of HCV from transfusions has dropped from about 10% in 1990 to about one case per 2 million units (McPhee et al., 2011).

Unfortunately, chronic carriers of HCV are usually unaware of their condition because they typically have little or no symptoms for many years. However, a significant number will develop serious liver disease later in life. The most common reason for a liver transplant is cirrhosis due to HCV. The second most common reason is alcohol-related cirrhosis, but many of these clients also have HCV (Everson & Weinberg, 2006). Clients may purchase a home test for HCV. Then a blood sample is sent to the laboratory for analysis.

A positive HCV-EIA test is confirmed by the use of a recombinant immunoblot assay (RIBA) that determines what antigens are causing an antibody reaction. The test has several antigen bands labeled as 5-1-1, c100-3, c33c, and c 22-3 and a control of superoxide dismutase (sod). If the person's antibodies react only against sod, the test is negative. Reactions to two or more of the antigen bands are reported as positive. Reactions to the antigens may necessitate further testing. The presence of antibodies against HCV does not imply protective immunity as do antibodies against HAV or HBV.

Further testing can be done with HCV-RNA assays to directly measure the virus in the blood. Methods using polymerase chain reaction (PCR) or a branched-chain DNA assay are used to determine the concentration of the virus and may be used as a marker for the effects of therapy, such as interferon. (See the discussion on viral loads for HIV, which uses these methods, too.) Several genotypes of HCV have been identified. Type 1 is the most common in the United States followed by Types 2 and 3. HCV is very common all over the world.

Preparation of Client and Collection of Sample

The laboratory needs 1 mL of serum and 2 mL of plasma for RIBA.

REFERENCE VALUE FOR ANTI-HVC AND RIBA
Negative titer

Clinical Significance

Chronic HCV infection is typically insidious for many years. Many clients with hepatitis C do not have jaundice, so the clue to diagnosis may be an elevated ALT level. The clinical signs and symptoms of acute hepatitis C are similar to those of hepatitis B but less severe. However, progression to chronic hepatitis and cirrhosis is more frequent with hepatitis C. Hepatitis C, like hepatitis B, is associated with the development of liver cancer. Approximately, 3–4 million Americans live with HCV, and the overwhelming majority are not aware of their infection. Clients who are positive for HIV are often coinfected with HCV (www.projectinform.org).

A combination of pegylated interferon and ribavirin is the standard treatment for HCV (Wilkins et al., 2010). The period of treatment is determined by the genotype and may last as long as 48 weeks for Type 1. An indicator of successful treatment is loss of detectable HCV-RNA in the serum. Research on the best treatment continues for persons with persistently elevated ALT levels (see Chapter 12), detectable HCV-RNA, and a liver biopsy indicating liver damage. (See Chapter 25 on liver biopsy.) Everson and Weinberg (2006) discuss the approved and experimental therapies for hepatitis C, including living donor liver transplants. Clients with chronic hepatitis C and cirrhosis may have ultrasounds (Chapter 23) for surveillance for liver cancer (McPhee et al., 2011).

Possible Nursing Diagnoses Related to Positive HCV Test

Deficient Knowledge Related to Prevention of Disease

At present, the most commonly recognized risk factors for HCV infection are use of contaminated needles, history of blood transfusions, hemodialysis, and health care employment.

Sexual spread of the disease and transmission to the newborn are relatively uncommon. No vaccine is available, so prevention involves avoiding contaminated blood and blood products. The American Liver Foundation (www.liverfoundation.org) has excellent information for patient education about hepatitis C and for other types of hepatitis, as does the Hepatitis Foundation International (www.hepfi.org).

Ineffective Health Maintenance

Treatments may also alter health maintenance and create activity intolerance. Interferon causes weakness and flu-like symptoms, and ribavirin can cause anemia and leukopenia. Clients may give themselves erythropoietin (EPO) (Chapter 2). Many clients also experience depression and anxiety that requires treatment (Wilson, 2005).

Support groups or lay publications may help the newly diagnosed client find answers to the many questions and fears brought on by the diagnosis. A healthy lifestyle should focus on decreasing stress levels, adequate sleep, and a balanced diet. The client needs to know that alcohol and some other drugs may further harm the liver, so they should be avoided. Vaccines for hepatitis A and B are advisable to protect the liver from other kinds of hepatitis.

HIV TESTING

Since the beginning of the AIDS epidemic, much research has been centered on studying the effects of HIV-1, which used to be called lymphadenopathy-associated virus (LAV) or human T-cell lymphotropic virus type III (HTLV-III).

Until 1988, only two types of tests were used to detect HIV-1 antibodies: a screening test performed with enzyme-linked immunosorbent assay (ELISA) and confirmation by the Western blot test, which uses electrophoresis, a process discussed in Chapter 10, to separate out component proteins of the virus. These proteins are transferred or blotted to a support medium. If antibodies to these specific viral proteins are present in the client's serum, mixing the medium with a sample of the client's serum causes a reaction. In 1989, the FDA licensed a latex agglutination test for HIV-1 antibodies that can give results in 5 minutes. This was the first test to use a protein engineered by DNA technology. A second virus that causes AIDS is HIV-2, which is endemic in West Africa but may also be found elsewhere. Further tests may be needed if HIV-2 is suspected. At present, a version of the Western blot remains the standard confirmatory test for HIV. The time between exposure to HIV and the appearance of antibodies is probably quite variable; a range of 12 days to 5 years has been reported in the literature. McPhee et al. (2011) noted that about 50% of people are positive within 22 days after HIV transmission and 95% are positive within 6 weeks.

Blood banks began using the test for antibodies against HTLV-III or HIV in 1985. The use of this screening test dramatically reduced the risk of transmission of AIDS by means of blood transfusions. Although heterosexual transmission is less likely than transmission through male homosexual activity, transmission of the AIDS virus is possible from men to women and vice versa. Although male-to-female transmission has been known for many years, many women with HIV do not receive an early diagnosis because they do not consider themselves at risk. In 1985, only 7% of the new AIDS cases were women. In 2006, 25.2% of the new cases were women.

The two major methods of transmission to women are heterosexual contact with an infected man and drug use (McPhee et al., 2011). The use of rapid HIV tests during labor and delivery has helped decrease transmission to infants, as treatment can be started immediately for those not tested earlier. Aggressive treatment for the mother and infant decreased transmission to less than 1% (Goldschmidt & Fogler, 2006). In developing countries, the perinatal transmission of AIDS is still a huge problem. More HIV-infected women are now planning to have children, so nurses must know current practice recommendations (Cibulka, 2006). (See Chapter 18 on HIV testing for pregnant women and newborns.) Now more than 90% of new pediatric infections occur in developing countries.

Major Changes in Guidelines for Testing for HIV

In 2006, the Centers for Disease Control and Prevention (CDC) proposed HIV screening for all citizens between 13 and 64 years of age because about a quarter of a million people in the United States do not know they have HIV. Clients can opt out of the offered test if they wish. These new guidelines were a significant break from the previous focus on offering testing only to those known to be at high risk. (In 2005, the recommendation was made to screen all pregnant women.) Other major changes were the dropping of mandatory pretest counseling sessions and the need for a separate written consent form. San Francisco was the first city to adopt the new policy. Clients now give oral, not written, permission for testing. Pretest counseling is still offered to those who want it, but it is no longer mandatory. The use of HIV testing as a routine assessment reduced the stigma of the test and makes it easier to offer in all settings. The National HIV/AIDS Clinical Consultation Centers website (www.nccc.ucsf.edu) has information on testing and updates on state laws for HIV testing.

Preparation of Client and Collection of Sample

A test for HIV antibodies requires 0.5 mL in a red tube. All results are confidential. Check for specific laboratory procedures and the latest legal requirements.

REFERENCE VALUE FOR HIV ANTIBODIES

Negative for antibodies to HIV

Western Blot HIV Test

A Western blot method that identifies antigens of HIV, including p24, gp41, and gp120/160, confirms a positive antibody test. The Western blot test uses electrophoresis as described earlier in this chapter. (The name of the test, developed in the West, is a play on the name of Southern blot, a technique to measure DNA developed by a man of that name. For further humor, the detection of a test for RNA is sometimes called Northern blot.) In the past, before nucleic acid test (NAT) was available, p24 antigen was used to screen donor blood for HIV.

RAPID TESTS FOR HIV AS POINT OF CARE

A rapid test for HIV-1 antibodies, using a finger stick, was first approved in 2002. Now there are three rapid tests that use blood from a finger stick and one that uses oral fluid. For the oral test, the clinician swabs the inside of the client's lip and places the swab inside a vial containing developing solution. If HIV antibodies are present, two reddish-purple lines appear in a window on the device. These tests deliver results in as little as 20 minutes with 99% accuracy (Wright & Katz, 2006). Positive tests are followed up with conventional testing. Negative tests can prompt education about safer sex. The ability to do this point-of-care testing has become very useful in emergency departments, clinics, and labor and delivery. However, these antibody-only tests miss approximately 10% of HIV infections, because they do not detect antigens. In 2010, an HIV antigen–antibody combination (Architect HIV Ag/Ab Combo Assay by Abbott) received FDA approval. This test detects the HIV p24 antigen and documents the direct presence of HIV.

HOME TESTS FOR HIV

In 1996, the FDA approved the collection of two home-sample testing kits for HIV. Clients purchase the commercial kit, perform a finger stick to obtain a blood specimen on filter paper, and mail the sample directly to the laboratory. (The laboratory uses the EIA and Western blot confirmation testing as described earlier.) Use of a code number for the specimen makes the testing anonymous. The client uses the code when calling a toll-free number for results. All callers who test positive or indeterminate are connected to a counselor who provides test results, counseling, and referrals. Education for the general public remains an important goal in helping people understand the ramifications of the epidemic. Debate continues about the pros and cons of individuals self-testing the rapid tests discussed earlier. The reader is encouraged to check for the recent updates on approval of these tests for home use.

Possible Nursing Diagnosis Related to Positive HIV Test

Ineffective Health Maintenance Related to a Positive HIV Test

In addition to psychological counseling, clients who have positive HIV tests need the most current information on drug therapy available to them, including participation in clinical trials for new promising drug therapy. To maintain health, clients also need concrete information on the importance of good nutrition and control of stress. Information about ways to express sexual needs without endangering others is important in helping the client maintain a balanced life.

Nurses are instrumental in helping both clients with positive HIV tests and those with AIDS lead lives as fulfilling and productive as possible. Maybe what is needed most when a client has a positive HIV test are positive-thinking nurses who are unsurpassed in giving compassionate and competent care to all. As life expectancy continues to increase in clients with

(Continued)

> ## Possible Nursing Diagnosis . . . *(Continued)*
>
> AIDS, the evolution of HIV infection into a chronic disease has made every nurse an HIV nurse (Bradley-Springer, Stevens, &Webb, 2010).
>
> Symptom management is an essential component of a comprehensive approach to the care of the person with HIV or AIDS, and nurses may be the ones to help the client cope with symptoms such as fatigue, anxiety, insomnia, and lack of appetite. Research has shown clients with HIV/AIDS use many types of resources to learn self-care (Chou et al., 2004). Another research focuses on the most frequently identified nursing diagnoses for clients with HIV/AIDS, such as risks of infection, activity intolerance, deficient knowledge, and a high frequency of psychosocial diagnoses (da Silva et al., 2006). As HIV has become a chronic (but still life-threatening) condition, some clients are aging with HIV and research needs to focus on this population (Vance, 2010).
>
> ### Risk of Injury Related to Drug Therapy
>
> Educating clients about their drugs and possible unwanted effects is an important nursing function. Covington (2005) and Deglin, Vallerand, and Sanoski (2011) discuss the recommended guidelines for administration of antiviral drugs. Although research has not yet found a way to eliminate HIV, newer types of drug therapy have transformed the disease into a manageable chronic condition. The use of highly active antiretroviral therapy (HAART) has decreased mortality rates but may create metabolic abnormalities and cardiovascular disease. Nurses are involved in research on ways to manage dyslipidemia and insulin resistance to these drugs (Delgado & Dort, 2010).

CD4 COUNTS

The client on antiretroviral therapy will have both the viral load and CD4 counts (Chapter 2) measured every 3–6 months. Treatment guidelines now recommend starting medications before the CD4 drops below 350–500. Current research suggests that individuals infected with HIV should begin immediate treatment instead of waiting until the CD4 count drops. (See www.projectinform.org for more details on treatment guidelines.) Therapy may include the protease inhibitors, introduced in 1996, combined with some of the other types of antiretrovirals such as zidovudine (AZT), the first antiretroviral. Over 20 drugs are currently available as antiretrovirals, and drugs come in combinations (3 or 4 drugs) so that the client does not need to swallow as many individual pills. Decreases in viral load and increases in CD4 counts are evidence of effective therapy (Deglin et al., 2011).

VIRAL LOAD TESTS

Commercial tests for viral loads of HIV in the serum became available in 1996 and, since then, have become very important for assessing the time to begin, change, or add therapy. Methods for determining the amount of HIV in the serum include the quantitative polymerase chain reaction (qPCR), a nucleic acid sequence-based amplification (NASBA) or nucleic acid testing (NAT), and the branched DNA assay (bDNA). These tests make multiple copies of the virus present in the serum. Viral loads below 10,000 copies are usually considered "low," and copies above 100,000 are considered "high." People with levels less than 10,000 copies seem to have a decreased risk of disease progression, while those with HIV-RNA copies greater than 100,000 are much more likely to progress to full-blown AIDS. Changes in the amount of copies are reported in logs, a shorthand way to express large numbers. For example, a change from 100,000 down to 10,000 is a 1-log drop. Newer versions of the tests for viral loads continue to become more sensitive so that as few as 50–75 copies may be detected (Wu, 2006). The reader is encouraged to contact the manufacturer of a specific test for the current sensitivity. After treatment some clients may have "undetectable" viral loads, but this does not mean that the virus is gone, as it is just below the sensitivity of the test.

HUMAN T-CELL LYMPHOTROPIC VIRUS TYPES I AND II

HTLV-I is a distinct retrovirus associated with adult T-cell leukemia. It has also been associated with tropical spastic paraparesis. Although distantly related to HIV, which used to be called HTLV-III, HTLV-I does not cause immunodeficiency syndrome. In 1989, the FDA approved three EIA test kits for use in screening blood supplies for HTLV-I. The tests for HTLV-I may also detect HTLV-II, a closely related retrovirus. However, some HTLV-II is missed, so several ELISA tests can be used. A nucleic probe with PCR is the best way to differentiate the two types. A combined assay for anti-HTLV-I/II is used mainly to screen blood donors.

WEST NILE VIRUS TEST

West Nile virus (WNV), an infection transmitted to humans primarily by mosquitoes, first emerged in the United States (New York) in 1999. In 2002, transmission of the virus from transfusions of blood products and organ transplantation was identified (Petersen & Epstein, 2005). By 2003, cases were reported all across the country. (For many years, WNV had been identified in other countries as a cause of encephalitis or meningitis.)

About 20% of the people with WNV are affected by a self-limited flu-like illness. Rarely, the more severe neurological form develops and can be fatal. Deaths have been more common in the older population (Avalos-Bock, 2005). Diagnostic tests are done on blood and cerebral spinal fluid. Treatment is symptomatic, but immunoglobulins may become a therapeutic option (McPhee et al., 2011). For primary prevention, nurses can teach clients how to protect themselves from mosquitoes and how to eliminate places where mosquitoes can breed (Overstreet, 2005).

Preparation of Client and Collection of Sample

For Blood, Stem Cell, and Organ Donor Screening (NAT)

Minimum of 5 mL to be collected in a lavender-topped tube.

Screening for Clients with suspected WNV

Two serum specimens are collected; first during the acute phase of the illness and the next 3–5 days after the acute specimen was sent. The blood (2 mL) collected in a red-topped tube can be stored or transported frozen with a cold pack to the health department. Cerebrospinal fluid (1–2 mL) may also be stored or transported frozen. Prior to sending specimens, the clinician must check with the health department for other requirements such as a completed West Nile Case History Form.

SEROLOGIC TESTS FOR SYPHILIS

Except for the common cold and flu, sexually transmitted diseases are the most common infectious diseases in the United States. Although chlamydia and herpes infections and gonorrhea are more common than syphilis, syphilis is more dangerous if left undetected and thus untreated. (See Chapter 16 for the tests for gonorrhea and chlamydia and herpes infections.)

Although the spirochete, *Treponema pallidum*, that causes syphilis may occasionally be identified from a syphilitic sore, or chancre, syphilis is more commonly diagnosed with a serologic test. Testing for syphilis may be divided into tests for screening and those for a confirmation of a positive screening test. The Venereal Disease Research Laboratory (VDRL) and rapid plasma reagin (RPR) are screening tests, whereas the test for treponemal antibodies called *Treponema pallidum* particle agglutination (TTPA) is confirmatory. The use of PCR is very useful to identify microbes in amniotic fluid and neonatal serum and spinal fluid (DeCherney et al., 2007). However, the PCR test is not widely available (McPhee et al., 2011).

Dark-Field Examination

A small amount of serum expressed from the base of a lesion is examined under a microscope. A dose of penicillin renders the dark field useless.

VDRL and RPR

The VDRL is named for the research laboratory that perfected this flocculation test for syphilis. The test measures a globulin complex called *reagin* that appears early in the course of syphilis. If the globulin complex reagin is present, an aggregation occurs that can be reported as either negative, weakly reactive, or reactive. The RPR uses the VDRL antigen, but it adds some carbon particles so that the flocculation can be seen on a plastic card.

The VDRL and variations of it are indirect tests for syphilis because they are tests for a reaction to a globulin, not to the spirochete itself. A person who has just contracted syphilis may not have had time to build up antibodies against *T. pallidum*, so these tests usually become positive 3–4 weeks after exposure. Because the screening tests react to abnormal globulins, other diseases, such as malaria; other infections; malignant tumors; and some connective tissue disorders may cause false-positive reactions.

TREPONEMA PALLIDUM PARTICLE AGGLUTIONATION (TTPA)

The TTPA may be used to confirm an infection with the spirochete that causes syphilis. It tests for the specific antibodies against *T. pallidum*.

Preparation of Client and Collection of Sample

The laboratory uses 4 mL of venous blood for STS. Alcohol may interfere with some tests.

Possible Nursing Diagnosis Related to Positive Serologic Test for Syphilis (STS)

Deficient Knowledge Related to Need for Screening and Follow-up with Sexual Contacts

If not detected in the early stages, syphilis may eventually spread, causing severe neurologic problems, blindness, and even death. The treatment of syphilis is extremely easy: penicillin by means of injection. Other antibiotics are used if the client is allergic to penicillin.

As a communicable disease, syphilis must be reported to the public health department either by the physician or through the laboratory. Public health departments have staffs who follow up with the sexual contacts of the client who has a positive STS. Clinicians unsure of local reporting requirements should seek advice from local health departments or state sexually transmitted disease programs. Nurses may take an active role in educating the public about the importance of screening people who may have been exposed to the disease. Nurses working with clients who have a positive STS can help impress on them the importance of early detection and early treatment of their sexual partners and the need for safer sex. Nurses must be nonjudgmental in their approach.

Because syphilis can be passed to a fetus, it is extremely important that a pregnant woman be treated for syphilis. (See Chapter 16 for information about other sexually transmitted diseases and pregnancy.) A nurse working in a prenatal clinic can explain to clients why an STS is done in early pregnancy. Screening maternal blood at delivery is also important and may be more effective than screening cord serum.

REFERENCE VALUES FOR STS

These tests should be negative.

Note that various conditions may cause false positives, as explained in the text. Also note that the tests are most strongly positive 4–6 weeks after exposure.

INFECTIOUS MONONUCLEOSIS (EPSTEIN–BARR VIRUS)

Infectious mononucleosis, caused by EBV, can be acquired from asymptomatic carriers as well as recently ill clients who may excrete the virus in saliva for many months. Young children infected from the saliva of playmates may have few symptoms (Hay et al., 2011). The classic triad of symptoms is fever, pharyngitis, and enlarged lymph nodes.

Rapid tests for infectious mononucleosis use a saline suspension of antigen. The mixture of the test material with a drop of the client's serum causes a coarse granulation if the client has infectious mononucleosis. The spot tests are rapid, specific, and sensitive as screening tests, and they are valuable in supporting a clinical diagnosis of infectious mononucleosis (Wu, 2006). Other criteria for diagnosing infectious mononucleosis include lymphocytosis and the presence of atypical lymphocytes in the serum (see Chapter 2 for a discussion of lymphocytes as part of a differential white blood cell [WBC] count).

Tests to confirm infectious mononucleosis, if needed, include tests for the Epstein–Barr nuclear antigen (EBNA) as well as for antibodies to the viral capsid antigen (VCA). These antibodies can be identified as either IgG or IgM (see Chapter 10).

Preparation of Client and Collection of Sample

The screening tests require 1 mL of blood. A WBC count with differential is also ordered.

Nursing Diagnosis for a Positive Test

Activity Intolerance Related to Fatigue

Nursing care for clients with infectious mononucleosis includes providing rest and other general measures to help them overcome a viral infection. Acetaminophen can be used for fever. There is no drug therapy for the disease. Infectious mononucleosis is sometimes called the *kissing disease*, because of transmission from saliva. Isolation is not necessary. Many people have antibody titers against the EBV. ALT levels (Chapter 12) and bilirubin levels (Chapter 11) are used to assess the degree of liver dysfunction. The spleen may remain enlarged for several weeks and fatigue may last several months.

STREPTOCOCCAL INFECTIONS

Definition and Purpose

Three tests are used to identify a recent infection with group A β-hemolytic streptococci:

1. Anti-streptolysin-O (ASO)
2. Anti-streptodornase-B or anti-deoxyribonuclease-B (anti-DNase-B)
3. Streptozyme test

Group A β-hemolytic streptococci produce several substances (antigens) that induce the formation of measurable antibodies in the serum. Because the aftermath of group A streptococci infections may be diseases such as rheumatic fever or glomerulonephritis, one or more of these three streptococcal antigen tests is used to help confirm that the client did have a streptococcal infection in the recent past. Rheumatic fever is becoming rarer because of early recognition and treatment of streptococcal infections such as strep throat. (See Chapter 16 on the importance of throat cultures to identify strep throat.)

Anti-streptolysin-O

The antibodies to streptolysin-O appear about 7–10 days after an acute streptococcal infection. The antibodies peak 2–4 weeks later, remaining high for weeks to months. The test may not always be elevated with streptococcal infections, and other disease conditions, such as liver disease, may make the test falsely positive.

Anti-streptodornase-B

Anti-DNase-B measures the antibodies formed against another of the streptococcal enzymes called *deoxyribonuclease-B*. It may be used in conjunction with the test for streptococcal antigens.

Streptozyme Test

This test, a commercial product, is more general than the ASO or anti-DNase-B. It measures antibodies against five different streptococcal enzymes: (1) streptolysin-O, (2) deoxyribonuclease-B, (3) hyaluronidase, (4) streptokinase, and (5) nicotinamide adenine dinucleotidase. This test is more sensitive than ASO titers (Hay et al., 2011).

Preparation of Client and Collection of Sample

These tests require venous blood. Record on the laboratory slip if the client is taking antibiotics because titers may not increase if the client has been taking antibiotics.

REFERENCE VALUES FOR TESTS FOR STREPTOCOCCAL INFECTIONS	
ASO titers:	
Preschool	1:85
Age 5–18 years	1:170
Adults	1:85
Anti-DNase-B titers:	
Preschool	1:60
Age 5–18 years	1:170
Adults	1:85
Streptozyme titers	<100 Streptozyme units

RUBELLA

Rubella (also called *3-day measles* or *German measles*) is usually of no clinical significance unless it occurs in a pregnant woman. Rubella may cause a miscarriage, or it may bring about congenital heart disease, cataracts, deafness, and brain damage in the fetus. Thus, it is important to assess whether women who are to become pregnant have an immunity against rubella.

Preparation of Client and Collection of Sample

The test requires venous blood, 0.5 mL, in an SST vacuum tube.

REFERENCE VALUES FOR RUBELLA

Titers ≥1:32 indicate immunity.

If tested by EIA, IgG: index >1.2 shows immunity.

IgM: index >1.09 is positive for acute infection.

Once a person has had rubella, an elevated titer of antibodies persists for many years or perhaps for life. Even a small number of antibodies indicates some immunity from the disease. Women who are not immune to rubella (i.e., who have no antibody titer) should be vaccinated before becoming pregnant.

Possible Nursing Diagnoses Related to Negative Rubella Titer

Deficient Knowledge Related to Need for Vaccine

The lack of a titer to rubella is clinically significant in women who may become pregnant. Since 1969, when the first rubella vaccine was licensed in the United States, there has been a mass immunization program for school-aged children. However, there are still women in their childbearing years who are susceptible to rubella. A single dose of rubella vaccine is recommended not only for children more than 12 months old but also for any woman who has no antibody titer for rubella and who may become pregnant.

Whether some action should be taken may be a disturbing question for a woman who contacts rubella during her pregnancy. If a pregnant woman is believed to have rubella, a rise in maternal rubella IgM is evidence of recent infection. The client needs to confer with the physician about possible damage to the fetus.

Health care workers must take all measures necessary to prevent susceptible pregnant women from contracting rubella. All health workers who might transmit rubella to pregnant women should be immunized against the disease.

Risk for Injury Related to Vaccine

Nurses should be aware that adult women who are given the vaccine should avoid pregnancy for 3 months. Giving the client information about reliable birth control may be necessary. Also, because the vaccine can cause some joint symptoms, particularly in adults, the possible side effects of the vaccine need to be explained. However, there are no reports of congenital rubella syndrome after inadvertent immunization of a pregnant woman (McPhee et al., 2011).

PARVOVIRUS B19 (ERYTHEMA INFECTIOSUM OR FIFTH DISEASE)

The term "fifth disease" got its name from a list of childhood infections that cause a rash or erythema. Rubeola, scarlet fever, rubella, and roseola were the first four, and the fifth was called erythema infectiosum before the causative agent (Parvovirus B19) was discovered in 1975. The disease is also called "slapped cheek" disease because of the appearance of rash on the cheeks. (Hay et al., 2011). The disease is almost always benign in healthy children but does cause a short-lived decrease in red blood cell production. This can cause a transient aplastic crisis (TAC) in clients with hemolytic anemia or who are immunocompromised. Transfusion therapy may be needed. This virus may also cause miscarriages in pregnant women, so they should avoid contact with children who have the disease. Both IgM and IgG antibodies can be measured. (Antibody testing may require special approval.) IgG persists for years and gives lifelong immunity. For complicated cases, diagnosis of current infection can be done with a DNA test.

TOXOPLASMOSIS

Toxoplasmosis (TPM or Toxo) is caused by infestation with the protozoan *Toxoplasma gondii*, which is found in raw or poorly cooked meat and in the feces of cats. The disease causes fatigue, fever, and lymph gland swelling. TPM can be treated with drugs, so usually the disease is not serious in an adult unless the host is immunocompromised, as in AIDS or after transplants. TPM can be passed to a fetus and cause neurologic damage and eye problems.

Preparation of Client and Collection of Sample

Check with the laboratory for the specific type of serologic test being used. Pertinent history includes whether the client has been exposed to cats, may be pregnant, or is immunosuppressed.

REFERENCE VALUES FOR TPM

IgM antibody titer is negative if <8 for an adult and <2 for an infant.

Infants may have an increased titer because of the transfer of antibodies from the mother. Infants need to be retested later.

Possible Nursing Diagnoses Related to Positive Titer

Deficient Knowledge Related to Danger for Pregnant Women

People should be aware that poorly cooked or raw meat can introduce organisms into the human body. Also, the importance of avoiding hand contamination from the feces of cats should be made common knowledge. Because cats are the host, the pregnant woman needs to be careful about handling the feces of a cat and certainly to avoid strange cats. A veterinarian can be contacted about the health status of a house cat. About 90% of mothers with acute TPM during pregnancy have no symptoms.

(Continued)

> ## Possible Nursing Diagnoses . . . *(Continued)*
>
> ### Anxiety Related to Unknown Diagnosis
>
> The presence of lymphadenopathy (enlarged lymph glands) and vague symptoms in an otherwise healthy person may suggest a viral infection. A client with suspected TPM may also undergo tests done for infectious mononucleosis. In contrast to infectious mononucleosis, there is no elevated HAT in TPM. (See earlier in this chapter for the discussion of the HAT.) Until the diagnosis is made by the physician, the client may be afraid that the lymph gland swelling is due to a malignant tumor and is likely to be very relieved to find out that the problem is an infection with a protozoan. In an immunosuppressed client, TPM may be a serious or even fatal disease unless treated early.

AMEBIASIS

Entamoeba histolytica is an ameba that causes amebic dysentery and hepatic abscesses. The ameba can be identified by means of microscopic examination. (See Chapter 16 for the technique used to obtain a stool culture for ameba.) The stool examination is the most definitive test for ameba, but it is technically difficult to obtain live ameba for direct examination. Serologic tests can identify antibodies to *E. histolytica*, which are present in 90–95% of clients with a hepatic abscess caused by the ameba and in 85–90% of clients with an intestinal infestation with *E. histolytica*. The medication used for treatment depends on the location of the infestation (Katzung, Masters, & Trevor, 2009).

Preparation of Client and Collection of Sample

The test requires venous blood. Check with the laboratory for the exact amount.

> ### REFERENCE VALUE FOR AMEBA
>
> Fourfold titer increase indicates infestation with the ameba. Antibody levels persist for several years after an active infestation.

> ## Possible Nursing Diagnosis Related to Increasing Titer
>
> ### Deficient Knowledge Related to Spread of Disease
>
> See Chapter 16 for the client teaching needed when a client must follow enteric precautions.

SEROLOGIC TESTS FOR LYME DISEASE

Lyme disease, named after a town in Connecticut, is caused by a spirochete transmitted by tick bites. A ring of redness (erythema migrans) may develop at the site of the tick bite within 3–30 days and may spread out to a diameter of 20 cm (Hay et al.,

2011). Laboratory confirmation requires identification of specific antibodies to the spirochete *Borrelia burgdorferi*. Antibodies are identified by EIA as a first step, with an index of 0.90 or lower considered negative and over 1.10 as positive. A positive or an equivocal finding of 0.91–1.09 is followed up by a second test of antibodies using the Western blot method described in the section on HIV testing. IgM antibodies appear within 2–4 weeks after the bite, and IgG antibodies appear later but last a long time. Use of serologic testing may be problematic because of a lack of specificity. Antibodies are not useful for evaluating the effectiveness of antibiotic therapy (Glatz et al., 2006). Consultation with an infectious disease specialist with experience in treating Lyme disease may be helpful for atypical cases (McPhee et al., 2011).

SEROLOGIC TESTS FOR *HELICOBACTER PYLORI*

H. pylori is highly correlated with duodenal and gastric ulcers. Serologic testing for IgG antibodies is available, and a point-of-care test detects IgG antibodies to *H. pylori* in 4 minutes. Clients with ulcers who are shown to have *H. pylori* infection are treated with antimicrobial agents in addition to other antiulcer drugs (Deglin et al., 2011). (See Chapter 27 on the use of endoscopy to detect and assess treatment of ulcers.)

Serologic tests do not denote ongoing infection. Noninvasive breath tests that measure C-urea can be used to indicate active infection with *H. pylori*. (See Chapter 24.)

HERPESVIRUS FAMILY

A primary infection with herpes simplex virus (HSV) (either HSV-1 for oral herpes or HSV-2 for genital herpes) may produce rising antibody titers. Sometimes these two viruses can be found in both locations. Transmission of the virus occurs when body fluid containing the virus is deposited directly on the mucosa of the other person. Because exposure to one of the herpesviruses is almost universal in the population, the serologic test for herpes is usually not useful for clinical management. However, the titers of HSV are useful in epidemiologic studies or for research. Clinical diagnosis of genital herpes is usually made on the basis of history and symptoms. The two specific tests to confirm HSV-2, the Tzanck test and viral cultures, are discussed in Chapter 16. Diagnosis is particularly important in pregnant women. Herpes in the infant can be very serious. Antiviral medications can control but not eradicate the virus from the body. EBV, CMV, and the varicella virus are also in the herpesvirus family and are discussed in this chapter. In 1986, human herpesvirus 6 (HHV-6) was isolated, and in 1990, HHV-7 was isolated. HHV-6 and, sometimes, a variant of HHV-7 are associated with roseola infantum, the most common cause of febrile seizures in infants (Hay et al., 2011). Since then, HHV-8 has also been isolated. PCR amplification is used to identify the type. (See Table 14–7.) Kaposi's sarcoma, the most common cancer associated with AIDS, was discovered to be caused by HHV-8 in 1996. Infection with HHV does not always lead to cancer, so other factors are involved. Exactly how HHV-8 is transmitted also remains unclear, even though it is endemic in some parts of the world. Research in Uganda, where HHV-8 is prevalent, gives evidence of transmission by blood transfusions (Hladik et al., 2006).

Table 14–7 Types of Human Herpesvirus (HHV) and Common Names

Type	Common Name
HHV-1	Oral herpes, herpes simplex type 1
HHV-2	Genital herpes, herpes simplex type 2
HHV-3	Varicella-zoster virus, chickenpox virus
	Recurrent infection causes shingles.
HHV-4	Epstein–Barr virus (EBV)
	Virus for infectious mononucleosis
HHV-5	Cytomegalovirus (CMV)
HHV-6	No common name
HHV-7	No common name
HHV-8	Kaposi's sarcoma herpesvirus (KSHV)

Note: See McPhee et al. (2011) foçr information about treatment options and client education.

CYTOMEGALOVIRUS TITERS

Cytomegalovirus (CMV), a type of herpesvirus found in almost all body secretions, can cross the placenta and be transferred in blood. Many adults have been exposed to the virus and thus have immunity. The virus may be dangerous for pregnant women because of damage to the fetus. The virus can cause cerebral malformation and necrosis of brain tissue (Hay et al., 2011). Immunosuppressed clients are highly susceptible to CMV infection. Clients with AIDS usually have high titers for CMV. Acute infection with the virus in the client with AIDS can lead to eye damage and blindness as well as cerebral damage. Drugs, such as foscarnet and ganciclovir, are used to treat CMV retinitis (Deglin et al., 2011).

REFERENCE VALUES FOR CMV

A fourfold or greater rise in titer between acute and convalescent samples is evidence of infection. A single IgM-specific titer of more than 1:8 is evidence of an acute infection.

Note: The CMV antigen can be detected with a DNA probe and electron microscopy, but both methods are expensive.

VARICELLA-ZOSTER ANTIBODY TITER

A varicella-zoster antibody screen is performed to see if the client has immunity to the herpes zoster virus that can cause both chickenpox (varicella) and shingles (herpes zoster). Titers are not so useful for determining acute infections. Vesicle scrapings can be used for viral culture (Chapter 16).

Preparation of Client and Collection of Sample

The laboratory needs 0.5 mL of serum.

> **REFERENCE VALUE FOR VARICELLA-ZOSTER ANTIBODY TITER**
>
> Negative finding means the client is susceptible to infections with the herpes zoster virus.

Clinical Significance

To curtail an epidemic of chickenpox in the clinical setting, it is useful to know which staff do not have an immunity to the herpes zoster virus, because they should not take care of patients who are believed to have shingles or chickenpox. The incubation period is 10–20 days after the initial exposure. However, the disease is infectious for 5 days before the rash and continues to be so until all the lesions have crusted over. A varicella vaccine (Varivax by Merck) became available in 1995 and is now recommended for all healthy children 12 months or older who have not had chickenpox (Hay et al., 2011). Clients who are immunosuppressed should be protected from patients or staffs who have negative titers and hence could become carriers of the virus if exposed. Health care workers with negative titers may be required to have the vaccine to prevent the spread of the disease to clients. Disseminated chickenpox can be fatal to an immunosuppressed person.

In 2005, a new and more potent version of the chickenpox vaccine became available for clients over age 60 years who have had chickenpox and whose immune system is not compromised. The vaccine boosts immunity and decreases the chance of shingles by half. If an attack occurs, the severity is lessened. Antiviral medications such as acyclovir may be used to reduce the severity when shingles is suspected (Deglin et al., 2011).

HANTAVIRUS

The hantavirus was first isolated from a field mouse near the Hantaan River in Korea many years ago. Today there are many types of this virus that can cause disease. The first hantavirus appeared in the United States in 1993 when an outbreak of acute respiratory disease occurred in the Southwest. By 2001, the hantavirus pulmonary syndrome had been reported in 31 states. This prompted public education about the danger of transmission from the infected secretions of rodents. Diagnosis of this rare disease is confirmed by the presence of IgM antibodies. Special forms are to be sent to the public health department.

FUNGAL ANTIBODIES: HISTOPLASMOSIS AND COCCIDIOIDOMYCOSIS

By use of the complement fixation (CF) or immunodiffusion (ID) techniques, the laboratory can identify antibodies that occur in response to fungal diseases, such as histoplasmosis or coccidioidomycosis. Histoplasmosis is found particularly in the Ohio Valley area, and coccidioidomycosis (valley fever or desert fever) is prominent in the San Joaquin Valley of California. Because many people who live in an area where a fungus is endemic may have positive serologic tests from past exposures, one titer is not enough to be diagnostic. A fourfold rise in titer is evidence of current infection. Although some types of fungus are endemic in certain areas, clients with the disease may be far from the origin. A travel history is mandatory when a fungal disease is suspected.

Skin testing and cultures may also be used to identify the particular fungus causing the systemic infection. (See Chapter 16 for some tips on cultures for fungus.) A positive skin test does not indicate that an infection is currently present, because the antibodies may be from past exposure. More diagnostically significant is conversion of a negative skin test to a positive one. Because skin tests can also cause a serologic test to become positive, they should be started after the blood is drawn for serologic tests for fungal antibodies.

FUNGAL ANTIGENS

Tests to identify antigens (rather than antibodies) for various fungi continue to be developed. Antigen tests are used for cryptococcosis and candidiasis, two fungi often found in immunocompromised clients.

Nursing Implications

The nurse should confer with the physician to see if the client presents any danger to other clients or to the staff. Refer to a nursing text for detailed information on the care of clients with fungal disease. Nurses may administer ordered skin tests for fungus. The technique for intradermal injection, the diluent strength of the antigen, and the times to read the results are clearly explained with the product information that accompanies the test material.

Preparation of Client and Collection of Sample

These tests require venous blood. Antibody tests should be drawn before any skin testing is done.

REFERENCE VALUES FOR FUNGAL ANTIBODIES AND ANTIGENS

Fourfold rise in antibody titer is evidence of infection. Specific antigens may be found in blood, urine, or cerebrospinal fluid.

IMMUNOLOGIC TESTS

The few tests discussed in this section are used primarily to assess for diseases such as systemic lupus erythematosus (SLE), rheumatoid arthritis (RA), or other autoimmune reactions. See Table 14–8 for a list of the common serologic tests used in immunology.

Table 14-8 Common Serologic Tests Used in Immunology

Test	Description
C-reactive protein	Measures an abnormal protein found in the serum in bacterial infections and inflammations. Compare with ESR in Chapter 2. See text for high-sensitivity cardiac CRP.
Complement activity	Measures activity of the complement system.
C3 and C4	Specific measurements of the amount of two of the complement factors
ANA	Measures antinuclear antibodies, which are often increased in SLE.
Anti-DNA	Other humoral antibodies, which are sometimes elevated in SLE
RF	Measurement of antibodies, which may be elevated in rheumatoid arthritis
Thyroid autoantibodies	Measurement of antibodies, which may be elevated in some types of thyroiditis

ANA, antinuclear antibodies; ESR, erythrocyte sedimentation rate; RF, rheumatoid factor; SLE, systemic lupus erythematosus.

C-REACTIVE PROTEIN ROUTINE AND HIGH SENSITIVITY (CARDIAC CRP)

The C-reactive protein (CRP) increases with inflammatory processes and with infections. Sometimes this test is used to monitor rheumatic fever or RA. Like the erythrocyte sedimentation rate (ESR), the CRP is a nonspecific test that indicates only an inflammation. CRP measurements are useful to monitor acute inflammations, but ESR may be the preferred test for chronic inflammation. (See Chapter 2 for the discussion of ESR as the other test used to monitor RA.)

Cardiac CRP

In the past few years, CRP has been used by researchers to predict the risk of myocardial infarctions and strokes because inflammation seems to be part of the pathology of atherosclerosis. Reduction of the incidence of first myocardial infarction associated with aspirin use appears to be directly related to the level of CRP.

Because nearly half of all myocardial infarctions occur in persons with normal lipid levels, researchers continue to look for other markers of risk such as homocysteine, fibrinogen, apolipoprotein A-I and B-100 and Lp (a) lipoprotein, as discussed in Chapter 9. Ridker et al. (2000) compared 12 markers for cardiovascular disease in women and found that a high-sensitivity C-reactive protein (hsCRP) was the strongest predictor of subsequent cardiovascular disease. These researchers concluded that the addition of CRP to lipid screening may provide an improved method of identifying clients at risk. Underlying tumor or inflammatory illnesses, including drug reactions and infections, may make the CRP unreliable as a cardiac marker. Now that CRP is known to be an independent predictor of future cardiovascular disease, research is focused on ways to lower the increased levels through medications or changes in lifestyle. One study suggests that dietary fiber may protect against high CRP (Ma et al., 2006).

A landmark study found that the use of a statin (rosuvastatin) significantly reduced the incidence of major cardiovascular events in healthy adults who had elevated hsCRP, but normal cholesterol levels (Ridker et al., 2008). Further research suggest that clinical outcomes improve in clients given rosuvastatin to drop the hsCRP to less than 2 mg/L and the LDL cholesterol to less than 70 mg/dL (Ridker et al., 2009). On the basis of the data, the FDA approved a new use of statin therapy for those with elevated hsCRPs and one other cardiovascular risk factor (Ridker, 2010). See Chapter 9 for more information on risk factors for cardiovascular disease.

Preparation of Client and Collection of Sample

The test requires 3 mL of venous blood.

REFERENCE VALUE FOR ROUTINE CRP

<10 mg/L may signify significant inflammatory disease.

REFERENCE VALUES FOR HIGH-SENSITIVITY C-REACTIVE PROTEIN (CARDIAC CRP)[a]

Risk	CRP mg/L
Low	<1.0
Average	1.0–3.0
High	3.0–10.0

[a]Noncardiovascular causes should be considered if values are 10 mg/L or higher on repeated measures (Wu, 2006).

ANTINUCLEAR ANTIBODIES

ANAs are γ-globulins found in clients with certain types of autoimmune diseases. ANAs are directed against components within the nucleus of the cell. Although they may be of various classes, most of the antibodies are of the IgA class (see Chapter 10). The test is typically used to rule out SLE because almost all clients with SLE have a positive ANA (Wu, 2006). However, the test is not specific for SLE because the test may also be positive in RA, scleroderma, carcinoma, tuberculosis, and hepatitis. ANA is elevated in approximately 90% of clients with Sjogren syndrome, so other tests are needed to identify specific autoimmune diseases (Pullen & Hall, 2010). Various drugs, such as quinidine and procainamide, may also cause an increased ANA titer.

Preparation of Client and Collection of Sample

The test requires 2 mL of serum, which should be sent to the laboratory immediately.

REFERENCE VALUES FOR ANA

Results may be expressed in units: 1–3, weakly positive; 3–6, positive; and above 6, strongly positive (Wu, 2006). Note that age and other factors may cause a weakly positive reaction even in clients without autoimmune disorders.

OTHER TESTS FOR SYSTEMIC LUPUS ERYTHEMATOSUS

Follow-up for Positive ANA

If the ANA test is positive, there are tests that can be used to determine which types of antibodies are present. Some common tests are anti-DNA, anti-Sm, and anti-Ro (www.labtestsonline.org). An immunoassay can detect four or six types of autoantibodies. These IgG antibodies are called extractable nuclear antigens (ENA). The lupus anticoagulant discussed in Chapter 13 may be present, as well as anti-cardiolipin antibodies. Other laboratory tests to help with diagnosis will be a CBC (Chapter 2) and platelet count (Chapter 13) to assess for anemia, leukopenia, and thrombocytopenia. These tests can help with the differential diagnosis of SLE, scleroderma, RA, and Sjogren syndrome. Clients with a chronic, multisystem autoimmune disorder such as SLE will most likely be on several types of drug therapy. Nurses can help clients learn to prevent flare-ups of SLE (Pullen, Brewer, & Ballard, 2009). Detailed information about tests for SLE and information on support groups can be obtained from the Lupus Foundation of America (www. lupus.org).

RHEUMATOID FACTOR

The RF is a test of abnormal proteins found in the serum of many clients with RA. Evidently the RF really consists of different types of IgM antibodies. (See Chapter 10 for the measurement of IgM.) Although the RF is present with other diseases, the highest levels are found in clients with RA, but the levels do not always correlate with the severity of the disease activity. Some "normal" people, particularly the elderly, may have the factor. Clients with tuberculosis, bacterial endocarditis, syphilis, and collagen diseases may have the RF.

Preparation of Client and Collection of Sample

The test requires 10 mL of clotted blood. A fasting sample is preferred.

REFERENCE VALUE FOR RF
<30 IU/mL

Possible Nursing Diagnosis Related to RF
Ineffective Health Maintenance A client with RA needs nursing care both during the acute stages and during remissions. Fatigue is common and affects many activities of daily living. Nurse practitioners may manage clients with this chronic disease. The best triad of treatment includes (1) physical therapy

(Continued)

> ## Possible Nursing Diagnosis . . . *(Continued)*
>
> and exercises, (2) emotional and psychological support, and (3) monitoring of drug therapy. A major role for the nurse practitioner caring for a client with RA is appropriate referral to a rheumatologist for a yearly evaluation of the medication regime. Current practice is to have early aggressive intervention with second-line agents that are disease-modifying antirheumatoid drugs rather than the first-line agents of nonsteroidal anti-inflammatory drugs previously used (Deglin et al., 2011; Katzung et al., 2009). The ESR (Chapter 2) and/or the CRP (Chapter 14) are used to follow the disease process.

THYROID AUTOANTIBODIES

In some types of thyroid disorders, the body produces antibodies against certain thyroid constituents. The end result is inflammation and destruction of the thyroid gland. Although the level of antibodies does not exactly correlate with the severity of the symptoms, identifying the probable cause of thyroid dysfunction is a help. (See Chapter 15 for a complete discussion on hypo- and hyperthyroidism, along with the tests used.) Relatives of clients with thyroid autoimmunity problems may also have high titers of thyroid antibodies. Because other diseases, such as the collagen diseases, may cause increased titers, the client may also undergo other types of antibody tests. In a patient with hypothyroidism, elevated thyroid antibodies support the diagnosis of autoimmune thyroiditis. An older test measured microsomal antibodies, but now a test has been defined to measure antibodies, specifically against thyroid peroxidase (TPO). Antibodies to TPO are the most common type of antibodies in thyroiditis, but 8–27% of the normal population also have the antibodies (Wu, 2006). See Chapter 15 on antithyroglobulin antibodies that are tested when thyroglobulin is used as a tumor marker for certain types of thyroid cancer.

Preparation of Client and Collection of Sample

The test requires 1 mL of serum. Because oral contraceptives may cause titers to become detectable, record whether the client is taking birth control pills.

REFERENCE VALUES FOR THYROID ANTIBODIES	
Thyroid peroxidase antibodies	Negative <0.80
	Equivocal >1.19
	Positive >2.00
Thyroglobulin antibodies	Titer <10

Note: Titers increase with age, particularly in some elderly, healthy women.

Questions

1. Which one of the following tests is routinely performed on a unit of donated blood?
   a. HAA (hepatitis A antigen)
   b. ANA (antinuclear antibodies)
   c. ASO titer (anti-streptolysin-O titer)
   d. HCV (hepatitis C virus)

2. A client has type AB blood. Theoretically, based on the ABO typing, he could receive any type of blood because he has which of the following?
   a. No A or B antigens
   b. No antibodies against A and B antigens
   c. Only antibodies against O
   d. Only AB antibodies

3. A client had a hemolytic transfusion reaction, possibly caused by incompatible blood. She had fever, chills, and low back pain. The transfusion was stopped, and the unit of blood was returned to the laboratory. The nurse should save a urine specimen for which reason?
   a. The urine may need to be checked for free hemoglobin
   b. Dehydration must be prevented
   c. A bilirubin test should be performed stat
   d. Circulatory overload may require use of a diuretic

4. A client who is Rh negative just delivered a healthy 8-lb (3.6-kg) baby boy who is Rh positive. She was given an injection of RhoGAM. She asks the nurse why she had the shot. Which of the following explanations by the nurse is accurate? "This shot
   a. Prevents you from having any problems with any other pregnancies because it eliminates the Rh factor."
   b. Gives you temporary antibodies against the Rh factor so that your body won't make any on your own, which could still be present if you have another Rh-positive pregnancy."
   c. Helps to eliminate any antibodies that you might have gotten from this pregnancy so that the next pregnancy will be normal."
   d. Helps your body to manufacture antibodies, so that if you have another pregnancy with an Rh-positive baby, there won't be any problems."

5. A positive Coombs' test indicates coating of erythrocytes by some type of globulin. Which of the following clinical situations is assessed with a Coombs' test?
   a. Hemolytic disease of the newborn
   b. Autoimmune thyroid disorders
   c. Systemic lupus erythematosus (SLE)
   d. Fungal infections

6. A client receiving renal dialysis three times a week has a positive report for HBsAg (hepatitis B surface antigen). He does not have any symptoms of hepatitis. Based on these data, which precaution should be instituted?
   a. None, because he has no evidence of clinical disease
   b. Administration of hepatitis B vaccine to the client
   c. Use of gloves when any blood-contaminated articles must be handled
   d. Administration of γ-globulin to staff who must work directly with him

7. The school nurse has been asked to provide some information about syphilis to a group of adolescent girls. Which of the following statements is *inaccurate*?
   a. A blood test for syphilis should be performed on anyone who had sexual contact with a person who has syphilis
   b. Syphilis is treated with a penicillin injection or with other antibiotics if the person is allergic to penicillin
   c. Syphilis is a communicable disease that must be reported to the health department
   d. A positive laboratory test for syphilis is always indicative of active infection

8. The current CDC recommendations for screening for HIV is to offer the test to which group of people?
   a. Sexually active adolescents
   b. Homosexual men
   c. Intraveneous drug users
   d. All people between age 13 and 64 years

9. A college freshman has had considerable lower abdominal discomfort and a low-grade fever. She is believed to have a repeat episode of pelvic inflammatory disease (PID). Which of the following may be used to assess for an acute inflammatory response?
   a. Heterophil antibody test and monospot test
   b. Anti-DNA, anti-Sm, and anti-Ro
   c. RF test
   d. C-reactive protein

10. ASO, anti-DNase-B, and streptozyme (the serologic tests for antibodies against group A β-hemolytic streptococci) would be the least useful for
    a. A child who has just been told she has "strep" throat
    b. A child who has symptoms of possible rheumatic fever
    c. A child who has acute glomerulonephritis
    d. A child who has a history of repeated sore throats and joint pain

11. A young female client wants to get pregnant, but she has a negative titer of rubella antibodies. What should she do before she becomes pregnant?
    a. Nothing, because a negative titer shows immunity to rubella
    b. Try to catch rubella by means of exposure to young children with measles
    c. Consult her physician about receiving the rubella vaccine if she becomes pregnant
    d. Ask her physician to give her the rubella vaccine now and practice birth control for at least 3 months

12. A client is to undergo a serologic test for toxoplasmosis. Which of the following is a significant factor in her health history in relation to the test for TPM?
    a. Has had a tick bite
    b. Just moved from the San Joaquin Valley
    c. Has a cat
    d. Likes raw fruits and vegetables

13. In the Ohio Valley area, where the fungus *Histoplasma capsulatum* is endemic, people who have positive skin and serologic tests for histoplasmosis are
    a. Highly susceptible to the fungus
    b. Always carriers of the fungal disease
    c. Always infected with the fungus
    d. Showing evidence of exposure to the fungus

14. Client teaching for a man who has tested positive for HCV would include all except
   a. Information about drugs that may damage the liver
   b. Reason to have vaccines for hepatitis A and hepatitis B
   c. Assurance that HCV does not cause chronic problems later in life
   d. Recommendation to avoid alcohol

References

Avalos-Bock, S. A. (2005). West Nile virus and the U.S. blood supply. *American Journal of Nursing, 105*(12), 34–37.

Bradley-Springer, L., Stevens, L., & Webb. A. (2010). Every nurse is an HIV nurse. *American Journal of Nursing, 110*(3), 32–39.

Chou, F., Holzemer, W., Portillo, C., & Slaughter, R. (2004). Self-care strategies and sources of information for HIV/AIDS symptom management. *Nursing Research, 53*(5), 332–339.

Cibulka, N. J. (2006). Mother-to-child transmission of HIV in the United States. *American Journal of Nursing, 106*(7), 56–64.

Covington, L. W. (2005). Update on antiviral agents for HIV and AIDS. *Nursing Clinics of North America, 40,* 149–165.

da Silva, M. R., Bettencourt, A., Michel, J., & Barbosa, D. (2006). Most frequently identified nursing diagnoses in HIV/AIDS patients. *International Journal of Nursing Terminologies and Classifications, 17*(1), 53.

DeCherney, A. H. Nathan, L. Goodwin, T. M. Lauter, N. (Eds.) (2007). *Current diagnosis & treatment: Obstetrics & gynecology* (10th ed.). New York: Mc Graw-Hill.

Deglin, J. H., Vallerand, A. H., & Sanoski, C. A. (2011). *Davis's drug guide for nurses* (12th ed.). Philadelphia: F. A. Davis.

Delgado, S. & Dort, K. (2010). HAART and its effects on the heart. *American Nurse Today, 5*(1), 50–53.

Dentinger, C. (2009). Emerging infections. *American Journal of Nursing, 109*(8), 29–33.

Everson, G. T., & Weinberg, H. (2006). *Hepatitis C: A survivor's guide* (4th ed.). New York: Hatherleigh Press.

Glatz, M., Golestani, M., Kerl, H., & Mullegger, R. (2006). Clinical relevance of different IgG and IgM serum antibody responses to *Borrelia burgdorferi* after antibiotic therapy for erythema migrans: Long-term follow-up study of 113 patients. *Archives of Dermatology, 142*(7), 862–868.

Goldschmidt, R. H., & Fogler, J. (2006). Opportunities to prevent HIV transmission to newborns. *Pediatrics, 117*(1), 208–209.

Hay, W. W., Levin, M. J., Sondheimer, J. M., & Deterding, R. (Eds.). (2011). *Current diagnosis and treatment: Pediatrics* (20th ed.). New York: McGraw-Hill.

Hladik, W., Dollard, S. C., Mermin, J., Fowlkes, A. L., Downing, R., Amin, M. M., et al. (2006). Transmission of human herpesvirus 8 by blood transfusion. *New England Journal of Medicine, 355*(13), 1331–1338.

Katzung, B., Masters, S. B., & Trevor, A. J. (Eds.). (2009). *Basic and clinical pharmacology* (11th ed.). New York: McGraw-Hill.

Knippen, M. A. (2006). Transfusion-related acute lung injury. *American Journal of Nursing, 106*(6), 61–64.

Ma, Y., Griffith, J. A., Chasan-Taber, L., Olendzki, B. C., Jackson, E., Stanek, E. J., et al. (2006). Association between dietary fiber and serum C-reactive protein. *American Journal of Clinical Nutrition, 83*(4), 760–766.

McAdams-Jones, D. (2009). What's causing this respiratory distress? *American Nurse Today, 4*(5), 28.

McPhee, S. J., Papadakis, M. A., & Rabow, M. W. (Eds.). (2011). *Current medical diagnosis and treatment* (50th ed.). New York: McGraw-Hill.

Overstreet, M. (2005). West Nile virus. *Nursing 2005, 35*(8), 64.

Petersen, L. R., & Epstein, J. (2005). Problem solved? West Nile virus and transfusion safety. *New England Journal of Medicine, 353*(5), 516–517.

Pullen, R., Brewer, S., & Ballard, A. (2009). Putting a face on systemic lupus erythematosus. *Nursing 2009, 39*(8), 25–28.

Pullen, R. & Hall, D. (2010). Sjogren syndrome: More than dry eyes. *Nursing 2010, 40*(8), 37–41.

Ridker, M. D., Hennekens, C. H., Buring, J. E., & Rifai, N. (2000). C-reactive protein and other markers of inflammation in the prediction of cardiovascular disease in women. *New England Journal of Medicine, 342*, 836–843.

Ridker, P., Danielson, E., Fonseca, F. Genest, J., Gotto, A., Katelein, J., et al., (2008). JUPITER Study Group. Rosuvastatin vascular events in men and women with elevated C-reactive protein. *New England Journal of Medicine, 359*(21), 2195–2207.

Ridker, P., Danielson, E., Fonseca, F. Genest, J., Gotto, A., Katelein, J., et al., (2009). Reduction in C-Reactive protein and LDL cholesterol and cardiovascular event rates after initiation of rosuvastatin: A prospective study of the JUPITER trial. *Lancet, 373*(9670), 1175–1182.

Ridker, P. M. (2010). Statin therapy for elevated hsCRP: What are the public health implications? *American Journal of Managed Care, 16*(8), 561–562.

Stringer, M., Ratcliffe, S., & Gross, R. (2006). Acceptance of hepatitis B vaccination in pregnant adolescents. *MCN: American Journal of Maternal Child Health Nursing, 31*(1), 54–60.

Toy, P., Popovsky, M., Abraham, E., Ambruso, D., Holness, L., Kopko, P., et al. (2005). Transfusion-related acute lung injury: Definition and review. *Critical Care Medicine, 33*(4), 721–726.

Vance, D. E. (2010). Aging with HIV: Bringing the latest research to bear in providing care. *American Journal of Nursing, 110*(3), 42–50.

Wilkins, T., Schade, R. R., Malcolm, J. K., & Raina, D. (2010). *American Family Physician, 81*(11), 1351–1357.

Wilson, T. R. (2005). The ABCs of hepatitis. *The Nurse Practitioner, 30*(6), 12–21.

Wright, A. A., & Katz, I. (2006). Home testing for HIV. *New England, Journal of Medicine, 354*(5), 437–440.

Wu, A. H. (Ed.). (2006). *Tietz clinical guide to laboratory tests* (4th ed.). St. Louis, MO: Saunders Elsevier.

Websites

www.hepfi.org (Hepatitis Foundation International.)

www.labtestsonline.org (Information on laboratory tests for blood transfusions and autoimmune diseases)

www.liverfoundation.org (American Liver Foundation.)

www.lupus.org (Update on tests for systemic lupus erythematosus.)

www.projectinform.org (Updates on medications, laboratory tests, and research on AIDS and HCV.)

www.sfhepbfree.org (Goal to make HBV screening part of basic care, especially for Asians in San Francisco.)

www.nccc.ucsf.edu (Updates on state laws for HIV testing.)

Answers

1. d, 2. b, 3. a, 4. b, 5. a, 6. c, 7. d. 8. d, 9. d, 10. a, 11. d, 12. c, 13. d, 14. c

Endocrine Tests

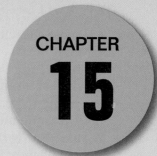

- Background Information — 375
- Pituitary Tumors — 378
- Growth Hormone or Somatotropin — 378
- Prolactin — 380
- Adrenal Cortex — 381
- ACTH–Adrenal Axis — 382
- Adrenocorticotropic Hormone — 382
- Cortisol Plasma Levels — 383
- Salivary Cortisol — 384
- Congenital Adrenal Hyperplasia — 388
- 17-Hydroxyprogesterone — 389
- Urinary Measurement of the Adrenal Cortex Steroid Pregnanetriol — 390
- Urinary Cortisol Levels — 390
- Aldosterone, Plasma, and Urine — 390
- Renin — 393
- Catecholamines, Vanillylmandelic Acid, and Metanephrines — 394
- Chromogranin A — 396
- Parathormone or Parathyroid Hormone — 396

- Thyroid Gland — 397
- Rapid Test for TSH — 398
- Thyrotropin or Thyroid-Stimulating Hormone — 399
- L-Thyroxine Serum Concentration (Total and Free T_4) — 400
- Triiodothyronine Serum Concentration (T_3) — 400
- Thyroglobulin Test — 405
- Gonadotropins and the Sex-Related Hormones — 405
- Follicle-Stimulating Hormone — 406
- Home Test for FSH — 406
- Luteinizing Hormone — 406
- Home Test for LH — 407
- Estradiol and Other Forms of Estrogen — 407
- Progesterone — 408
- Pregnanediol (Progesterone Metabolite) — 408
- Estrogen and Progesterone Receptors in Breast Cancer — 408
- Testosterone and Other Androgens — 409

OBJECTIVES

1. Explain the concepts of negative feedback, circadian rhythms, and ectopic hormone production.
2. Give examples of how laboratory tests are used to assess the relation between the anterior pituitary gland and other endocrine glands.
3. Determine the appropriate nursing diagnoses for a client with increased or decreased serum cortisol levels.

4. Devise a teaching plan for parents who have a child with adrenogenital syndrome.

5. Identify the characteristic clinical manifestations of increased and decreased levels of serum aldosterone, including changes in renin activity.

6. Explain the purpose of 24-hour urine specimens for vanillylmandelic acid (VMA) and metanephrines.

7. Describe the clinical effect of an increased level of parathyroid hormone (PTH) and the most important nursing intervention needed.

8. Explain the usefulness of thyroid-stimulating hormone (TSH) and free thyroxine (T_4) index in evaluating clients with hyper- or hypothyroidism.

9. Determine the appropriate nursing diagnoses for clients with increased or decreased serum thyroid hormones.

10. Explain why infants who may have hypothyroidism (cretinism) need immediate medical evaluation and treatment.

11. Identify the key nursing diagnoses when a client has altered levels of the sex hormones.

The brief discussions of the negative feedback system, circadian rhythms, ectopic hormone production, and other physiologic information in this chapter should help the reader understand the tests performed to measure hormone levels.

Except for ectopic hormone production (discussed later), each hormone is produced by a specific endocrine gland, and each has a specific function or functions. These functions are briefly discussed in relation to the tests for each hormone.

Table 15–1 gives an overview of the endocrine glands, the hormones produced by each gland, and how the hormones are tested with specific laboratory tests of blood and urine samples. The releasing factors (discussed in the following section) are not included in this table because they are not usually measured.

Table 15–1 Commonly Measured Hormones

Source of Hormone	Name of Hormone	Tests Used to Assess Hormone Levels
Anterior pituitary gland	Growth hormone (GH) or somatotropin (STH)	Serum GH levels
	Adrenocorticotropin (ACTH)	Serum ACTH levels; see section on adrenal gland for ACTH suppression and stimulation tests.
	Thyroid-stimulating hormone	Serum TSH levels; see section on tests of thyroid gland.
	Follicle-stimulating hormone (FSH) (one of the gonadotropins)	Serum and urine FSH levels; see section on sex hormones.
	Luteinizing hormone (LH), sometimes called interstitial-cell-stimulating hormone (ICSH) in male (the other gonadotropin)	Serum and urine levels; see section on sex hormones.
	Prolactin (PRL)	Serum prolactin
	Melanocyte-stimulating hormone (MSH)	Serum MSH not usually measured directly; see discussion about increase of MSH with cortisol lack.

Source of Hormone	Name of Hormone	Tests Used to Assess Hormone Levels
Posterior pituitary gland	Antidiuretic hormone (ADH) or arginine vasopressin (AVP)	Not commonly measured; see Chapter 4 on serum and urine osmolality.
	Oxytocin	Not measured as diagnostic test; oxytocin is used in obstetrics as a drug to induce labor.
Adrenal cortex	Glucocorticoids (cortisol as principal one)	Plasma and urine cortisol; 17-hydroxy-corticosterolds (17-OHCS) or Porter–Silber test; see also ACTH tests.
	Mineralocorticoids (aldosterone as principal one)	Serum and urine aldosterone levels; tests for renin activity; see Chapter 5 for serum levels of sodium and potassium.
	Sex hormones (androgens, progesterone, and estrogen)	Pregnanetriol in urine
Adrenal medulla	Norepinephrine	Catecholamines in urine; metanephrines in urine;
	Epinephrine	vanillylmandelic acid (VMA) in urine; norepinephrine and epinephrine are not commonly measured in serum; pharmacologic tests not commonly performed.
Parathyroid	Parathyroid hormone (PTH)	Serum PTH; serum and urine calcium and phosphate levels; see Chapter 7.
Thyroid	Calcitonin	Calcitonin not commonly measured; see Chapter 7 on serum calcium
	L-thyroxine (T_4) and triiodothyronine (T_3)	Free T_4; free T_4 index; total T_4; T_3; TSH levels
Pancreas	Insulin Glucogen	See Chapter 8 for tests of glucose metabolism.
Testes	Androgens	Serum testosterone; see urine test for androgens.
	Estrogen and progesterone in minute amounts	Serum estradiol; see also tests for FSH and LH.
Ovaries	Estrogens	Serum estradiol; serum and urine estradiol in pregnancy (see Chapter 18) Serum progesterone.
	Progesterone	Pregnanediol in urine
	Androgens in minute amounts	Testosterone; see also tests for FSH and LH.

BACKGROUND INFORMATION

Releasing Factors That Stimulate Anterior Pituitary Gland

The central nervous system is closely connected to the endocrine system because some releasing factors from the hypothalamus are carried to the pituitary gland through the venous system that connects the hypothalamus and the pituitary gland. Because *hypophysis* is another name for the pituitary gland, this venous system is called the *hypophyseal portal system*. These releasing factors from the hypothalamus stimulate the pituitary gland to release certain hormones. For example, thyrotropin-releasing factor (TRF) is sent from the hypothalamus to the pituitary gland. The pituitary gland is thus stimulated to release TSH, which in turn acts on the thyroid gland to produce T_4 and T_3.

Negative Feedback System for Endocrine Functioning

The anterior pituitary gland secretes hormones that act on specific target organs to cause the release of other hormones. For example, the pituitary gland releases adrenocorticotropic hormone (ACTH), which then stimulates the adrenal gland to produce cortisol. When the cortisol reaches a certain level in the bloodstream, continued secretion of ACTH from the pituitary gland is suppressed. In other words, a high level of cortisol turns off the secretion of ACTH. Conversely, a low level of serum cortisol is a stimulus for the increased production of ACTH. This interplay, in which the increased level of one hormone causes a decrease in the level of the other hormone, is called *negative feedback*. The hormones from the adrenal cortex, thyroid gland, ovaries, and testes all have negative feedback systems with hormones from the anterior pituitary gland. Understanding negative feedback is important because tests for the suppression or stimulation of hormones are based on the physiologic principle that levels of one hormone should change the level of another hormone.

Other Methods to Control Hormone Production

Not all hormones are controlled with a negative feedback system through the pituitary gland. For example, PTH is regulated by the serum calcium and phosphorus levels (see Chapter 7). A high level of serum calcium causes a suppression of PTH from the parathyroid gland. A decrease in the serum calcium level causes an increased production of PTH.

The intricate balance between too much and too little of a hormone is one of the wonders of the human body. In a healthy state, all hormones are kept within a precise range that can fluctuate as body needs change. All hormones are interrelated to some degree, so changes in the one hormone may affect the level of others, although not in as direct a manner as in negative feedback.

Circadian Rhythms and Other Rhythms

A change in the levels of a hormone every 24 hours is called a *circadian* (around the day) *rhythm*. For example, cortisol is higher in the morning than in the evening. Although cortisol seems to be relatively independent of the sleep pattern, growth hormone is strongly bound to the sleep pattern. In addition to cortisol and growth hormone, aldosterone, prolactin, TSH, testosterone, luteinizing hormone (LH), and follicle-stimulating hormone (FSH) all vary considerably during each 24-hour period. Because the hormones do fluctuate, more than one blood sample or one urine specimen may be needed for an accurate reflection of an individual client's hormone level.

The female hormones, estrogen and progesterone, are, of course, on another rhythm that must also be taken into account in comparing reference values.

Rhythms that are longer than circadian (24-hour) rhythms are termed *infradian rhythms.* In adult women, the menstrual cycle is an infradian rhythm, because the variations in FSH and LH are on a monthly, not a daily, cycle. Besides the sex hormones, other hormones may fluctuate with menstrual cycles. In women, therefore, various hormones must be considered in relation to the menstrual cycle.

Ectopic Hormone Production

Most elevations of serum hormone levels are due to an overproduction by the specific endocrine gland. They can also occur if there is production of the hormone from a nonendocrine source. Hormones from nonendocrine sources are called *ectopic hormones* because they come from the wrong place or originate outside the normal pathway. For example, some benign and malignant tumors manufacture hormones similar to the hormone produced by the endocrine gland. ACTH, melanocyte-stimulating hormone (MSH), gonadotropins, antidiuretic hormone (ADH), and PTH are common ectopic hormones.

In some malignant conditions, hormone tests may be performed to see if some of the symptoms are due to ectopic hormone production. For example, a tumor that produces PTH may cause symptoms of hypercalcemia. (See Chapter 7 for a discussion of hypercalcemia.)

Screening Tests and Definitive Tests for Primary and Secondary Imbalances

In general, screening tests for hormone imbalances are performed by measuring the concentration of the hormone in the serum. If the serum level is greater or lesser than the reference values, more definitive tests are completed to find out if the problem is in the gland itself. If the disorder is due to a problem in the gland itself, the disorder is called *primary.* If the endocrine imbalance is due to other causes, such as pituitary dysfunction, the endocrine disorder is termed *secondary.* For example, if hypothyroidism is due to malfunction of the thyroid gland, the disorder is called *primary hypothyroidism.* If the hypothyroidism is due to pituitary insufficiency, the disorder is called *secondary hypothyroidism.* Laboratory tests that use drugs to stimulate or to suppress hormone production are useful in determining if the disorder is primary or secondary (Table 15–2).

Table 15–2 Screening and Definitive Tests of Hormone Function

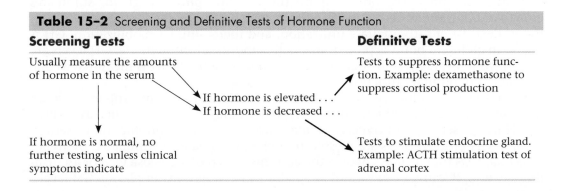

Screening Tests	Definitive Tests
Usually measure the amounts of hormone in the serum	Tests to suppress hormone function. Example: dexamethasone to suppress cortisol production
If hormone is elevated . . .	
If hormone is decreased . . .	
If hormone is normal, no further testing, unless clinical symptoms indicate	Tests to stimulate endocrine gland. Example: ACTH stimulation test of adrenal cortex

PITUITARY TUMORS

Pituitary tumors are classified as either hyperfunctional or nonfunctional on the basis of their effects on hormone production. The most common symptom of nonfunctional pituitary tumors is bitemporal hemianopsia caused by pressure on the optic nerve. The client has impaired vision in either the right or the left side of both eyes. Symptoms of hyperfunctional tumors vary greatly depending on the type or types of hormones released. The most common syndrome is due to overproduction of prolactin, which can cause galactorrhea and changes in menses. A transphenoidal approach is often used for resection of these tumors. Microsurgery techniques via a transnasal endoscopic approach can remove an adenoma and preserve function in most cases (McPhee, Papadakis, & Rabow 2011).

Possible Nursing Diagnoses Related to Pituitary Disorders

Anxiety Related to the Disease

Emotional problems with mood changes are likely to be a part of most disorders of the pituitary gland. Some of the symptoms are directly related to the hormonal imbalance, whereas others may be brought on by the delay before an accurate diagnosis is made. Because it is not unusual for an emotional condition associated with the pituitary gland to be misdiagnosed for several years, a sense of bitterness and anger may complicate the efforts to help the client deal with the problems of the disease. After the diagnosis is established, clients and their significant others may need help to deal with surgical or other planned treatment.

Disturbed Body Image

Various pituitary disorders cause physical changes such as acromegaly, dwarfism, or obesity. Clients may need help accepting the physical changes that may or may not be remedied with therapy. For example, acromegaly may necessitate reconstruction of the bones of the face. The physical changes may also affect sexual functioning, an issue sometimes overlooked.

GROWTH HORMONE OR SOMATOTROPIN

Growth hormone (GH), produced by the anterior pituitary gland, stimulates growth of bone and other tissue. GH affects metabolism by increasing protein synthesis, decreasing carbohydrate utilization, and increasing fat mobilization. GH is higher in children, but it is present in small amounts all through life. GH levels are performed to evaluate lack of growth of a child. For adults, GH is measured as one assessment of pituitary function.

Several factors influence the production of GH. Diets low in protein cause an increased production of the hormone. Hypoglycemia also causes an increased surge of GH in the serum, and hyperglycemia causes a decreased production of serum. Because GH production is suppressed by hyperglycemia and stimulated by hypoglycemia, tests for GH may involve the administration of a glucose load or an insulin injection. Because exercise and sleep also cause variations in plasma GH levels, the activity of the client and the timing of specimen collection are important to note. (For reasons that are still unknown, GH levels increase during sleep.)

Preparation of Client and Collection of Sample

For definitive testing, GH levels are drawn after the client has been given drugs such as L-dopa, clonidine, insulin, or others (Wu, 2006). Several serum blood samples are drawn after the administration of a drug to see how much the GH increases.

In clients with GH excess, a glucose load may be given to demonstrate that the GH cannot be suppressed. The procedure may consist of a glucose tolerance test (GTT) with simultaneous glucose and GH measurement. (See Chapter 8 for the procedure for GTT.)

REFERENCE VALUES FOR GH	
Cord Blood	8–41 ng/mL
Infants	2–10 ng/mL
Children	1–16.4 ng/mL with variations related to age
Adults: Men	0–4 ng/mL
Women	0–18 ng/mL
Aged: Men	1–9 ng/mL
Women	1–16 ng/mL

In adults, the usual values may be so low that the hormone cannot be detected. Stimulation with L-dopa may increase GH to measurable levels.

Values are based on World Health Organization references as reported by Wu (2006).

Increased GH Serum Level

Clinical Significance

Severe malnutritional states cause a prolonged elevation of GH. Various types of tumors, either benign or malignant, can cause excess secretion of GH. In children, an abnormal increase of GH causes *gigantism*. Increased GH after puberty brings about a distortion of bony structures because the bones are stimulated to grow after closure of the epiphyses. Growth hormone excess in the adult creates *acromegaly*.

Possible Nursing Diagnosis Related to Increased GH

Deficient Knowledge Related to Treatments

A client with a pituitary tumor may undergo radiation or surgical therapy to remove the tumor. (See earlier discussion of general nursing diagnoses.) An important point to remember in relation to increased GH levels is that hyperglycemia may be a clinical problem. (See Chapter 8 for more discussion of hyperglycemia and appropriate nursing diagnoses.) Medications such as cabergoline, octreotide, and lanreotide may be prescribed for clients who cannot be treated successfully with surgery (McPhee et al., 2011).

Decreased GH Serum Level

Clinical Significance

Lack of GH is due to hypofunction of the pituitary gland, which can result from a tumor, from trauma, or from an unknown cause. In children, a lack of GH causes *dwarfism*. In adults, although the lack of GH does not cause clinical symptoms, it may be associated with deficiencies of other pituitary hormones, so symptoms are related to the other deficiencies. Hence, a measurement of GH may be used to help in assessing the presence of hypopituitarism in the adult.

Sheehan's syndrome is a type of hypopituitarism that sometimes occurs after a complicated delivery with bleeding and shock. During the postpartum period, a thrombus may occur in the hypophyseal vessels, which causes destruction of the pituitary gland. Symptoms of a deficiency may occur months or years later.

Possible Nursing Diagnosis Related to Decreased GH

Deficient Knowledge Related to Replacement Therapy

In a child, a lack of GH is treated medically with injections of GH so that the child develops normally. In 1985, the U.S. Food and Drug Administration (FDA) approved the manufacture of GH by means of gene splicing. (This was the second product of recombinant DNA technology to be approved for human use. The first was insulin, approved in 1982.) Children who are very short may be given a trial of GH (Hay et al., 2011). Parents need detailed instructions about the injections and follow-up care. In infants, a lack of GH may cause an immediate problem by causing hypoglycemia. Older clients with a lack of GH may show symptoms of hypoglycemia only if they are fasting. Adults are not usually given injections of GH, but they may need replacement of other pituitary hormones, all of which can be replaced by means of parenteral injection. Also, hormones from specific glands, such as thyroid, may be given. The nursing implications for specific hormone therapy are briefly covered in the discussion of each hormone. (See also the two general nursing diagnoses discussed earlier.)

PROLACTIN

Prolactin (PRL), a hormone from the anterior pituitary gland, normally increases during pregnancy and the subsequent lactation period. Tumors of the pituitary gland, drugs, or other variables can result in increased PRL secretion. Women have an abnormal secretion of breast milk and suppression of menstruation (amenorrhea–galactorrhea syndrome). Some women may not realize they have galactorrhea until a milking pressure is applied to the breast. Other symptoms, such as headaches and weight gain from sodium retention, may occur. Men may experience impotence because excess PRL has a negative feedback to the pituitary gland, suppressing gonad function.

An enlarging tumor can cause visual problems because of pressure on the optic chiasm. The impairment of vision is particularly noted in pregnant women who have a pituitary tumor because the pituitary gland increases in pregnancy.

If the increased secretion is a result of a tumor, the lesion is usually benign and can be removed surgically. Bromocriptine is a drug used for short-term therapy (Deglin, Vallerand, & Sanoski, 2011). Some drugs, such as tranquilizers, can mimic the PRL tumor syndrome, and thus treatment is elimination of the causative factor. Magnetic resonance imaging (MRI) (see Chapter 21) can be used to evaluate the effect of drug treatment on the size of the tumor.

Preparation of Client and Collection of Sample

Test requires 2 mL of serum. Stimulation and suppression tests may help with assessment in some cases (Wu, 2006).

REFERENCE VALUES FOR PROLACTIN

Adult: Men	0–15 ng/mL
Women	0–20 ng/mL
	Increases up to 40 ng/mL in luteal phase
	Postmenopausal 0–15 ng/mL
Pregnant women	1st trimester: <80 ng/mL
	2nd trimester: <160 ng/mL
	3rd trimester: <400 ng/mL
Newborn	<500 ng/mL

Nursing Diagnoses Related to Increase or Decrease of Prolactin Levels

See the general nursing diagnoses for pituitary disorders discussed earlier.

ADRENAL CORTEX

The adrenal cortex secretes three types of hormones (Table 15–3):

1. The glucocorticoids. The glucocorticoid usually measured in the plasma is cortisol. Free cortisol can also be measured in the urine. Various metabolites of the glucocorticoids can be measured in the urine as 17-hydroxycorticosteroid (17-OHCS).

2. The mineralocorticoids. The mineralocorticoid measured in the serum is aldosterone.

3. The sex hormones. The sex hormones produced by the adrenal cortex include the androgens, progesterone, and estrogen. Both males and females have the male hormones (androgens, such as testosterone) and the female hormones (progesterone and estrogen). Measurement of androgens becomes important when there is hyperplasia of the adrenal gland, which increases the production of the sex hormones. A urine test, 17-ketosteroid (17-KS), is one way to determine an increase of sex hormones from the adrenal gland.

Table 15–3 Effects of Three Types of Hormones from Adrenal Cortex

Hormone	Effect
Glucocorticoids (cortisol)	Effects on metabolism of carbohydrates, fats, and proteins Suppresses immune responses
Mineralocorticoids (aldosterone)	Effect on fluid and electrolyte balance Increased retention of sodium and water Decreased retention of potassium
Sex hormones (androgens, progesterone, and estrogen)	Affect secondary sex characteristics but not as substantially as hormones from ovaries and testes

ACTH–ADRENAL AXIS

Production of cortisol by the adrenal cortex is controlled by the ACTH–adrenal axis. Because ACTH and cortisol are related by a negative feedback system, the pituitary is stimulated to produce ACTH when the plasma cortisol level is low. ACTH then increases production of cortisol by the adrenal cortex. The increasing plasma cortisol level becomes the stimulus for the pituitary gland to discontinue the high levels of ACTH production. Homeostasis is maintained by the increases and decreases of ACTH, which balance cortisol in the serum. ACTH also increases production of the sex hormones by the adrenal cortex, but this effect is usually not clinically significant except in some adrenogenital syndromes. (Androgen excess is discussed in the section on the clinical significance of decreased cortisol levels.) ACTH has little or no effect on the serum levels of the third type of adrenal cortex hormones, the mineralocorticoids or aldosterone. Aldosterone is controlled by the renin–angiotensin system, which is explained in the section on aldosterone.

ADRENOCORTICOTROPIC HORMONE

A measurement of ACTH helps determine whether the lack of serum cortisol is due to hypofunction either of the adrenal cortex or of the pituitary gland. The administration of drugs such as dexamethasone or metyrapone is used to stimulate or to suppress the production of ACTH. Each of these tests is discussed briefly with a summary of the clinical significance of the findings.

Preparation of Client and Collection of Sample

The baseline specimen, for which the laboratory needs 5 mL of plasma, is usually collected in the morning. The specimen should be put on ice and sent to the laboratory immediately. The blood should not come in contact with glass. The collection tube may contain EDTA or heparin.

REFERENCE VALUE FOR ACTH

6–76 pg/mL

ACTH Stimulation Test with Metyrapone

Metyrapone interferes with the normal production of cortisol by blocking some enzymatic actions, so compound S is not converted to cortisol. Because of negative feedback, a fall in plasma cortisol level should cause an increase in the level of circulating ACTH. If clients have pituitary insufficiency, however, ACTH level is *not* increased, even with the blockage of cortisol production by metyrapone. Because several ACTH levels may be drawn after the administration of metyrapone, nurses must check with the individual laboratory for the exact timing of the specimens. Phenytoin interferes with the test because the drug has a variety of endocrine effects. Estrogen compounds also interfere with the test.

ACTH Suppression Test: Dexamethasone Suppression Test

Normally high plasma corticosteroid levels suppress the formation of ACTH (the negative feedback concept again). Dexamethasone, a potent corticosteroid that suppresses the formation of ACTH, is given as a test to determine whether the client continues to produce large amounts of cortisol after ACTH is suppressed. Clients with a hyperactive adrenal cortex (Cushing's syndrome) do continue to have high serum cortisol levels because the suppression of pituitary ACTH does not affect the hyperactive adrenal gland.

For screening purposes, 1 mg of dexamethasone is given orally at 11 PM (a client who weighs more than 200 lb [90 kg] takes a larger dose) to suppress ACTH formation. A sample for serum cortisol measurements is drawn the next morning at 8 AM. The plasma levels of cortisol should drop below 5 µg/100 mL. Urine levels of cortisol and other metabolites also may be measured. (These tests are discussed later.) For confirmation of the results, the dexamethasone dosage may be increased and given for several days.

Use of ACTH (Cosyntropin) to Stimulate Cortisol Production

Clients with suspected diseases of the adrenal cortex can be given a test dose of ACTH to determine whether ACTH causes an increased production of cortisol in the serum. A synthetic type of ACTH, called *cosyntropin*, may be given intravenously as a diagnostic test. A lack of response to cosyntropin indicates primary hypofunctioning of the adrenal cortex.

CORTISOL PLASMA LEVELS

Cortisol, the glucocorticoid found in the largest concentration in the serum, is the one usually measured to gain information about the functioning of the adrenal cortex. Plasma cortisol has a diurnal variation, its levels being higher in the morning than in the evening. Baseline readings can be taken in the morning with the client at rest. The timing of the cortisol levels with suppression and stimulation are determined by the procedure of the particular laboratory.

Preparation of Client and Collection of Sample

The laboratory needs 1 mL of plasma. The specimen is usually drawn in the morning after the client has been fasting. Evening samples may also require about 3 hours of fasting. Water is allowed. Because activity increases the level, the client needs to be supine for 2 hours before the test.

REFERENCE VALUES FOR SERUM CORTISOL

8 AM (client at rest) 5–25 µg/dL

8 PM <10 µg/dL

1. There are no age or sex differences, but pregnancy causes an increase. Obese people do have higher levels. Activity also increases levels.
2. Dexamethasone suppression should decrease cortisol levels to <5 µg/100 mL.
3. Cosyntropin stimulation should increase 8 AM cortisol levels at least 18 µg/100 mL.

SALIVARY CORTISOL

Salivary cortisol reflects the unbound cortisol in the serum. A sample obtained at midnight is a highly specific and sensitive test to detect high cortisol levels in an adult.

Preparation of Patient and Collection of Sample

Collect saliva in the special kit provided by the manufacture. Instruct the client to refrain from brushing their teeth or rinsing their mouth prior to the specimen collection. The specimen may be kept at room temperature for 2 weeks, refrigerated for 4 weeks, and frozen for 8 weeks.

REFERENCE VALUES*

11 PM <0.3–4.3 nmol/L

7 AM 4.7–32.0 nmol/L

*See www.acllaboratories.com for more information on collection kits.

Increased Serum Cortisol Level

Clinical Significance

An increase in cortisol can be either ACTH dependent or ACTH independent. A pituitary tumor can cause an increase of ACTH, which causes an increased cortisol level. This type of cortisol increase is ACTH dependent, and it is sometimes called *Cushing's disease*. Increases of serum cortisol from other causes are called *Cushing's syndrome*. (Cushing was an American endocrinologist who first described the characteristic signs and symptoms of cortisol excess.)

Plasma cortisol levels increase independently of the pituitary gland when there is hyperplasia of the adrenal cortex. Hypersecreting tumors of the adrenal cortex may be malignant or benign.

Some nonendocrine malignant tumors can secrete ACTH, which can result in increased serum cortisol levels (see earlier discussion on ectopic hormones). Cushing's syndrome, or high plasma cortisol levels, can be caused by the administration of corticosteroids over a long period of time.

The specific medical treatment of elevated cortisol levels depends on the cause. The client may undergo a battery of tests to determine whether there is a tumor of the pituitary gland or of the adrenal gland.

If Cushing's syndrome is due to exogenous cortisol administration, the dosage of cortisone may be decreased. Sometimes difficult medical decisions must be made regarding the continuation of cortisone therapy. The problems caused by the disease must be weighed against the untoward effects of the therapy. Short-term use of corticosteroids is quite common for many conditions including prenatal use (Deglin et al., 2011).

Possible Nursing Diagnoses Related to Increased Serum Cortisol Level

Risk for Infection

Nurses must recognize that clients with cortisol elevations do not have a normal response to infections. Cortisol impairs antibody production and cellular immunity, qualities that are beneficial in the treatment of abnormal inflammatory responses but detrimental in the presence of an infection. Such clients may have little elevation of temperature or other responses to a bacterial invasion. So they must be taught to avoid possible sources of infection.

Imbalanced Nutrition

Cortisol stimulates the formation of glucose from other substances, such as protein (gluconeogenesis), and it interferes with the action of insulin. Clients may thus have problems with hyperglycemia. (See Chapter 8 for nursing implications for hyperglycemia.) Weight gain may be a problem, so a typical eating plan for a client with Cushing's syndrome would be a low-sodium, high-protein, low-carbohydrate, and low-calorie diet.

Risk for Injury Related to Poor Wound Healing

Increased levels of cortisol tend to make the skin fragile. Wound healing is delayed. For a postoperative client taking corticosteroids, dehiscence of wounds is a potential problem. Thus, inspection of the skin and measures to promote skin integrity and wound healing are important when there are known or suspected high cortisol levels.

Risk for Injury Related to Loss of Calcium from Bone

High levels of cortisol cause a reduction in protein stores. If cortisol levels are elevated for more than 6 months, the matrix of the bone may be damaged and calcium may be released, leading to osteoporosis. Guidelines recommend that clients who require more than 3 months of corticosteroid therapy should have calcium supplements, vitamin D, and other medications to prevent bone loss. Periodic measurements of bone mineral density are also recommended for clients on long-term steroid therapy (see Chapter 21). In a study of over

(Continued)

Possible Nursing Diagnoses . . . (Continued)

6,000 clients on long-term corticosteroids, less than half (42%) had bone density testing (Curtis et al., 2005). Nurses need to help clients understand the need for preventive measures to decrease the risk of osteoporosis, and ways to prevent falls, because fractures may occur. Sometimes long-term steroid therapy leads to joint replacements because of the slow erosion of bone.

Risk for Bleeding Related to Development of Gastric Ulcers

Increased cortisol levels cause an increased secretion of hydrochloric acid (HCl) and pepsinogen. There is also an inhibition of collagen formation and of other protective proteins in the gastric mucosa. The exact cause of gastric ulcers is not known, but ulcers are a risk when cortisol levels are high. Any signs of gastrointestinal bleeding should be reported at once. (See Chapter 13 for guaiac tests for occult gastrointestinal bleeding.)

Risk for Excess Fluid Volume

Depending on the level of cortisol increase, clients may have sodium retention and potassium excretion. (See the discussion on the effects of aldosterone.) The increased sodium and water retention may lead to elevated blood pressure, weight gain, and edema. (See Chapter 5 for the nursing implications for clients with hypernatremia or hypokalemia.)

Disturbed Body Image

Elevated cortisol levels cause a round, full face ("moon face") and a redistribution of fat deposits. Clients may have a "buffalo hump" on the back. Their trunks are obese, and their wasted muscles make the extremities thin. Females may become masculinized with unwanted hair because of some androgenic effects. Acne may occur. Treatment helps correct most of these body changes, but clients need help to cope with their altered body images.

Ineffective Coping of Family Related to Changes in Mood

Increased cortisol levels tend to cause hyperactivity. Clients may need to be cautioned about too much activity. The client may have dramatic mood changes. Euphoria is often present, and psychotic behavior may occur. The family may need help in learning to deal with such wide mood changes.

Decreased Serum Cortisol Level

Clinical Significance

A subnormal level of cortisol in the plasma is known as *Addison's disease*. (One way to remember that Addison's disease involves a lack of cortisol is to remember that in Addison's disease, one must *add* some cortisone.) The lack of cortisol in the serum may be due to primary hypofunction of the adrenal cortex, or it may be secondary to hypofunctioning of the pituitary gland. Infections may invade the adrenal cortex. Once the most common cause of adrenal insufficiency was tuberculosis, but now it is autoimmune destruction. Adrenal insufficiency can be a complication of acquired immunodeficiency syndrome (AIDS) (McPhee et al., 2011).

Long-term administration of high doses of corticosteroids causes suppression of ACTH production and a resulting inactivity of these clients' own adrenal glands. There is some atrophy of the adrenal cortex, so the glands do not respond normally to the need for more cortisone in stress. The inability of the adrenal cortex to increase production of cortisol during stress may cause a collection of symptoms known as *addisonian crisis*. If cortisol drugs are not withdrawn gradually (tapered off), the client may have a lowered cortisol level before the adrenal glands can begin to function normally again. (See the section on congenital adrenocortical hyperplasia for an explanation of cortisol lack in newborns and young children.)

Clients with borderline adrenal cortex functioning may not have problems until they are faced with a stressful situation, such as a surgical procedure or some other physical or psychological trauma. Insufficiency occurs when at least 90% of the adrenal glands are destroyed. Once the symptoms of a lack of cortisol and aldosterone are recognized and confirmed, replacement therapy is started. Until the hormones are replaced, or when the need is greater than the supply, these clients may have problems related to the lack of cortisol and aldosterone.

Possible Nursing Diagnoses Related to Decreased Serum Cortisol Level

Deficient Fluid Volume Related to Lack of Retention of Sodium and Water

A lack of cortisol and of the mineralocorticoid aldosterone causes low serum sodium levels, which may lead to hypovolemia. Thus, clients with a lack of cortisol tend to become dizzy, and they may faint if they leave bed rapidly (postural hypotension). In more advanced cases, the lack of sodium retention can lead to hypovolemia severe enough to cause shock. (See Chapter 5 for the nursing implications for clients with hyponatremia.)

Risk for Altered Cardiac Output Related to Retention of Potassium

Cortisol and, even more so, aldosterone cause sodium retention and potassium excretion. So in Addison's disease, when cortisol is low, not only is the serum sodium low, but the serum potassium rises. The serum potassium may or may not be high enough to cause symptoms. Certainly the client should not be given additional potassium. (See Chapter 5 for the nursing implications for hyperkalemia.)

Risk for Injury Related to Hypoglycemia with Fasting States

Clients with a lack of cortisol are less able to maintain a normal blood sugar when there is no continual replacement of glucose. Thus, clients with suspected cortisol deficiency may have symptoms of hypoglycemia if they fast. (See Chapter 8 for the signs, symptoms, and treatment of hypoglycemic episodes.)

Ineffective Coping Related to Inability to Handle Stress (Addisonian Crisis)

Clients with slightly low cortisol levels may have no symptoms until faced with stress: They cannot cope with a crisis. The client needs to be protected not only from physical stress, such

(Continued)

Possible Nursing Diagnoses . . . (Continued)

as infections, but also from psychological stress, such as high levels of anxiety. In either case, because the adrenal cortex cannot produce enough cortisol and aldosterone, the person has an addisonian crisis. The symptoms of an addisonian crisis are the extreme of the problems already described. Clients experience shock due to the lack of sodium and water in the plasma, and their serum potassium levels increase. They have pain, nausea, and vomiting. Circulatory collapse and death can occur. Treatment of an addisonian crisis includes the intravenous administration of hydrocortisone along with the replacement of sodium, chloride, and water.

Disturbed Body Image

On the whole, a lack of cortisol does not cause as many changes in body image as does an excess of cortisol. One characteristic of a lack of cortisol is pigmentation of the skin because the lack triggers the release of MSH. The exact reasons for the increase in MSH are not well understood. It is hypothesized that the lowered cortisol triggers the pituitary gland to produce not only more ACTH but also MSH. Clients can be told that the darkening of the skin fades when the cortisol level is brought back to normal.

If the cortisol lack is associated with a lack of androgens, there may not be many changes because most sex hormones are produced by the gonads. However, if only cortisol is lacking, the adrenal cortex may be stimulated to increase the production of androgens. This increase causes a collection of symptoms known as *adrenogenital syndrome*, which causes the masculinization of females. (See the section on androgen levels.) In infants and children, congenital hyperplasia of the adrenal glands caused by cortisol lack causes many body changes, as described in the section on adrenogenital syndrome.

Deficient Knowledge Related to the Need for Lifelong Replacement Therapy

Clients with a lack of cortisol take cortisone supplements. Most of the dose is usually given in the morning because this is in keeping with the normal rhythm of the hormone. Clients should be taught to take the cortisone replacement with food or antacid.

A mineralocorticoid may also be needed; fludrocortisone is one that is taken orally (Deglin et al., 2011). Mineralocorticoid replacement is needed only when clients are deficient in aldosterone as well as in cortisol.

These clients need to be aware of need for extra cortisone in times of stress. They may also keep parenteral hydrocortisone for emergency replacement. They may be taught to double their doses for minimal stress and triple them for great stress, such as a surgical procedure. Clients should carry a syringe with a 100-mg dose of injectable hydrocortisone and a medical alert tag (or a card) that indicates they have Addison's disease and should be given the injection if they are seriously injured or incapacitated (Holcomb, 2006; Radovich, 2010). Also parents need to know when to give extra medication to children. (See the discussion on congenital adrenal hyperplasia.)

CONGENITAL ADRENAL HYPERPLASIA (CAH)

A congenital lack of certain enzymes can decrease production of cortisol and sometimes of mineralocorticoids. At least six different inherited genetic defects cause decreased synthesis of cortisol, and some of these defects also cause a lack of mineralocorticoids (Hay et al., 2011). About 95% of cases of CAH are due to a lack of the enzyme 21-hydroxylase. A lack of this enzyme, an autosomal recessive disease, causes a lack of cortisol and the mineralcorticoid aldosterone. The classical CAH can be detected through newborn screening (see 17-hydroxyprogesterone discussed later). The National Adrenal Diseases Foundation discusses the role of molecular genetic testing for prenatal use, and for confirming a diagnosis (www.nadf.us).

The lack of cortisol causes an increased production of ACTH and hyperplasia of the adrenal glands. Even when the adrenal glands enlarge, they do not produce more cortisol because of the genetic defect in manufacturing cortisol. However, the adrenal cortex is stimulated to produce more androgens and the precursors of hydrocortisone. In an infant, although the increase in estrogens is not apparent, the increase in androgens causes masculinization of girls and signs of early puberty in boys. In addition to the genetic defect that causes a lack of manufacture of cortisol, there may be an associated inability to produce aldosterone. Children who also lack aldosterone are called *salt losers* because they are unable to retain sodium and water.

Nursery nurses need to examine each newborn's genitalia for any abnormalities. Sometimes girls are incorrectly assumed to be boys. Infants may experience failure to thrive and milk intolerances. Salt losers may have a very poor appetite, frequent vomiting, and other symptoms of severe fluid and electrolyte imbalance.

Another type of CAH is sometimes called nonclassical or late onset. Some children may seem normal at birth but show symptoms of very early puberty. In these children, diagnosing the lack of cortisol is important so that the increased androgen level does not create secondary sex characteristics. Girls may need surgical treatment to repair an enlarged clitoris or fused vagina. The parents need reassurance that normal sexual function can be expected later. Treatment with cortisol and, if necessary, with a mineralocorticoid reduces the level of ACTH and thus the hyperplasia of the adrenal cortex causing the excess of androgens.

17-HYDROXYPROGESTERONE (17-OHP)

A precursor of cortisol, 17-hydroxyprogesterone (17-OHP) is markedly elevated in congenital adrenal hyperplasia (CAH). A number of states screen for CAH in newborns by using blood collected on filter paper. The test may be indicated when an infant has ambiguous genitalia or when a young female has symptoms of masculinization or a boy has early puberty. The 17-OHP may also be used to monitor CAH treatment (see www.labtestsonline.org for more details). 17-OHP is also used to evaluate adrenal or ovarian tumors that have endocrine activity (Wu, 2006).

Possible Nursing Diagnosis Related to Congenital Adrenal Hyperplasia

Deficient Knowledge Related to Emergency Replacement Therapy

Children with a cortisol lack and their parents need careful instruction on how to manage the replacement of cortisol. It is recommended that families always keep a plastic syringe, two

(Continued)

Possible Nursing Diagnoses ... (Continued)

needles, and an ampule of hydrocortisone in their automobiles and homes for emergency injections. Parents are told that a dose of hydrocortisone given unnecessarily does not harm the child, but a delay in giving a dose could be fatal. Older children can be taught to recognize symptoms that indicate a need for more hydrocortisone.

URINARY MEASUREMENT OF THE ADRENAL CORTEX STEROID PREGNANETRIOL

Free urinary cortisol, as well as various metabolites of the adrenal cortex hormones, such as pregnanetriol, can be measured in 24-hour urine specimens. In general, the urinary excretion of steroid increases when the serum levels of the steroids increase and decrease when steroids are low in the serum. Sometimes creatinine in the urine sample is measured to ensure that the volume of urine is normal.

See Chapter 3 for details on urine collection. The nurse should check with the laboratory to see if any preservative is needed. The urine specimens are kept cold to decrease bacterial growth. These urine specimens may be ordered as part of tests of ACTH suppression or ACTH stimulation.

URINARY CORTISOL LEVELS

This test, which measures cortisol itself rather than the metabolites, has become the usual test for evaluating adrenal hyperfunction, or Cushing's syndrome. Some drugs, such as spironolactone or quinacrine, interfere with the results. Low levels do not necessarily mean adrenal hypofunction.

REFERENCE VALUE FOR URINARY CORTISOL

20–70 μg/24 hr or 25–95 ng/mg of creatinine

Note: Increased in pregnancy and with oral contraceptives.

ALDOSTERONE, PLASMA, AND URINE

Aldosterone, a hormone produced by the adrenal cortex, is a mineralocorticoid. Increases in aldosterone cause an increase in the extracellular fluid (ECF) volume because aldosterone increases the reabsorption of sodium and chloride while increasing the excretion of potassium and hydrogen ions.

A decrease in ECF causes increased production of aldosterone through stimulation of the renin–angiotensin system. A decreased flow of blood through the kidney is a stimulus for the production of renin, a hormone secreted by the kidney. Renin, when secreted into the bloodstream, acts on angiotensinogen to form angiotensin. (Angiotensinogen is formed in the liver and circulates in the plasma.) Angiotensin then stimulates the adrenal cortex to increase production of aldosterone. Thus, a

Table 15–4 Renin–Angiotensin Control of Aldosterone and Tests That Measure Aldosterone-Producing Ability of Adrenal Cortex

Decrease of Na in plasma. (Measurement of Na levels.)	
↓	
Increased production of renin by kidney. (Measurement of renin activity.)	Aldosterone causes increase of Na in plasma and decrease in K. (Measurement of K levels, aldosterone levels in serum and urine.)
↓	↑
Renin converts angiotensinogen into angiotensin I, which through enzyme action becomes angiotensin II.	→ Angiotensin II stimulates production of aldosterone by adrenal cortex.

K, potassium; Na, sodium.

drop in ECF volume is corrected by the final action of retaining more sodium and water in the plasma. Conversely, an increased ECF volume is a signal for less production of renin. Without renin, angiotensinogen is not converted to the active form of angiotensin, so the adrenal cortex decreases production of aldosterone. Less aldosterone means less sodium (and water) retention, so the ECF volume is decreased to normal again. (See Table 15–4 for a simple diagram of the regulation of aldosterone and the related laboratory tests.)

Preparation of Client and Collection of Sample

The client needs to eat a conventional diet with the usual intake of sodium and potassium. The client may be instructed to eat a specific sodium diet of 100–200 mEq (mmol). With more sodium in the diet, the reference values are lower. The dietitian must plan the diet if a specific sodium intake is to be followed before the urine and plasma samples are collected.

The laboratory needs 3 mL of plasma or serum for the specimen. The plasma specimen is taken after the client has been resting in the supine position for at least 2 hours. Samples may also be obtained in an upright position for comparison. The peak concentration of aldosterone is in the early morning sample. A 24-hour urine specimen may also be collected, and it needs to be kept cold. (See Chapter 3 on 24-hour urine collection.)

REFERENCE VALUES FOR ALDOSTERONE

Plasma levels	With normal sodium intake	
	7 AM recumbent	2–9 ng/dL
	9 AM upright	2–5 × supine
Urinary excretion for 24 hr	2.3–21 μg/24 hr	

Pregnancy levels are three- to fourfold higher.

Note: In addition to direct measure of aldosterone levels, serum and urine levels of sodium and potassium are measured. (See Chapter 5 on electrolyte measurements in serum and urine.)

Increased Aldosterone Levels in Serum and Urine (Hyperaldosteronism)

Clinical Significance

Increased levels of aldosterone can be either primary or secondary. In primary hyperaldosteronism, a tumor of the adrenal cortex or adrenal hyperplasia (Conn's syndrome) causes increased secretion of aldosterone. The renin level in the serum is low because the increased production of the hormone is not caused by the renin–angiotensin mechanism. (The test for renin is discussed next.)

Secondary hyperaldosteronism is a much more common clinical problem than the primary condition. In secondary hyperaldosteronism, the oversecretion of aldosterone is due to continuous activity of the renin–angiotensin system. This constant stimulation of the system occurs when perfusion to the kidneys is not adequate. For example, clients with heart failure (HF) often have poor renal perfusion. A lack of pressure in the juxtaglomerular apparatus causes the kidney to secrete more renin because the kidneys interpret the lack of perfusion as a lack of ECF. Renin activates angiotensin, which stimulates aldosterone production. Unfortunately, in CHF, the ECF is already in abundance. So the increased aldosterone level, as a response to poor renal perfusion, does not correct the underlying problem. With secondary hyperaldosteronism, the renin level is therefore high.

Not all cases of increased aldosterone are so simple. Sometimes drugs, such as oral contraceptives, cause an increase in aldosterone levels, although the exact mechanism is not well understood. Clients with severe liver dysfunction, such as cirrhosis, tend to have elevated aldosterone levels, which are partly related to poor renal perfusion. Also, if a failing liver can no longer metabolize aldosterone, levels of serum aldosterone remain higher for longer periods.

Possible Nursing Diagnoses Related to Increased Aldosterone Levels

Risk for Injury Related to Hypertension and Hypokalemia

Increased aldosterone levels tend to cause an elevation of serum sodium levels and a decrease of serum potassium levels. In primary aldosteronism, many clients do not have edema even though a sodium excess occurs. This lack of edema is probably because ECF volume is controlled by several factors. Hypertension and hypokalemia are the two most outstanding characteristics of primary aldosteronism. Monitoring the blood pressure and electrolytes is important. (See Chapter 5 on the nursing implications of hypokalemia.)

Risk for Excess Fluid Volume Related to Retention of Sodium

If the increased aldosterone level is due to secondary causes, edema is usually a clinical problem. (See Chapter 5 for a discussion of the nursing implications when a client has edema and needs to follow a restricted sodium diet.) Diuretics may be particularly useful for secondary hyperaldosteronism. The type of diuretic often used is spironolactone because this drug is an aldosterone-blocking agent. Spironolactone is a steroid compound that presumably acts by competing with aldosterone for cellular receptor sites in the tubules. Thus, it promotes sodium and water excretion without a loss of potassium (Deglin et al., 2011).

Decreased Aldosterone Levels
Clinical Significance
The decrease in aldosterone is often part of a generalized hypofunctioning of the adrenal gland. The causes of Addison's disease are discussed in the section on cortisol deficiencies. In CAH, the infant lacks an enzyme needed to manufacture cortisol from cholesterol, and this deficiency may or may not be associated with a deficiency of aldosterone. In the most common type of genetic defect that causes a lack of cortisol, about one-third of clients are also deficient in a mineralocorticoid or aldosterone. The lack of aldosterone gives the symptoms of "salt wasting" seen in some genetic defects and in Addison's disease. Hay et al. (2011) discuss various enzyme deficiencies that can cause decreased aldosterone levels in CAHs.

Possible Nursing Diagnosis for Decreased Aldosterone Levels

Deficient Fluid Volume Related to Hyponatremia

Clients with decreased aldosterone levels are unable to maintain normal serum sodium and potassium levels and thus can experience hypovolemic shock and hyperkalemia. (See the discussion on addisonian crisis in the section on low cortisol levels.) They must therefore have salt, water, and mineralocorticoid replacement. If they lack aldosterone, clients take fludrocortisone orally to ensure mineralocorticoid activity. These medications are continued for life. Because a lack of mineralocorticoid activity also may be part of the adrenogenital syndrome, children who experience salt wasting as part of their congenital problem must undergo mineralocorticoid replacement. Children born with a severe lack of mineralocorticoids may die, however, before the defect is recognized.

RENIN

Renin is an enzyme produced by the juxtaglomerular apparatus in response to decreased blood flow through the kidneys. A change from the recumbent position to upright also causes an increased production. A high-sodium diet causes a decrease in renin. Thus, diet and the position of the client must be taken into account when using reference values for renin activity. The test for renin is used in the differential diagnosis of hypertension.

Preparation of Client and Collection of Sample
Because the values of renin are normally higher in the morning, the test is performed early in the day. The client is usually in the supine position when the blood is drawn, but blood also may be drawn with the patient upright for comparison. The laboratory needs 4 mL of plasma, which is put into a tube with EDTA as an anticoagulant (lavender vacuum tube). The specimen should be iced. Also note the sodium content of the diet, which should be controlled for several days. Diuretics, estrogens, oral contraceptives, and antihypertensive drugs should be withheld for several days before the test.

CATECHOLAMINES, VANILLYLMANDELIC ACID, AND METANEPHRINES

The adrenal medulla secretes epinephrine and norepinephrine, both of which are essential in assisting the body for the "fight-or-flight" response to stress. These two hormones, called the *catecholamines*, are usually measured in 24-hour urine samples, but plasma samples also can be tested. Dopamine, also a catecholamine and the precursor of the other two, may be measured in the serum and urine.

Catecholamines are broken down into intermediate metabolites, which are called *normetanephrine* and *metanephrines*. Laboratories may also measure these intermediate metabolites in the urine. The main product of catecholamine breakdown is an acid called vanillylmandelic acid (VMA). Because the VMA test is easier to perform than the other urine tests for catecholamines, the laboratory may use the VMA as the screening procedure.

Preparation of Client and Collection of Specimen

All the tests for the metabolites of the catecholamines require that the urine remain acid with a pH of 3 or less. Usually 12 mL of HCl is added to the 24-hour specimen bottle. Clients should be warned about the strong acid in the bottle. The usual procedure for collecting urine for 24 hours is followed (see Chapter 3).

The client needs to be relatively free of stress. Vigorous exercise causes an elevation of catecholamines. Blood pressure, height, and weight should be recorded on the laboratory slip.

A multitude of drugs can lead to confusing results. Drugs that act via the sympathetic nervous system, such as some antihypertensives, and antidepressants make the test invalid. Ideally, the client should not take any drugs for 5 days before the test. However, nurses must check to see which drugs can be given, and whether or not certain foods must be withheld for 24 hours prior to the procedure.

REFERENCE VALUES FOR CATECHOLAMINES AND METABOLITES IN URINE

Dopamine	65–400
Epinephrine	1.7–22.4
Norepinephrine	12.1–85.5
Metanephrines	0.0–0.9
Vanillylmandelic acid (VMA)	1.4–6.5

Note: All results are µg/24-hr urine specimen.

Increased Catecholamines in Urine

Clinical Significance

Mild elevations of the catecholamines and of their metabolites can be caused by stress such as operations, burns, or childbirth. (No endocrine response can be effectively evaluated during stress.) A marked increase in the catecholamines has two main causes: The first, a tumor of the adrenal medulla, called a *pheochromocytoma*, causes a marked elevation in catecholamines. Pheochromocytomas are sometimes hereditary, and even clients who have no family history of the disease may be carriers of mutations that lead to the disease (Daub, 2008). The second comes from certain types of malignant tumors, called *neuroblastomas*, which arise from primitive sympathetic tissue. Other tests, such as scans, help pinpoint the presence of a tumor.

Possible Nursing Diagnoses Related to Increased Catecholamines

Anxiety and Altered Cardiac Output Related to the Effects of Increased Catecholamines

Clients with elevated catecholamines have symptoms reflective of the stimulating effects of epinephrine and norepinephrine. Often, their symptoms are attributed to other causes. Some of the outstanding symptoms are increased blood pressure and pulse. Because clients may feel jittery and notice heart palpitations, their symptoms may be wrongly ascribed to an anxiety attack. The surge of catecholamines may be intermittent, so that during an attack the blood pressure may become high and the client can have pounding headaches, nausea, and vomiting. The high levels of epinephrine can cause hyperglycemia and glycosuria, and the client may be believed to have diabetes. (See Chapter 8 on symptoms of hyperglycemia.)

Nurses should carefully monitor the blood pressure and pulse of any client with suspected catecholamine increase caused by pheochromocytoma or a childhood neuroblastoma. A blood or urine sample taken during or soon after an attack may demonstrate the presence of high levels of catecholamines.

Deficient Knowledge Related to Drug Therapy and an Impending Surgical Procedure

Symptoms can be controlled with α-adrenergic blocking drugs, but the definitive treatment is an operation for isolated tumors. Some clients are treated with drugs for weeks before the operation, whereas other clients undergo surgical treatment soon after the diagnosis is made (Katzung, Masters, & Trevor, 2009). Multifocal lesions require long-term medical treatment for hypertension.

Catecholamine Deficiency

Clinical Significance

Even when the adrenal medulla is hypofunctional or destroyed by disease or surgical intervention, the client does not have any symptoms of catecholamine deficiency because catecholamines are also produced by the autonomic nerve endings.

CHROMOGRANIN A

Chromogranin A (CgA) is a type of protein found in neuroendocrine cells. Serum levels are often increased in carcinoid tumors, pheochromocytomas, and neuroblastomas. This test may be particularly useful if the neuroendocrine tumors are not secreting the hormones discussed earlier. Specimen requirements and reference values vary because the laboratory may use several different types of assays (Wu, 2006).

PARATHORMONE OR PARATHYROID HORMONE

Parathormone is produced by the parathyroid glands—the only hormone secreted by these glands. The parathyroid glands, usually four in number, are located in the vicinity of the thyroid gland. Unlike that of many of the other hormones, the level of PTH is not under the influence of the pituitary gland.

The function of PTH is to control serum calcium and phosphorus levels (Table 15–5). A lowered serum calcium level is a stimulus for the release of more PTH to keep the serum calcium level normal. PTH works in various ways to keep a constant serum calcium level and a correspondingly normal phosphorus level:

1. It works in concert with vitamin D to stimulate calcium and phosphorus absorption via the intestinal mucosa.
2. It causes mobilization of calcium from the bone.
3. It causes increased excretion of phosphorus in the urine.

An abnormal elevation or decrease in PTH always changes serum calcium and phosphorus levels. (See Chapter 7 for a detailed discussion of the effects of PTH on serum calcium and phosphorus levels. Note that phosphorus is measured as phosphate in the serum.)

Preparation of Client and Collection of Sample

The client should be fasting. Collect a morning sample. The laboratory needs 1 mL of serum, which should be kept on ice in all cases or, if it must be sent a distance, frozen. (Samples are often shipped because the test is difficult to conduct in most laboratories.) PTH is stable for only 2 hours at room temperature.

REFERENCE VALUE FOR SERUM PTH (INTACT MOLECULE)
10–60 pg/mL

Table 15–5 Effects of Parathormone (PTH) on Serum Calcium and Serum Phosphorus

$\uparrow$ PTH causes $\uparrow$ Ca $\downarrow$ P

$\downarrow$ PTH causes $\downarrow$ Ca $\uparrow$ P

Increased PTH Serum Level
Clinical Significance
Tumors of a parathyroid gland, which are usually benign, cause increased secretion of PTH. A persistently low serum calcium level or a high phosphate level causes a secondary rise in PTH. Additionally, malignant tumors from nonendocrine sources can secrete PTH. (See the discussion on ectopic hormones.) Many clients with hyperparathyroidism have little or no symptoms, so the diagnosis is found on routine chemistry panels that show a high calcium level. Some clients may have renal stones or abdominal and bone pain (McPhee et al., 2011).

Because an elevated PTH causes an increased serum calcium level and a decreased serum phosphate level, the nursing diagnoses are based on these imbalances. (See Chapter 7 for the nursing implications when a client has hypercalcemia.) If the client has an adenoma, surgical intervention can restore the balance.

Decreased PTH Serum Level
Clinical Significance
Decreased levels of PTH can be due to trauma to the parathyroid glands during a thyroidectomy. Infections or other trauma may affect the parathyroid gland. Tumors of the gland usually cause an increase in hormone production, but some tumors may cause decreased function of the gland. Because the levels of PTH are normally low in the serum, a low level may not be helpful in diagnosis.

The symptoms and clinical manifestations of a lack of PTH are reflected in low serum calcium levels and in high phosphate levels. Severe hypocalcemia causes tetany. (See Chapter 7 for a detailed description of tetany and nursing diagnoses for hypocalcemia.)

A lack of PTH is treated with administration of vitamin D and calcium salts. (See Chapter 7 on the treatment of low serum calcium levels and possible client teaching.) PTH, available as recombinant human parathyroid hormone (rh PTH), increases bone mass and strength. These injections have been approved for use in the treatment of osteoporosis (Katzung et al., 2009).

THYROID GLAND
The thyroid gland secretes three hormones: triiodothyronine (T_3), L-thyroxine (T_4), and calcitonin. Calcitonin lowers the plasma calcium level by inhibiting mobilization of calcium from the bone. (See Chapter 7 on the role of calcitonin in the regulation of calcium levels.) Calcitonin levels are measured only for known or suspected cases of medullary carcinoma of the thyroid. Because this type of cancer is often inherited, the calcitonin test may be used to screen family members at risk (Wu, 2006). See Chapter 15 on tumor markers. The other two of these hormones, T_3 and T_4, are forms of thyroxine, and they are usually called the *thyroid hormones*. (T_3 contains *three* iodine atoms and T_4 contains *four* iodine atoms in a molecule.) An adequate intake of iodine is necessary for the continual formation of T_3 and T_4. As with the other hormones, protein intake also must be normal. In many countries, table salt has been iodized so that people have an adequate intake of iodine.

Most of the output of the thyroid is in the form of T_4; only a small amount is in the form of T_3, but T_3 is much more potent than T_4. Both T_4 and T_3 can be measured directly. Also, the amount of T_4 can be calculated with other tests, such as the Free T_4 Index. Each of these tests is discussed individually later in this section. The thyroid hormones, T_4 and T_3, have several functions:

1. They potentiate the effects of epinephrine and decrease the serum cholesterol level.
2. They are necessary for normal development of the central nervous system.
3. They stimulate growth and normal metabolism in all cells.

Tests to Diagnose Thyroid Disease

Although there are several different tests for diagnosing hyper- and hypothyroidism, estimation of the free thyroxine (free T_4) and the thyroid-stimulating hormone (TSH) are the two principal laboratory tests. In some cases, the patient may also have radioactive iodine (RAI) uptakes or thyroid scans, both of which are discussed in Chapter 22. Cancer of the thyroid is suggested by cold nodules on a thyroid scan, not by serum laboratory tests. Some types of thyroid inflammation are associated with increased amounts of antibodies. Chapter 14 discusses the test for thyroid antibodies.

Because the thyroid hormones increase the metabolism of cholesterol, clients with hyperthyroidism tend to have low serum cholesterol levels, and clients with hypothyroidism tend to have high serum cholesterol levels. (See Chapter 9 on cholesterol tests.) The elevated cholesterol associated with hypothyroidism will be reduced by 20–30% when the client is treated with thyroid replacement.

Screening for Thyroid Disease in Asymptomatic Clients

Subclinical or mild hypothyroidism (defined as normal thyroid hormones with an increased TSH) is relatively common but may be misdiagnosed. Various organizations have developed guidelines for screening for hypothyroidism in asymptomatic clients. More than 10% of women over 65 years are diagnosed with hypothyroidism, a rate 10 times than that of men (Mauk, 2005). In addition to age, clients may have other reasons for testing, including a history of certain autoimmune diseases such as type 1 diabetes (see Chapter 8) or pernicious anemia (see Chapter 2). Clients on certain medications such as lithium (see Chapter 17) or amiodarone will need thyroid monitoring.

Pregnant women are screened at the first prenatal visit (see Chapter 18) as hypothyroidism is a relatively common condition during pregnancy (Kooistra et al., 2006).

RAPID TEST FOR TSH

Thyrotest is a rapid immunoassay similar to a pregnancy test. The test requires two drops of blood and 5 drops of diluent. However, no special training is required to perform the procedure. (See CLIA waived tests in Chapter 1). Usually this test is performed in a health care setting and is 95.5% accurate (www.thyrotest.com). Clients may also buy tests for home use that measures TSH.

THYROTROPIN OR THYROID-STIMULATING HORMONE

The production of T_4 and T_3 is controlled by TSH from the anterior pituitary gland. TSH is released from the pituitary in response to the thyrotropin-releasing hormone (TRH) in the hypothalamus. Thus, like most of the other anterior pituitary hormones, TSH is sensitive to nervous response from the hypothalamus. Measurement of TSH is useful in determining whether hypothyroidism is due to primary hypofunction of the thyroid gland or due to secondary hypofunction of the anterior pituitary gland. In sophisticated endocrine evaluations, TRH from the hypothalamus can be measured. High doses of corticosteroids and dopamine infusions can suppress TSH levels.

Higher-than-normal levels of TSH have been used for a long time to help diagnose primary hypothyroidism. In the past, TSH was not useful in the diagnosis of hyperthyroidism because some clients with normal thyroid function (euthyroid) had such low levels of TSH that the levels were barely detected. More sensitive assays did away with this limitation.

Preparation of Client and Collection of Sample

The laboratory requires 2 mL of serum. The client does not need to be fasting.

REFERENCE VALUE FOR TSH

0.5–5.0 µU/mL

Note: Thyrotropin has a diurnal variation with the lowest levels at about 10 AM and the highest levels at about 10–11 PM. Acutely ill clients may have different patterns.

Increased or Decreased TSH

Clinical Significance

One purpose of measuring TSH is to evaluate the possibility of pituitary failure as the cause of hypothyroidism. A low TSH is an indication for further investigation of pituitary disorders. Primary hypothyroidism, caused by insufficiency of the thyroid gland itself, is a much more common cause of hypothyroidism. In primary hypothyroidism, the TSH level becomes greatly elevated in an attempt to stimulate the failing thyroid gland. For many years, TSH has been used to confirm primary hypothyroidism in newborns. Although elevated TSH suggests a treatable condition, follow-up for adults may be problematic. Researchers linking laboratory and pharmacy databases identified several quality control issues, including lack of communication to clients about the abnormal TSH results, undertreatment or delays in therapy adjustment, and lack of client adherence to treatment (Schiff et al., 2005). The very sensitive TSH is also used to monitor the treatment of hypothyroidism. Increased levels of circulating thyroid hormone decrease the amount of TSH secreted from the anterior pituitary gland. This is another example of the negative feedback concept discussed at the beginning of this chapter.

L-THYROXINE SERUM CONCENTRATION (TOTAL AND FREE T$_4$)

T_4, the thyroxine with four iodine atoms, is the most abundant of the thyroid hormones. The test for total T_4 measures both free thyroxine and the portion carried by the thyroid-binding plasma proteins. The free part of T_4 can also be measured and values vary depending on method. Although free T_4 is generally preferred to total T_4 for assessing thyroid function, the total T_4 is used for pregnant women, as it remains stable at about 1.5 times the nonpregnant value.

Preparation of Client and Collection of Sample

The laboratory requires 1 mL of plasma. Fasting is recommended. If the client is taking a thyroid preparation, this should be recorded on the requisition slip. Many drugs (e.g., propranolol and phenytoin) may interfere with the test results.

REFERENCE VALUES FOR L-THYROXINE (TOTAL T$_4$)	
Adult	4.5–10.9 µg/dL Values vary according to different laboratory methods.
Pregnant women	Causes an increase, as do oral contraceptives.
Infants	Up to 16.5 µg/dL
Children	Up to 15.0 µg/dL (declines with age)
Aged	Values maintained, but decrease in plasma protein lowers values.

REFERENCE VALUE FOR FREE T$_4$ (ACTUAL ASSAY)
0.8–2.7 ng/mL (varies with method)

Decreases and Increases in T$_4$

Clinical Significance

The hormone is increased in hyperthyroidism and decreased in hypothyroidism. The nursing diagnoses for these two conditions are summarized later in this chapter.

TRIIODOTHYRONINE SERUM CONCENTRATION (T$_3$)

T_3 is more biologically active than T_4, but both hormones have similar actions in the body. T_3 is not usually used in confirming the diagnosis of suspected hypothyroidism because other tests can demonstrate hypofunction of the thyroid gland. Sometimes, however, a client may have clinical signs of thyrotoxicosis with a normal T_4. Measurement of the T_3 is then needed because T_3 may be elevated in thyrotoxicosis, while other thyroid tests are still in the normal range.

Preparation of Client and Collection of Sample

The preparation and collection instructions are the same as those for the T_4 test.

REFERENCE VALUES FOR TOTAL TRIIODOTHYRONINE (T_3)

Adult	60–181 ng/dL
Pregnancy and oral contraceptives	Tend to increase the values
Infants and children	Have higher values

Note: A decrease in plasma proteins causes lowered values.

Increased Serum Thyroid Levels

Clinical Significance

Table 15–6 shows which of the common tests of thyroid function are usually elevated in hyperthyroidism. An excess of thyroid hormone can result from inflammation, tumors, or autoimmune disorders of the thyroid gland. Often the cause of the hyperthyroidism is unknown (i.e., it is idiopathic). A hyperthyroid state associated with goiter and a bulging of the eyes (exophthalmos) is called *Graves' disease*, which is considered the most fully developed hyperthyroid state and is the most common. It sometimes follows an infection, physical stress, or emotional crisis. Holm et al. (2005) found that smoking, not alcohol intake or physical activity level, was associated with risk of Graves' hyperthyroidism in women. Hyperthyroidism is rare in infants, but it does occur in children and particularly in adolescents. Hyperthyroidism is much more common in girls than in boys. Once hyperthyroidism is definitely diagnosed, treatment may include the use of antithyroid drugs, therapy with radioactive iodine, or surgical intervention. Propylthiouracil and methimazole decrease the production of thyroid hormones. Treatment with either propylthiouracil or methimazole will usually last 12–18 months (Simmons, 2010). β-Adrenergic blockers help control tachycardia and are used with other treatments for all types of hyperthyroidism. The goal of treatment is to bring the client back to a euthyroid, or normal thyroid, balance. The client needs help from the nurse and from others in learning to cope with the manifestations of hyperthyroidism.

Table 15–6 Tests of Thyroid Function

Test	Hypothyroidism	Hyperthyroidism
TSH (thyroid-stimulating hormone)	↓ or ↑ (see text)	↑ or ↓ (see text)
T_4 (L-thyroxine) total and free	↓	↑
T_3 (triiodothyronine)	Not usually performed	↑
RAI (radioactive iodine uptake)	↓	↑
Thyroid scans (see Chapter 22)	Used to identify nodules, not hypo or hyper states per se	
Antithyroid antibodies (see Chapter 14)	Used to help diagnose Hashimoto's thyroiditis	

Possible Nursing Diagnoses Related to Increased Serum Thyroid Levels

Risk for Altered Cardiac Output Related to Tachyarrhythmias

In general, most of the symptoms of hyperthyroidism are due to the accelerated metabolism that results from an excess of circulating thyroid hormones. These clients have tachycardia and often arrhythmias, such as atrial fibrillation. Even their resting pulses may be more than 90 beats per minute. Extreme thyrotoxicosis can even cause high-output cardiac failure. The high pulse decreases as the thyroid gland is brought under control. However, the pulse should be monitored to gauge how well clients can tolerate activity so that they are not overtaxed. β-Blockers, such as propranolol, may be ordered to decrease symptoms until the hyperthyroidism is controlled.

Imbalanced Nutrition: Less than Body Requirements Related to Increased Metabolism

These clients' increased metabolism makes them hungry most of the time. They need a well-balanced diet with extra calories, as well as between-meal snacks. Extra fluids are needed because of the diaphoresis. Stimulants, such as caffeine, should be avoided. The client should be weighed periodically to see that weight loss is not continuing. If diarrhea is a problem, the client should avoid foods that tend to aggravate the hyperactive bowel.

Risk for Imbalanced Body Temperature Related to Ineffective Thermoregulation

Clients with hyperthyroidism have heat intolerance, so they should be protected from high environmental temperatures. The room should be kept cool, and additional fluids should be offered to prevent hyperthermia. A thyroid storm can occur after an operation if the thyroid hormones are released in increased amounts. Antipyretics are not as helpful as they are with fevers related to hypothalamic control. Usually acetaminophen is ordered instead of aspirin, as aspirin may increase T_3 and T_4 serum levels (Holcomb, 2009). Measures such as a cooling blanket are useful. Abrupt withdrawal of antithyroid medication can also lead to thyroid storm, so clients need to know the importance of complying with a medication regimen.

Insomnia Related to Hyperactivity and Increased Metabolic Rate

Clients with hyperthyroidism often have insomnia. They need a quiet, relaxing environment and perhaps sedatives to sleep. (Sedatives are contraindicated for clients with hypothyroidism.)

Disturbed Body Image Related to Exophthalmos

Exophthalmos is an abnormal protrusion of the eye that sometimes occurs with hyperthyroidism when lymphocytes and mucopolysaccharides collect behind the eyeball. This collection may be unilateral or bilateral. Lid swelling, eye pain, and damage to the optic nerve may occur. Most cases of Graves' ophthalmopathy respond to symptomatic treatment, such as protective eyedrops, special glasses, and an eye patch for diplopia. Treatment for severe cases may include glucocorticoids and even radiation or surgery. Control of the hyperthyroidism usually improves the eye problems.

Ineffective Coping

Family, coworkers, and friends may find it difficult to understand the actions of a client who has symptoms of hyperthyroidism. Nurses may be helpful by explaining in simple terms why these clients fuss about heat, noise, or what may seem like small irritations. Control of a hormone imbalance is not always achieved in a short time. It may take months to gain adequate balance.

Decreased Serum Thyroid Levels

Clinical Significance

The findings of the several tests to confirm the diagnosis of hypothyroidism are summarized in Table 15–6. In adults, the presence of severe hypothyroidism is called *myxedema*. The failure of the thyroid gland to produce thyroid hormones is usually a primary dysfunction of the gland itself. However, hypothyroidism can also result from a lack of TSH (as discussed in the section on TSH). Diets deficient in iodine also cause a lack of thyroid hormone and an enlargement of the thyroid gland (goiter). Hashimoto's thyroiditis occurs when the body produces antibodies that destroy an enzyme needed to produce T_3 and T_4. This is the most common cause of hypothyroidism in areas of the world where iodine levels are sufficient. This type of hypothyroidism may be detected by measurement of antiperoxidase or antithyroid antibodies (see Chapter 14).

Many clients in an intensive care unit have low serum T_4 levels but no symptoms of hypothyroidism, so this is called the *sick, low-T_4 euthyroid syndrome*. The T_4 returns to normal after recovery from the illness.

In congenital hypothyroidism, the lack of the thyroid hormone can cause cretinism. Lack of thyroid in newborns causes growth failure and mental retardation. The symptoms of hypothyroidism may not be present at birth because the infant has some thyroid hormones from the mother. (See Chapter 18 on newborn screening.) In addition to newborns, other populations particularly susceptible to hypothyroidism are elderly people; postpartum women; people with autoimmune diseases, such as type 1 diabetes mellitus or Addison's disease; and those who have had treatment for hyperthyroidism in the past. Clients with hepatitis C as well as clients receiving medications such as amiodarone have a higher rate of hypothyroidism (McPhee et al., 2011).

Possible Nursing Diagnoses Related to Decreased Serum Thyroid Levels

Altered Health Maintenance Related to Need for Lifelong Replacement Therapy

Hypothyroidism in Infants. Nurses must be aware of the symptoms of hypothyroidism in newborns and in adults, because nurses may be involved in case finding. Case finding in infants is important because mental retardation occurs if the infant is not treated within 2–3 months

(Continued)

Possible Nursing Diagnoses . . . (*Continued*)

after birth, and sometimes the effects of lack of thyroid may not be prominent at birth because the infant has some thyroid hormones from the mother. Some of the outstanding characteristics of a lack of thyroid in a newborn are protruding tongue; a broad, flattened nose; a protruding abdomen with an umbilical hernia; and a generalized muscle hypotonia. The baby has a hoarse cry and may be a poor feeder. The heart rate is slow.

Once hypothyroidism is diagnosed, treatment is begun with thyroid replacement. The medication helps the infant grow and develop normally. The parents need careful teaching about the importance of lifelong administration of the hormone and normal patterns of growth and development.

Older Children and Adults. Symptoms of hypothyroidism, or myxedema, in clients beyond infancy are due to the slowing of metabolism that occurs with insufficient thyroid hormone. These clients may have only slight symptoms, so the disease may be overlooked. They typically have fatigue, lethargy, and intolerance to cold. Their hair is coarse and their skin is very dry. They gain weight on a limited diet. Constipation may be a problem. Blood pressure and pulse are low. Clients may have memory impairment or a definite slowness in mental ability. Thyroid replacement eradicates these symptoms. The client needs to know the signs of overdosage of the drugs. (See the discussion on the symptoms of hyperthyroidism.) A resting pulse greater than 90 beats per minute is an indicator of possibly too much thyroid replacement. Clients should be taught to check their own pulse. Any improvement in the way thyroid is commercially prepared can cause a need for less medication as the drugs become more potent (Katzung et al., 2009). The condition of the clients with excessive or insufficient thyroid replacement may be difficult to clinically recognize, so laboratory monitoring is important to prevent adverse drug effects.

Altered Comfort Related to Cold Intolerance and Slowness of Thought

Clients with hypothyroidism have a cold intolerance, so the environment needs to be warm. The nurse can provide extra clothing, such as heavy socks. The environment must also be warm in the psychological sense. These clients may be slower in activity, so others must let them proceed at their own pace. The clients may need help to adjust to fast-moving situations. Because inactivity may produce more lethargy and dullness, sensory stimulation is needed. In the home setting, the family may need help making the environment warm, relaxed, and relatively quiet for the client.

Imbalanced Nutrition: More than Body Requirements

Clients may need to follow a diet that is low in calories to prevent weight gain. The nurse should see that the diet contains all the essential nutrients and vitamins. Clients can be assured that when their thyroid level is returned to normal, their excess poundage should be easier to lose. (In fact, thyroid pills have been used as a type of diet pill. Thyroid pill intake by a client who is euthyroid is not a physiologically sound way to lose weight.) Plenty of fluids and fiber in the diet help to decrease the problem of constipation.

Risk for Injury Related to Intolerance for Sedatives and Opioids

Because these clients have a slower-than-normal metabolism, sedatives and opioids may have a profound effect. These types of drugs should be used with caution, if at all.

Risk for Injury Related to Lack of Medication

After clients have been on thyroid replacement for a while, they may decide to discontinue their medication because of cost, inconvenience, or a belief that they no longer need to take the medicine every day. Clients who do not take their thyroid replacement are at risk for development of a myxedema coma, which may be brought on by a stress or illness. The client will need treatment for clinical shock and possible mild hyponatremia and hypoglycemia. Intravenous infusions of levothyroxine and liothyronine are available (Deglin et al., 2011).

Disturbed Body Image

Clients may be distressed by their rough skin and coarse hair. They may need to use hair conditioners and plenty of skin lotion to keep their skin and hair attractive looking. These skin and hair problems fade as the hormonal balance is restored.

Deficient Knowledge Related to Symptoms of Fatigue and Depression

Clients may experience fatigue and depression before thyroid tests become markedly abnormal. Assessment of reasons for fatigue may include TSH screening.

THYROGLOBULIN TEST

Thyroglobulin, made by the thyroid gland, is the storage form of the thyroid hormones. A thyroglobulin test is used as a tumor marker after a total thyroidectomy for differentiated carcinoma of the gland. Levels of thyroglobulin should drop to very low or undetectable levels after the gland is removed. An elevated level several months after surgery merits whole-body scanning with I^{131} (see Chapter 22) to identify tumors in the thyroid bed or beyond. Some clients have antibodies to thyroglobulin (see Chapter 14), and these may interfere with testing, so the laboratory will test for these antibodies at the same time.

Thyroglobulin may also be measured in clients with thyroiditis or symptoms of hyperthyroidism.

GONADOTROPINS AND THE SEX-RELATED HORMONES

The sex-related hormones include the gonadotropins from the anterior pituitary gland (FSH and LH) and estrogen, progesterone, and the androgens from the ovaries, testes, and adrenal cortex. Both the ovaries and testes produce progesterone, estrogen, and the androgens but in markedly different proportions in males and females.

Infertility, the lack of development of secondary sex characteristics, and changes in sexual characteristics or sexual functioning are common reasons for measuring the sex hormones.

FOLLICLE-STIMULATING HORMONE

FSH from the anterior pituitary gland controls the growth and maturation of the ovarian follicles in women for ovulation. FSH also controls the secretion of estrogen in women. In women, a high FSH is the most reliable indicator of the ovarian failure of menopause. In men, FSH stimulates the testes to produce sperm.

Preparation of Client and Collection of Sample

There is no special preparation of the client. The laboratory needs 5 mL of serum or plasma for the blood test. The same sample can be used for LH.

REFERENCE VALUES FOR FSH

Adult: Men	4–15 mU/mL
Women	4.6–22.4 mU/mL pre- or postovulatory; 13–41 mU/mL midcycle peak
Prepubertal: Boys	2–10 mU/mL
Girls	3–7 mU/mL
Postmenopausal women	30–170 mU/mL

HOME TEST FOR FSH

A home test for FSH has been approved by the FDA. The client should use a first-morning-voided urine specimen. The testing vial detects FSH levels above 25 IU/L. The manufacturers note that using this test, a woman can monitor herself during the perimenopausal years and detect the beginning of menopause. The clients are advised to discuss the results with their physicians. Nurses need to educate clients that a change in menses during the menopausal years should not be dismissed as being normal until the client is examined by a health care provider.

LUTEINIZING HORMONE

LH is the second gonadotropic hormone secreted by the anterior pituitary gland. In women, LH, along with FSH, is necessary for ovulation to take place. After ovulation, LH stimulates the ruptured follicle to secrete increasing amounts of progesterone. In men, LH stimulates the production of androgens, which are important in determining the secondary sex characteristics. LH in men is sometimes referred to as the interstitial-cell-stimulating hormone (ICSH). In men, LH may be measured if serum testosterone levels are low.

REFERENCE VALUES FOR LH

Adult: Men	3–18 mU/mL
Women	2.4–34.5 mU/mL pre- and postovulatory; 43–187 mU/mL midcycle peaks
Children	2–12 mU/mL
Postmenopausal women	30–150 mU/mL

Preparation of Client and Collection of Sample

The requirement of 3 mL of blood or plasma for LH is the same as for FSH, and both tests can be performed on the same specimen.

HOME TEST FOR LH

Various test kits are available to measure the surge of LH as a signal of ovulation. See Chapter 28 on tests for fertility.

Changes in FSH and LH Serum Levels

Clinical Significance

FSH and LH levels are measured to see whether clients with hypogonadism have a primary gonad problem or a secondary problem of pituitary insufficiency. Pituitary insufficiency may be first manifested by a lack of function of the testes or ovaries. LH and FSH are low if the failure of the gonads is due to pituitary insufficiency (secondary hypogonadism). The levels of FSH and LH in serum and urine are high if the failure of the gonads is primary failure of the ovaries or testes. Increased levels of FSH are also used to verify that a woman is undergoing menopause.

ESTRADIOL AND OTHER FORMS OF ESTROGEN

Different forms of the estrogens, including estradiol, estrone, and estriol, can be measured. Estriol is the estrogen present in largest amounts at pregnancy. (See Chapter 18 for the use of estriol as a test of fetal well-being during pregnancy.) Because estrogens are produced not only by the ovaries but also by the adrenal cortex and testes, estradiol levels may be useful to assess pathologic conditions in all three glands.

The level of estradiol is increased in men who have testicular or adrenal tumors. In women, the increased estradiol arises from estrogen-secreting ovarian tumors. Decreases of estradiol in women, or a lack of increase during a menstrual cycle, can be due either to ovarian failure or to pituitary insufficiency. Other factors, such as anorexia nervosa, may also cause decreases in estradiol. Hepatic and renal failure can cause abnormal increases of estrogens in the serum. Women may show no symptoms when estrogens are increased. Men may exhibit feminizing signs, such as enlarged breasts, when any of the estrogens is increased.

Preparation of Client and Collection of Sample

For estradiol, collect 5 mL in a red-topped tube. Include the date of last menstrual period (LMP). Values vary considerably as to ranges considered normal.

REFERENCE VALUES FOR SERUM ESTRADIOL	
Men	<50 pg/mL
Women	
Follicular phase	50–145 pg/mL
Midcycle	112–143 pg/mL
Luteal phase	50–241 pg/mL
Postmenopausal	<59 pg/mL

PROGESTERONE

In women of childbearing age, progesterone is low during the first part of the menstrual cycle (follicular phase). When LH is increased at the time of ovulation (luteal phase), there is a resulting surge of progesterone for several days. Progesterone remains elevated in early pregnancy. Progesterone levels are used to document the occurrence of ovulation. Progesterone is also secreted by the adrenal glands, so progesterone levels may be elevated in neoplasms of either the ovaries or the adrenal glands.

Preparation of Client and Collection of Sample

The laboratory needs 2 mL of serum in a red-topped tube. Include the date of LMP and trimester of pregnancy.

REFERENCE VALUES FOR SERUM PROGESTERONE	
Men	0–1.0 ng/mL
Women	
Follicular phase	0–1.5 ng/mL
Luteal phase	2–30 ng/mL
Postmenopausal	0–1.5 ng/mL
Pregnant women	Peaks in third trimester to as high as 200 ng/mL

PREGNANEDIOL (PROGESTERONE METABOLITE)

Pregnanediol is the principal form of progesterone in the urine. (Pregnanetriol is another urine test performed to evaluate adrenocortical function. See the discussion earlier in this chapter.) In women, the level of pregnanediol in the urine rises rapidly after ovulation and steadily during pregnancy.

REFERENCE VALUES FOR URINARY PREGNANEDIOL	
Children	0.4–1.0 mg/24-hr specimen
Men	0.5–1.5 mg/24-hr specimen
Women	
Pregnant, 28–32 weeks	27–47 mg/24-hr specimen
Nonpregnant	0.5–7.0 mg/24-hr specimen
Luteal phase	2.0–7.0 mg/24-hr specimen
Postmenopausal	0.3–1.5 mg/24-hr specimen

ESTROGEN AND PROGESTERONE RECEPTORS IN BREAST CANCER

Estrogen (ER) and progesterone (PR) receptors are measured routinely in biopsy specimens of breast tumors because they have important implications for therapy and prognosis. Clients who have estrogen- and progesterone-positive tumors tend to have a better prognosis, and they are much more likely to respond to anti-hormone medications such as tamoxifen and aromatase inhibitors that decrease estrogen levels. An individual's response to endocrine therapy depends on several factors, but typical response rates are as follows:*

ER positive	PR positive	75–80%
ER positive	PR negative	40–50%
ER negative	PR positive	25–30%
ER negative	PR negative	10% or less

*www.labtestsonline.org

HER-2/neu receptors are present in some breast cancer cells. A medication that is an antibody to this type of receptor, trastuzumab, is discussed in Chapter 10 under tumor markers. Breast cancers lacking all three of these receptors are called "triple negative" and, until recently, have been treated with chemotherapy (McPhee et al., 2011). Medications that specifically target "triple negative" breast cancer are in several clinical trials. Clinicians and clients can call 1 (800) 4-CANCER to obtain up-to-date information about clinical trials for breast cancer and other information about cancer and diagnostic testing, or use the website www.cancer.gov.

TESTOSTERONE AND OTHER ANDROGENS

The male sex hormones, the androgens, are produced by the adrenal cortex, the testes, and the ovaries. The most powerful of the androgens, testosterone, comes mainly from the testes. Men with increased testosterone levels do not have any symptoms. In boys before puberty, there is precocious development of secondary sex characteristics. In women and girls, there is masculinization. Polycystic ovary syndrome (PCOS), an endocrine disorder that affects women of reproductive age, causes increase in androgens and steady levels of estrogen and LH (McPhee et al., 2011). Increased insulin resistance, obesity, infertility, and a risk for diabetes are associated with this syndrome. The adrenogenital syndrome, which occurs because of a lack of cortisol and an abundance of androgens, is discussed earlier in this chapter. In men, a lack of testosterone, which can be due to primary failure of the testes or secondary to pituitary insufficiency, causes feminization. To evaluate impotence, serum testosterone is ordered before the gonadotropins.

Preparation of Client and Collection of Sample

The laboratory needs 4 mL of serum.

REFERENCE VALUES FOR SERUM TESTOSTERONE (TOTAL)	
Men	270–1,070 ng/dL
Women	6–86 ng/dL
Adolescent males	>100 ng/dL
Some laboratories use 250 ng/dL as the lower limit in men.	

Possible Nursing Diagnoses Related to Imbalances in Sex Hormones

Disturbed Body Image

Hormones are potent in shaping and altering secondary sex characteristics. For example, a woman who has an increase of testosterone has more facial hair, more muscle mass, and a deeper voice. One of the key nursing implications for clients undergoing sex hormone changes caused by pathologic conditions is to help them cope with the disturbance in their body images. Alterations in sexual characteristics are corrected if the hormone balance can be established. The mood changes and depression may be due to both hormonal influences and the effect of the physical changes. Nurses can help these clients reduce the effect of the unwanted characteristics. Even details such as helping a woman find a place to have unwanted hair removed can mean a great deal.

Specific Interventions for Malignant Tumors. Several of the tumors that cause masculinizing features in women or feminizing features in men are malignant. Nurses must be aware of the specific nursing care guidelines related to the pathophysiologic features of the tumor. Some types of cancer are treated with hormone therapy, which causes an imbalance of sex hormones and permanent changes in body image.

Ineffective Sexuality Pattern Related to Hormonal Changes

A client may need professional counseling to deal with problems related to sexual functioning. The emphasis for any sex-hormonal change is to help the client deal with a decreased sexual self-concept. If hormone tests are being performed as part of an infertility evaluation, the nurse needs to be sensitive to the anxiety of the couple who has not been able to conceive a child. (See Chapter 28 for diagnoses related to infertility.)

Ineffective Family Coping Related to Precocious Puberty in Children

The problem of mistaken sexual identity in newborns is discussed in the section on congenital adrenal hyperplasia. (See the section on cortisol.) Masculinization of a girl or precocious puberty in either sex is disturbing for the child and, probably much more so, for the parents. Endocrine problems in children are usually treated by specialists who can also help parents, who may be alarmed by the changes in their child. A visiting nurse may be helpful in assessing the adjustment of child and family to these changes. School nurses can be instrumental, too, in recognizing children who may need counseling to deal with the physical and psychological problems of early maturity. Precocious puberty is more common in girls than in boys, and more girls have a benign slow progression that may not need intervention (Hay et al., 2011). Some girls are capable of reproduction at 8 or 9 years of age.

Ineffective Health Maintenance Related to Use of Anabolic Steroids for "Sports Doping"

Anabolic steroids are sometimes abused by athletes to enhance their performances. Therefore, laboratory studies may be ordered to evaluate the possible presence of these drugs. Clearly, the adverse effects of these drugs make their use inadvisable for sports (Katzung et al., 2009).

Questions

1. Which of the following illustrates the concept of a negative feedback system for control of serum cortisol?
   a. An increase of serum cortisol when ACTH secretion is increased
   b. A decreased level of serum cortisol when ACTH secretion is decreased
   c. A decreased secretion of ACTH when serum cortisol is increased
   d. An increased secretion of ACTH when serum cortisol is increased

2. A client has an elevated serum cortisol level with a tentative diagnosis of Cushing's syndrome caused by an adrenal cortex tumor. Which nursing action would be most needed?
   a. Observing and noting any gastric distress, because gastric ulcers may develop
   b. Assessing for fluid deficit and high serum potassium levels (hyperkalemia)
   c. Taking the pulse every 4 hours to assess for bradycardia
   d. Encouraging physical activity to counteract lethargy and boredom

3. A client has a lower-than-normal serum cortisol level. Which nursing action would be appropriate for this client with a diagnosis of Addison's disease?
   a. Informing the client that his increased skin pigmentation will not fade away, although cortisol hormonal replacement is adequate
   b. Checking the blood sugar level because hyperglycemia is a potential problem
   c. Helping the client prevent postural hypotension by teaching him to get out of bed slowly
   d. Encouraging compliance with a restricted sodium diet

4. A young child has been referred to an endocrinologist because he has an enlarged penis and secondary sex characteristics. His serum sodium was low, and his serum potassium was elevated. A 24-hour urine for 17-ketosteroids (17-KS) was elevated. The increased elevation of serum androgens in congenital adrenal hyperplasia is due to a basic lack of which of the following?
   a. ACTH production
   b. Cortisol production
   c. Gonadotropic hormones
   d. Testosterone

5. An elderly client has heart failure with secondary aldosteronism. An elevation of the mineralocorticoid aldosterone would cause which of the following symptoms?
   a. BP of 90/60 mm Hg
   b. Serum potassium of 5.8 mEq/L
   c. Pitting edema of the ankles
   d. Polyuria (urine output of 2,500 mL in 24 hours)

6. Urine testing for metanephrine and catecholamines are two of the screening tests for tumors of the
   a. Adrenal cortex
   b. Adrenal medulla
   c. Pituitary gland
   d. Parathyroid gland

7. An increased level of parathormone (PTH) causes an increased serum level of which of the following?
   a. Sodium
   b. Potassium

c. Phosphorus
d. Calcium

8. A middle-aged client has been admitted to the hospital because of suspected hyperthyroidism. Which of the following nursing actions would be appropriate in caring for her?
   a. Seeing that she has a low-calorie diet
   b. Keeping her room slightly warmer than usual
   c. Encouraging her to increase her activity level
   d. Checking an apical pulse when vital signs are taken

9. A client has come to the clinic to begin tests for hypothyroidism because symptoms were noted by a home care nurse who was visiting the family. Which of the following symptoms is characteristic of a client with suspected hypothyroidism?
   a. Agitation
   b. Diarrhea
   c. Intolerance to cold
   d. Weight loss

10. The most important nursing information for clients with alterations in sex hormones is to be aware that they often need help in coping with which of the following?
    a. Decreased appetite and weight loss
    b. Changes in secondary sex characteristics
    c. Changes in energy level
    d. Physical stress, such as an infection

References

Curtis, J. R., Westfall, A. O., Allison, J. J., Becker, A., Casebeer, L., Freeman, A., et al. (2005). Longitudinal patterns in the prevention of osteoporosis in glucocorticoid-treated patients. *Arthritis & Rheumatism, 52*(8), 2485–2494.

Daub, K. F. (2008). Pheochromocytoma, not you everyday diagnosis. *American Nurse Today, 3*(7), 9–11.

Deglin, J. H., Vallerand, A. H., & Sanoski, C. A. (2011). *Davis's drug guide for nurses* (12th ed.). Philadelphia: F. A. Davis.

Hay, W. W., Levin, M. J., Sondheimer, J. M., & Deterding, R. (Eds.). (2011). *Current diagnosis and treatment: Pediatrics* (20th ed.). New York: McGraw-Hill.

Holcomb, S. S. (2006). Do the clues add up to Addison's disease? *Nursing 2006, 39*(3), 64hnl–64hn3.

Holcomb, S. S. (2009). Thyroid storm. *Nursing 2009, 36*(3), 72.

Holm, I. A., Manson, J., Michels, K., Alexander, E., Willett, W., & Utiger, R. (2005). Smoking and other lifestyle factors and the risk of Graves' hyperthyroidism. *Archives Internal Medicine, 165,* 1606–1611.

Katzung, B., Masters, S. B., & Trevor, A. J. (Eds.). (2009). *Basic and clinical pharmacology* (11th ed.). New York: McGraw-Hill.

Kooistra, L., Crawford, S., van Baar, Brouwers, E., & Pop, V. (2006). Neonatal effects of maternal hypothyroxinemia during early pregnancy. *Pediatrics, 117*(1), 161–167.

Mauk, K. L. (2005). Rooting out hypothyroidism in the elderly. *Nursing 2005, 35*(12), 65–66.

McPhee, S. J., Papadakis, M. A., & Rabow, M. W. (Eds.). (2011). *Current medical diagnosis and treatment* (50th ed.). New York: McGraw-Hill.

Radovich, P. (2010). Primary adrenal insufficiency: Elusive and potentially life-threatening. *American Nurse Today, 5*(3), 37–39.

Schiff, G. D., Kim. S., Krosnjar, N., Wisniewski, M. F., Bult, J., Fogelfeld, L., et al. (2005). Missed hypothyroidism diagnosis uncovered by linking laboratory and pharmacy data. *Archives Internal Medicine, 165*, 574–577.

Simmons, S. (2010). A delicate balance: Detecting thyroid disease. *Nursing 2010, 40*(7), 22–29.

Wu, A. H. (Ed.). (2006). *Tietz clinical guide to laboratory tests* (4th ed.). St. Louis, MO: Saunders Elsevier.

Websites

www.acllaboratories.com (Information on salivary cortisol collection kits.)

www.cancer.gov (Information on triple negative breast cancer.)

www.labtestsonline.org (Information on 17-hydroxyprogesterone and breast cancer receptor sites.)

www.nadf.us (National Adrenal Diseases Foundation for Information on Addison's Disease and Congenital Adrenal Hyperplasia.)

www.thyrotest.com (Information on rapid diagnostic screen for hypothyroidism.)

Answers

1. c, 2. a, 3. c, 4. b, 5. c, 6. b, 7. d, 8. d, 9. c, 10. b

CHAPTER 16

Culture and Sensitivity Tests and Rapid Tests for Infections

- Classification of Bacteria at Microscopic Examination 415
- Culture Growths 415
- Culture and Sensitivity Tests 417
- β-Lactamase Assay 418
- Minimal Inhibitory Concentration 418
- Minimum Bactericidal Content or Minimum Lethal Concentration 419
- Collecting Specimens for Culture 420
- Urine Cultures 423
- Blood Cultures 425
- Sputum Cultures and Acid-Fast Bacillus 427
- Wet Mounts of Sputum Specimens 428
- QuantiFERON-TB Gold Test 429
- Rapid Test for Tuberculosis 430
- Throat Cultures 430
- Nasal Swabs and Nasopharyngeal Cultures 431
- Wound Cultures 432
- Eye Cultures 434
- Vaginal and Urethral Smears 434
- Rapid Tests for Gonorrhea and Chlamydia 435
- Rapid Tests for Trichomonas and Bacterial Vaginosis 436
- Vaginal Self-Test for Detecting pH Changes 436
- Vaginal and Rectal Cultures to Prevent Transmission of Neonatal Group B Streptococci Disease (Perinatal GBS) 439
- Cultures of Cerebrospinal Fluid and Other Fluids 442

OBJECTIVES

1. Describe the classification system used by the laboratory to identify bacteria.
2. Interpret the clinical significance of culture and sensitivity (C&S) and minimal inhibitory concentration (MIC) reports.
3. Identify the general nursing implications when a client has cultures ordered for a possible bacterial infection.
4. Describe in detail the various ways urine is collected for urine cultures.
5. Explain the procedures used to obtain blood cultures, as well as the timing of preliminary and final reports.
6. Describe what the nurse should teach the client to obtain a useful sputum specimen.
7. Explain why it may be important to perform throat cultures for children with sore throats.
8. Describe the correct procedure to obtain a wound culture and what should be taught to the client.

9. Describe how gonorrhea and other sexually transmitted infections (STIs) are detected by smears and cultures.
10. Describe the proper procedure for collecting a stool specimen for laboratory examination.

The first part of this chapter provides background information about the classification of bacteria and about how the laboratory performs cultures and sensitivity testing on clinical specimens. Nursing implications for culture collection are outlined. In addition, the nurse's role in caring for clients with infections is reviewed. The last part of the chapter outlines the purpose, procedure, and preparation of the client for each common type of culture.

CLASSIFICATION OF BACTERIA AT MICROSCOPIC EXAMINATION

Bacteria can be classified into three groups according to the following criteria:

1. Whether the bacteria take a Gram stain
2. The shape of the bacteria—round (cocci), rod-shaped (bacilli), or spiral-shaped (spirilla)
3. Whether the bacteria thrive with oxygen (aerobic) or without oxygen (anaerobic)

The distribution of cocci in pairs (diplococci), in a string (streptococci), or in a cluster (staphylococci) helps the microbiologist classify bacteria. A preliminary stain may not identify the exact bacteria, but it can help with a presumptive diagnosis and help rule out what the bacteria are not. For example, if the Gram stain shows gram-negative diplococci, gonorrhea is most likely the causative organism. If the Gram stain reveals gram-negative rods, the infection may be caused by organisms such as *Escherichia coli* or *Pseudomonas*. Table 16–1 shows the classification of some of the common bacteria identified in laboratory specimens.

The laboratory technician also records other details, such as the number of different bacteria present, to estimate the probability of an infection. Gram stains are scanned for polymorphonuclear neutrophils (PMNs), which are present in infection, and for squamous epithelial cells, which are present in mucosal contamination. The technician also is able to see that the specimen is grossly contaminated with normal flora.

Gram stains may be useful for the presumptive identification of gonorrhea in endocervical smears in women and urethral smears in men and for meningitis in cerebrospinal fluid (CSF). Gram stains of stool and urine may or may not be helpful. In several specimens, such as sputum smears, the usefulness of a Gram stain is controversial.

CULTURE GROWTHS

A stain is only a presumptive identification of bacteria. A culture allows the bacteria to grow and to multiply so that the exact organism can be identified by various methods of analysis. The laboratory usually takes 2 or more days to make a final identification of the organisms present in a specimen. For some specimens, it may

Table 16–1 Examples of Common Bacteria Found in Cultures

Organism	Culture in Which Commonly Found
Aerobic	
Gram-positive cocci	
Staphylococcus aureus (coagulase-positive)	Blood, wound, sputum
Streptococcus (β-hemolytic)	Throat, wound, sputum
Streptococcus pneumoniae (pneumococcus)	Sputum, CSF in adult
Gram-negative cocci	
Neisseria meningitidis (meningococcus)	CSF, throat
Neisseria gonorrhoeae (gonococcus)	Urethra, endocervix, throat
Gram-negative rods or bacilli	
Escherichia coli (many strains)	Urine, blood, wound
Proteus	Urine, sputum, wound
Enterococcus	Blood, sputum, wound
Pseudomonas	Sputum, urine, wound
Salmonella	Stool
Shigella	Stool
Anaerobic	
Gram-positive cocci	
Anaerobic streptococci	Wound, stool, vagina
Gram-positive bacillus	
Clostridium group	Wound, stool
Gram-negative bacillus	
Bacteroides	Wound, stool
Acid-fast bacillus	
Mycobacterium tuberculosis	Sputum, gastric contents, CSF

CSF, cerebrospinal fluid.

Information compiled from several references.

take 6–10 days. The growth on the culture takes about 24 hours. The laboratory must then use various tests to determine the species of bacteria present. Various methods, such as the addition of sugars, are used to identify different strains of a species. These tests to identify a type of bacteria may take another 24 hours or more.

The amount of growth on the culture varies with the organism. For example, some bacteria, such as *E. coli*, reproduce every 20 minutes. At the other extreme, the organism that causes tuberculosis, *Mycobacterium tuberculosis*, reproduces only about once a day. Thus, a final report of a culture for tuberculosis may take 1–6 weeks. (See the section on sputum collection for acid-fast bacillus [AFB] for a faster way to detect *M. tuberculosis* by nucleic acid probe.)

Anaerobic Cultures

Unless there is a specific order to the contrary, bacterial cultures are usually performed under aerobic conditions because most disease-causing organisms require oxygen. However, if the client may have an infection with an anaerobic organism, the specimen must be cultured without oxygen. For an anaerobic specimen, the nurse should call the laboratory to obtain the needed container for anaerobic transport, or a syringe with the needle capped with a cork may be used for transport. The specimen should be sent to the laboratory immediately. With blood cultures, the routine is to put the blood specimens into two different containers so that both anaerobic and aerobic cultures can be performed. Two laboratory requisitions should be sent with the two specimens so the laboratory is aware of the need to perform both types of culture.

Cultures for Fungus

Cultures for fungus require specific preparations with India Ink, KOH (potassium hydroxide), or PAS (periodic acid Schiff) stain. With swabs moistened with saline solution, small scrapings may be taken from a lesion. The nurse should consult with the laboratory on exactly how to collect the specimen.

The cultures for fungus take a long time to grow, and they must be handled carefully because the spores from the fungus can get into the air. For most of the systemic fungal diseases, such as histoplasmosis, various serologic tests are performed (see Chapter 14 on serologic tests). Skin tests are also used to identify clients who have antibodies against certain fungal infections (see Chapter 10 on cellular immunity).

Cultures for Viruses

The laboratory identification of viral diseases is usually performed with serologic tests because a culture of a virus requires a living cell culture, which demands the services of a specialized laboratory. Some viruses have been identified by means of electron microscopy, but the positive identification of certain viruses is still performed only at large medical centers. Specimens for virus isolation should be collected in the first 4 days of illness. Almost all viruses are extremely labile outside the human host, so the specimen should be put in the special viral-holding medium supplied by the laboratory. Viral testing is expensive, so the laboratory may require a detailed clinical history of the client for approval of the test. Newer tests to screen for viral infections utilize antigen detection by immunologic methods such as viral loads of HIV and other viruses. (Serologic titers for some viral diseases and viral loads of HIV and hepatitis C virus [HCV] are discussed in Chapter 14.)

CULTURE AND SENSITIVITY TESTS

Sometimes, in addition to knowing the exact organism causing the infection, it is necessary to demonstrate if the organism is sensitive to a certain antibiotic. In regard to culture and sensitivity (C&S), *sensitivity* refers to the ability of the antibiotic to inhibit the growth of the bacteria. *Sensitivity* has an entirely different connotation when describing the reaction of a client to an antibiotic. A client who is allergic to a drug is said to be *sensitive* or *hypersensitive* to the drug. Sensitivity of the *client* to the drug is undesirable, whereas sensitivity of the *organism* to the antibiotic is essential. If the antibiotic does not inhibit growth of the bacteria, the organism is said to be *resistant* to the antibiotic.

The most common way that a laboratory checks the sensitivity of organisms to specific antibiotics is to put disks of paper impregnated with antibiotics in a culture. Laboratories may list the test as a Kirby–Bauer susceptibility test. If the growth of an organism is retarded, the report is an *S* for *sensitive* or *susceptible*. If the antibiotic disk does not retard the growth of the specific bacteria in the culture, the report is *R* for *resistant*. An *I* on a report means that the results are in an *intermediate* zone or

Table 16–2 Example of Sensitivity Report (Shortened List)

Drug	*Escherichia coli*	*Pseudomonas ceruginosa*
Amikacin	S	S
Ampicillin	R	R
Gentamicin	S	S
Methicillin	R	R
Penicillin G	R	R
Tobramycin	S	S

S, sensitive; R, resistant.

inconclusive of growth retardation. Some laboratories place an intermediate growth into the resistant category. Usually, the laboratory uses only one member of an antibiotic family because sensitivity differences are usually minor.

The purpose of conducting C&S is to ensure that the client is receiving the correct antibiotic for the particular organism causing the infection. For example, suppose a client were receiving ampicillin. If a report showed the organisms to be resistant to ampicillin but sensitive to other antibiotics, the physician must change the antibiotic order. (See Table 16–2 for an example of a C&S report that necessitates notification of the physician before the next dose of ampicillin is given.) C&S is particularly useful when a client is not responding to therapeutic dosages of antibiotics. A routine sensitivity for every culture may not be needed and could be an unnecessary health cost. In addition, note that several microorganisms can be tested by DNA probes, as discussed later in this chapter.

β-LACTAMASE ASSAY

Some bacteria become resistant to some of the penicillins and cephalosporins because the bacteria produce enzymes that make the drugs ineffective. These enzymes, the β-lactamases, affect a certain structure in the antibiotic known as the β-*lactam ring*. The first of these enzymes was called *penicillinase* because it made penicillin ineffective as an antibiotic. Several types of β-lactamase assays are performed, and most tend to be accurate, particularly when a positive reaction is reported. A positive reaction means that the offending organism is resistant to many of the penicillins and the first- and second-generation cephalosporins. Like C&S, which takes longer, a β-lactamase assay helps with the choice of the most effective and least expensive drug for a particular infection.

MINIMAL INHIBITORY CONCENTRATION

Minimal inhibitory concentration (MIC) is a report of the concentration of an antibiotic that inhibits the growth of the organism. Venous blood containing the microorganism is put into liquid culture mediums, each containing an antibiotic at a specified concentration. Table 16–3 shows the range of testing for some antibiotics. The concentration of the antibiotic that inhibits the growth of the microorganism in vitro is then noted. The MIC helps the clinician choose antibiotics that are

Table 16–3 Ranges Tested for Minimal Inhibitory Concentration (MIC) by Laboratory

Antibiotics (Range Tested)	Representative Adult Dose (G)	Approximate Blood Levels (μg/mL)	Approximate Urine Levels (μg/mL)
Clindamycin (0.25–16)	p.o. 0.15–0.3 q6h IV 0.3–6 q6–8h	2–4 4–8	30–90 45–240
Erythromycin (0.25–16)	p.o. 0.25–0.5 q6h IV 0.3 q4–6h	1–4 10–20	(5%)
Methicillin (0.25–16)	IV 1–2 q4h	10–40	
Penicillin (0.06–4)	(p.o. 0.25–0.5 q6h) IV 1–2 mL q4h	1.5–4.0 20–40	300–450 3,000–5,000
Ampicillin (0.12–8, gram-positive) (0.25–16, gram-negative)	p.o. 0.25–1.5 q6h IV 1–2 q4h	1.5–4.0 15–30	50–100 200–400
Cephalothin (1–64)	p.o. 0.25–0.5 q6h IV 1–2 q4h	2–15 25–85	300–1,000 800–2,000
Gentamicin (0.25–16)	IM,IV q8–12h (3–5 mg/kg per day)	5–10	65–300
Tetracycline (0.25–16)	p.o. 0.25–5 q6h IV 0.5 q6–12h	1.5–4.0 10–20	200–800 600–1,000
Carbenicillin (8–512)	p.o. 1 q6h IV 4 q4h	5–10 125–175	350–14,000 2,000–10,000
Chloramphenicol (0.5–32)	p.o. 0.25–0.5 q6h IV 0.5–1 q6h	1.5–4.0 10–20	200–700 500–1,400
Kanamycin (1–64)	IV,IV 5 q12h (15 mg/kg per day)	15–20	100–200
Tobramycin (0.25–16)	IM,IV q8–12h (3–5 mg/kg per day)	5–10	65–300
Amikacin (1–64)	IM,IV q8–12h (15 mg/kg per day)	16–21	700–830

clinically appropriate and cost-effective. For an organism to be considered sensitive to an antibiotic, attainable blood levels should be at least two to four times the MIC. For urinary tract infections (UTI), the dose of antimicrobial agent in the urine needs to be 10 times the MIC.

For example, if for organism X the MIC is reported as 4.0 μg/mL for methicillin, one uses the information in Table 16–3 to determine if methicillin would be effective. If the approximate blood level is only 4.0, the drug would not be effective. For intravenously administered methicillin, the obtainable blood levels are much higher (10–40 μg/mL), and thus it would be considered an appropriate antibiotic. However, the MIC that is effective in vitro (test tube) may not always correlate well with the effectiveness in vivo. Blood levels vary according to body fat, and hepatic and renal functioning.

MINIMUM BACTERICIDAL CONTENT OR MINIMUM LETHAL CONCENTRATION

The minimum bactericidal content (MBC) or minimum lethal concentration (MLC) denotes the concentration of antibiotic needed to actually kill an organism. The technique is an in vitro one as described for MIC. End reports for the MBC may note either 99%, 99.9%, or 100% colonies killed. Not a routine test, the MBC may be used to assess debilitated clients with leukopenia or to eradicate bacterial endocarditis or meningitis (Katzung, Masters, & Trevor, 2009) (See Chapter 2 for decreased white blood cell [WBC] count.)

COLLECTING SPECIMENS FOR CULTURE

General Nursing Implications

Specific information about each common type of culture is covered in the second half of this chapter. This section presents general guidelines for the collection of all specimens for bacterial culture.

Collect Specimens Before Giving Antibiotics

If possible, cultures should be collected before administration of the antibiotic is begun. If the client is already taking antibiotics, the laboratory should be notified, because techniques to counteract the effect of the antibiotic, such as adding enzymes, may be performed, or special collection tubes are used.

Use the Correct Specimen Container

All specimens must be collected in a sterile container, and anaerobic specimens must be collected in oxygen-free containers. Some cultures, such as throat cultures, may be transferred to the culture medium immediately. The nurse should call the laboratory if there is any doubt about the type of culture medium to be used. For example, the laboratory has specific cultures for blood, and it may be desirable to have the blood transferred to the culture medium as soon as it is drawn. In other settings, the laboratory may prefer to receive blood in tubes and make the transfer to the culture medium in the laboratory. If the specimen is not placed in the correct medium, it is useless.

Know How Much of the Specimen Is Needed

For example, the laboratory can perform a culture on only a few milliliters of sputum, so it is useless to keep the container longer to try to obtain a larger amount. Table 16–4 lists the amounts needed for each type of specimen. Information on the amount needed for each type of specimen is also covered with the discussion on the specific test.

Do Not Expose Others to the Infectious Material

Meticulous handwashing before and after obtaining a culture is essential. The nurse must make sure that the outside of the specimen container does not become contaminated with the contents inside it. All containers are placed inside special bags for transport to the laboratory.

Make Sure That the Specimen Is Properly Labeled

The laboratory requisition must be filled out correctly. A specimen that is not properly identified is useless. If the specimen is for an outpatient, making sure that the home phone number of the client is available is important. Information required

Table 16–4 Amounts Needed for Culture and Tips for Collection

Type of Culture	Amount Needed	Special Notes
Urine	2–3 mL in sterile container (if also for urinalysis, send 15–30 mL)	Must be clean-catch or catheterized specimen so that it is not contaminated by perineal flora
Blood	10 mL by venipuncture; keep in syringe or put into culture at bedside—5 mL aerobic, 5 mL anaerobic	Be sure it is not contaminated with skin flora; special skin cleansing needed
Sputum	2–3 mL in sterile container	Sputum, *not* saliva
Throat	One swab put in prepared culture (Culpak)	Touch back of throat only
Nasopharyngeal	One swab in test tube	Swab gently
Wound	One swab in test tube; may use syringe for anaerobic specimens	Clean skin around wound first—see text on chronic wounds
Eye	One swab	Be careful not to touch cornea
Vaginal	One swab; if anaerobic, need special container	Need cervical specimen for gonorrhea
Urethral	One swab	See text for other ways to detect gonorrhea in men
Stool	1-inch lump (walnut size) or 20 mL if diarrhea	See text for special techniques
CSF, pleural fluid, peritoneal fluid	1 mL—aerobic and anaerobic	Need to notify lab that CSF is coming; CSF, pleural, or peritoneal fluid is collected in other tubes for other types of analysis

CSF, cerebrospinal fluid.

Information compiled from several references.

on the laboratory slip includes the client's name and other identification, such as medical record number, hospital room number, or clinic site. The type and *source* of the specimen, as well as the date and time collected, are essential. Other details, such as the need for an anaerobic report or whether the client is on antibiotics, should be recorded.

Send the Culture to the Laboratory As Soon As Possible

All cultures should be sent to the laboratory immediately, but some specimens, such as urine, can be refrigerated if there is a delay in transporting the specimen. Some commercial kits contain an ampule of transport medium that keeps samples moist for as long as 72 hours. For some specimens, such as a culture of CSF, the laboratory needs to be called before the culture is sent, so that the personnel are available to begin immediate examination of the fluid when it arrives at the laboratory. In the hospital setting, cultures are not usually collected on the evening or the night shift unless the laboratory provides 24-hour service. If specimens are collected in a home, the nurse must check with the laboratory to see how the specimen can be transported without causing the death of the organism to be cultured.

General Nursing Diagnosis When Cultures Are Ordered

Risk for Injury Related to Transmission of Infectious Material

Universal precautions, first introduced in 1987, heightened the awareness of the risks to health-care workers who are careless with blood and body secretions. Currently, there are two levels of precautions: (1) standard precautions combine the major features of the universal precautions and apply to every client, and (2) transmission-based precautions (airborne, droplet, and contact) apply to clients who have documented diseases that are transmitted by one of these methods.

Even with the emphasis on standard precautions, staff may need to be reminded that the spread of microorganisms is best controlled by handwashing after every physical contact with every client. *Some staph infections are staff induced.* Compliance with handwashing remains an issue (Hughes, 2006). Thus, when clients are known to have a positive culture, it behooves the nurse to see if proper handwashing is occurring and to give feedback to those who are break-ing technique. Consultation with an infection control nurse may be needed. In the home setting, family members need to be taught how to protect themselves from the spread of infection.

Assessing for Signs and Symptoms of Infection. Often the nurse may be the first one to detect that the client may be getting an infection. For example, a nurse in a nursing home may notice that the urine in a drainage bag has a foul odor. A pediatric nurse may notice that the lungs of a child have crackles and that the child has a fever. A nurse making a home visit may notice that a wound appears inflamed and sore to the touch.

Although fever is usually present in infections, in some clients, particularly the elderly, fever may be absent and the WBC count and differential normal. (See Chapter 2 for a discus-sion of the "shift to the left" as a characteristic sign of a developing bacterial infection.) Elderly clients who describe "not feeling good" or who are confused or lethargic may need a com-plete physical examination to rule out the possibility of an unnoticed infection. The two most common infections of clients in nursing homes are UTI and pneumonia. In newborns, the WBC count may not be elevated, but an increase in the erythrocyte sedimentation rate (ESR) and the bands (see Chapter 2) may be important in screening for newborn sepsis. CRP (Chapter 14) is also used to screen newborns for infection.

Assisting the Client to Combat Infection. Too often health professionals consider that the administration of antibiotics is the only way to treat infections, but a holistic approach to the treatment of an infection includes more. Increased fluids, a diet adequate in protein and other nutrients, and plenty of rest are other ways to help the body combat a bacterial inva-sion. Adults may need antipyretic drugs to reduce the fever, if the fever is high or the client is uncomfortable. Aspirin or acetaminophen may be prescribed to reduce fevers in adults. Aspirin is not used with children because of the association with Reye's syndrome. A moder-ate increase in temperature is considered useful in helping the body mobilize the defense against bacterial invasion. The elevated temperature may improve the efficiency of leukocytes and may impair the growth of some microorganisms. The natural defenses of the body against infection need to be encouraged along with the proper use of antibiotics and antipyretics. The use of the 23-valent pneumococcal vaccine can help prevent outbreaks of pneumonia in the elderly (Goldrick, 2005). Some studies have supported the health attributes of yogurt in combating diarrhea and vaginal infections that may accompany antibiotic use, but some stud-ies have not supported the efficacy of yogurt (Eckert, 2006). Stress reduction should also be employed, so the body is free to mobilize against the infection.

Recognizing Situations That Allow the Growth of Opportunistic Organisms. Poor techniques by health professionals are not always to blame when clients have an infection in the hospital or nursing home. Always present in our environment are opportunistic pathogens, which do not usually cause an infection unless the resistance of the host is low. Reducing all possible pathogens in an environment may be difficult. For example, food is not sterile. Salad is a notorious source of organisms, and even pepper has been shown to carry potential pathogens. Opportunistic organisms such as *Pneumocystis carinii* (now called *Pneumocystis jiroveci*) are commonly present but cause pneumonia only in immunosuppressed clients, such as those with acquired immunodeficiency syndrome (AIDS). Clients who are immunosuppressed need extra careful observation for any signs of infection.

URINE CULTURES

General Indications

For routine microscopic urinalysis, the findings that suggest UTI are the presence of a large number of WBCs and bacteria in the urine. Two screening tests for UTI, nitrites and leukocyte esterase (LE), are discussed in Chapter 3. For nonpregnant women, treatment with antibiotics can be given without a culture if there are no signs suggestive of pyelonephritis, vaginitis, or chlamydial urethritis and the client has not had more than one other UTI in the past year. In pregnant women, treatment for UTI is important to prevent pyelonephritis. If the UTI does not respond quickly to medication, the culture may be needed to determine the appropriate therapy. The most common organism causing such infections is *E. coli*. Other gram-negative rods, such as the *Proteus* or *Pseudomonas* groups, are occasionally present in UTI.

The Centers for Medicare and Medicaid Services (CMS) will not reimburse a facility for catheter-associated urinary tract infections (CAUTI) unless the condition was present on admission. Therefore, many facilities have changed practice to reduce the use of urinary catheters (Harris, 2010).

Female clients are particularly susceptible to UTI because of the short length of the urethra and the possible contamination from perineal organisms. ("Honeymoon" cystitis often occurs when sexual activity introduces organisms into the urinary tract.) Girls are also much more likely to have UTI than are boys. Catheterization procedures for either sex increase the risk for UTI.

Preparation of Client and Collection of Sample

Ideally, urine for cultures should be the early morning specimen because the urine is concentrated. However, urine can be collected at any time for the culture. Most laboratories consider a clean-catch, midstream urine the best for a culture. The laboratory needs only 1 mL to grow the culture, so the urine can be transmitted in a syringe if the specimen is removed from a Foley catheter. (See discussion on Foley specimens, later in this chapter.)

There are various diagnostic kits for urine cultures. Clients may be taught to use these at home. (See Chapter 1 for a discussion of diagnostic kits.)

Clean-Catch or Midstream Specimens

The problem in collecting urine for C&S is that the urine may be contaminated with the bacteria normally present in the perineal area. Current practice is to use simple soap and water to clean the perineal area. Women should use a tampon to prevent menstrual fluid or vaginal secretions from contaminating the urine specimen.

The urine is collected midstream, so it contains fewer of the bacteria that reside on the perineal surfaces near the urinary meatus. To collect a midstream specimen, the client must be able to stop the urine flow after it is begun and then urinate into a sterile cup or directly onto a dipstick for culture. Women hold the labia apart so that the urinary meatus is clear. If the client is unable to clean the area, the nurse can clean around the meatus. (A nonsterile glove can be used to protect the nurse who washes the perineal area.) In an uncircumsized male client, the foreskin must stay retracted during the procedure.

Collecting Urine by Direct Catheterization

The danger of infection as a result of catheterization is a reason to try to obtain urine by means of clean-catch whenever possible. If catheterization is necessary to collect a urine specimen, sterile technique must be followed.

Collecting Urine from a Foley Catheter

Urine taken from a drainage bag is never suitable for a culture because the urine is not fresh. Foley catheter drainage tubes have a special sample port for inserting a needless syringe to remove a few milliliters of urine for tests. The tube below the area may be bent back on itself or clamped so that urine collects near the port. The sample port should be cleaned with alcohol if a needle must be inserted. It is important for microscopic urinalysis to remove the needle from the syringe before emptying the urine from the syringe into the specimen cup. Forcing urine through the needle breaks up cells.

Collecting Urine in Children

A sterile cotton ball can be placed in the diaper of an infant. Another technique is to clean the perineal area and attach a sterile collection bag around the meatus. This procedure is easier with male infants. For older children, meatal cleaning and midstream collection may be no more effective than simply having the child void into a sterile container.

REFERENCE VALUES FOR URINE CULTURES

Urine is sterile in the bladder, but it becomes contaminated with organisms normally present in the perineal area. The amount of organisms is counted and usually interpreted as follows:

<10,000 organisms/mL	Unlikely UTI, probable contamination
10,000–100,000 organisms/mL	Probable UTI, particularly if urine specimen is from a catheter
>100,000 organisms/mL	Definite UTI

Note: These numbers exclude the presence of normal genital flora such as lactobacilli.

In low-grade pyelonephritis, the urine culture may be negative even though bacteria are present in the pelvis of the kidney.

Possible Nursing Diagnosis Related to Positive Urine Culture

Deficient Knowledge Related to Preventive and Therapeutic Measures for Urinary Tract Infection

The key measure to assist a client in overcoming a UTI is to keep the urine as dilute as possible so that bacteria cannot multiply rapidly. Keeping the urine acidic may also be helpful for some bacterial infections. See Chapter 3 for more discussion on UTI and dipsticks. The client needs to know exactly how much fluid should be consumed each day. Caffeine may irritate the bladder. The clinician may prescribe sulfa drugs or antibiotics, such as ampicillin, depending on the causative organism for the UTI, and the client should know the possible side effects of the drugs. In addition, the nurse should make sure that the client knows ways to prevent infections in the future by continuing adequate fluid intake. Also, some women are not aware that wiping the perineal area should be front to back so that the intestinal bacteria are not transmitted to the meatus. Avoiding bubble baths and nylon pants is another preventive measure often suggested. Sexual intercourse and use of a diaphragm and spermicide are the two behavioral factors most consistently associated with UTI in otherwise healthy adult women.

Virtually all clients with long-term use of catheters do have bacteriuria, but cultures are not routinely performed unless the client has symptoms. Proper catheter care is a concern in extended care facilities. Nurses have an important role in reducing the risk of infection of indwelling catheters by promoting excellent catheter care. Research has shown that an increase in cases of UTI is one of the adverse outcomes when there is a less amount of RN direct care of residents for long-term care. Nurses in all settings need to carefully assess the need for a Foley catheter. Wenger (2010) describes a "nurse-driven protocol" that empowers nurses to remove Foley catheters when they are unnecessary.

BLOOD CULTURES

General Indications

Blood cultures are ordered when a client is believed to have septicemia. In many localized infections, a few bacteria may enter the bloodstream (bacteremia), but they are usually not sufficient to cause symptoms of sepsis (septicemia). A client with septicemia is usually severely ill with fever, chills, and other signs of serious infection. Newborns may have no symptoms. The spikes of fever may be related to the release into the bloodstream of more bacteria. So sometimes blood cultures are ordered to be performed when the client has another spike in temperature.

Bacteria can enter the bloodstream from infections in soft tissues; from contaminated intravenous lines, such as those used for hyperalimentation; or even from simple surgical procedures, such as tooth extraction or instrumentation with endoscopes, particularly cystoscopes. Bacteremia in elderly clients can result from pneumococcal pneumonia. In adults, the most common organisms causing septicemia are gram-negative rods, such as *E. coli* or *Aerobacter* species, which can enter the bloodstream because of UTI or instrumentation of the urinary tract. *Staphylococcus aureus* may also cause septicemia. In newborns, *E. coli* and β-hemolytic streptococci are two frequent causes of septicemia. In newborns, sepsis is often a result of prolonged labor and early rupture of the membranes (more than 24 hours before delivery), maternal infection (proved or suspected), and neonatal aspiration. Another reason for blood cultures is to assess for listeriosis, an infection transmitted by contaminated food with the *Listeria monocytogenes* bacterium (Snow, 2009).

If meningitis is suspected in children, blood cultures are drawn and antibiotics started even before a lumbar puncture (Chapter 25) is done (Hay et al., 2011). In adults also, blood cultures are not used alone. For example, the criteria for the diagnosis of endocarditis include blood cultures with an echocardiogram (Chapter 23) as well as other well-defined signs and symptoms (Fink, 2006).

Preparation of Client and Collection of Sample

In most instances, blood samples for blood culture are drawn on two separate occasions and from two different sites to increase the chance of detection of any organisms.

Usually, 10–20 mL is obtained from one venipuncture. Half the specimen is put into a culture for anaerobic bacteria and the other half into a culture for aerobic bacteria. Pediatric specimens may require only 3–5 mL and newborns even less. For infants, a heel stick may be performed to obtain blood for a culture. Some laboratories have the person who draws the blood add the blood directly to the culture media. Other laboratories prefer that the blood sample be sent directly to the laboratory and that the transfer to the culture be made by the bacteriologic technician. Blood culture bottles also come with an antibiotic absorbing resin that is useful for clients who have received antibiotics before the cultures were drawn.

The main problem with blood cultures is that the specimen is often contaminated with bacteria from the environment. The skin is specially prepared before the venipuncture is performed. The current evidence-based guidelines consist of thorough cleansing with chlorhexidine (Meyers & Reyers, 2011). The skin over the vein must not be touched after preparation is completed. If the skin over the vein is probed, the person drawing the blood uses a sterile glove. The transfer of the blood sample to the culture medium must also be a sterile procedure. Lactate levels are also ordered when blood cultures are performed (see Chapter 6).

REFERENCE VALUES FOR BLOOD CULTURES

Any bacteria in the blood are clinically significant. Yet, because there is always the possibility of contamination from the skin, the bacteriologist may make an interpretation of possible contaminants if certain skin bacteria are present in small amounts. At least three cultures in 24 hours may be ordered to determine if bacteria are actually in the blood. A final diagnosis from a blood culture may take several days. However, if the laboratory identifies the presence of certain pathogens, even in small amounts, it issues a preliminary positive report so that the physician can order appropriate antibiotics. *E. coli* is a common pathogen in both adults and children. Other pathogens may be *S. aureus* and various streptococci. Some fungi, such as *Candida* and *Cryptococcus,* grow in routine blood culture medium.

Central Line Infection

Septicemia can result from use of an indwelling intravenous catheter, particularly a central venous catheter used to deliver hyperalimentation fluids. The high glucose content of hyperalimentation fluids supports bacterial growth. To avoid removal of the catheter, a blood specimen from a peripheral vein and one directly from the catheter can be submitted for culture (Wu, 2006). Since January 2010, a Joint Commission National Patient Safety Goal requires hospitals to implement evidence-based practice guidelines to reduce catheter-related bloodstream infections. "Care bundles" (groupings of best practices) have been developed for central venous catheter care (Hatler et al., 2010).

Possible Nursing Diagnosis Related to Positive Blood Culture

Risk for Injury Related to Septic State

Clients with septicemia often have low resistance to infection because they are already critically ill from other causes. Most of the appropriate nursing care is that given to acutely ill clients. Septic shock may occur and be fatal.

Nurses need to be aware that sepsis starts with a systemic inflammatory infection response syndrome (SIRS). A client with SIRS will have at least two of these signs.

1. Core temperature below 96.8°F (36°C) or above 100.4°F (38°C)
2. Heart rate above 90
3. Respiratory rate above 20 or a $PaCo_2$ less than 32 mm Hg (See Chapter 6)
4. WBC less than 4,000 or greater than 12,000 or immature neutrophils (bands) greater than 10% (See Chapter 2)

Practice guidelines recommended by the Surviving Sepsis Campaign call for a "bundle" on interventions to halt the progress of sepsis to septic shock (Powers & Burchell, 2010).

Laboratory findings, which may signify the need for more interventions, are hyperglycemia (Chapter 8), increased liver function tests (Chapter 12), thrombocytopenia and increased D-dimer (Chapter 13), hyperbilirubinemia (Chapter 11), and elevated lactate levels (Chapter 6). Medical surgical nurses need to be able to interpret this data, which may require additional training in the use of a surveillance system to organize all the data for an individual client (Dodge, 2010).

SPUTUM CULTURES AND ACID-FAST BACILLUS

General Indications

Sputum cultures are often ordered when a client has lung congestion (crackles), elevated temperature, and other signs of a probable respiratory infection. Respiratory infections cause an increased secretion of respiratory secretions or sputum. Sputum originates in the bronchi, not in the upper respiratory tract. Different bacteria cause the sputum to be greenish, yellowish, or rust colored. The sputum may have a foul smell.

Almost all the bacteria that cause respiratory infections are normally present in the upper respiratory tract in small amounts. In healthy people, these organisms, such as *Klebsiella* or *Staphylococcus,* do not cause disease because they are present in small amounts. Yet when an organism has a chance to grow quickly because of stagnant respiratory secretions, the client can experience pneumonia. Postoperative clients and those who are immunosuppressed are at high risk for pneumonia. Infectious pneumonia is a problem among elderly clients who have both acute and chronic illnesses. Unfortunately, the identification of a bacterial organism does not prove that the organism is an actual respiratory pathogen. About half the time the cause of both community-acquired and nosocomial (hospital-acquired) pneumonia cannot be determined by culture (McPhee, Papadakis, & Rabow, 2011). If certain infections, such as *Legionella*, are suspected, a preliminary urine test may be done as a screening tool. A simple urinary antigen screen for one type of *Legionella* has led to the detection of many unrecognized cases. However, the urine test detects only one species and serotype of *Legionella*, so a culture may be needed to identify other species and serotypes (Todd, 2005). *P. carinii*, now called *P. jiroveci*, a fungus that is seen in clients with AIDS or other severely immunocompromised states, cannot readily be cultured, but newer techniques have improved the sensitivity of the test. Induced sputum cultures may be obtained after nebulization therapy. Sometimes specimens are obtained by bronchoscopy (Chapter 27).

If tuberculosis is suspected, a special type of culture for this AFB culture is done. PCR or a DNA probe may also be used. These tests may also be noted as nucleic acid amplification (NAA) tests. See the section on rapid tests for tuberculosis.

Preparation of Client and Collection of Sample

The laboratory needs only a few milliliters of sputum for a culture. Sputum, however, is not the same thing as saliva. The sputum specimen must be from the bronchial tree, not simply saliva from the mouth. Having clients rinse out their mouths before the sputum is obtained is a good idea, so that the sputum is not contaminated with saliva and mouth bacteria. An early morning specimen is ideal because the sputum is concentrated then. Early morning sputum also tends to be plentiful if the client has been sleeping through the night and the secretions have pooled.

Sputum from the bronchial tree can be obtained in several ways. If at all possible, the client should be allowed to cough up the sputum. If the client is unable to cough, suctioning can be performed with a special catheter that allows some of the secretions to be caught in a special reservoir. Sputum cultures are also obtained with a bronchoscope.

If the purpose is to determine the presence of the AFB that causes tuberculosis, the culture should be performed on at least three different days. Other cultures besides sputum may be needed to detect tuberculosis in other sites. Sometimes the delayed diagnosis of tuberculosis can be related to the fact that nonpulmonary clinical presentations account for 15% of active cases (Jackson, 2006). See the text on a new blood test to screen for latent TB, which may improve detection rates.

Nurses can help reduce the spread of tuberculosis by identifying clients who have a productive cough and possible TB. In addition to sputum specimens, the client will need a chest x-ray (Chapter 20).

WET MOUNTS OF SPUTUM SPECIMENS

The first laboratory examination of a sputum specimen is a wet mount. If a large number of epithelial squamous cells are observed, no further testing is conducted, because these cells indicate the specimen is oropharyngeal secretion. Another specimen of sputum, not saliva, must be obtained. A wet mount may also be used to detect a large number of eosinophils. Sputum eosinophilia is associated with asthma and other nonbacterial pulmonary diseases.

REFERENCE VALUES FOR SPUTUM CULTURES

The laboratory reports the predominant organism or organisms present in the sputum. Common pathogenic organisms include *Streptococcus pneumoniae*, *S. aureus*, and *Haemophilus influenzae*. Various gram-negative bacilli may also cause respiratory infections. The culture for these common bacteria is completed in 24–48 hours.

A culture for tuberculosis (AFB culture) grows very slowly. It may take 1–6 weeks to obtain a final report. (See text for NAA tests.)

Possible Nursing Diagnoses Related to Positive Sputum Culture

Ineffective Airway Clearance

Clients need encouragement to perform deep breathing and coughing exercises. They may also need intensive respiratory therapy by suctioning or postural drainage. The nurse needs to make sure that hydration is adequate because without adequate fluids the sputum becomes tenacious.

Deficient Knowledge Related to Spread of Disease to Others

Teaching clients to cover their mouths or cough into their sleeves when coughing seems common sense, but the nurse may have to remind clients. The nurse also needs to teach clients how to safely dispose of sputum that is excreted. If clients are coughing up large amounts of sputum, cleaning an emesis basin is easier if the basin is first lined with tissues. Otherwise, sputum tends to become encrusted in the basin. As a rule, clients with most types of pneumonia are not isolated. However, depending on the type of organism in the sputum, respiratory isolation might be justified.

Ineffective Management of Therapeutic Regimen for TB

Because incomplete treatment of TB is a community health hazard, clients need careful follow-up to see that they take a multidrug regimen for the prescribed amount of months. Local health departments can provide this follow-up, including daily visits for direct observation therapy (DOT). DOT, although expensive and time consuming, is cheaper than treating multi-drug-resistant TB (Shalo, 2010). Unfortunately, TB and multi-drug-resistant TB rates are increasing in other countries (Nelson, 2010)

QUANTIFERON-TB GOLD TEST

In 2005, the FDA approved the first blood test to detect latent and active TB. This blood test can be used in the place of a tuberculin skin test (TST). Like the TST, a positive result of the quantiFERON-TB gold test (QFT-G) must be followed up by a physical examination, chest x-ray (Chapter 20), and the smear, culture, and NAA discussed earlier to diagnose active disease.

The QFT-G test uses the ELISA method (discussed in Chapters 1 and 14) to detect the reaction of the client's WBCs to two antigens secreted by all *Mycobacterium tubercular* strains as well as those by *Mycobacterium bovine* (Todd, 2006c). The client's blood sample is collected no more than 12 hours before testing to ensure that the lymphocytes remain viable when the laboratory runs the test. Results are ready within 24 hours.

An advantage of QFT-G over the TST is that the blood test is one-step testing with faster results. Also, previous use of the Bacillus Calmette-Guérin (BCG) vaccine does not create a false-positive result as it may do with skin tests. Although the blood test saves time for clinicians, it does require more time by microbiology staff and is more costly. More information on this test is available from the Centers for Disease Control at www.cdc.gov.

RAPID TEST FOR TUBERCULOSIS

In 2011, the World Health Organization endorsed a new rapid test that can detect tuberculosis in two hours. The test can also determine if the bacillus is resistant to rifampin (www.labtestsonline.org).

THROAT CULTURES

Throat cultures are the only reliable means of differentiating strep throats from viral sore throats. Most sore throats are caused by viruses; only about 10–15% of them in children are caused by group A β-hemolytic streptococci. Yet identifying whether the patient has group A β-hemolytic streptococci is important because rheumatic fever and glomerulonephritis may follow untreated infections. Streptococci are classified according to the antigens. Some are not considered particularly pathogenic, whereas group A β-hemolytic strep is. (See Chapter 14 on the streptococcal antigen–antibody tests of anti-streptolysin-O, anti-streptodornase-B, and streptozyme.) Occasionally, a throat culture for gonorrhea may be performed if the client has been engaging in oral sex with a partner who has gonorrhea.

Certain clinical signs and symptoms should alert nurses to the possibility that a sore throat is indeed a bacterial infection rather than a viral one. For bacterial infections

1. Temperatures are higher than with viral infections
2. Symptoms usually occur more abruptly and the client seems more ill
3. The patches on the throat are often distinctive
4. The WBC count is characteristically elevated—not so with viral infections (see Chapter 2 on the significance of the WBC count in bacterial infections)

Preparation of Client and Collection of Sample

Throat cultures are performed with a swab that is immediately placed into a test tube or kit with a special medium for the growth of bacteria. The client's tongue is depressed with a tongue blade, and a flashlight is used to visualize the inflamed area of the throat. The sterile swab is rubbed over each tonsilar area and the posterior pharynx without touching the lips or tongue. Any white patch should be cultured. The results of throat cultures take 24–48 hours. Special test kits for strep throat show a positive reading in 7 minutes (as a stat test) or 70 minutes as a batch test.

REFERENCE VALUES FOR THROAT CULTURES

The diagnosis of strep throat is based on finding group A β-hemolytic streptococci. Other possible pathogens, such as *H. influenzae, Corynebacterium diphtheriae,* gonococci, or meningococci, can be identified with culture.

Possible Nursing Diagnoses Related to Positive Test for Group A Streptococci

Deficient Knowledge Related to Needed Treatment

If streptococci are the cause of the sore throat, penicillin or erythromycin is most often prescribed. Clients sometimes stop taking antibiotics after they begin to feel better. Yet antibiotic therapy for strep throat must be continued as prescribed, regardless of how well the client feels. For some drugs, 5 days of therapy may suffice (Hay et al., 2011). Either the physician or the nurse may have to explain to the parents that undertreating strep throat increases the possibility of the later development of rheumatic fever.

Health Maintenance Management to Reduce Community Spread

Clients with strep throat are not isolated because the disease is considered noninfectious a few hours after antibiotic therapy is begun. Other family members should be tested because about half of siblings and nearly one-fourth of parents of a child with strep throat also have the organism. Because streptococci are transmitted in droplets from the respiratory tract, an infected client should not cough or breathe on others. The nurse may become involved with follow-up contacts for other family members. In a school, the nurse or public health nurse can be effective in both detecting and preventing the spread of strep throat in a population. Preventing strep infections helps prevent rheumatic fever. (See Chapter 14 on the streptococcal antigen tests used to assess for previous acute infections with streptococci.)

NASAL SWABS AND NASOPHARYNGEAL CULTURES

General Indications

Nasopharyngeal cultures are performed to screen for *Bordetella pertussis, Candida albicans, Candida diphtheriae, Neisseria meningitidis, H. influenzae,* and others. Nasal cultures may be performed to identify carriers of organisms, such as *S. aureus,* that are also called *coag-positive.* However, many adults have this organism in the nasopharynx. The differentiation between carrier state and infection is often difficult because some pathogens do transiently appear in the normal human pharynx. Health workers in areas such as newborn nurseries or operating rooms may have nasal cultures to screen out potential sources of spread. The frequency and targeting of surveillance culturing vary but are always part of the epidemiological follow-up in outbreaks or when a new resistant organism such as vancomycin-resistant *S. aureus* (VRSA) appears (Todd, 2006a).

Methicillin-resistant *S. aureus* (MRSA) has been classified as a hospital-acquired infection, but it can also occur in the community. Nurses should help educate the public about ways to prevent spread of this organism (Noble, 2009).

Rapid Tests for Influenza

The two types of influenza that commonly infect humans are A and B. The exact strain varies each season, and these influenza viruses can also mutate to entirely new strains such as the Influenza A H1N1 (swine flu), which became a pandemic in 2009. A school nurse in New York was the first link in a chain that led to the influenzas when she alerted public health authorities to the symptoms she was seeing in her students (Jacobson, 2009). A molecular test for detection of this novel virus has been developed. Viral cultures are also done, but results take 3–10 days (www. labtestsonline.org).

A rapid test for influenza uses mucus from a nasal swab dipped into a testing vial. Mucus can also be sneezed into the vial or collected by a nasal wash. The result, positive or negative, is ready in about 10 minutes. A positive test eliminates the need for antibiotics or other follow-up tests such as cultures or lumbar punctures. A negative test indicates the need to continue with other tests to rule out the cause of the symptoms. A respiratory syncytial virus (RSV) test, discussed next, may be the next step. This test costs about $15 compared to $150 for a culture.

Rapid Test for Respiratory Syncytial Virus

Nasopharyngeal swabs or washes may also be used for rapid antigen detection of RSV in children. Results may be available in about 20 minutes. RSV is the most important cause of respiratory tract infection in young children. This common virus is especially dangerous for premature infants and children or adults who are immunocompromised. Infection can spread to the lower respiratory tract (bronchiolitis) and the alveoli (pneumonia) and can cause severe respiratory distress. Treatment is mainly supportive, but ribavirin may be used in severe cases (Coffman, 2009). The American Academy of Pediatrics recommends that high-risk infants and children up to age 2 be protected with palivizumab, a monoclonal antibody for RSV (Hay et al., 2011).

WOUND CULTURES

General Indications

An infected wound is usually obvious even to the untrained eye. The characteristic signs are redness, heat, and swelling. There may also be drainage that contains pus (purulence) and that may have a foul odor. If the wound cannot drain, the infection can cause pain and swelling, such as in an abscess. The wounds of surgical clients should be inspected daily for any sign of infection. Clients with burns are also susceptible to infections of the open skin areas. All chronic wounds contain some bacteria, and this may not be all bad because low levels of bacteria can stimulate the inflammatory phase of wound healing (Calianno & Jakubek, 2006).

Preparation of Client and Collection of Sample

A specimen for a wound culture may be obtained by swab, aspiration with a needle and syringe, or tissue biopsy. Most experts agree that swab cultures are the least reliable method because of contamination from skin flora. After cleaning the wound, a swab is rolled on the wound base hard enough to get fluid out of the tissue. Aspiration of wounds is usually a better technique. It is important to reach an area of viable tissue because more microorganisms survive there than in the exudate. The wound may be irrigated with normal saline solution to eliminate the exudate. The saline solution is soaked up with sterile gauze, and the wound is massaged slightly to provide fresh drainage, which is aspirated. Contents from aspiration usually are collected in an anaerobic container. All air must be expressed from the syringe before the specimen is injected into the container. An anaerobic container also can be used for aerobic collection. Tissue biopsy, most often used for clients with burns or long-standing decubitus ulcers, is analyzed for bacterial growth per gram of tissue. Debrided tissue may be used, but it is viable tissue that supports the colonization of pathogens. Included with all specimens should be the location of the wound and the clinical diagnosis, such as cellulitis, furuncle, abscess, or decubitus ulcer.

REFERENCE VALUES FOR WOUND CULTURES

Common organisms found in wounds are *S. aureus*, group A streptococci, gram-negative bacilli, and fungi. If the wound is deep and hence not in direct contact with the air, anaerobic bacteria, such as clostridia or anaerobic streptococci, may also thrive.

Possible Nursing Diagnosis Related to Positive Wound Culture

Risk for Injury Related to Spread of Infection

If the wound is completely covered and is not draining to the outside, simple wound precautions are needed. Sometimes staff tend to become careless in using sterile technique when the client has a wound infection. A break in sterile technique is shrugged off as being not important because "the client already has an infected wound." This kind of thinking is not justifiable because no matter how infected a wound may be, adding other organisms is possible. Dressing changes of an infected wound require the same careful sterile technique as do wounds that are not already infected.

If the wound is draining enough that the dressings become soaked, the client may become a source of infection to others. So more extreme isolation procedures may need to be carried out. Refer to the specific policies of the institution. In the home, the nurse needs to teach the client how to avoid transmitting the infection to others. Because proper wound healing requires good nutrition, the dietary needs of the client should be assessed. (See the ideas discussed earlier in this chapter about ways to increase a person's resistance to infection.)

EYE CULTURES

Although the eye does contain some bacteria, the bathing of the eye with tears usually keeps the actual count of bacteria low. An infected eye is easy to see even by an untrained person. Because of the need to treat most eye infections with topical antimicrobial agents, the laboratory may routinely use a Kirby–Bauer disk to test the organisms found for susceptibility to drugs such as neomycin and chloramphenicol.

Preparation of Client and Collection of Sample

A sterile swab is used to collect some of the purulent matter from the eye. The client should be told to look up while the nurse gently pulls down the cheek. The swab can be placed on the conjunctiva. *Not touching the cornea with the swab is important.* After the specimen is collected, it is put into a sterile culture tube.

REFERENCE VALUES FOR EYE CULTURES

S. aureus and *P. aeruginosa* are two bacteria that may cause eye infections. In newborns, infections can be transmitted during passage through the birth canal. To prevent this transmission of gonorrhea or other infections, state laws require delivery room personnel to instill an antibiotic ointment in every newborn's eyes.

Possible Nursing Diagnosis Related to Positive Eye Culture

Deficient Knowledge Related to Care for Eye Infection

Clients should be taught not to wipe the infected eye. They must also avoid transmitting the infection to the other eye. Dark glasses may offer some comfort to clients if they need to be outdoors. Clients also may need instructions on the proper way to instill eye drops. For example, clients may not know how to put pressure on the lacrimal duct to prevent the drop from entering the nasal cavity.

VAGINAL AND URETHRAL SMEARS

The vagina normally contains bacteria such as *Lactobacillus, Staphylococcus*, and *E. coli* and some yeast. Most commonly, vaginal infections are due to *Trichomonas vaginalis* or to the fungus *C. albicans*. Smears of the discharge may detect the causative agent. If gonorrhea is suspected in a female client, an endocervical smear is performed. In male clients, smears or cultures of the drainage from the urethra may be performed for gonorrhea or other organisms. Also in male clients, centrifuged urine may be cultured for gonorrhea. See the section on NAA tests.

Cultures in Children

Vaginal cultures are done on all girls and penile cultures on all boys who are victims of sexual assault. Oral and anal cultures may be done for both sexes. In situations that may involve legal action, the nurse must follow the chain of custody for samples, as discussed in Chapter 17.

Preparation of Client and Collection of Sample

Vaginal and Endocervical Smears

To obtain a vaginal smear or culture, the swab must be inserted well into the vagina. Check with the laboratory regarding any special techniques needed for smears, such as a wet saline swab for *Trichomonas* or KOH for *Candida*. The client or the nurse needs to hold the labia apart so that the swab does not touch the outer lips. If the nurse must separate the lips of the vagina, a nonsterile glove should be used. An endocervical specimen, necessary for suspected gonorrhea or chlamydia, requires the use of a speculum as for other pelvic examinations. Only water is used to lubricate the speculum. Excess cervical mucus is wiped off with a dry cotton ball, and then a cotton-tipped swab is inserted in the endocervical canal for 30 seconds to absorb any organisms. Two specimens are put on one special culture medium. (If an anal specimen is collected, it is put on a separate culture medium.)

Urethral Smears in Male Clients

Collection of urethral smears in male clients is often performed at the time the physician is examining the client because of discharge from the penis. The exudate is collected on a swab, which is rolled, not rubbed, on a slide. A special loop swab can be gently inserted into the urinary meatus to obtain exudate. If the client has no discharge from the penis, a urine specimen may be centrifuged to obtain a smear or culture for possible gonorrhea.

REFERENCE VALUES FOR VAGINAL, ENDOCERVICAL, AND URETHRAL SMEARS

The presence of pathogens on a smear is considered diagnostic. A culture may or may not be needed to confirm the identification of certain organisms, such as fungus (*Candida*) or protozoan (*Trichomonas*), that may be causing vaginitis.

RAPID TESTS FOR GONORRHEA AND CHLAMYDIA

The use of NAA test or DNA probe (see Chapter 1) is a newer way to identify some microbes. Commercial kits are available that can detect both gonorrhea and chlamydia from one swab or from a urine sample. For chlamydia, urine samples are as useful as samples collected directly from the cervix or urethra. For gonorrhea, urine samples may have a false-negative result for women, so swabs of the cervix may still be needed (Cook et al., 2005). These molecular probe assays are much faster and more sensitive than traditional cultures. In addition, these assays can detect nonviable organisms, so quick transportation is not important. Urine samples should be refrigerated, but specimens may be stored for a week. The use of urine samples and the lack of urgency for transport to the laboratory make it possible to do widespread screening in various locations. Because the assays detect nucleic acids, not viable organisms, the tests are not useful to determine effective treatment. If these tests are not available, smears and cultures are used for screening.

RAPID TESTS FOR TRICHOMONAS AND BACTERIAL VAGINOSIS

Rapid tests for *trichomonas* and bacterial vaginosis are done with a vaginal swab placed in a testing vessel for 10 minutes. Color changes indicate the presence of an infection. Eckert (2006) described guidelines for treatment of three kinds of vaginitis and noted that point-of-care tests may be useful when a microscope is not available. Cost may be a factor in their use for routine screening.

VAGINAL SELF-TEST FOR DETECTING pH CHANGES

Researches have developed the use of a diagnostic panty liner to ascertain vaginal acidity as help in identifying vaginal infections (Geva et al., 2006). The pH is greater than 4.5 in infections with *trichomonas* and bacterial vaginosis and 4.5 or less in infections with *Candida*. Clients may also perform their own vaginal pH testing by using swabs and a pH test to decide on over-the-counter treatment with an antifungal or to see a physician (Kulp et al., 2008).

Clinical Significance of Positive Smears or Cultures

Gonorrhea

About half the cases of pelvic inflammatory disease (PID) in women are due to infection with *gonorrhoeae*. Gonorrhea produces no symptoms in up to 80% of women, and many men may be asymptomatic for up to 45 days. Although a smear may be diagnostic for men with gonorrhea, women need a culture because the smear may not allow differentiation between other vaginal flora and gonorrheal organisms. The sample for the culture must be taken from the endocervical canal, not from the vagina. Oropharyngeal and rectal smears and cultures must be performed if the person has had oral or anal sex with an infected person.

Chlamydia

Chlamydia is a bacteria-like microbe with some of the characteristics of a virus. The disease may have few symptoms and often is found with other STDs. If left untreated, the disease may cause sterility because of chronic inflammation in the urogenital tract. The use of the urine test discussed earlier makes the screening relatively easy.

Herpes

The genital type of herpes is caused by a virus called herpes simplex virus 2 (HSV-2). (HSV-1 causes cold sores in the mouth and can also cause genital ulceration.) Exudate from the lesions present during an acute episode of herpes infection can be examined with a microscope. A herpes culture takes several days, but an antibody test can detect active herpes in 4 hours. For the test of herpes, a specimen can be obtained by scraping the vesicle, but the ideal way is aspiration of fluid from an intact vesicle. A tuberculin syringe with a 28-gauge needle is used.

After an initial outbreak, stress reduction and general good health habits may keep the virus in remission. Reoccurrences are more likely with type 2 or if the first episode was severe. To reduce risk of transmission, clients should be advised to use barrier methods and to avoid sexual contact when the client has active sores or feels an outbreak coming on. Several antiviral drugs are available to treat outbreaks. Daily use of acyclovir to suppress genital herpes has been effective and without unwanted effects for many clients (Katzung et al., 2009). Because there is no cure, clients may need referral to a support group for people living with herpes.

Human Papilloma Virus

Another sexually transmitted infection is human-papilloma virus (HPV). Vaccines have been developed to prevent HPV. See the discussion in Chapter 25 on pap smears to detect cervical and anal cancers.

Trichomonas

T. vaginalis is a protozoan that grows optimally under anaerobic conditions. Sometimes a wet smear may be performed to detect the active protozoa in a drop of vaginal discharge or in a drop of urine from a male client. Culturing of urogenital discharges can reveal protozoa even if direct microscopic examination seems normal. The most common symptoms are itching and a foul-smelling yellow-green discharge. See the rapid tests discussed earlier.

Moniliasis or Other Yeast Infections

C. albicans and, less frequently, other species of *Candida* may be normally present in vaginal secretions. These yeast-like fungi may become invasive under conditions that favor their rapid growth. Predisposing factors for rapid growth of fungi include long-term antibiotic therapy, pregnancy, oral contraceptives, diabetes, and wearing nonventilating pants. The vaginal discharge viewed with a microscope on a wet mount using KOH preparation shows many budding yeast cells and may be diagnostic. The main symptoms are itching of the vaginal area with a discharge that is usually odorless, whitish, and sometimes thick (like cottage cheese).

Bacterial Vaginosis

Bacterial vaginosis may be caused by *Gardnerella*, *Corynebacterium*, or *Haemophilus* species. It may be called nonspecific or anaerobic vaginitis. Bacterial vaginosis may be diagnosed after the other pathogens have been ruled out. The pH of secretions helps with ruling out some organisms: *Gardnerella* and *Trichomonas* species occur with a pH above 4.5 and *Candida* with a pH less than 4.5. The normal pH of the vagina is usually 3.8–5.0. Because vaginosis is an overgrowth of organisms without an inflammatory process, a slide will not have a high number of WBCs as do those for trichomoniasis and candidiasis. Symptoms usually include a foul-smelling, thin, white or colored discharge with little or no itching. See the rapid tests discussed earlier.

Toxic Shock Syndrome

Toxic shock syndrome (TSS) is a rare disease believed to be caused by toxin-producing strains of the bacterium *S. aureus*. Clients believed to have TSS undergo blood and urine cultures as well as a vaginal culture to detect a focal staph infection. The use of high-absorbency tampons may be linked to an increased incidence, but a rise of the syndrome in 1983, after use of high-absorbency tampons declined because of published warnings, has not been explained. Nonmenstrual cases of toxic shock syndrome can originate from various infected sites and are as common now as menstrual cases (McPhee et al., 2011). Because of the possible association with tampon use, manufacturers of tampons now include detailed information about the symptoms of TSS in their product information folders. Early symptoms may be fever and a rash. Abnormal laboratory reports include leukocytosis with pronounced left shift (Chapter 2), elevated BUN and creatinine (Chapter 4), severe acidosis (Chapter 6), hypocalcemia (Chapter 7), hyperbilirubinemia (Chapter 11), elevated CPK (Chapter 12), and thrombocytopenia (Chapter 13). Treatment involves the use of antibiotic therapy and treatment of the circulatory collapse that may occur from the release of enterotoxins.

Possible Nursing Diagnoses Related to Positive Vaginal or Urethral Smear or Culture

Deficient Knowledge Related to Sexual Transmission of Disease

Syphilis, gonorrhea, chlamydia, and AIDS are reportable diseases in every state. HIV infection and chancroid are reportable in many states. (See Chapter 14 for serology tests for syphilis and HIV.) Partner notification may differ from state to state. Clinicians must know the state and local reporting requirements, which may be done by the laboratory or by the provider of health care. Although the sexual contacts of these clients need to be examined for case finding, clients may not wish to name their sexual partners. The nurse can be sensitive to their needs and yet also impress on them the importance of the disease as a public health problem.

Other diseases, such as trichomoniasis, do not require reporting, but the spread from person to person is also of concern. Women may be reinfected by a male partner unless he, too, is cultured and treated (the ping-pong effect). Thus, treatment of any STD involves not only the client but also the person or persons who have been and who will be sexual partners of the client. At present, herpes infection cannot be cured, but the disease is infectious only when it is active. The nurse can help set a climate that is conducive to assisting these clients help themselves and others by learning about safer sexual practices. Clients need factual information on how to best proceed as a sexual being and how to live with a chronic STD.

Deficient Knowledge Related to Treatment

Female clients may need specific instructions on how to insert vaginal suppositories or to administer douches, if medicine is ordered in these forms. Again, the nurse must foster a climate that helps clients feel comfortable about discussing intimate details. Excellent literature and videotapes for patient teaching are available free of charge from the pharmaceutical companies that manufacture vaginal medications.

VAGINAL AND RECTAL CULTURES TO PREVENT TRANSMISSION OF NEONATAL GROUP B STREPTOCOCCI DISEASE (PERINATAL GBS)

Group B streptococcus (GBS) or *Streptococcus agalactiae,* the leading bacterial infection in newborns, may cause death or permanent disabilities in newborns. The infant may acquire this infection by vertical transmission from the birth canal of the mother who is colonized with GBS. Therefore, prenatal screening of pregnant women for GBS is recommended between 35 and 37 weeks' gestation. The screening for GBS colonization involves the collection of cultures from the distal vagina and the anorectal area. Women who test positive for GBS colonization are given intrapartum antibiotics to prevent transmission to the newborn. This screening approach should prevent more cases of GBS transmission to neonates. However, studies to compare the screening approach to a more limited approach based on known risk factors are not available to evaluate the cost, practicality, and efficiency of the two methods (Hay et al., 2011). See Chapter 18 for more discussion on approaches to testing in pregnancy.

Stool Cultures

Many normal bacteria live in the feces. In fact, a large percentage of the weight of feces is bacteria. Most of the organisms in the intestine are many types of gram-negative bacilli. *E. coli* is a common normal inhabitant in adults, but it can also be a pathogen. *E. coli* (especially serotype 0157:H7) may lead to the hemolytic–uremic syndrome. Studies identify subgroups of clients with bloody diarrhea and positive stool cultures to see what interventions prevent this complication. In 2006, an *E. Coli* outbreak from contaminated spinach spread to 26 different states and Canada, causing at least 31 cases of renal failure and several deaths.

Cultures may be used to detect an outbreak of food-borne illness. More attention is being paid to keeping food safe as an increase in imported foods has resulted in a rise in food-borne illness. Preventing food- and water-borne illnesses is particularly important for clients who are immunocompromised.

Bacterial cultures of stool are routinely checked for *S. aureus, Salmonella, Shigella,* and other enteropathogens. If anaerobic organisms are suspected, such as *Clostridium botulinum,* an anaerobic culture also is performed. A microscopic examination to detect the presence of fecal blood, leukocytes, and organisms can be performed in 30 minutes. A test for fecal leukocytes differentiates infectious from noninfectious colitis.

In addition to cultures for bacteria, stool specimens may also be collected to identify parasites that can be protozoa or worms (helminths). Protozoa are more common in most areas than are helminths, unless there is a history of travel to the tropics or a heavy influx of immigrants. If the laboratory is checking for protozoa such as *Entamoeba histolytica,* the nurse must collect several specimens over a period of days. Because protozoan parasites have cyclical life spans, multiple collections increase the chance of spotting a parasite. The use of enzyme immunoassay (EIA) has made it possible to screen for *Giardia* in one stool specimen. If the laboratory is still using the traditional microscopic examination, three specimens are required. (See Chapter 14 for a serologic test performed for amebae.) For helminths, a single stool specimen is usually sufficient.

Infant botulism, first identified in 1976, differs from the food-borne botulism seen in adults and older children because the spores germinate in the infant's intestinal tract. The organism, or more likely the toxin, can be identified in the stool. *Clostridium difficile* can be identified by the toxin in the stool. *C. difficile* infection is associated with recent antibiotic use, particularly use of third-generation cephalosporins. Newer strains are discussed later under clinical significance.

Two other methods of collecting stool specimens for examination involve cellophane tape and a rectal swab. The cellophane tape may be pressed over the perineal area to pick up pinworms, which are very small intestinal worms. Rectal swabs are sometimes performed for *Shigella* infection and for gonorrhea, if this disease is suspected. Yet few organisms live in the rectal wall; the mass of bacteria or parasites is in the feces.

Preparation of Client and Collection of Sample

For bacterial or protozoan cultures, a walnut-sized piece of feces is all that is needed. Diarrheal stool can also be cultured; only about 15–20 mL is needed, and the rest of the stool is discarded. The specimen should be sent to the laboratory immediately. Check with the laboratory for the time span permissible.

The client must defecate into a clean bedpan. Urine in the bedpan may kill some of the growth. A tongue blade can be used to transfer the small amount of stool to the stool container. Commercial kits contain small spoons inside a specimen container. When handling the bedpan, the nurse should wear disposable, nonsterile gloves. Because parasites or bacteria may often be harbored in mucus or in streaks of blood, some of this material should be included in the sample. The stool specimen is put into a waxed container with a tight-fitting lid. It is important not to contaminate the outside of the specimen container. Clients may collect a stool specimen at home. If so, they need to be taught how to collect the specimen properly and how to wash their hands properly so that the outside of the container is not contaminated. (Enteric diseases are spread by oral–fecal transmission.) A plastic bag or newspaper can be taped under the toilet seat so the client can sit on the toilet.

If a rectal swab or cellophane tape is used to collect material from the rectal area, the nurse should wear a glove when touching the perineal area. A sterile cotton-tipped swab is inserted 1 inch (2.5 cm) into the anal canal. The swab should be moved side to side and left for 30 seconds for absorption of organisms. Record on the laboratory slip whether the client is taking antibiotics because these drugs can change the flora in the intestines. Also, the use of antacids may change the pH of the stool and affect bacterial growth.

If the fat content of the stool is to be measured because of malabsorption problems, the *entire* stool for 1–3 days is sent to the laboratory. The client follows a 100-g fat diet. A wax container should not be used to collect the sample.

REFERENCE VALUES FOR STOOL CULTURES

The laboratory may issue a preliminary report of probable findings of *Salmonella* or *Shigella* so that enteric precautions can be started. Parasites or worms may be immediately identified at examination. The two important protozoan infections in the United States are amebiasis and giardiasis. Immunosuppressed clients may have an infection with *Cryptosporidium* or other uncommon organisms.

Clinical Significance of C Difficile

C. difficile was first identified as normal flora in the gastrointestinal tract in the 1930s. The name was chosen because of the difficulty in culturing this spore-forming gram-positive anaerobic bacillus. In the past several years, *C. difficile* has become important as a cause of antibiotic-related pseudomembranous colitis. Colonoscopy (Chapter 27) may help diagnose pseudomembranous colitis. Clients may develop diarrhea up to 6–8 weeks after antibiotic therapy. Fever, pain, and a markedly elevated WBC (e.g., 50,000 mm^3) may be present. Toxins are released from the organism. Toxin A, an enterotoxin, can cause hemorrhage and fluid leakage in the gut. Toxin B is a very potent cytotoxin that decreases cellular protein synthesis. Not all cases are related to previous use of antibiotics as it may infect otherwise healthy people in the community. Recent reports suggest that the rate and severity of *C. difficile*–related disease has increased because a previously uncommon strain of *C. difficile* with variations in toxin genes has become more resistant to the antibacterial fluoroquinolones (McDonald et al., 2006). None of the commonly used tests can differentiate between the strains.

Laboratory tests include a stool culture assay for toxins A and B. Culture is not recommended because it is both costly and slow and does not identify toxicogenic strains. ELISA and PCR (Chapter 1) are newer methods of testing. Stopping antibiotic therapy will be enough treatment for some clients but most will need oral vancomycin or metronidazole (Grossman & Mager, 2010). Cholestyramine is used as an adjunct to treatment because it binds up the toxins. For refractory cases, nontoxigenic *C. difficile* strain may be administered to compete with the toxigenic strain (Oriola, 2006).

Clinical Significance of Vancomycin-Resistant Enterococcus (VRE)

Many types of enterococci live in the GI tract and stool, and perirectal–rectal cultures can determine if a person is colonized with them. Colonization does not mean the same as an infection. However, VRE colonization does pose a risk factor for the development of wound or urine infections. Bacteremia can occur, particularly in seriously ill clients. VRE, like other enterococci, generally does not cause respiratory infections. The identification and control of VRE requires surveillance studies.

Once VRE is discovered, the infection control nurse should be notified so appropriate education is given to the client and staff. Using contact precautions is very important for both *C. difficile* and VRE because both are capable of remaining viable on environmental surfaces.

Clinical Significance of Salmonella Infections

Two main clinical syndromes associated with infections from the various serotypes of *salmonella* are typhoid fever and the non-typhoid form known as food poisoning. Poultry contaminated with *salmonella* is a major avenue of transmission. Nurses need to educate clients about safe kitchen practices. Immunocompromised clients may want to purchase eggs pasteurized in the shell (Todd, 2006d).

Clinical Significance of the Rotavirus

The rotavirus is one of the several viruses that can cause gastroenteritis. Diarrhea can lead to death in infants and young children. A rapid test can detect the rotavirus antigen in a stool specimen (Snow, 2010).

The use of rotavirus vaccine has caused a significant decline in diarrhea-related deaths. In 2006, Mexico became one of the first countries worldwide to use the vaccine in its national program (Richardson et al., 2010).

Possible Nursing Diagnoses Related to Positive Stool Culture

Deficient Knowledge Related to Spread of Infection to Others

Depending on the type of pathogen in the stool, the nurse must make sure that the client does not spread the pathogens to others. Isolation is usually not required if clients can wash their hands properly and if the feces can quickly be flushed into the sewage system. Stool precautions are not needed for botulism, *C. perfringens* infection, or staph food poisoning. The nurse should be aware that the collection of stool and the focus on the anal area are often a source of embarrassment for the client. (Saving a stool is frowned on since the age of 2 years and the anal stage.) The client should not be made to feel "unclean" because of the extra precautions needed to protect others. Children are prone to spread disease because of poor hygiene. In fact, giardiasis has been called *daycare diarrhea*. Positive cultures for *C. difficile* have been obtained from hospital rooms up to 40 days after a client's discharge. The organism has been isolated from toilet seats, shelves where bedpans are stored, and numerous other locations. The organism also has been cultured from the hands of personnel caring for clients with *C. difficile* infection. Contact isolation should be used for presumed as well as confirmed cases. Alcohol does not kill spores, so handwashing should also include soap and water to mechanically remove spores (Todd, 2006b).

Deficient Knowledge Related to Effect of Drugs

Once appropriate therapy has been started, clients need follow-up stool samples to evaluate the effectiveness of the therapy. Some of the drugs used for intestinal pathogens cause gastrointestinal symptoms, so it is important that clients know what may be expected from the drug and what may be an indication that therapy is not being effective. Later stool samples may show a second type of pathogen present.

CULTURES OF CEREBROSPINAL FLUID AND OTHER FLUIDS

Specimens of CSF are obtained by means of lumbar puncture. CSF is sterile, and it is collected under sterile conditions. Various organisms may be responsible for meningitis, including *H. influenzae, N. meningitidis*, and *S. pneumoniae*. The first is common in infants and the last in adults. West Nile Virus (Chapter 14) may also be identified in CSF.

The laboratory performs an immediate smear to see if any organisms exist. The laboratory should be notified that CSF is going to the laboratory so that immediate analysis can begin. Specific identification of the organism may take 48–72 hours, although rapid tests can distinguish viral from bacterial meningitis in a shorter time. (See Chapter 25 on the procedure for lumbar puncture and tests on CSF.)

Cultures of Pleural Fluid, Peritoneal Fluid, and Joint Fluid

Pleural fluid, obtained by means of thoracentesis, can be cultured for possible bacterial growth, as can peritoneal fluid obtained at paracentesis (see Chapter 25). Joint fluid from a joint aspiration may also be cultured after preliminary Gram stains. The role of the nurse in carefully marking the specimens and sending them to the laboratory is discussed in the beginning of this chapter. Careful labeling is necessary for *all* specimens. If a urine specimen is not labeled correctly, it is usually possible to obtain another specimen, but it may be much less feasible to obtain a second specimen of any fluid that requires an invasive technique.

Questions

1. The laboratory reports a large number of gram-negative rods are present on the preliminary stain of a urine specimen. Which one of the following organisms is thus ruled out?
   a. *Escherichia coli*
   b. *Proteus* species
   c. *Neisseria gonorrhoeae*
   d. *Pseudomonas* species

2. A client's urine was sent to the laboratory for a C&S (culture and sensitivity). The report notes an S next to all the listed antibiotics except penicillin, which is marked with an R. An R next to the penicillin indicates
   a. Penicillin is the right drug for the urine infection
   b. The client is resistant to penicillin
   c. Penicillin must be increased to obtain a successful urine level
   d. The organisms in the culture were resistant to penicillin

3. Common bacteria that cause hospital-acquired infections are staphylococci and gram-negative rods. Which nursing action would be the most effective way to prevent these infections?
   a. Administering all prescribed antibiotics on time
   b. Emphasizing handwashing before and after caring for every client
   c. Isolating all clients with fevers of undetermined origin (FUO)
   d. Culturing all open wounds

4. An elderly client has undergone cultures of blood, urine, and sputum because of a persistent fever and general malaise. In planning care for the client, the nurse in the nursing home should
   a. Assess the fluid intake and determine how much fluid by mouth should be taken daily
   b. Move the client to a private room for isolation
   c. Encourage more activity to keep the client stimulated
   d. Use aspirin as needed to keep the temperature normal

5. Which of the following is a correct statement about the collection of urine for urine cultures?
   a. The meatus of a male client requires more cleaning than does the meatus of a female client
   b. A disinfectant is always used to clean the genital area before a clean-catch is performed
   c. A clean-catch urine specimen requires that the urine be caught in midstream
   d. Only a catheterized urine specimen is suitable for urine culture

6. The client has been having fever and chills from an unknown cause. He is to have blood cultures drawn twice. The nurse should be aware of which of the following?
   a. The skin over the venipuncture site must be prepared with an iodine solution to reduce contamination by skin flora.
   b. Two blood samples can be drawn at the same time if the specimens are drawn from two different sites.
   c. Blood cultures should not be drawn after a spike of fever or a chill.
   d. A positive confirmation of a diagnosis can be made in 24 hours.

7. Which of the following laboratory tests is very useful in identifying sepsis from a bloodstream infection?
   a. A low blood sugar
   b. A high lactate level
   c. A low bilirubin level
   d. A high platelet level

8. A client is to have a sputum specimen obtained because of a productive cough and fever. Which of the following instructions by the nurse is correct to tell the client?
   a. "Save as much sputum as you can in the next 2 hours because the laboratory needs at least an ounce (30 mL) of sputum."
   b. "Discard the first specimen in the morning because the secretions will not be fresh."
   c. "Saliva will be all right for a specimen if it hurts to cough deeply."
   d. "Rinse out your mouth before obtaining the specimen so bacteria from the mouth will be less numerous."

9. A client is to provide sputum specimens three times for AFB. If the preliminary report is positive, she will be on respiratory isolation to prevent the spread of
   a. Tuberculosis
   b. *Legionella pneumophila*
   c. Influenza
   d. *Pneumocystis carinii*

10. A 10-year-old client has come to see the school nurse for a sore throat. The concern for correctly identifying the cause of the sore throat is important because rheumatic fever or glomerulonephritis sometimes occurs after infection with which organism?
    a. Any of the staphylococci
    b. Group A β-hemolytic streptococci
    c. *Staphylococcus aureus*
    d. Any of the streptococci

11. A client has a Penrose drain inserted into an abdominal stab wound that is inflamed and draining around the drain. Which of the following measures would be the most appropriate for the nurse to obtain a specimen for wound culture?
    a. Swab the end of the Penrose drain
    b. Swab the base of the wound
    c. Use a needle and syringe to aspirate fluid
    d. Obtain a tissue biopsy specimen

12. A client with diabetes appears to have an eye infection. Which of the following actions by the visiting nurse is inappropriate?
    a. Using a sterile swab to collect some exudate and putting the swab into culture medium supplied by the laboratory
    b. Lightly touching the cornea with the swab to obtain the specimen

   c. Instructing the client not to rub his eye with his fingers

   d. Showing the client how to rinse off the exudate without contaminating the other eye

13. A 17-year-old client is concerned that he may have gonorrhea. He asks the nurse in the clinic how gonorrhea can be detected. The nurse should explain to him that the test for gonorrhea involves which of the following?

   a. Drawing blood by venipuncture for a serologic test

   b. Obtaining some secretions from the end of the penis

   c. Both urine and blood tests

   d. Only a finger stick for a blood sample

14. A client is to have a stool specimen collected because of a possible *Salmonella* infection. He just had a bowel movement in the bedside commode. Which action by the nurse is appropriate?

   a. Send a small portion of the stool in a waxed container to the laboratory

   b. Discard the stool because it was diarrhea rather than formed stool

   c. Use sterile gloves to transfer all the stool to a sterile container and send it to the laboratory

   d. Send the entire stool in a waxed container to the laboratory

References

Calianno, C. & Jakubek, P. (2006). Wound bed preparation: The key to success for chronic wounds, Part II. *Nursing 2006, 36*(3), 76–77.

Coffman, S. (2009). Late preterm infants and risk for RSV. *MCV, 34*(6), 378–384.

Cook, R. L., Hutchison, S., Østergaard, L., Braithwaite, R., & Ness, R. (2005). Systematic review: Noninvasive testing for *Chlamydia trachomatis* and *Neisseria gonorrhoeae*. *Archives of Internal Medicine, 142*(11), 914–925.

Dodge, M. (2010). SIRS: A systematic approach for medical surgical nurses to stop the progression to sepsis. *MEDSURG Nursing, 19*(1), 11–15.

Eckert, L. O. (2006). Acute vulvovaginitis. *New England Journal of Medicine, 355*(12), 1244–1252.

Fink, A. M. (2006). Endocarditis after valve replacement surgery. *American Journal of Nursing, 106*(2), 40–52.

Geva, A., Bornstein, I., Dan, M., Shoham, H., & Sobel, J. (2006). The VI-sense-vaginal discharge self-test to facilitate management of vaginal symptoms. *American Journal of Obstetrics and Gynecology, 195*(5), 1351–1356.

Goldrick, B. A. (2005). Infection in the older adult. *American Journal of Nursing, 105*(6), 31–34.

Grossman, S. & Mager, D. (2010). *Clostridium difficile*: Implications for nursing. *MEDSURG Nursing, 19*(3), 155–158.

Harris, T. A. (2010). Changing practice to reduce the use of urinary catheters. *Nursing 2010, 40*(2), 18–20.

Hatler, C., Hebden, J., Kaler, W., & Zack, J. (2010). Walk the walk to reduce blood stream infections. *American Nurse Today, 5*(1), 26–31.

Hay, W. W., Levin, M. J., Sondheimer, J. M., & Deterding, R. (Eds.). (2011). *Current diagnosis and treatment: Pediatrics* (20th ed.). New York: McGraw-Hill.

Hughes, N. L. (2006). Handwashing. *American Journal of Nursing, 106*(7), 96.

Jackson, M. M. (2006). Delayed diagnosis: The tuberculosis tragedy. *American Journal of Nursing, 106*(4), 13.

Jacobson, J. (2009). School nurses nationwide respond to influenza A (H1N1) outbreaks. *American Journal of Nursing, 109*(6), 19.

Katzung, B., Masters, S. B., & Trevor, A. J. (Eds.). (2009). *Basic and clinical pharmacology* (11th ed.). New York: McGraw-Hill.

Kulp, J. L., Chaudhry, S., Wiita, B., & Bachmann, G. (2008). The accuracy of women performing vaginal pH self-testing. *Journal of Women's Health, 17*(4), 523–526.

McDonald, L. C., Killgore, G. E., Thompson, A., Owens, R. C., Kazakova, S. V., Sambol, S. P., et al. (2006). An epidemic, toxin gene-variant strain of *Clostridium difficile. New England Journal of Medicine, 353*(23), 2433–2441.

McPhee, S. J., Papadakis, M. A., & Rabow, M. W. (Eds.). (2011). *Current medical diagnosis and treatment* (50th ed.). New York: McGraw-Hill.

Meyers, F. E. & Reyers, C. (2011). Blood cultures: 5 steps to doing it right, *Nursing 2011, 41*(3), 62–63.

Nelson, R. (2010). Drug resistant tuberculosis: Are rates declining or increasing? *American Journal of Nursing, 110*(10), 55–57.

Noble, D. B. (2009). Patient education on MRSA prevention and management: The nurses' vital role. *MEDSURG Nursing, 18*(6), 375–378.

Oriola, S. (2006). *C. difficile*: A menace in hospitals and homes alike. *Nursing 2006, 36*(8), 14–15.

Powers, K. A. & Burchell, P. L. (2010). Sepsis alert: Avoiding the shock. *Nursing 2010, 40*(4), 34–38.

Richardson, V., Hernandez-Pichardo, J., Quintanar-Solares, M., Esparza-Agular, M., Johnson, B., Gomez-Altamirano, C. M., et al. (2010). Effect of rotavirus vaccination on death from childhood diarrhea in Mexico. *The New England Journal of Medicine, 362*(4), 299–305.

Shalo, S. (2010). The war on tuberculosis. *American Journal of Nursing, 110*(7), 20–22.

Snow, M. (2009). On the lookout for listeriosis. *Nursing 2009, 39*(7), 59.

Snow, M. (2010). Rounding up rotavirus. *Nursing 2010, 40*(5), 56.

Todd, B. (2005). Legionella pneumonia. *American Journal of Nursing, 105*(11), 35–38.

Todd, B. (2006a). Beyond MRSA: VISA and VRSA. *American Journal of Nursing, 106*(4), 28–30.

Todd, B. (2006b). *Clostridium difficile*: Familiar pathogen, changing epidemiology. *American Journal of Nursing, 106*(5), 33–35.

Todd, B. (2006c). The QuantiFERON Gold test. *American Journal of Nursing, 106*(6), 33–37.

Todd, B. (2006d). The increasing risk of *salmonella* infections. *American Journal of Nursing, 106*(7), 35–37.

Wenger, J. E. (2010). Reducing rates of catheter associated urinary tract infection. *American Journal of Nursing, 110*(8), 40–46.

Wu, A. H. (Ed.). (2006). *Tietz clinical guide to laboratory tests* (4th ed.). St. Louis, MO: Saunders Elsevier.

Website

www.cdc.gov (Updates on tests for infectious diseases.)
www.labtestsonline.org (Updates on tests for H1N1 and rapid test for tuberculosis.)

Answers

1. c, 2. d, 3. b, 4. a, 5. c, 6. a, 7. b, 8. d, 9. a, 10. b, 11. c, 12. b, 13. b, 14. a

Therapeutic Drug Monitoring and Toxicology Screens

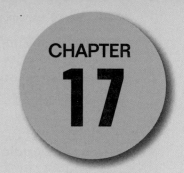

- Pharmacogenetic Testing for Drug Therapy   448
- Reasons for Monitoring Plasma Drug Levels   448
- Reasons for Not Monitoring   450
- Antibiotics: Aminoglycosides   452
- Antibiotics: Vancomycin   453
- Immunosuppressive Agents: Cyclosporine and Sirolimus   454
- Anticonvulsants   454
- Mood Stabilizer: Lithium Carbonate   457
- Tricyclic Antidepressants   457
- Bronchodilators: Theophylline Products   458
- Digoxin   459
- Antiarrhythmic Drugs   460
- Salicylates: Acetylsalicylic Acid   462
- Acetaminophen   463
- Blood Alcohol (Ethanol)   464
- Transdermal Monitoring of Alcohol Levels   465
- Barbiturates   466
- Toxicology Screens in Blood and Urine   466
- Saliva-Based Drug Tests   468
- Home Drug Test Kits   468
- Lead   468

OBJECTIVES

1. Discuss reasons for monitoring serum, urine, and saliva drug levels.
2. Describe how plasma peak and trough levels are used to monitor aminoglycoside levels.
3. Name four anticonvulsants that are sometimes monitored with serum levels and indicate the clinical symptoms of each that may indicate toxicity.
4. Identify the antipsychotic drug that must be monitored with serum drug levels to avoid toxicity.
5. Describe possible nursing diagnoses related to toxicity from antidepressants and other drugs.
6. Identify the two main clinical problems that may develop if a client has a serum theophylline level above the therapeutic range.
7. Identify which cardiac drugs are most commonly monitored with serum drug levels, along with the key nursing implications for each drug.
8. Describe clinical situations in which acetylsalicylic acid (ASA) serum levels are useful.

9. Identify the important facts that emergency department nurses should know about blood levels of alcohol and other depressant drugs.
10. Identify the usual medication history of a client who abuses drugs.
11. Describe current protocols for screening for lead poisoning in young children.

In clinical practice, the line between therapeutic effects and toxic effects may be narrow. The cardinal principle of experimental toxicology, first expressed by a 16th-century physician and alchemist, is that only the *dose* differentiates between a poison and a remedy. For example, digoxin in the correct dosage for an individual is therapeutic, but if the dose is increased even slightly, the drug may be extremely toxic. Measurements of arsenic, carbon monoxide, or lead (all poisons) are traditional examples of toxicologic tests.

Although any drug can be measured in the serum, this chapter focuses on drugs that are commonly measured and that have clinical significance for the nurse. Some general reasons for monitoring drugs, some of the pitfalls of using drug levels as assessment tools, and the general nursing implications when drug levels are used are discussed at the beginning of this chapter. Tests for specific drugs, along with any needed precautions about collection of the sample and about the specific nursing implications, are listed separately in the second part of this chapter.

PHARMACOGENETIC TESTING FOR DRUG THERAPY

In late 2004, FDA approved a DNA genetic test (AmpliChip CYP450) by Roche that analyzes two genes in the cytochrome P450 system that can markedly influence metabolism of drugs. Based on this analysis, the test classifies the client as poor, intermediate, extensive, or ultra rapid metabolizer of drugs. The majority of people are extensive metabolizers who have normal enzyme activity and thus handle standard drug doses well. Other people metabolize drugs at a slower or more rapid rate, so dosages should be adjusted accordingly or other drugs should be prescribed. Use of a medication regimen tailored to a specific genotype can prevent adverse reactions and optimize the correct dose of drugs such as antidepressants, beta blockers, chemotherapeutic drugs, or codeine for the client (Lea, 2005). At the present time, genotyping to guide medication selection and dosage is not in widespread use, but research is ongoing (Rebsamen et al., 2009). Some genetic tests for warfarin and clopidogrel are discussed in Chapter 13.

REASONS FOR MONITORING PLASMA DRUG LEVELS

When the Rate of Metabolism of a Drug Has a Wide Interindividual Variation

For some drugs, such as theophylline, the rate of metabolism may vary greatly, depending on metabolic variations in the individual. The dosage of theophylline must be tailored to fit the particular individual. For example, if a smoker becomes a nonsmoker, the theophylline dose may have to be decreased. Serum theophylline concentrations can be measured to make sure that the dosage is maintaining the correct serum level.

When Saturation Kinetics Occur

For some drugs, such as phenytoin, an increase in dosage beyond a certain point does not increase the effectiveness of the drug because the body is saturated. The actual pharmacokinetics of a drug may be very complex, and they are used to determine the serum level considered therapeutically effective.

When the Therapeutic Ratio of the Drug Is Close to the Toxic Level

If a drug leaves considerable leeway between its therapeutic effect and its toxic effect, careful monitoring with serum levels is usually not considered necessary. Lithium, however, is a good example of a drug that has a narrow margin of safety and that must be monitored.

When Signs of Toxicity Are Difficult to Recognize Clinically

Serum levels of certain drugs help detect or prevent toxicity that might otherwise not be noticed because of other clinical problems. An antiarrhythmic drug, such as quinidine, may depress the myocardium and cause symptoms that could be wrongly attributed to a worsening of the underlying cardiac disease rather than to the toxicity of the drug.

When Gastrointestinal, Hepatic, or Renal Disease Is Present

If gastrointestinal (GI) problems are present, any oral medication may have an erratic drug absorption. (Usually the drug would be ordered for parenteral administration to avoid this problem.) If hepatic disease is present, drugs that are metabolized by the liver—and almost all are—are not cleared from the serum normally. (See Chapter 12 on alanine aminotransferase [ALT] levels to assess liver damage.) Finally, because most drugs are excreted in the urine, renal disease means a problem with excretion. For example, the aminoglycoside antibiotics, if given at all, must be carefully monitored with serum levels when renal disease is present. (See Chapter 4 for assessment of renal function.)

When Drug Interactions Result from the Use of Several Drugs

Clients with epilepsy may take two types of anticonvulsants, both of which can cause central nervous system symptoms, such as lethargy and depression. It may not be at all clear which drug or combination of drugs is causing the toxic effects. A serum level of the drugs helps pinpoint the culprit.

When Noncompliance Is Suspected

Noncompliance means that a client is not taking a drug as ordered. The reasons for not taking a drug can be varied, including simple misunderstanding of the need. Clients for whom certain drugs are prescribed may be overly afraid of side effects, so they reduce the amount of drug prescribed or they "forget" to take the pill at certain times. Sometimes when clients are admitted to the hospital, they have a toxic reaction to a drug, such as digoxin, because in the hospital they are given it routinely every day as ordered. At home, the administration may not be on schedule. A home health nurse can be of assistance in visiting clients at home to determine whether noncompliance is a reason for erratic serum drug levels.

When an Overdose of an Unknown Substance or Substances Has Occurred

Therapeutic drugs, such as aspirin or barbiturates, are often taken in toxic amounts either accidentally (poisoning) or deliberately as a suicidal gesture. With drug experimentation, the client may have inhaled, ingested, or injected a variety of different drugs. The laboratory can screen serum, urine, and gastric contents to identify the chemicals present. In chronic poisoning with heavy metals, such as lead, the laboratory can identify the toxic substances in both the serum and the urine.

To Detect Abuse of Drugs for Legal Prosecution

The legal implications of the blood alcohol test are discussed in the section on alcohol tests. Other legal problems are discussed in the section on opiate abuse.

REASONS FOR NOT MONITORING

Although there are many reasons to monitor drugs, there are also reasons not to monitor them. One good reason is cost. If the drug is not particularly toxic and if the client responds well to the usual prescribed dosage, a serum drug level is unnecessary. For some drugs, the effect of the drug on other laboratory tests is more important than the actual serum level of the drug. For example, if the client is taking anticoagulants, either partial thromboplastin time (PTT) (for heparin) or prothrombin time (PT with INR) (for warfarin) is used to monitor the dosage of the respective anticoagulants. (See Chapter 13 on tests for coagulation.) If the client is undergoing insulin therapy, blood glucose levels are used to monitor drug effects, not the insulin level per se. (See Chapter 8 on glucose.)

Use of Laboratory Tests to Monitor for Unwanted Effects of Drugs

In addition to monitoring for the therapeutic effects of medications, laboratory tests may be needed to prevent adverse effects. For example, baseline levels of creatinine (Chapter 4) and potassium (Chapter 5) are needed for many drugs such as digoxin, diuretics, and potassium supplements, but Simon et al. (2005) found that clients who are prescribed certain cardiovascular medications did not always get the needed baseline monitoring. In other research studies, standard recommendations for creatinine, electrolytes, and tests such as ALT (Chapter 12) to monitor liver function or CBC (Chapter 2) to monitor hematological effects were often not followed at the initiation of therapy (Raebel et al., 2005). Lapses in laboratory monitoring of clients who are taking chronic medications have also been documented as a common problem (Hurley et al., 2005). Better tracking tools such as computerized reminders for prescribers and clients may help.

Caution in Interpretation

Because serum drug levels reflect only the amount of the drug in the plasma at a given time, the level may not reflect the actual physiologic activity of the drug. Laboratory tests of serum drugs measure both bound and unbound parts of the drug. A client with less albumin in the serum may thus have a larger amount of free drug in the serum. It is the free or unbound drug that is biologically active and is related to the amount of plasma proteins available for binding. (See Chapter 10 on the measurement of albumin.)

General Nursing Implications

Correct Sample Timing: Peaks, Troughs, and Steady States

Serum samples of drug levels may be ordered as peak levels, as trough levels, or after obtaining a steady state. For serum drug levels, peak times refer to measurements of the highest level of drug reached in the serum; trough times represent the lowest levels. Some laboratories may refer to the trough levels as residuals.

The *steady state* of a drug refers to the time when the plasma level has been stabilized with a maintenance dose. For some drugs, a steady state is not obtained for several days. A practical way to estimate the steady state is to multiply the half-life by 5, which gives the approximate time to reach 97% of the steady-state value. Each drug has its own distribution time and volume of distribution (VD) to the tissues. Some drugs have a small VD, which means they remain in the serum. Other drugs have a large VD, which means they are distributed to the tissues.

Controversy exists about whether peak or trough levels are better indicators of toxicity for specific drugs. In general, the peak is a determination of the rate of absorption of the drug, whereas the trough is a measurement of the drug's rate of elimination. A time table for drawing peak and trough levels for tobramycin is shown in Table 17–1.

Peak and trough levels of serum drug levels are meaningless unless it is known when the drug was given, the amount given, and the route. Knowing what other drugs are being taken by the client is also important, because they may interfere with some tests. If the client is being assessed for a steady state of the drug, make note not only of this information but also of the daily dosage that has been maintained for a certain period. (Also, question the client and make sure that the ordered dosage was, in fact, the dosage being taken at home.) In summary, the laboratory needs the following information:

1. The exact timing of the last dose of the drug
2. The exact amount of the drug given

(Continued)

3. The route of the drug (peak times change dramatically between oral and parenteral administration)
4. How long the client has been taking a certain dosage (if the client is being assessed for a steady-state level)
5. Other medications that may interfere with the specific test (check with the individual laboratory to determine this)

The information gained by serum drug levels is used primarily by the physician, who readjusts the dosage if needed. Nurses need to be aware of the reference values used in a particular setting, so that deviations from normal can be reported before another drug dosage is given. For example, if a trough level shows a range as high, or nearly as high, as the expected peak, continuing with the drug may be dangerous. Contacting the physician before the next dose of the drug is administered would be wise. Unless the information from the laboratory report is used in a timely way, the serum drug levels are only an expensive academic exercise that has no benefit to the client.

ANTIBIOTICS: AMINOGLYCOSIDES

Serum antibiotic levels are not routinely measured if the antibiotic is not usually toxic, if the infection is responding appropriately, and if the client does not have liver or renal dysfunction. For example, because penicillin and cephalosporins have a much wider range between therapeutic doses and toxic doses than do the antibiotics that are classified as aminoglycosides, clients taking penicillin or cephalosporins are not monitored with serum antibiotic levels.

All aminoglycosides have a central amino sugar—hence the name *aminoglycoside* (sugar). These antibiotics are used for serious infections with gram-negative bacteria, such as *Escherichia coli* and *Pseudomonas* species. (See Chapter 16 on cultures and sensitivities.) The aminoglycosides that are commonly monitored with serum levels are gentamicin, tobramycin, and amikacin (Deglin, Vallerand, & Sanoski, 2011).

Preparation of Client and Collection of Sample

The laboratory needs 1 mL of serum. Usually, blood samples for peak levels of antibiotics are drawn 30–60 minutes after completion of intravenous infusion of an antibiotic.

Table 17–1 Peak and Trough Levels

Timing of Medication	Peak to Be Drawn 30 Minutes After IV Infusion Completed	Trough to Be Drawn 5 Minutes Before Next Dose
Tobramycin 80 mg in 100 mL of D_5W q8h intravenously over 1 h		
8 AM–9 AM	Draw sample at 9:30 AM	Draw sample at 3:55 PM

Note: Check with individual laboratory for peak time for other drugs.

See Chapter 4 on serum creatinine levels also used to monitor drug nephrotoxicity.

The trough or residual level is measured immediately before the next dose of antibiotic is due. The nurse should check with the laboratory about exact trough and peak times. Table 17–1 gives an example of the timing of levels for tobramycin.

REFERENCE VALUES FOR AMINOGLYCOSIDES

Gentamicin, tobramycin	Peak, 4–8 µg/mL
	Trough, <2 µg/mL
Amikacin	Peak, 15–25 µg/mL
	Trough, <8 µg/mL

Possible Nursing Diagnoses for Aminoglycosides

Risk for Injury Related to Dizziness or Hearing Loss

The nurse needs to be aware that the aminoglycosides may cause nerve damage (neurotoxicity). The eighth cranial nerve is often affected by this group of antibiotics. Ototoxicity manifests itself mainly as vestibular dysfunction, but loss of hearing can occur and can be irreversible (Katzung, Masters, & Trevor, 2009). Involvement of the vestibular branch causes a lack of equilibrium. The client should be examined for any dizziness or lack of balance. Clients should also be examined for any hearing impairment.

Risk for Impaired Urinary Elimination

Aminoglycosides may cause renal damage (nephrotoxicity). Nephrotoxicity is more likely if renal function is not normal. Blood urea nitrogen (BUN) and creatinine tests are often used to monitor renal function while the client is taking aminoglycosides. (See Chapter 4 on BUN and creatinine.) The client must remain well hydrated, and the intake and output records must be carefully maintained.

ANTIBIOTICS: VANCOMYCIN

Oral vancomycin is not well absorbed, so it is not used for systemic infections. However, it has been useful for some GI infections, such as those caused by *Clostridium difficile* (see Chapter 16). Because of the development of vancomycin-resistant enterococci (VRE), other drugs may be used to treat *C. difficile*. Intravenous vancomycin is used for serious gram-positive infections that do not respond to less toxic antibiotics, such as penicillin or cephalosporins. Although not an aminoglycoside, vancomycin can also cause damage to the eighth cranial nerve (ototoxicity) and to the kidneys (nephrotoxicity).

Preparation of Client and Collection of Sample

The laboratory needs 1 mL of serum. Trough levels are drawn 30 minutes before the next intravenous dose is started. Peak levels have no clinical significance.

IMMUNOSUPPRESSIVE AGENTS: CYCLOSPORINE AND SIROLIMUS

As a potent immunosuppressive agent, cyclosporine has dramatically increased the success rate of organ transplants. In addition to having serum cyclosporine levels measured periodically, the client undergoes renal function tests (see Chapter 4 on BUN and serum creatinine) and liver function tests (see Chapter 12 on ALT). Unwanted effects include nephrotoxicity, increased hair growth, and transient liver dysfunction (Katzung et al., 2009). Hyperlipidemia (Chapter 9) and hyperglycemia (Chapter 8) may also occur. Sirolimus, another immunosuppresant, may be given in combination with cyclosporine and corticosteroids (Chapter 15).

Preparation of Client and Collection of Sample

Cyclosporine adheres tenaciously to plastic, so samples should not be drawn from any catheter that has been used for infusion of the drug. Blood samples for both cyclosporine (2 mL) and sirolimus (3 mL) are collected in lavender-topped tubes. Cyclosporine levels may be drawn at 12 and/or 24 hours after dosage. Sirolimus levels are drawn just before the next dose.

REFERENCE VALUE FOR CYCLOSPORINE AND SIROLIMUS

Therapeutic levels 12 hours after dose of cyclosporine

Renal transplant	100–400 mg/mL
Cardiac transplant	100–300 mg/mL
Bone marrow transplant	100–250 mg/mL
Therapeutic level for sirolimus	12–14 mg/mL (trough levels)

Note: References are from Wu (2006). Other sources may have different values.

ANTICONVULSANTS

Phenytoin

Phenytoin is the most common drug used to treat various types of epilepsy. It may be used alone or in combination with other anticonvulsants discussed in this section. Phenytoin is also used as an antiarrhythmic agent for certain types of cardiac irregularities. (See the section on antiarrhythmic drugs.)

Fosphenytoin, a prodrug formulation, becomes active phenytoin in the body. A significant advantage of fosphenytoin is that it is water soluble and can be administered intramuscularly as well as intravenously.

Clients may have serum phenytoin levels measured to determine the proper dose for long-term therapy. It takes at least 1 week to achieve stable serum phenytoin levels.

Serum levels are related to certain side effects. In general, nystagmus (involuntary rapid movements of the eyeballs) appears when serum phenytoin levels are greater than 20 µg/mL. Gait ataxia occurs at about 30 µg/mL, and constant lethargy occurs when the level is about 40 µg/mL.

Preparation of Client and Collection of Sample

The laboratory needs 1 mL of serum. Record the time of the last dose, the route, and the amount of phenytoin. Caffeine, theophylline, probenecid, warfarin, and quinidine interfere with the results.

REFERENCE VALUES FOR PHENYTOIN	
10–20 µg/mL	As an anticonvulsant*
10–18 µg/mL	As an antiarrhythmic

*Some clients remain free of seizures at serum levels below 10 µg/mL and others may need above 20 µg/mL to control seizures (Roach & Roach, 2005).

Free Phenytoin

Phenytoin is strongly bound to albumin, so when the client has a low serum albumin level (Chapter 10), the amount of active or "free" phenytoin is increased in the bloodstream and may lead to toxicity. Thus, an algorithm for monitoring phenytoin uses the albumin level and its ratio to total phenytoin to determine if the free phenytoin test is appropriate. In clients with hypoalbuminemia or significant renal disease (Chapter 4) or hyperbilirubinemia (Chapter 11), the free phenytoin is more accurate for monitoring.

REFERENCE VALUE FOR FREE PHENYTOIN
1–2 µg/mL

Valproic Acid

Valproic acid, an oral anticonvulsant, is also used to treat bipolar affective disorder (Deglin et al., 2011). Because valproic acid has a short biologic half-life, the time of the last dose and the time of the sampling must be considered carefully when judging the clinical effect from a certain concentration. Liver toxicity can occur. (See Chapter 12 on liver enzymes.)

Preparation of Client and Collection of Sample

The laboratory needs 0.5–1.0 mL of venous blood in a green-, gray-, lavender-, or blue-topped tube. A steady state is achieved in 2–3 days. There may be some fluctuation of serum values even with a steady state.

REFERENCE VALUE FOR VALPROIC ACID

Therapeutic range   50–100 µg/mL

Note: Free valproic acid is about 2.5–11 µg/mL (Wu, 2006).

Phenobarbital

Phenobarbital is a long-acting barbiturate (see later discussion of barbiturate panel) that is sometimes used in conjunction with other anticonvulsants.

Preparation of Client and Collection of Sample

The laboratory needs 1 mL of serum. Because phenobarbital is long acting and cumulative, the client's daily dose should be recorded. A tolerance to high levels of phenobarbital can develop if the increase is gradual. A steady state may take 8–15 days for children and 10–25 days for adults. Phenobarbital has interactions with many other drugs.

REFERENCE VALUES FOR PHENOBARBITAL

Therapeutic range   For anticonvulsant control 15–50 mg/L
Newborn   Levels > 40 mg/L may cause apnea

Carbamazepine

Carbamazepine, used for seizure control, can itself cause seizures if the serum level is greater than the therapeutic range. The most widely feared side effect is bone marrow depression, which is rare but can occur. Clients need monitoring with a complete blood count (CBC) (Chapter 2) and platelet counts (Chapter 13). Carbamazepine is also used as a mood stabilizer and for relief of chronic pain.

Preparation of Client and Collection of Sample

The laboratory needs 0.5 mL of serum. It takes about 2 weeks for carbamazepine to reach a steady state. Many drugs can interfere with this test.

REFERENCE VALUE FOR CARBAMAZEPINE

Therapeutic range   4–12 mg/mL

Possible Nursing Diagnosis for Anticonvulsant Therapy

Risk for Injury Related to Gait Disturbance or Seizure Activity

Most of the anticonvulsants in higher-than-therapeutic levels in the bloodstream can lead to ataxia, gait disturbances, dizziness, and drowsiness. Attention to safety is warranted. Injury from seizures is also a possibility, so clients need to carry identification about their seizure disorder and instruct significant others how to manage a seizure. Clients need to maintain a seizure calendar that documents the occurrence and type of all seizures and bring it to each healthcare appointment. Over the years, there is less of a tendency for fully controlled seizures to return, and it is likely that lower serum levels will continue to be effective (Hay et al., 2011).

MOOD STABILIZER: LITHIUM CARBONATE

Lithium is a psychotherapeutic agent used to treat the manic state of some types of bipolar disorder (manic depressive disorder). When the dosage is being adjusted, blood samples are drawn one to two times a week. Blood for the serum level may be drawn 8–12 hours after the drug is given. After a therapeutic dosage has been established, the client may have serum lithium levels measured every 2–3 months (Deglin et al., 2011).

Preparation of Client and Collection of Sample

The laboratory needs 1 mL of serum. Lithium samples are drawn 8–12 hours after dosage. Record the amount, route, and time of the last dose on the laboratory request.

REFERENCE VALUE FOR LITHIUM

Therapeutic range	0.5–1.5 mEq/L or 0.5–1.5 mmol/L (SI units)

Possible Nursing Diagnosis for Lithium Levels

Risk for Injury Related to Toxicity or Adverse Reactions

Lithium toxicity is a very serious problem. In some clients, particularly the elderly, neurotoxicity can develop even with normal serum levels. Hence, clients must be assessed for such symptoms as diarrhea, vomiting, muscle weakness, and lack of coordination. An important nursing implication is to make sure that these clients have normal amounts of salt because lithium toxicity may be greater if serum sodium levels are low. Diuretics should not be used. (See Chapter 5 on diets with high sodium content.) Hypothyroidism (Chapter 15) is one of the chronic adverse reactions.

TRICYCLIC ANTIDEPRESSANTS

The tricyclic antidepressant drugs represent a frequent and serious problem in both unintentional and intentional overdosage. These drugs may take as long as 1 month to relieve depression, and dosage adjustments vary from person to person. The laboratory may measure both the drug and its active metabolite and report the sum of the active drugs. Some of the active metabolites are also available as primary drugs. For example, desipramine is an active metabolite of imipramine and nortriptyline of amitriptyline. Most clients on antidepressants do not need serum monitoring unless the clinical response has been disappointing. High blood levels are not more effective than moderate levels and may cause more unwanted effects (McPhee, Papadakis, & Rabow, 2011).

Preparation of Client and Collection of Sample

The laboratory needs 3 mL of serum in a red-topped tube. For once-a-day dosages, the specimen should be drawn about 10–14 hours after dosage. For divided doses, the specimen can be drawn 4–6 hours after the last dosage. The steady state is obtained about 1 week after therapy is begun, but clinical improvement may not be noted for *several* weeks. Many drugs may interfere with the test.

REFERENCE VALUES FOR ANTIDEPRESSANTS	
Imipramine	150–250 ng/mL
Desipramine	50–300 ng/mL
Amitriptyline	80–250 ng/mL
Nortriptyline	50–150 ng/mL
Doxepin	110–250 ng/mL

Note: See Wu (2006).

Possible Nursing Diagnosis for Antidepressants

Risk for Injury Related to Possible Adverse Reactions of Antidepressant Drugs

A client taking antidepressant drugs needs careful assessment for adverse reactions, which can include cardiotoxicity and orthostatic hypotension. Clients who take these drugs are suffering from clinical depression, so usual client teaching may be difficult. Significant others must be educated about ways to decrease problems from long-term use. Deglin et al. (2011) recommends baseline and periodic electrocardiograms (ECGs) for elderly clients, clients with heart disease, and children being treated with imipramine for enuresis. See Chapter 24 on ECG.

BRONCHODILATORS: THEOPHYLLINE PRODUCTS

Theophylline and its derivatives, such as aminophylline and dyphylline, are used as bronchodilators. Once used as a primary drug for asthma, theophylline is now used only if other drugs such as the corticosteroids and β-2-agonists are not effective. The low cost of theophylline is an advantage (Katzung et al., 2009).

Because high serum levels of theophylline can result in life-threatening cardiac arrhythmias and seizures, the safest approach to individualize dosages of theophylline or theophylline products is to monitor serum levels. Clients who have abnormal liver function, have congestive heart failure (CHF), or are very young or very old may need very close monitoring of serum theophylline levels.

Preparation of Client and Collection of Sample

The laboratory needs 3 mL of serum. Since theophylline and caffeine are xanthines, the client should not have coffee, colas, tea, chocolate, or any other source of caffeine for several hours before the serum specimen is drawn. After a steady state is achieved, serum peak levels should be drawn 30 minutes after intravenous dosage, 2 hours after a regular oral dosage, and 5 or more hours after the slow-release forms are given.

Possible Nursing Diagnosis for Theophylline Levels

Risk for Injury Related to Overdosage

Nurses should be aware of early clinical symptoms of theophylline overdose; because theophylline is a xanthine, as is caffeine, some of the early symptoms of theophylline toxicity resemble a "coffee jag." Clients may have tachycardia with skipped beats. They may also be nervous and jittery, with tremors of the hands. Headache, dizziness, and vomiting may signal toxicity. The dosage of theophylline must be adjusted to prevent development of dangerous cardiac arrhythmias or seizures.

REFERENCE VALUES FOR THEOPHYLLINE

Therapeutic range	10–20 µg/mL
Risk of toxicity	>20 µg/mL

DIGOXIN

Digoxin, a cardiotonic agent used to treat CHF, slows the heart rate and thus may also be used in the treatment of atrial fibrillation, atrial flutter, and paroxysmal atrial tachycardia (Deglin et al., 2011). Digoxin has a long half-life, and thus serious toxicity can occur over time.

Preparation of Client and Collection of Sample

The laboratory needs 1 mL of serum. The dosage route and time of the last dose should be included on the requisition. Amiodarone, verapamil, and quinidine can increase serum digoxin levels by 100%, so dosage adjustments are necessary to prevent toxicity (McPhee et al., 2011).

REFERENCE VALUES FOR DIGOXIN

Therapeutic range	
Digoxin	0.8–1.5 ng/mL for CHF[a]

[a]Slightly higher therapeutic ranges (1.5–2.0 ng/mL) may be desirable for treating atrial fibrillation (Wu, 2006).

> ## Possible Nursing Diagnosis for Digoxin
>
> ### Risk for Injury Related to Digoxin Toxicity
>
> To prevent digoxin toxicity, the key nursing implication is to monitor the client's pulse before digoxin is given. Digoxin, or other digitalis products, should be withheld and the physician notified if the adult's pulse is less than 60 beats per minute or a new irregularity is noted. Usually, a pulse less than 70 beats per minute is the guideline for children, but this criterion varies depending on age. Clients should be taught to take their own pulses because once digoxin is begun, it is usually continued on a long-term basis. Other symptoms of digitalis toxicity—such as nausea and vomiting, diarrhea, headaches, and visual disturbance—are also used to signal digitalis toxicity because toxicity can occur with normal serum levels. An ECG also helps the clinician determine whether there is a toxic effect from digoxin. However, the symptoms of mild toxicity from digoxin may not be readily detected with clinical assessment or ECG data. A measurement of serum levels of digoxin therefore aids in determining whether symptoms are due to a higher-than-necessary digoxin level.
>
> Other laboratory tests important in assessing for digoxin toxicity are the serum potassium, magnesium, and calcium levels. The nurse needs to be aware that a low serum potassium or magnesium and a high serum calcium level tend to increase the risk of digitalis toxicity, even though the serum digoxin levels are not high. (See Chapter 5 on potassium level and Chapter 7 on magnesium and calcium levels.) Because digoxin is excreted by the kidneys, clients with poor renal function are prone to digitalis toxicity. (See Chapter 4 on tests of renal function: BUN and creatinine.)

ANTIARRHYTHMIC DRUGS

Quinidine

Quinidine is an alkaloid obtained from the bark of the cinchona tree. Hence, toxicity from quinidine products is sometimes referred to as *cinchonism*. Because quinidine depresses the excitability of the heart, it is used as an antiarrhythmic drug. Serum quinidine levels help the clinician adjust the dosage to the correct amount for the individual client. In fact, quinidine is the antiarrhythmic drug most often monitored with serum levels. Because the toxicity may not be readily apparent or may be attributed to other causes, serum levels can be used to ascertain whether a client's drug level is in a therapeutic range.

Preparation of Client and Collection of Sample

The dosage, the time of the last dose, and the route should all be recorded on the lab requisition. The laboratory needs 1 mL of serum. Concurrent use of phenytoin or barbiturates may lower the serum quinidine level.

REFERENCE VALUES FOR QUINIDINE

Therapeutic range	2–5 µg/mL
Toxic range	>6 µg/mL

> ## Possible Nursing Diagnosis for Quinidine
>
> ### Risk of Injury Related to Adverse Effects of Drug
>
> Nurses should be aware that quinidine, a class I-A antiarrhythmic drug, can cause bradycardia and hypotension, so vital signs must be monitored. A few clients experience a syndrome called *quinidine syncope* because of a disorganized type of ventricular tachycardia (*torsade de pointes*). (See Chapter 24 on ECG assessments of arrhythmias.) Diarrhea and nausea are the most common noncardiac adverse reactions to quinidine. Headache, dizziness, and tinnitus, which may signify the development of cinchonism, should be reported immediately to the healthcare provider. As with all antiarrhythmic drugs, client teaching is crucial.

Procainamide and NAPA

Procainamide is usually given orally for long-term prevention of arrhythmias. As with quinidine products, serum levels help prevent toxicity such as myocardial depression. Some laboratories also measure N-acetyl procainamide (NAPA), the active metabolite of procainamide.

Preparation of Client and Collection of Sample

The dosage, the route, and the time of administration of the last dose should be recorded on the laboratory request. The level is usually drawn just before the next dose is given.

> ### REFERENCE VALUES FOR PROCAINAMIDE AND NAPA
>
> | | |
> |---|---|
> | Procainamide therapeutic level | 4–10 µg/mL |
> | NAPA therapeutic level | 2–8 µg/mL |

> ## Possible Nursing Diagnosis for Procainamide
>
> ### Risk for Injury Related to Adverse Effects of Drug
>
> Monitoring of vital signs is essential to assess for adverse cardiovascular effects of this class I-A antiarrhythmic. Note that all antiarrhythmics may also be proarrhythmic. (See Chapter 24 on monitoring for arrhythmias.) Like quinidine, procainamide can also cause diarrhea and other GI symptoms. Because the drug may also cause a lupus-like syndrome, the client may have antinuclear antibody (ANA) titers (Chapter 14) drawn periodically.

Phenytoin

Although phenytoin is more commonly used as an anticonvulsant, it is also sometimes used to control cardiac arrhythmias, such as those caused by digitalis toxicity. (See the reference values in the section on anticonvulsant drugs.)

Lidocaine

Lidocaine is given intravenously for the immediate control of premature ventricular contractions (PVCs). Because lidocaine is usually given only on an intermittent basis when the need arises, lidocaine levels are seldom measured. If clients have a continuous lidocaine drip, there may be a need to monitor serum levels if arrhythmias persist or if lidocaine toxicity is suspected.

Preparation of Client and Collection of Sample

Note the concentration of the drug and the rate of intravenous administration on the laboratory request. Lidocaine samples of 2 mL may be collected in a serum separator tube (SST), but green-, blue-, gray-, or lavender-topped tubes are also acceptable.

REFERENCE VALUES FOR LIDOCAINE

Therapeutic ranges

    Lidocaine   1.5–5.0 mg/L

Possible Nursing Diagnosis for Lidocaine

Risk for Injury Related to Adverse Effects or Toxicity

Although unwanted cardiac effects are less likely than with the class I-A antiarrhythmic medications quinidine and procainamide, vital signs must be closely monitored as must the ECG when lidocaine is given intravenously. (See Chapter 24 on ECG monitoring.) Overdosages of lidocaine and tocainide, which are class I-B antiarrhythmics, tend to cause central nervous system depression, which can lead to slurred speech, confusion, and even convulsions.

SALICYLATES: ACETYLSALICYLIC ACID

Acetylsalicylic acid (ASA) is used as an antipyretic, as an analgesic, as an anti-inflammatory agent, and as an anti-platelet. ASA is used as a regular medication for clients who are at risk for thromboembolic episodes. See Chapter 13 for tests for aspirin resistance. ASA is a component of many over-the-counter (OTC) pain relievers. ASA poisoning is the most common type of poisoning in children. Adults may also take ASA or ASA-containing drugs in a suicidal gesture. In an overdose, the laboratory can screen a serum sample to see whether ASA is the culprit. (If an overdose has occurred, gastric contents and urine specimens should be sent to the laboratory, if available.)

Mild intoxication, or salicylism, causes a ringing in the ears (tinnitus) and gastric upsets. Because ASA acts as a respiratory stimulant, the hyperventilation that may result from aspirin overdose can cause respiratory alkalosis with a metabolic acidosis. (See Chapter 6 on acid–base balance.) Large doses of ASA also may cause GI bleeding, which is due to the irritant effect on the gastric mucosa and due to interference with coagulation factors.

Preparation of Client and Collection of Sample

The laboratory needs 2 mL of plasma, collected in a heparin (green-topped) or EDTA (lavender-topped) tube. In the case of an overdose, urine, vomitus, or gastric lavage should be saved for laboratory analysis.

REFERENCE VALUES FOR SALICYLATES	
Toxic range	
Children and adults	>30 mg/dL
Older than 60 years	>20 mg/dL

ACETAMINOPHEN

Serum levels are not necessary when acetaminophen is routinely used as an antipyretic and analgesic. Serum levels are measured if an overdose has occurred because toxic levels may cause liver damage. The overdose may be accidental or intentional. Accidental overdosage has become a problem because many pain and flu medications contain acetaminophen and people may not be aware that they should never take more than 4 grams of acetaminophen in 24 hours. Research has shown that even 4 grams daily in some healthy people is associated with increased ALT levels (Watkins et al., 2006). Nurses need to inform clients about the warning labels on medications containing acetaminophen. See www.liverfoundation.org for more information about acetaminophen. The level of the drug in the serum, 4 or more hours after ingestion, determines the need for acetylcysteine therapy to protect the liver. Times may vary if extended-release acetaminophen tablets were taken or if there was co-ingestion of drugs that delay gastric emptying such as opioids or anticholinergics. The current protocol for treatment of acetaminophen poisoning is oral N-acetylcysteine based on the serum levels of acetaminophen and elevation of liver enzymes. Oral acetylcysteine is as effective as the IV form, but smells like rotten eggs, so many clients are unable to tolerate it (Lopez, 2009). Information about dosage calculation of the IV form is available at www.acetadote.net. Follow-up care includes monitoring the liver enzyme ALT (Chapter 12) for several days. (See Chapter 6 on lactic acid in drug-induced liver failure.)

Preparation of Client and Collection of Sample

Collect 1 mL of serum in an SST. Record time of ingestion and amount of drug ingested, if known. Samples drawn 4 and 12 hours after ingestion are used for treatment decisions. Acetaminophen is also part of a coma panel.

REFERENCE VALUES FOR ACETAMINOPHEN	
Therapeutic	10–20 mg/L
Toxic (4 hours after ingestion)	>150 mg/L
Toxic (12 hours after ingestion)	>40 mg/L

BLOOD ALCOHOL (ETHANOL)

Ethanol, or grain alcohol, is the type of alcohol in alcoholic beverages. Ethanol, undoubtedly the most commonly abused drug, may often be one of the drugs involved in an overdose. As part of a toxicology screen, the laboratory may perform an alcohol panel that, in addition to ethanol, includes methanol (wood alcohol), isopropyl (rubbing alcohol), and acetone (an alcohol-related compound). A serum osmolality test (Chapter 4) may also be used to screen for ethanol or methanol. Alcohol and related toxic compounds may be ingested by drinking undrinkable solutions, such as cleaning fluids, shaving lotions, or disinfectants. Methanol is particularly dangerous because it can result in convulsions, blindness, and possibly death.

In addition to determining the cause of a coma, blood alcohol tests are also used to determine whether a driver was intoxicated at the time of a collision. The drawing of the blood specimen must be performed in a medically suitable environment according to the legal requirements of the state. (Breath analyzers are used at the scene of the collision, so nurses are not involved in obtaining samples.) Nurses who are trained in venipuncture may draw the blood for alcohol blood samples when the client is brought to the emergency department for medical treatment. The reluctance to involve hospital staff in drawing blood for legal evidence is based on the fact that the people drawing the blood may not know the exact legal ramifications of the procedure and that they will probably be subpoenaed to testify in a court case. Although it is permissible for qualified nurses to draw blood for the alcohol test, it is important that they understand the legal ramifications of the procedure and the policy for nurses in a particular institution. Blood may be drawn without consent in some states if it is drawn in a legally and medically accepted manner. A refusal to allow blood to be drawn may have legal consequences. Healthcare providers must be aware of their current state statutes regarding testing procedures.

Legal Definitions of Intoxication

The 21-year-old minimum drinking age has been the nationwide law since 1986, but until recently the blood alcohol concentration (BAC) to define illegal driving under age 21 varied from state to state. Organizations such as Mothers Against Drunk Drivers (MADD), founded in California in 1980, have been instrumental in getting these laws changed. In 1995, Congress passed legislation that required by 1999 all states would adapt "zero tolerance" laws for drivers under 21. The logic was that since drinking is illegal for anyone younger than 21, no alcohol is tolerated for these drivers. MADD is now working on legislation to require ignition devices or in-car breathalyzers, which require convicted drunk drivers to prove that they are sober before their car will start. See www.MADD.org for states that have enacted laws for the use of these devices.

Until 2000, each state continued to define the legal limit of BAC for intoxication in drivers over age 21. Less than 20 states had as low a level as 0.08%. Most were set at 0.10%. Due again to the lobbying from MADD, a federal bill, passed in 2000, made 0.08% BAC the national standard for conviction of driving under the influence (DUI) of alcohol.

Relation of Alcohol to Other Laboratory Tests

In addition to the usual symptoms of alcohol intoxication, a client who abuses alcohol may have severe hypoglycemia, because alcohol tends to inhibit the formation of glucose. (See Chapter 8 for symptoms and treatment of hypoglycemia.) Alcohol-induced hypoglycemia carries a high mortality if not identified and corrected. The mortality is particularly high for children. High blood alcohol levels are also an important cause of secondary hyperlipidemia. (See Chapter 9 on serum triglyceride levels.) If ethanol levels are not readily available, the ethanol concentration may be estimated by calculating the osmolar gap, as discussed in Chapter 4 on serum osmolality.

Preparation of Client and Collection of Sample

The client should give consent for collection of a blood specimen, but blood may be drawn without consent in some states if it is drawn in a legally and medically accepted manner. Be aware of the legal ramifications, state requirements, and the individual hospital's policy. No alcohol, such as alcohol wipes, should be used to obtain the blood specimen. Iodine or an aqueous germicidal solution such as benzalkonium can be used. Tinctures should not be used, because they have an alcohol base. The specimen should be refrigerated if it cannot be sent to the laboratory immediately. See information about chain-of-custody protocol under the section on toxicology screens.

REFERENCE VALUES FOR BLOOD ALCOHOL LEVELS

Ethanol or ethyl (grain) alcohol

0.00%	Legal limit, under age 21
0.08%	Legal limit, over age 21
0.30–0.40%	Marked intoxication
0.40–0.50%	Severe toxic effects with alcoholic stupor[a]
≥0.50%	Coma and death possible

Methanol or methyl (wood) alcohol

25 mg/dL	Toxic level
80–115 mg/dL	Lethal

[a]Clients who chronically abuse alcohol may be awake with these levels.

TRANSDERMAL MONITORING OF ALCOHOL LEVELS

Rehabilitation programs for clients recovering from alcohol abuse may use assessments such as laboratory tests for GGT and CDT (Chapter 12) and MCV (Chapter 2) to identify continuing alcohol use. Another way to validate the success or failure of an alcohol rehabilitation effort is monitoring at home by an electronic device worn 24/7 by the client. Secure continuous remote alcohol monitor (SCRAM) is a lightweight, tamper-resistant, and water-resistant ankle bracelet to monitor and record the amount of alcohol permeating through the skin. A modem in the client's home, using radio frequency signals, sends the stored data from the bracelet to SCRAMNET by a standard telephone line (www.alcoholmonitoring.com).

BARBITURATES

The barbiturates are used as anticonvulsants and infrequently as sedatives or hypnotics. Phenobarbitol is sometimes used in assisted suicide and to execute condemned criminals. The most severe effect of overdose with barbiturates is respiratory failure followed by circulatory collapse. Because the various barbiturates are often used in overdoses, the laboratory runs a barbiturate panel when clients are comatose from an unknown cause. The barbiturates usually measured include the following:

1. Short-acting—pentobarbital and secobarbital
2. Intermediate-acting—amobarbital
3. Long-acting—phenobarbital

A smaller amount of the short-acting barbiturates, as opposed to a larger amount for the long-acting barbiturates, causes coma. A toxicology screen for barbiturate overdose also includes an analysis of urine samples and, if requested, gastric contents. Any vomitus or gastric lavage products should be saved for laboratory analysis.

Preparation of Client and Collection of Sample

The laboratory needs 5 mL or less of serum, depending on the method used. Note any drugs that the client may have taken. Theophylline, for example, can cause a false elevation of the barbiturate level, as can valproic acid.

REFERENCE VALUES FOR BARBITURATES

Short-acting barbiturates	Coma level at about 5 mg/L
Long-acting barbiturates	Coma level at about 40 mg/L

Note: See the section on anticonvulsants for the measurement of therapeutic levels of phenobarbital.

TOXICOLOGY SCREENS IN BLOOD AND URINE

The following drugs may be tested for serum or urine screening:

1. Opioids (codeine, morphine, etc.)
2. Phenothiazines (prochlorperazine, chlorpromazine, etc.)
3. Tricyclic antidepressants (imipramine, amitriptyline, etc.)
4. Stimulants (amphetamines, methylphenidate, etc.)
5. Benzodiazepines (diazepam, etc.)
6. Phencyclidine (PCP)
7. Cocaine (as benzoylecgonine metabolite)
8. Marijuana (THC)

9. Nicotine (measured as serum or urinary cotinine)
10. Barbituates
11. Methaqualone
12. Propoxyphene
13. Methadone
14. MDMA (Ecstasy)

As a result of the Joint Commission patient safety issues, many clinical agencies may require drug screening for employees and other healthcare workers, such as nursing students who engage in providing care to clients.

Preparation of Client and Collection of Sample

A urine sample of 50–100 mL is needed for a complete toxicology screen. Check with the individual laboratory. A large amount of blood, 20–30 mL, collected in several types of tubes is needed for a comprehensive drug screen or coma panel. These serum panels are expensive and may require specific approval from the laboratory. Individual screens of drugs may be performed if the type of drug is known.

Gastric secretions and urine are the best samples for broad qualitative studies. Blood samples should be saved for possible quantitative testing, but blood is not a good specimen for screening for many common drugs. Urine is a good medium for drug testing and storage because there are very few active proteins or enzymes in urine that degrade the drug. Many drugs are stable in urine when frozen, for many years. A regional poison control center should be consulted to help select testing and treatment methods. Individual poison control centers can be reached by dialing 1-800-222-1222. This hotline is provided by the Nationwide Poison Control Center. Healthcare providers need to realize that toxicology screens become part of a permanent medicolegal record and may be important in suspected cases of homicide, assault, or child abuse.

Chain-of-Custody Protocol

Nurses must be aware of needed checks and precautions to prevent substitution or tampering with a sample. Specimens must be sealed and signed by the client and the healthcare provider collecting the sample. Chain-of-custody forms are used to document and ensure sample integrity from collection, through transport to the laboratory, and during analysis and reporting.

Possible Nursing Diagnosis Related to Increased Drug Levels, Including Alcohol

Disturbed Sensory Perception

The focus for nursing intervention is to promote a sense of reality by explaining environmental stimuli and also reducing those stimuli. Because the altered perceptions may be frightening, the client needs reassurance of safety and protection by healthcare workers. Long-term management of drug abuse necessitates other nursing diagnoses based on the individual client's needs and coping methods.

SALIVA-BASED DRUG TESTS

Saliva can be used to screen for drugs of abuse. This oral fluid (OF) analysis is sometimes called the "lollipop" method because the client puts the stick with the testing swab in the mouth for 2–3 minutes until the swab is saturated with saliva. The swab is placed in a testing cradle that registers the bars as negative or positive. Current saliva tests can test for most drugs of abuse. The ease of the test as point-of-care testing and the near-inability to cheat (the healthcare provider remains with the client) are advantages over urine screening. Several recent studies support the utility of the saliva test, but the gold standard for detecting recent marijuana use is urinalysis (Yacoubian & Wish, 2006).

HOME DRUG TEST KITS

The FDA sanctions drug testing for "personal use" as long as the kit meets performance standards. In the beginning, home drug test kits had to have a prepaid laboratory option to confirm "positive" test results as false-positive results may occur. Some kits are available without the follow-up option, so they cost less. For example, one kit tests for the six drugs most commonly offered to youngsters aged 11–18. The advertisements do make the point that test kits must be used with love and communication in order to achieve the goal of no drug use.

LEAD

Among children, lead toxicity is second only to malnutrition as a public health problem in the United States. Exposure to lead is an occupational hazard for some adults. Lead poisoning in children is mostly from contaminated house dust, and prevention programs are ongoing to educate families about risks in older houses (Brown et al., 2006). Lead freely crosses the placenta and can affect the developing fetus (Cleveland et al., 2008a). Children also ingest lead by chewing on toys or jewelry that contain lead or drinking from pottery that has a lead base. Also lead toxicity secondary to retained bullet fragments has been documented for both adults and children (Coon et al., 2006). The client usually has a variety of chronic symptoms, such as abdominal pain, weakness, and eventually neurologic dysfunction, with the potential for permanent brain damage. Because lead interferes with the normal synthesis of red blood cells, clients have anemia and characteristic changes in the peripheral blood smear (Chapter 2). However, many children do not look or feel sick even though they have lead levels that are associated with developmental defects. Public health departments and consumer groups have been active in promoting blood screening for all children at risk. Free testing is available in most communities. Levels should be measured at 12 months and 24 months of age with follow-up measurements as needed.

Preparation of Client and Collection of Sample

The laboratory needs 2 mL of blood. It is important that all the blood-drawing equipment be free from lead or lead particles. Special collection tubes are used that are lead free. Prior to the specimen collection, the area should be cleaned with soap and water to remove any lead dust. A complete history is needed concerning the client's exposure to toxic chemicals. Most public health surveys have a definite assessment guide that is to be followed when interviewing clients. The possible exposure of other people in the client's environment must be considered. Industrial pollution also is a public health problem. The traditional lead test takes 2 weeks. A newer rapid test gives results in 3 minutes.

REFERENCE VALUES FOR BLOOD LEAD LEVELS

In 1991, the Centers for Disease Control and Prevention (CDC, 1991) lowered the cutoff level for defining lead poisoning in children from 25 to 10 µg/dL. The previous levels were from a 1985 recommendation. When a large proportion of children have blood levels greater than 10 µg/dL, community-wide childhood lead poisoning activities are warranted (Hay et al., 2011). However, no blood level of lead is safe for children (Heavey, 2008).

Possible Nursing Diagnosis for Lead Poisoning

Impaired Health Maintenance Related to Unhealthful Environment

For many years, nurses have been involved in lead screening (Brown et al., 2006; Cleveland et al., 2008b). The client most likely to experience lead poisoning is a child who lives in a poorly maintained home with peeling paint. Lead was banned as an ingredient in interior paints in 1978, but older houses may still contain particles that children ingest. In addition to the ban on lead in paints, environmental lead contamination in the United States has been lessened by the use of unleaded gasoline and a reduction in the amount of lead used in food and drink containers.

The treatment of lead poisoning is a process called chelation. Either intravenous or newer oral medications are used to bind the lead so that it is removed from the body via urine. Chelation should be considered for all children whose lead levels are above 45 µg/dL (Hay et al., 2011).

Questions

1. Serum levels of drugs may be needed when the risk of toxicity from a drug is increased. A factor that increases the toxicity of most drugs is
   a. Change in drug from a brand name to a generic
   b. Use of intramuscular or oral route rather than intravenous
   c. Hepatic dysfunction
   d. Increased urine output caused by increased intake of fluids

2. The nurse should be aware that the type of antibiotics that are commonly monitored by serum levels are the
   a. Penicillins
   b. Cephalosporins

    c. Aminoglycosides

    d. Tetracyclines

3. A teenager has epilepsy controlled by phenytoin. A serum phenytoin level drawn today was 23 µg/mL. Because this is slightly above the therapeutic range of 10–20 µg/mL, the client may begin to show a symptom of early phenytoin toxicity, which is

    a. Severe lethargy

    b. Cardiac arrhythmias

    c. Gait ataxia

    d. Nystagmus (involuntary rapid movements of the eyeballs)

4. A psychiatric client is being observed in a mental health clinic. Which of the following drugs requires monitoring with serum levels?

    a. Chlorpromazine

    b. Lithium carbonate

    c. Fluphenazine

    d. Thioridazine

5. A client is receiving aminophylline 20 mg/h by the intravenous route for treatment of an acute asthmatic attack that did not respond to β-2-agonists. Because aminophylline is a theophylline derivative, serum theophylline levels have been measured. The latest level of 30 µg/mL is considerably higher than the desired therapeutic range of 10–20 µg/mL. The nurse needs to make assessments of the client and be prepared for

    a. Cardiac arrhythmias and seizures

    b. Bronchospasms and dyspnea

    c. Renal and hepatic failure

    d. Hypertension crisis and stroke

6. A young teenager recovering from an asthmatic attack is being discharged with instructions to take a theophylline suspension every 6 hours. His parents need to be taught that early symptoms of overdose of theophylline may be similar to which of the following?

    a. Deep sleep

    b. Overuse of coffee

    c. Another asthmatic attack

    d. Cold or flu

7. An elderly client is taking digoxin 0.25 mg/day because of congestive heart failure (CHF). He is being visited by a community health nurse. Which of the following information in the client's health history should alert the nurse that this client should be closely watched for digoxin toxicity?

    a. Large intake of sodium in the diet, refusal of visit from dietitian

    b. Slightly low serum calcium level caused by a possible endocrine problem, evaluation in progress

    c. Poor renal function as evidenced by increased serum creatinine level

    d. History of noncompliance with physician's orders

8. A client has a serum quinidine level of 6 mg/L, which is higher than the therapeutic range of 1.0–4.0 mg/L. Because there may be possible toxic effects of the quinidine, the nurse should assess and record which of the following?

    a. Level of consciousness every 2 hours

    b. Blood pressure and pulse every 2 hours

    c. Lack of appetite or other gastrointestinal symptoms

    d. Hourly urine output

9. In relation to blood alcohol levels, the emergency department nurse should know that
   a. Alcohol should be used to wipe the skin before the blood specimen is drawn
   b. A blood alcohol of 0.01% is considered legal evidence of intoxication
   c. A chain-of-custody protocol must be followed
   d. The person who draws the blood cannot be subpoenaed to testify in a court case

10. A public health nurse is preparing to speak to a community group about the problem of lead poisoning. Which of the following should be included in the talk?
    a. Screening of all children should be done at birth and repeated in 6 months
    b. Prevention is crucial because there is no treatment of lead poisoning
    c. Children with lead poisoning may not feel or act sick
    d. Elderly people are at the greatest risk for lead toxicity

References

Brown, M. J., McLaine, P., Dixon, S., & Simon, P. (2006). A randomized, community-based trial of home visiting to reduce blood lead levels in children. *Pediatrics, 117*(1), 147–153.

Cleveland, L. M., Minter, M. L., Cobb, K. A., Scott, A. A., & German, V. F. (2008a). Lead hazards for pregnant women and children: Part 1. *American Journal of Nursing, 108*(10), 40–50.

Cleveland, L. M., Minter, M. L., Cobb, K. A., Scott, A. A., & German, V. F. (2008b). Lead hazards for pregnant women and children: Part 2. *American Journal of Nursing, 108*(11), 40–48.

Coon, T., Miller, M., Shirazi, F., & Sullivan, J. (2006). Lead toxicity in a 14-year-old female with retained bullet fragments. *Pediatrics, 117*(1), 227–230.

Deglin, J. H., Vallerand, A. H., & Sanoski, C. A. (2011). *Davis's drug guide for nurses* (12th ed.). Philadelphia: F. A. Davis.

Hay, W. W., Levin, M. J., Sondheimer, J. M., & Deterding, R. (Eds.). (2011). *Current diagnosis and treatment: Pediatrics* (20th ed.). New York: McGraw-Hill.

Heavey, E. (2008). Lead poisoning in children: Still a threat. *Nursing 2008, 38*(12), 17–18.

Hurley, J. S., Roberts, M., Solberg, L. I., Gunter, M. J., Nelson, W. W., Young, L., et al. (2005). Brief report: Laboratory safety monitoring of chronic medications in ambulatory care settings. *Journal of General Internal Medicine, 20*(4), 331–333.

Katzung, B., Masters, S. B., & Trevor, A. J. (Eds.). (2009). *Basic and clinical pharmacology* (11th ed.). New York: McGraw-Hill.

Lea, D. H. (2005). Tailoring drug therapy with pharmacogenetics. *Nursing 2005, 35*(4), 22–23.

Lopez, D. P. (2009). Acetaminophen poisoning. *American Journal of Nursing, 109*(9), 48–51.

McPhee, S. J., Papadakis, M. A., & Rabow, M. W. (Eds.). (2011). *Current medical diagnosis and treatment* (50th ed.). New York: McGraw-Hill.

Raebel, M. A., Lyons, E. E., Andrade, S. E., Chan, K. A., Chester, E. A., Davis, R. L., et al. (2005). Laboratory monitoring of drugs at initiation of therapy in ambulatory care. *Journal of General Internal Medicine, 20*(12), 1120–1126.

Rebsamen, M. C., Desmeules, J., Daali, Y., Chiappe, A., Diemand, A., Rey, C., et al. (2009). The ampliChip CYP_{450} test: Cytochrome P_{450}2D6 genotype assessment and phenotype prediction evaluation of the AmpliChip CYP_{450} test. *The Pharmacogenomics Journal, 9*, 34–41.

Roach, A. & Roach, E. (2005). How to assess phenytoin levels. *Nursing 2005, 35*(11), 18–19.

Simon, S. R., Andrade, S. E., Ellis, J. L., Nelson, W. W., Gurwitz, J. H., Lafata, J. E., et al. (2005). Baseline laboratory monitoring of cardiovascular medications in elderly health maintenance organization enrollees. *Journal of American Geriatrics Society, 53*(12), 2165–2169.

Watkins, P. B., Kaplowitz, N., Slattery, J. T., Colonese, C. R., Colucci, S. V., Stewart, P. W., et al. (2006). Aminotransferase elevations in healthy adults receiving 4 grams of acetaminophen daily: A randomized controlled trial. *Journal of American Medical Association, 296*(1), 87–93.

Wu, A. H. (Ed.). (2006). *Tietz clinical guide to laboratory tests* (4th ed.). St. Louis, MO: Saunders Elsevier.

Yacoubian, G. S. & Wish, E. (2006). A comparison between instant and laboratory oral fluid analysis among arrestees. *Journal of Psychoactive Drugs, 38*(2), 207–210.

Websites

www.acetadote.net (Information on medication used to treat acetaminophen toxicity.)

www.alcoholmonitoring.com (Transdermal monitoring of alcohol levels.)

www.liverfoundation.org (American Liver Foundation for information on effects of drugs on liver.)

www.MADD.org (Information on laws requiring interlocks for convicted drunk drivers.)

Answers

1. c, 2. c, 3. d, 4. b, 5. a, 6. b, 7. c, 8. b, 9. c, 10. c

Tests Performed in Pregnancy, the Newborn Period, and for Genetic Screening

- Pregnancy Tests 475
- Urine Pregnancy Tests 475
- Serum HCG Levels 476
- α-Fetoprotein 478
- Prenatal Screening for Down Syndrome: Serum Markers 478
- Dimeric Inhibin A 480
- Pregnancy-Associated Plasma Protein A 480
- HIV Screening 480
- Group B Streptococcus Screening 481
- Sickle Cell Anemia 481
- Thalassemia (Cooley's Anemia) 483
- Tay–Sachs Disease 484
- Canavan Disease 484
- Gaucher Disease 484
- Inherited Thrombophilia During Pregnancy and Postpartum 485
- Tests for Preeclampsia 485
- Estriol Levels 485
- Biochemical Marker for Preterm Labor—Fetal Fibronectin 486
- Newborn Screening 486
- Phenylketonuria 487
- Hypothyroidism 489
- Galactosemia 489
- Tests for Cystic Fibrosis 489
- Helping the Family of a Child with a Genetic Defect 490
- Cord Blood Banking and Stem Cell Research 491
- Use of DNA Samples for Genetic Testing and Identification 491

OBJECTIVES

1. Identify how a normal pregnancy changes the values of common laboratory tests in relation to prepregnancy values.
2. Explain the basic immunologic principle of tests for pregnancy.
3. Explain which of the autosomal recessive genetic diseases are commonly tested with screening programs for certain ethnic groups.
4. Explain why phenylketonuria (PKU), galactosemia, hypothyroidism, and sickle cell are screened with routine tests for newborns even though the infants appear healthy.
5. Explain the use of the combination of human chorionic gonadotropin (HCG), α-fetoprotein (AFP), and serum estriol for prenatal screening.
6. Compare the types of tests for cystic fibrosis, including DNA probes.

7. Discuss the impact of the Human Genome Project on the field of genetic counseling and the role of the nurse.

8. Describe the appropriate nursing functions for a community health nurse who is working with a family that has a child with a genetic defect.

Previous chapters have described some tests important in pregnancy (Table 18–1). Appendix C summarizes the expected changes in laboratory values in a normal pregnancy and a list of references for values in pregnancy. Appendix A lists expected changes in newborns. Although integration of content from all clinical settings is emphasized in this book, some tests pertain *only* to the pregnant or the newborn state. This chapter, therefore, focuses on common laboratory tests that are unique in maternal–child health settings.

Interwoven with all these advanced methods of testing is the nurse's involvement with the client as a person. The premise of this chapter is that pregnancy and childbirth should be joyous and healthy events. If tests must be used for a pregnancy, the health professionals must make sure that such tests are as nonthreatening as possible. The focus is what is normal about the pregnancy, not what may be abnormal.

Table 18–1 Routine Tests Done During Pregnancy

Name of Test	Assessment	Location in Book
Hgb-Hct	Anemia	Chap. 2 on CBC
Urinalysis	Possible urinary tract infection (UTI) and other conditions	Chap. 3 on routine urinalysis nitrites and LE
Urine for protein	Possible toxemia	Chap. 3 on proteinuria
Blood glucose at 24–28 weeks' gestation	Possible diabetes	Chap. 8 on diabetes and pregnancy
Rh typing and unexpected antibody screen	Possible hemolytic disease of newborn (HDN)	Chap. 14 for Rh factor in pregnancy
STS	Possible syphilis	Chap. 16 on syphilis and pregnancy
Rubella titer (*before* pregnancy)	Immunity to 3-day measles	Chap. 14 on why rubella titers are measured *before* pregnancy
Sickle cell	Also need to test father for trait	Chap. 28 on follow-up
Hepatitis B surface antigen	HBV carrier	Chap. 14 on HBV and pregnancy
Triple screen	Anencephaly, spina bifida, open ventral wall defects, trisomy 21, and trisomy 18	This chapter
Culture for GBS	Colonization with group B streptococcus	This chapter and Chap. 16

Note: If tests for hypothyroidism are done, note that reference values are 1.5 times those for nonpregnant state (see Chapter 15). Other tests, such as those for cytomegalovirus (CMV), AIDS, herpes (Chapter 14), chlamydia, and gonorrhea (Chapter 16), may be conducted if the pregnant woman is at risk for these infections. See Chapter 25 on HPV and Pap smears.

PREGNANCY TESTS

Although pregnancy has early presumptive signs and symptoms, such as amenor-rhea, nausea and vomiting, and skin changes, the positive signs occur later. Any one of the following signs is both legal and medical proof of pregnancy: (1) fetal heart-beat, (2) palpation of fetal outline, (3) recognition of fetal movements by someone other than the mother, and (4) ultrasonographic demonstration of the fetus.

In the modern world, few, if any, women are willing to wait a few months to know for sure if they are pregnant. The desire to know as soon as possible is strong, both for the woman who desires a child and for the woman who may choose to terminate a pregnancy. A pregnancy test and ultrasonography (Chapter 23) are also important if the client is believed to have an ectopic pregnancy, because immediate surgical intervention is needed (DeCherney et al., 2007). The rate of ectopic preg-nancies increases as the rate of pelvic inflammatory disease increases.

All pregnancy tests are based on detecting the presence of human chorionic gonadotropin (HCG) in the urine or serum of a pregnant woman. HCG, produced by the trophoblast cell component of the fetal placental tissue, can be measured as subunits of α and β. The α subunit is identical with that of luteinizing hormone (LH), follicle-stimulating hormone (FSH), and thyroid-stimulating hormone (TSH). The β subunit is unique for HCG and thus is a more sensitive test for pregnancy. HCG is present in the serum within 6–10 days after implantation, peaks in 12–14 weeks, and remains elevated during entire pregnancy. HCG is also produced by some types of tumors of the testes or placenta. (See the quantitative test for HCG.) Although HCG can be measured directly in the serum to detect pregnancy, most pregnancy tests rely on detection of HCG in the urine.

URINE PREGNANCY TESTS

Biologic Tests For Pregnancy

The older pregnancy tests used animals to test for pregnancy: Some of the wom-an's urine was injected into mice, rabbits, or frogs, and various changes in the ani-mals were evidence that HCG was present. For example, HCG in the injected urine causes ovarian changes in rabbits (Friedman test) and in mice (Aschheim–Zondek [AZ] test). In frogs (Galli–Mainini test), sperm are found in the frog's urine if the injected urine contains HCG. With the advent of immunologic techniques, these older, biologic tests for pregnancy are only of historical interest.

Immunologic Tests for Pregnancy

Pregnancy tests now use monoclonal antibodies specific for HCG. A solution con-taining these antibodies is mixed with a small amount of urine. The presence of HCG causes a change in urine color.

Home Pregnancy Tests

Kits that can be used at home to detect pregnancy were introduced in 1976. Various manufacturers make the tests, which are widely advertised to the public. Some of these tests can detect pregnancy as early as 5 days before the expected period. All the tests recommend a second test if the first test is negative and if menses does not begin within a week. A second test may be needed because the urine did not have enough HCG yet, or because the woman may have miscalculated her period. If the test is positive, the woman can visit her physician or clinic to receive definite confirmation of the pregnancy.

All the kits emphasize that the kit does not replace the advice or care of a physician or midwife. If repeated tests are negative, the woman has saved the expense and time of consulting the healthcare system. Advertisements for the kits also make the point that a pregnancy test at home provides a way for a couple to learn the good news together. A test at home means no waiting for appointments and no suspense in waiting for an answer. A home pregnancy test (HPT) may be a way for a woman to establish from the beginning that the baby belongs to her—not to a health professional. However, health professionals express concern that a woman may not perform the test correctly and thus function under the false assumption that she is not pregnant, continuing to take medicines that could be dangerous to the fetus Adolescents who use HPT may be more likely to obtain false-negative results because of developmental issues and greater variation in menstrual cycles.

Preparation of Client and Collection of Sample

A first voided morning sample is ideal because the urine is concentrated. Some tests require a few drops of urine, and some are one step, performed with a stick placed in the urine stream. The absorbent tip is recapped, and results are read in 3 minutes. Multiple-step tests take longer. All these pregnancy tests have an accuracy of about 99% if the test is performed exactly as outlined by the manufacturer.

SERUM HCG LEVELS

HCG Qualitative Pregnancy Tests

The laboratory can detect small amounts of HCG in the serum. There is some cross-sensitivity with LH and other pituitary hormones if the total HCG is measured. To reduce cross-sensitivity, the laboratory measures the β subunit of HCG.

Preparation of Client and Collection of Sample

The test requires 0.5 mL of serum.

REFERENCE VALUES FOR HCG PREGNANCY TEST

Laboratory usually reports as a qualitative test of either positive or negative.

An inconclusive finding should be repeated on another sample.

Negative	<5 IU/L
Inconclusive	5–20 IU/L
Positive	>20 IU/L

HCG Qualitative Test for Pregnancy: Needed Follow-Ups

A positive test for pregnancy requires follow-up health care, and so should a negative result if the client is relieved that she is not pregnant. One study (Daley et al., 2005) found that 77% of urine pregnancy tests were negative in teenage clients. These researches stressed that a negative pregnancy test is an opportunity for some discussion about unintended pregnancies and information on contraception and prevention of sexually transmitted infections.

HCG Quantitative Test

The HCG level can be increased by some tumors, such as a hydatidiform mole (a benign adenoma) of the placenta, a choriocarcinoma (malignant) of placenta-like tissue, or some types of testicular carcinoma. If any of these conditions is suspected, the β subunit of HCG helps to confirm a diagnosis. Serial HCG levels are also used to monitor the response to surgical therapy or chemotherapy. In some cancers of the testes, the β subunit of HCG can be used as a tumor marker, as can α-fetoprotein (AFP) (see Chapter 10). HCG levels help with the assessment of an ectopic pregnancy as levels tend to show only a slow rise or a drop compared to a normal pregnancy. HCG levels are also used to monitor the status of an implanted fertilized ovum. Falling levels suggest fetal loss.

HCG, in combination with AFP and serum unconjugated estriol, is used for prenatal screening, as discussed later in this chapter. High levels of HCG are associated with Down syndrome.

Preparation of Client and Collection of Sample

The test requires 0.5 mL of serum.

REFERENCE VALUES FOR HCG QUANTITATIVE (β CHAIN SPECIFIC)		
Tumor marker	Males: less than 3 IU/L	
	Females: less than 6 IU/L	
	Weeks	IU/L
Normal pregnancy	3–4	9–130
	4–5	75–2,600
	5–6	850–20,800
	6–7	4,000–100,200
	7–12	11,500–289,00
	12–16	18,300–137,00
	16–29	1,400–53,000 (second trimester)
	29–41	940–60,000 (third trimester)

Note: Values vary depending on methods used. Note that trends are more useful than any one reading.

α-FETOPROTEIN

AFP is made by the liver of the embryo. If the fetus has a neural tube defect, the protein leaks out to the amniotic fluid. Between 15 and 20 weeks of pregnancy, AFP may be measured in the mother's blood. AFP was the first screening test of the pregnant woman's blood as a check for genetic defects in the child (Table 18–2).

High levels of AFP in pregnant women do not always indicate a problem with neural tube defects because the fetal age may be incorrectly estimated, the woman may be bearing twins, or the rise could be caused by other reasons that are not yet well understood. If the AFP blood screening test is abnormal, a repeat is done. If the test is positive on the second blood sample, the woman undergoes ultrasonography. If there is still doubt about the possibility of a defect, amniocentesis is performed. (See Chapter 28 for a detailed discussion on screening for neural tube defects. See Chapter 10 for discussion of AFP as a tumor marker.)

Low values of AFP may also be clinically significant because less AFP is present when the fetus has Down syndrome. (See the discussion on triple screen.)

Preparation of Client and Collection of Sample

The laboratory needs 4 mL of serum in a serum separator tube (SST). The sample must be drawn between 15 and 20 weeks' gestation. Check state laws regarding notification of client about the results. Since 1986, the standard of care has been to offer all pregnant women the maternal serum alpha-fetoprotein screening (MSAFP) and document if they refuse it.

GENERAL REFERENCE VALUES FOR MATERNAL SERUM[a]	
Week 19–21	2.1–9.6 µg/dL
31–33	8.4–34.4 µg/dL
37–40	6.3–16.5 µg/dL

[a]Check with AFP screening centers for specific values for the critical levels for 15–20 weeks' gestation.

Clinical Significance

Although this test is sensitive to the conditions mentioned earlier, it is not highly specific, so there are a high number of false-positive results. See Chapter 28 for more discussion about the anxiety related to follow-up testing such as amniocentesis.

PRENATAL SCREENING FOR DOWN SYNDROME: SERUM MARKERS

Maternal serum AFP levels tend to be lower than normal if the fetus has Down syndrome. Therefore, in 1984, maternal serum AFP, already in use as a screening test for neural tube defects, began to be used as a screening test for Down syndrome. In the late 1980s, two additional maternal serum markers, an elevated HCG and a decreased unconjugated estriol level, were discovered to be associated with Down syndrome. The combined use of all three tests has made prenatal screening for

Table 18-2 Common Genetic Diseases That May Be Detected with Screening

Defect	Detected in Carrier States in Blood Samples of Both Parents	Screening of Maternal Blood After Woman Is Pregnant[a]	Types of Screen Amniocentesis[b]	Fetal Blood Sampling (Research Studies)	Comments
Sickle cell anemia	X		X	X	Most common in black families. May be difficult to diagnose accurately in fetus or newborn, but new tests on cord blood are being tried.
Tay–Sachs disease	X		X		Most common in Jewish families of Eastern European origin. Wide-scale testing is conducted in Jewish populations.
Neural tube defects		X	X	X	Genetic defect that can be screened in maternal blood by use of AFP. Can occur in any pregnancy.
Cystic fibrosis	X		? or X	X	Gene can now be identified; also see sweat test. More common in Caucasians. Many mutations of gene.
Galactosemia			X		Tests of newborns required by law in all states.
Hemophilia			? or X	X	Sex-linked gene. Amniocentesis cannot determine if disease is present but can do so indirectly by showing sex of fetus.
Down syndrome		X	X		Incidence increases with maternal age. See text for use of HCG, AFP, and serum estriol as a screen for Down syndrome. Most common reason for amniocentesis is to check for Down syndrome.
Thalassemia (β)	X		X	X	Most common in families of Mediterranean descent. Screening of carriers not commonly performed on large-scale basis.
PKU	X		X	X	More common in Caucasians. All states require newborn testing.

[a]Nucleated cells of fetal origin have been reported to be present in most pregnancies, so researchers are developing techniques to use DNA diagnosis on fetal cells in maternal blood samples

[b]See Chapter 28 for a discussion on amniocentesis and chorionic villus biopsy.

Table 18–3 Screening Tests for Down Syndrome

First trimester	PAPP-A free beta-HCG, and ultrasound of neck of fetus to detect nuchal translucency
Second trimester	Alpha-fetoprotein, total HCG, estriol, and dimeric inhibin A

Note: See Malone et al. (2005) for research on the two times for testing. All pregnant women may be offered these tests regardless of age. See Chapter 28 for follow-up diagnostic tests of chorionic villus sampling (CVS) and amniocentesis and Chapter 23 for fetal sonograms.

Down syndrome more specific. The triple screen can identify women who may be carrying a fetus with anencephaly, spina bifida, open ventral wall defects, trisomy 21 (Down syndrome), and trisomy 18. The results of this triple screen are considered useful for decision making by both younger and older pregnant women. Clients with positive results are offered genetic counseling and follow-up tests, such as ultrasound (Chapter 23) and amniocentesis (Chapter 28). Current practice is to offer the triple screen between 15 and 18 weeks' gestation.

More recently, dimeric inhibin A has been added to the original triple screen. The four-marker test or quadruple test is used in the second trimester. (See Table 18–3 to compare this with another type of first-trimester screening.) Both methods have high rates for detection and low rates of false positives (Malone et al., 2005).

DIMERIC INHIBIN A

Inhibin is the major peptide regulator of FSH in both sexes. During pregnancy, it is synthesized by the placenta and reaches a plateau at about 14–30 weeks. Subunits include inhibin A and inhibin B. Addition of dimeric inhibin A enhances the rate of detection of Down syndrome.

PREGNANCY-ASSOCIATED PLASMA PROTEIN A

Serum levels of free β-HCG and pregnancy-associated plasma protein A (PAPP-A) combined with an ultrasound measurement of the amount of fluid collected behind the fetal neck (nuchal translucency) are used to screen for Down syndrome in the first trimester.

The sampling time for PAPP-A is only 10–14 weeks' gestation because after this time the power of discrimination seems to be lost. Malone et al. (2005) compared first-trimester screening with the quadruple screening done in the second trimester to detect Down syndrome. Clients can be reassured that both methods have high rates of detection of Down syndrome with low false positives. Clients who test positive may be offered CVS at 10–12 weeks' gestation and/or amniocentesis, as discussed in Chapter 28.

HIV SCREENING

Perinatal transmission of HIV is the major cause of AIDS in children, and rates of transmission may vary from 13% to 32% depending on the retroviral strain. In the mid-nineties, clinical trials demonstrated that the use of zidovudine significantly reduced the rate of HIV transmission to the fetus. Thus, nurses became aware of the need to educate clients about the importance of HIV testing as treatment was available to help stop the spread of the epidemic to the next generation. Under current federal guidelines, healthcare providers are to give extensive counseling to all pregnant women about the risk of AIDS and the benefits of testing. McPhee, Papadakis, and Rabow (2011) noted that the two principal modes of HIV infection in women are heterosexual activity (62%) and injection drug use (32%). Studies have shown that when pregnant women are approached in a sensitive manner, most will consent to prenatal testing for HIV. Women often learn of their positive HIV status when they become pregnant; nurses can help them decide about options (Lachat, Scott, & Relf, 2006). In addition to zidovudine, other antiretroviral drugs are now used to decrease HIV maternal–fetal transmission and to treat AIDS (Deglin, Vallerand, & Sanoski (2011). Now improvements in rapid HIV tests used in labor and delivery give clinicians a last-minute opportunity to prevent transmission to the infant. (See Chapter 14 for details on rapid HIV testing in labor and delivery.)

GROUP B STREPTOCOCCUS SCREENING

All pregnant women should be screened for Group B streptococci (GBS) during 35–37 weeks' gestation. (See Chapter 16 for collection of rectal and vaginal cultures.) Nurses who work with pregnant clients need to explain when GBS screening is needed, and nurses who work with newborns need to be aware of the results of GBS screening, whether the mother has been treated with antibiotics, and what needs to be observed in the newborn.

SICKLE CELL ANEMIA

Sickle cell anemia results from an autosomal recessive gene that produces an abnormal type of hemoglobin (Hgb) called *hemoglobin S* (HgbS). (See Chapter 2 for tests on Hgb.) HgbS does not function as normal Hgb. The red blood cells have a sickle form, particularly when they are exposed to low oxygen concentrations or if the person is dehydrated. The abnormal cells are hemolyzed at an increased rate. The capillaries can become occluded by these sickled cells. In addition to the sickle cell gene that causes sickle cell anemia (called the beta-globin genotype), there are other genotypes such as sickle-hemoglobin C disease and two types of sickle beta-thalassemia that cause sickle cell disease. In order to have sickle cell disease, the client must have two autosomal recessive genes, but other modifier genes may also be important in determining the severity of the disease (Kenner, Gallo, & Bryant, 2005).

A person can either be a carrier of or have sickle cell disease. If the person has only one recessive gene for the sickle cell trait, she or he is a carrier who has the trait. A person with the sickle cell trait usually has no symptoms, although exposure to very low oxygen concentrations may cause minimal symptoms. However, the effect of the trait, if any, is being studied because in the past, some people with the trait were denied jobs, such as piloting planes. If only one parent is a carrier, there is no difficulty. If both parents are carriers, they face the one-in-four risk, for each pregnancy, that their child will have the disease. As shown in Table 18–4, the risk is

Table 18–4 Probability of Autosomal Recessive Genetic Diseases When Both Parents Are Carriers

Mother		Father	
↓		↓	
ND		ND	
NN	DD	ND	DN
1:4 have two normal genes, so no disease or carrier state.	1:4 have two defective genes, so have disease	2:4 (or 1:2) have one normal and one defective gene, so will be carriers of the trait	
25% of all children born to couples who are carriers	25% of all children born to couples who are carriers	50% of all children born to couples who are carriers	

N, normal gene; D, defective gene.

Note: Autosomal recessive diseases discussed in this chapter include the following: (1) PKU, (2) cystic fibrosis, (3) sickle cell anemia, (4) Tay–Sachs disease, (5) thalassemia (Cooley's anemia), and (6) Gaucher disease.

Sex-linked recessive traits occur in different patterns. See the text for a discussion of hemophilia, which is transmitted by X chromosome.

also one in four that the child will not receive the trait from either parent, and the chance is one in two that the child will be a carrier. The carrier state is estimated to be present in about 8–10% of American blacks.

Screening programs that target a specific racial or ethnic group do not identify all infants with the disease, because healthcare professionals cannot always identify a client's racial or ethnic background on the basis of physical appearance, surname, or self-report. Hence, the recommendation is for universal screening of newborns for sickle cell disease so that no infant is subjected to early death because screening was not performed. The collection method for blood for sickle cell screening is a heel stick. Like other routine newborn screening procedures for phenylketonuria (PKU), galactosemia, and hypothyroidism, the blood sample is put on filter paper for transportation to the laboratory. Blood samples obtained from the umbilical cord or directly from a venipuncture are also acceptable, but collection is more expensive and the specimen is difficult to transport. The blood sample must be collected before any transfusions are given.

Although sickle cell disease is not curable, identifying newborns with the disease makes it possible for them to receive preventive vaccines for pneumonia, which can be lethal in children with sickle cell disease. Additionally, prophylactic penicillin may be started and continued until at least 5 years of age (Hay et al., 2011).

Hydroxyurea, an antineoplastic drug, may be used as a palliative drug for sickle cell vaso-occlusive crisis (Deglin et al., 2011). Stroke remains as one of the complications of sickle cell disease, so Doppler ultrasound (Chapter 23) is used to identify at-risk clients. These high-risk clients may be helped by long-term blood transfusions, but iron overload, marked by elevated ferritin levels (Chapter 2), may be an unwanted effect. However, discontinuation of transfusion results in a high rate of reversion to abnormal blood-flow velocities as shown on Doppler studies (Adams & Brambilla, 2005).

The American Sickle Cell Anemia Association has updates on treatment at www.ascaa.org.

THALASSEMIA (COOLEY'S ANEMIA)

Thalassemia, like sickle cell anemia, is transmitted by autosomal recessive genes. Several variations of the defect can occur. Both the carrier state (thalassemia minor) and the presence of two recessive genes (thalassemia major) can be detected with Hgb electrophoresis (see Chapter 2). In the United States, the thalassemia genes are most predominant in people of Mediterranean, Asian-Indian, Southeast Asian, and Chinese ancestry. Thalassemia minor, characterized by mild hypochromic, microcytic anemia, does not require therapy but does have implications for genetic counseling. Thalassemia major (Cooley's anemia) is a potentially fatal disease because the bone marrow cannot produce enough Hgb to sustain life. The mainstays of treatment have been regular blood transfusions and the removal of iron with deferoxamine, an iron-chelating agent. These infusions are given subcutaneously for 8–12 hours every night. The chelated iron is excreted in the urine and makes it red, orange, or tea colored. An oral iron chelator, deferasirox, was approved by the FDA in 2006. Chronic blood transfusions can lead to iron overload and organ damage because each transfused unit contains 200–250 mg of iron. Clients on multiple blood transfusions over a long period of time need information on avoiding foods high in iron. New technology is being used in clinical trials to obtain noninvasive measurements of liver iron and cardiac iron. A ferritometer may measure liver iron. The measurement of cardiac iron (T2*) is done by a special analysis of an MRI (Chapter 21). The only available cure for beta-thalassemia major is a bone marrow transplant from a matched sibling. The Cooley Anemia Foundation has more information on treatments at www.cooleysanemia.org.

In recent years, there has been great progress in determining the pathologic molecular structure of the different forms of thalassemia. Detection of the carriers and the prenatal diagnosis with amniocentesis (Chapter 28) of the more severe forms have been accompanied by a reduction in the number of new cases. Many children, however, continue to be born with the disease, particularly in the developing world.

Possible Nursing Diagnoses

Ineffective Coping Related to Chronic Illness

Both sickle cell anemia and thalassemia major are chronic conditions for which there is no cure. The child and the family need help coping with the disease. Families who have one child with the disease may greatly fear another pregnancy. (See the discussion at the end of this chapter.)

The cornerstone of treatment of children with serious chronic conditions is enrollment in a program that provides family education with comprehensive outpatient care and early treatment of acute complications. Nurses may function as case managers for a group of clients in addition to giving direct care. Information about management of these diseases can be obtained from the national organizations. (See the websites in the reference list.)

Activity Intolerance Related to Anemia

Children with hemolytic anemias have a lowered Hgb and hematocrit (Hct), elevated reticulocyte counts, and, in some cases, abnormal red blood cells on a peripheral smear. (See Chapter 2 for a discussion on activity intolerance and other nursing diagnoses for a client with anemia.)

TAY–SACHS DISEASE

Tay–Sachs disease, another inherited autosomal recessive condition, is most commonly found in Ashkenazi Jews of Eastern European origin. As with all other recessive diseases, both parents must have the gene to produce a child with the disease. The classic form of Tay–Sachs disease demonstrates a deficiency in an enzyme known as hexosaminidase A. The lack of this enzyme causes mental retardation, flaccid muscles, and death by 3–4 years of age. At present, there is no treatment. Some variants of this disease may proceed more slowly.

There is a simple blood test to screen for carriers of Tay–Sachs disease, and it requires only a venous blood sample. The carriers of the recessive gene have lowered levels of the enzyme hexosaminidase A. The Tay–Sachs test is performed on couples to see whether both are carriers. If needed, the Tay–Sachs test can then be carried out on amniotic fluid (Chapter 28 on amniocentesis). Unless both parents have the gene, however, there is no need to test the amniotic fluid because the infant will not have the disease. Preconception tests and/or prenatal testing for both Tay–Sachs and Canavan, discussed next, are standard screenings offered to Jewish women (McPhee et al., 2011).

CANAVAN DISEASE

Canavan disease, an inherited degenerative disease of the brain, is caused by a deficiency in the enzyme aspartoacylase, which leads to a chemical imbalance that destroys the myelin. At present, there is no treatment. Like Tay–Sachs (1 in 30) discussed earlier, the defective gene is much more common in Jewish people (1 in 40) of Eastern and Central European (Ashkenazi) descent. Premarital and/or preconception testing has dramatically reduced these relatively common autosomal recessive genetic diseases among the Jewish population (Callister, 2006).

GAUCHER DISEASE

Gaucher (pronounced as Go-shay) disease is the most common inherited disease in Ashkenazi Jews. Like Tay–Sachs, it is autosomal recessive, but unlike Tay–Sachs, it is treatable. The deficiency of the enzyme glucocerebrosidase or acid-β-glucosidase can be corrected by intravenous infusions. The natural enzyme is modified to allow uptake of the enzyme by lyosomes in the cells. Symptoms, which may occur soon after birth or much later, include anemia, bleeding or bruising, fractures, and enlarged liver and spleen. Confirmation of diagnosis is achieved by measuring the enzyme in white blood cells or by a skin culture. Enzyme replacement therapy with imiglucerase or velaglucerase leads to an increase in hemoglobin and platelets and a decrease in the size of the liver and spleen although the spleen usually stays enlarged. A volumetric MRI (Chapter 21) is used to assess the size of the liver and spleen. PCR amplification can identify the gene mutation in carriers. Carriers are symptom free, so prenatal testing may be needed if there is a family history. The National Gaucher Foundation (www.gaucherdisease.org) has information on local support groups and updates on treatment.

INHERITED THROMBOPHILIA DURING PREGNANCY AND POSTPARTUM

Approximately half of the cases of venous thrombosis during pregnancy and postpartum are due to an inherited condition such as a factor V Leiden mutation, protein C or S deficiencies, and several other genetic mutations. (See Chapter 13 for a discussion on these tests).

TESTS FOR PREECLAMPSIA

Preeclampsia, characterized by pregnancy-induced hypertension (140/90 or higher) and proteinuria (more than 300 mg in a 24-hour urine collection) (see Chapter 3), occurs after 20 weeks' gestation. In the past, edema was considered the third marker, but may not always be present. Rapid weight gain with edema of the face and hands is more significant than edema of the lower legs, as this is common during pregnancy. Cases may be mild to severe. If seizures occur, preeclampsia becomes eclampsia. Sibai (2005) notes that the onset of seizures may be antepartum (38–53%), intrapartum (18–36%), or postpartum (11–44%). Researchers have found that one of the hallmarks of severe preeclampsia is the HELLP syndrome.

> H   Hemolysis indicated by a falling HCT (see Chapter 2) and elevated bilirubin (see Chapter 11)
>
> EL   Elevated Liver enzymes (see Chapter 12 on AST, ALT, and LDH)
>
> LP   Low Platelet count (see Chapter 13)

Preeclampsia usually resolves within 48 hours after childbirth. If the fetus is too immature for delivery, the condition must be treated with bed rest and, if needed, medications such as magnesium sulfate (see Chapter 7) and antihypertensives (DeCherney et al., 2007).

For a long time, preeclampsia (formerly called toxemia), one of the hypertensive disorders of pregnancy, has been one of the three leading causes of maternal death. (Hemorrhage and infection are the other two causes.) New research has shown that even if the women's blood pressure returned to normal after delivery, she may be at high risk for cardiovascular disease later in life. Therefore, teaching about how to control risk factors for heart disease may be appropriate (Fedorka & Heasley, 2008).

ESTRIOL LEVELS

During pregnancy, the fetus and the placenta function as a unit to produce estrogens, of which estriol (E_3) is the principal estrogenic compound. (See Chapter 15 for a discussion on other tests of estrogen compounds.) Estriol levels begin to increase about the eighth week of pregnancy and continue at high levels to term. Consistently high levels of estriol indicate a normally functioning fetal–placental unit.

BIOCHEMICAL MARKER FOR PRETERM LABOR: FETAL FIBRONECTIN

Fibronectin, an oncofetal glycoprotein produced by trophoblasts, seems to function as an important component for adherence of the placenta to the uterine wall. Thus, increasing levels may signify a separation of the placenta from the uterine wall. The fetal fibronectin (fFN) test was approved by the FDA in 1995. (Other types of fibronectin are present in the body and may be measured for other reasons, so this test is specified fetal.) Many studies have shown the usefulness of fFN in high-risk pregnancies. The test is not used as routine screening in pregnant women as it does not help predict preterm labor in asymptomatic women (Wu, 2006).

Preparation of Client and Collection of Sample

A vaginal exam with a speculum is needed to collect a cervical sample of fFN. Semen, douches, and other factors may invalidate the results.

REFERENCE VALUES FOR fFN	
Fibronectin	>50 ng/mL

Clinical Significance

If a woman has a negative report, she may be advised to repeat the test at a 2-week interval depending on her assessed risk status. Negative tests can help prevent unnecessary treatment for preterm labor. The presence of fFN during weeks 24–34 of a high-risk pregnancy, along with symptoms of preterm delivery, documents a possibility of the need for a preterm delivery. However, the majority of clients with positive results will successfully continue the pregnancy because the placenta can heal a small disruption (Wu, 2006). Although there may be a genetic link to preterm labor, current tests can identify the condition only once it begins (Giarratano, 2006).

NEWBORN SCREENING

For many newborns, the symptoms of serious inborn errors of metabolism are evident at birth. Nurses who work with newborns need to be on the alert for any symptoms or signs that require medical assessment. The following characteristics may be noted by healthcare workers and sometimes by parents:

1. Unexplained metabolic alterations in electrolytes with acidosis or dehydration
2. Progressive downhill course with central nervous system deterioration
3. Unexplained renal or cardiac failure
4. Unexplained large viscera
5. Abnormal urine odor
6. Marked change in features, large tongue, coarse features
7. Thrombocytopenia, neutropenia, or anemia
8. Renal colic or calculus
9. Idiosyncratic or unusual reaction to drugs

Different inborn errors of metabolism, of course, cause different symptoms. For example, the only symptom of PKU is a musty odor of the urine, which may not be noticed. Several other inborn defects give urine an odor that has been described as smelling like rotten cabbage, sweaty feet, stale fish, or burned sugar.

Although some genetic diseases produce symptoms at birth, others do not. Some of these "hidden" defects can cause serious damage if treatment is not begun early. Many tests can be performed to detect genetic abnormalities in the newborn.

The first newborn screening test, PKU, has been available since 1962. At the present time, all the states screen for congenital hypothyroidism, PKU, galactosemia, and hemoglobinopathies, biotinidase deficiency, congenital adrenal hyperplasia (Chapter 15), maple syrup urine disease, and cystic fibrosis.

The dramatic expansion in testing in the United States has led to concern about the number of false positives and the impact on families who are told that their child has a disease when they do not (Tarini, Christakis, & Welch, 2006).

An information sheet is given to all new parents that explains in simple terms the reason for the tests. If the parents do not wish their child to have the tests, they must sign a statement relieving the physician and hospital of any liability for damages that may result from the lack of early detection. Parents are told that if they refuse the tests now, they can request the tests from a physician or a public health nurse later. The nurse can often be useful in further explaining how these tests are beneficial in helping the newborn get off to the best start possible.

The reader is encouraged to go on the web to the National Newborn Screening and Genetics Resource Center (htpp://genes-r-us.uthscsa.edu) to see what tests are currently done in a particular state. Until all screening is standardized, nurses must be aware of state regulations where they practice and understand the confusion that parents may have about what is available. Some families may opt to obtain supplemental screening from commercial companies. These programs are offered in cooperation with a local hospital or birth center. Results are given to the healthcare provider.

The Human Genome Project, begun in 1988, has located all human genes and their sequence. One of the early benefits of the project was the identification of defective genes responsible for about 4,000 known inherited disorders. Advances in DNA-based diagnostic procedures (Chapter 1) make it possible to screen for these newly found genes. As more testing becomes possible, society must decide whether the benefits are worth the costs. As noted earlier, any *mandatory* tests for newborns not only must be accurate and suitable for mass screening, but also must detect diseases that can be controlled if early treatment is begun. Informed consent, legal liability, and quality assurance have been issues for many years.

Twomey (2006) noted that the significance of a positive result in a newborn screening is not limited to the health of the baby but also affects other family members who may carry the gene. He cautions that nurses must be aware of the ethical concerns about the implications of testing other family members.

PHENYLKETONURIA

Phenylalanine is an amino acid found in all protein foods. An infant with PKU has a buildup of phenylalanine in the serum caused by the lack of an enzyme needed for the normal metabolism of this amino acid. Because the phenylalanine spills into the urine, the condition is called *phenylketonuria*. PKU is dangerous because the high levels of phenylalanine in the serum can cause brain damage. Originally, screening tests for PKU were performed on the urine, but the blood test (Guthrie test) is more valuable. PKU is much more common in Caucasians than in other groups.

Preparation of Client and Collection of Sample

The serum level may be abnormally elevated within 24 hours after the infant begins a milk diet. If the infant is not taking milk well, the test should be delayed. The laboratory needs to know the date and time of birth as well as the date and time of the first milk feeding.

The usual procedure is to perform the PKU 24–48 hours after birth. If the baby is breastfeeding, a second PKU may be performed after the milk supply is abundant. A screening test for PKU is performed on capillary blood drawn from a heel stick. (Chapter 1 describes the procedure for heel sticks for infants.) Serum levels are monitored if there is a positive first test. Some babies may have increased phenylalanine levels caused by immaturity of the liver. Not all infants with elevated serum phenylalanine levels have PKU. Prenatal diagnosis of PKU is often possible with DNA probes. Molecular approaches are also replacing serum measurements of phenylalanine to determine carrier status (Hay et al., 2011).

For serum phenylalanine, 1 mL of serum should be put in a plastic vial containing sodium fluoride (NaF) as a preservative.

REFERENCE VALUES FOR PHENYLALANINE

Serum phenylalanine	<4.0 mg/dL

Note: See Wu (2006) for low birth weight values and other tests to determine variants.

Possible Nursing Diagnoses Related to PKU

Imbalanced Nutrition

The treatment of PKU consists of limiting the intake of phenylalanine to a level appropriate for each child. (There are several varieties of PKU.) Products such as Lofenalac contain the essential amino acids with only a small amount of phenylalanine.

A restricted diet tailored to the serum levels of phenylalanine makes it possible for the child to develop normally without mental retardation. The nurse may have a role in helping the family meet the dietary needs of a child with PKU. In the past, children with PKU were continued on the restricted diet until around age 8, but researchers began to question if this was sufficient. Now current practice is to keep the client with classical PKU on phenylalanine restriction throughout life (Hay et al., 2011).

Anxiety Related to Planning for Future Pregnancies

PKU is an autosomal recessive genetic disease. So if a couple has one child with the disease, they have a one-in-four chance of having another child with the disease (Table 18–3). PKU can be detected with amniocentesis. Parents may choose to have a second child, however, even with the known risk, if they see that a first child is progressing well with dietary control. (See the discussion on genetic counseling at the end of this chapter.)

Deficient Knowledge Related to Danger of PKU for Newborn

When a woman who has PKU becomes pregnant, there is some risk that her infant will be harmed unless the woman follows the PKU diet before and during pregnancy. Some women may have forgotten they ever followed a special childhood diet or were never told the reason why. Therefore, all women who have PKU need to be educated about the problems of maternal PKU and referred to a PKU clinic. For women with PKU who have gone off their diets, the current recommendation is to begin dietary phenylalanine restriction at least 3 months prior to conception.

HYPOTHYROIDISM

The pilot program for screening for hypothyroidism in newborns began in the United States in 1972. The screening of more than 1 million infants resulted in the recommendation to use the thyroxine (T_4) filter paper test for screening and a follow-up of TSH for the 3–5% of low T_4 results. The T_4 filter paper test requires only a drop of capillary blood. (See Chapter 1 for the discussion about heel sticks of infants.)

The tests used for hypothyroidism are discussed in Chapter 15. See the sections on hypothyroidism of the newborn for the symptoms of the disorder, on the medical treatment, and on the nursing implications.

GALACTOSEMIA

The urine test used to screen the inborn metabolism of galactose is discussed in detail at the end of Chapter 8, where the treatment of the disease and the nursing diagnoses are also covered. Like other screening tests of the newborn, galactosemia screening tests can be performed by means of a heel stick to obtain capillary blood for filter paper. (Chapter 1 discusses heel sticks of infants.) Deficiency of the enzyme galactose-1-phosphate uridyl transferase in red blood cells establishes the diagnosis.

TESTS FOR CYSTIC FIBROSIS

Cystic fibrosis (CF) is a hereditary disease, caused by an autosomal recessive gene that affects the exocrine glands of the body. Because in this disease the mucous glands produce very thick mucus, the older name was mucoviscidosis. The thick mucus is the most troublesome in the lungs. The other problem in CF is the partial destruction and malfunction of the exocrine glands in the pancreas. Because CF also affects exocrine glands, such as the sweat glands, tests for its detection are based on determining the amount of sodium (Na) and chloride (Cl) in the sweat. The CF gene mutation test identifies mutations in CFTR, a gene on chromosome 7. There are many mutations in this gene, but only a few are common and these make up the standard panel. Infants or children who test positive on sweat tests can be given this panel of tests as can older people who want to know if they have the gene mutation.

All 50 states, and the District of Columbia, now require newborn screening for CF.

Possible Nursing Diagnosis for CF

Ineffective Airway Clearance

For a child with CF, the malabsorption problems may be partially overcome by the use of oral preparations of pancreatic enzymes. The problem with mucus in the lungs requires diligent and daily respiratory care. The primary cause of death in CF is cardiorespiratory failure. In 1980, the life expectancy was about 18 years, and by 2000, it had risen to 32.5 years. More recently, the survival age has increased to 37 years, and more adults with cystic fibrosis want to start families (Lomas & Fowler, 2010). A plan of care focused on pulmonary and nutritional health can definitely slow the progress of the disease. Lung transplants are an option. See the Cystic Fibrosis Foundation (www.cff.org) for updates on treatment.

HELPING THE FAMILY OF A CHILD WITH A GENETIC DEFECT

General Nursing Diagnoses

Grieving Related to Loss of "Ideal" Infant

A family who has a child with a genetic defect needs help and encouragement to adjust to the changes that the disease requires. Because hypothyroidism can be controlled with the administration of thyroid hormone, and galactosemia and PKU can be made less severe by dietary restrictions, the family can be assured of a relatively healthy child. Still, the family needs time to mourn the "loss" of the perfect child. Skirton (2006) described the experiences of parents whose child was referred for a possible genetic diagnosis. Parents in the study benefited from being told that the parents and siblings may also be examined. The greatest stressor was waiting for the results. Another stressor was guilt. Even after the diagnosis of a genetic mutation, parental guilt persisted. Nurses have a major role to play in informing and supporting clients before, during, and after a genetic referral.

Risk for Ineffective Family Coping Related to Chronic Illness

In the case of defects such as sickle cell anemia, thalassemia major, and cystic fibrosis, parents have no assurance that the child will be healthy. When a child is born with any disorder, treatable or not so treatable, nurses are in a position to focus their attention on the total needs of the family. They can, for example, be part of a team that conducts follow-up studies with the family. Five methods of assistance used by nurses and other health professionals to help families cope are as follows:

1. Offering support, including the role of a listener
2. Guiding the parents, which involves use of available resources
3. Teaching so that all family members understand the disease
4. Providing physical care during bouts of illness
5. Providing an environment that promotes personal development to meet the demands of the situation

> Surely the development of nursing needs to progress to match the technical advances that make it possible for children with defects to receive sophisticated medical intervention. Medical technology has certainly made it possible to increase the quantity of life. Nurses have a role of helping to improve the quality of life. Nursing research has shown that the quality of life for children with CF may be improved by teaching them social skills and problem solving related to their chronic disease (Christian & D'Auria, 2006).
>
> **Deficient Knowledge Related to Risk of Future Pregnancies**
>
> One final important point in helping a family to adjust to the birth of a child with a genetic defect is the availability of genetic counseling to help the couple make a decision about future children. During the presentation of genetic information, families often first experience denial of the problem, followed by anger and blame. The desirable final phase is integration and insight into the problem. The couple can then make their own decision about future pregnancies. (See Chapter 28 on amniocentesis and chorionic villus biopsy.)

CORD BLOOD BANKING AND STEM CELL RESEARCH

One of the newer decisions that parents must make is whether to store blood extracted from the newborn's umbilical cord. The chance that the donor would ever use the blood is very small. If parents of newborns arrange to have cord blood obtained for a private bank, labor and delivery staff need to be aware that this is an outside service and the healthcare provider performing the delivery is usually responsible for the collection. A written policy should be in place, and safety products specifically designed for cord blood collection should be used. Parents may also choose to donate to a public cord blood bank. These donations can be made available to anyone who may need a blood stem cell transplant (www.marrow.org). Additionally, the donated blood is used by researchers. There is no cost for donating to a public cord blood program. More information is available at www.nationalcordbloodprogram.org.

Parents interested in donating cord blood to a private or public cord bank are encouraged to speak to their prenatal healthcare provider early in the pregnancy.

USE OF DNA SAMPLES FOR GENETIC TESTING AND IDENTIFICATION

DNA, present in every cell, is unique for each individual. Although the tests for DNA analysis are sophisticated, the collection of the sample can be simple. A sample of skin cells can be obtained by inserting a cotton swab into the mouth and rubbing it against the inside cheek (buccal swab). The swab is then placed in a specially treated vial or put on a slide for transportation to a laboratory that can do DNA assay (see Chapter 1).

Another simple collection technique is to use filter paper to collect blood from a heel stick (infant) or finger stick (child or adult). Whole blood, tissue samples, cultured cells, and hair follicles can also provide DNA for analysis. In addition to immediate testing, samples can be stored for future use when new genetic tests become available. Clients are able to get DNA direct testing from private laboratories that advertise on the Internet. Some common genetic screens available to the public are those for alpha-1-antitrypsin (Chapter 10), breast/ovarian cancer (Chapter 10), blood-clotting disorders (Chapter 13), colon cancer (Chapter 13), cystic fibrosis (Chapter 18), hemochromatosis (Chapter 2), and infertility and pregnancy losses (Chapter 28).

Clients and families who have questions about genetic diseases need to be referred for a genetics consultation. Because family history is such a powerful screening tool for genetic disease, the U.S. Department of Human and Health Services developed the *U.S. Surgeon General's Family History Initiative*. Since 2004, Thanksgiving has been designated as National Family History Day to help families focus on creating a family history. More information and a computerized tool for developing a family history are available at www.genome.gov.

In addition to detecting genetic disease, DNA samples are also useful in identifying the genetic makeup of a child to help determine the biological parents. (See Chapter 17 for a discussion about chain of custody when samples are taken for legal reasons.)

Yet another use of DNA is DNA "fingerprinting." Parents of young children may buy DNA identification kits for about $15.00. (Some businesses give them away as an inducement for their products.) Instead of, or in addition to, keeping a set of fingerprints of their children, parents can store DNA information in case the child is ever missing. While foot printing was once used as the standard identification for newborns, many institutions now use footprints only as mementos for parents.

Another recent application of DNA testing is genealogical tests offered by commercial companies. These tests help a person trace the mystery of his or her personal ancestry and their relationship to other racial and ethnic lines.

Questions

1. A client who is 2 months pregnant, has come to the clinic for her first prenatal visit. Which of the following tests would be routine for this first visit?
   a. Blood glucose and serum electrolytes
   b. Urinalysis and hematocrit
   c. CMV titers and HIV status
   d. α-Fetoprotein levels

2. The month after a client underwent a hysterosalpingogram, she missed her period. When menses still had not occurred after 2 weeks, she bought a home pregnancy test kit. If she is pregnant, then
   a. The human chorionic gonadotropin (HCG) in her urine will react with sensitized cells in the test sample
   b. The test will be negative because it is only 14 days after an expected period
   c. The HCG antibodies in her urine will agglutinate the HCG in the test sample
   d. The gonadotropins LH and FSH may cause a false-negative result because the test is the direct agglutination type

3. A quantitative HCG measurement may be used to follow the course of
   a. Preterm labor
   b. Testicular cancer
   c. Breast cancer
   d. Preeclampsia

4. All the following are autosomal recessive genetic diseases. For which one is a screening test performed on Jewish people of Eastern European origin?
   a. Sickle cell anemia
   b. Thalassemia
   c. Tay–Sachs disease
   d. PKU

5. A client and his wife are both carriers of the autosomal recessive genes for sickle cell anemia. They have one child who has sickle cell anemia. What is the probability that a second pregnancy will produce a child who does not receive the defective gene from either parent (i.e., no sickle cell anemia or even sickle cell trait)?
   a. One-in-four chance
   b. One-in-two chance
   c. All children will have the trait
   d. Risk cannot be stated because one child has the disease

6. An expanded α-fetoprotein screening that also includes tests for HCG and serum unconjugated estriol is offered to pregnant women to screen for
   a. Down syndrome
   b. Neural tube defects
   c. Fetal maturity
   d. Endocrine disorders

7. Which of the following is not a rationale for conducting PKU, galactosemia, and hypothyroid screening on all newborns?
   a. Mass screening tests for all three disorders are accurate, technically easy to do, and considered cost-effective
   b. All three genetic defects cause mental retardation if treatment is not begun within weeks or months after birth
   c. All these diseases may cause symptoms within a day or two after birth
   d. All three diseases can be effectively controlled by dietary restrictions or hormone replacement

8. Which of the following is an inappropriate role for the home care nurse who is working with a family who has a child with a genetic defect?
   a. Helping the family find and use available community resources
   b. Teaching the family about the effects of the disease
   c. Encouraging the family not to risk having another child
   d. Assisting with physical care if the child is ill

References

Adams, R. J. & Brambilla, D. (2005). Discontinuing prophylactic transfusions used to prevent stroke in sickle cell disease. *New England Journal of Medicine, 353*(26), 2768–2769.

Callister, L. C. (2006). Global genetics: Worldwide considerations. *MCN: American Journal of Maternal Child Nursing, 31*(3), 202.

Christian, B. J. & D'Auria, J. (2006). Building life skills for children with cystic fibrosis: Effectiveness of an intervention. *Nursing Research, 55*(5), 300–307.

Daley, A. M., Sadler, L. S., Leventhal, J. M., Cromwell, P. F., & Reynolds, H. D. (2005). Negative pregnancy tests in urban adolescents: An important and often missed opportunity for clinicians. *Pediatric Nursing, 31*(2), 87–89.

DeCherney, A. H., Nathan, L., Goodwin, T. M., & Lauter, N. (Eds.). (2007). *Current diagnosis & treatment: Obstetrics & gynecology* (10th ed.). New York: Mc Graw-Hill.

Deglin, J. H., Vallerand, A. H., & Sanoski, C. A. (2011). *Davis's drug guide for nurses* (12th ed.). Philadelphia: F. A. Davis.

Fedorka, P. D. & Heasley, S. W. (2008). Preeclampsia: the little known truth. *American Nurse Today, 3*(2), 9–11.

Giarratano, G. (2006). Genetic influences on preterm labor. *MCN: American Journal of Maternal/Child Nursing, 31*(3), 169–176.

Hay, W. W., Levin, M. J., Sondheimer, J. M., & Deterding, R. (Eds.). (2011). *Current diagnosis and treatment: Pediatrics* (20th ed.). New York: McGraw-Hill.

Kenner, C., Gallo, A., & Bryant, K. (2005). Promoting children's health through understanding genetics and genomics. *Journal of Nursing Scholarship, 37*(4), 308–314.

Lachat, M. F., Scott, C., & Relf, M. (2006). HIV and pregnancy: Considerations for nursing practice. *MCN: American Journal of Maternal/Child Nursing, 31*(4), 233–242.

Lomas, P. H. & Fowler, S. B. (2010). Parents and children with cystic fibrosis: A family affair. *American Journal of Nursing, 110*(8), 30–37.

Malone, F. D., Canick, J. A., Ball, R. H., Nyberg, D. A., Comstock, C. H., Bukowski, R., et al. (2005). First trimester or second trimester screening, or both, for Down's syndrome. *New England Journal of Medicine, 353*(19), 2001–2011.

McPhee, S. J., Papadakis, M. A., & Rabow, M. W. (Eds.). (2011). *Current medical diagnosis and treatment* (50th ed.). New York: McGraw-Hill.

Sibai, B. M. (2005). Diagnosis, prevention, and management of eclampsia. *Obstetrics and Gynecology, 105*(2), 402–410.

Skirton, H. (2006). Parental experience of a pediatric genetic referral. *MCN: American Journal of Maternal/Child Nursing, 31*(3), 178–184.

Tarini, B. A., Christakis, D., & Welch, H. (2006). State newborn screening in the tandem mass spectrometry era: More tests, more false-positive results. *Pediatrics, 118*(2), 448–456.

Twomey, J. G. (2006). Issues in genetic testing of children. *MCN: American Journal of Maternal/ Child Nursing, 31*(3), 156–163.

Wu, A. H. (Ed.). (2006). *Tietz clinical guide to laboratory tests* (4th ed.). St. Louis, MO: Saunders Elsevier.

Websites

genes-r-us.uthscsa.edu (National Newborn Screening and Genetics Resource Center for information on newborn screening in each state.)

www.ascaa.org (American Sickle Cell Anemia Association for support groups in each state.)

www.cff.org (Cystic Fibrosis Foundation for updates on cystic fibrosis.)

www.cooleysanemia.org (Information on treatment for thalassemia.)

www.gaucherdisease.org (Updates from National Gaucher Foundation.)

www.genome.gov (Information on National Family Day and forms for creating a family history.)

www.marrow.org (National Marrow Donor Program for updates on transplants.)

www.nationalcordbloodprogram.org (Information on the largest and oldest public cord blood banking.)

Answers

1. b, 2. a, 3. b, 4. c, 5. a, 6. a, 7. c, 8. c

CASE STUDIES

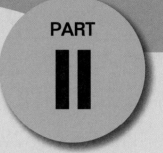

PART

II

Practice Interpretation of Laboratory Data

The following four case studies are presented:

- Mrs. Rita Rios, 38 years of age
- Sally Jamison, 14 years of age
- Mr. Jack Lee, 77 years of age
- Max Goldstein, 2.5 years of age

These case studies give the reader an opportunity to practice interpreting laboratory data and using the data to formulate possible nursing diagnoses. The reader may select from the nursing diagnoses presented with each case study, although this is not meant to be an exclusive list of possibilities. (Reference values for the laboratory tests are found in Appendix E.) A discussion of the laboratory data follows each case presentation. Interpretation of each test is completed, and some suggested nursing diagnoses are given. Page numbers are listed in the discussion so the reader can refer quickly to the text for further elaboration on each test and possible nursing diagnoses.

RITA RIOS

Rita Rios, 38 years of age, was admitted last evening with possible pneumonia. She had completed a course of chemotherapy last week for cancer of the pancreas. She appears malnourished and states that she has no appetite. She is being maintained on intravenous fluids of D_5 0.45 NaCl with 20 mEq KCl/150 mL/h. Her urine is orange, and her skin is slightly jaundiced. Current vital signs are as follows: BP 130/80, P 130, R 28, T 102°F (39.2°C). The night nurse reports that Mrs. Rios keeps removing the O_2 cannula. The current laboratory results are as follows:

1. Hgb 8 g; Hct 25%; RBC 3 million/mm³; MCV and MCH both low
2. WBC 4,000 per mm³ with 25% neutrophils and 5% bands (absolute count of neutrophils is thus 1,200)
3. Platelets 30,000/mm³; PT 20 seconds (control 12 seconds); INR 1.68
4. Urinalysis: positive for nitrites, leukocyte esterase, glucose, and bilirubin
5. BUN and serum creatinine WNL (within normal limits)
6. Lytes: K 3.0 mEq/L; chlorides slightly elevated, 115 mEq/L
7. ABGs: pH 7.52; $Paco_2$ 30 mm Hg; Pao_2 60 mm Hg; bicarbonate 20 mEq/L
8. FBS 190 mg/dL
9. Bilirubin: total 5 mg/dL; indirect 0.5 mg/dL; direct 4.5 mg/dL
10. Alkaline phosphatase 150 U/L; GGTP 135 U/L

What Are the Priority Nursing Diagnoses for This Client?

- Ineffective airway clearance?
- Ineffective breathing pattern?
- Anxiety?
- Activity intolerance?
- Sensory perceptual alterations?
- Risk for injury? Infection? Bleeding?
- Imbalanced nutrition?
- Deficient fluid volume? Actual or risk?
- Altered cardiac output?
- Disturbed body image?

Discussion of Laboratory Data for Rita Rios

1. The values for Hgb, Hct, and RBC indicate anemia, most likely related to the malignant disease and the client's malnourished state. The anemia is not from acute blood loss alone because the low MCV and MCH are indicative of a microcytic, hypochromic anemia (see Chapter 2, p. 36). Chronic blood loss and iron deficiency are common reasons for changes in these two erythrocyte indices. Possible nursing diagnoses related to this chronic anemia would be *imbalanced nutrition requirements* for *iron* and *protein*, *risk for activity intolerance*, *risk for infection*, and possible *sensory perceptual alteration* related to feeling chilly. If iron supplements are prescribed later, Mrs. Rios may have *deficient knowledge* regarding side effects (see Chapter 2, p. 30).

2. Mrs. Rios has neutropenia, not an unexpected side effect of chemotherapeutic drugs. The priority nursing diagnosis related to a lack of neutrophils is the *risk for infection* (Chapter 2, p. 50, discusses neutropenia).

3. Mrs. Rios also has thrombocytopenia, which is a possible side effect of the chemotherapy. The PT is increased and the percentage is decreased; both show a lack in some of the coagulation factors manufactured by the liver. The changes in PT may be due to the obstructive jaundice (see the bilirubin levels) or less likely liver dysfunction from metastatic disease. Whatever the reason, these abnormal coagulation tests indicate that Mrs. Rios has a *risk for bleeding* (see Chapter 13, p. 305, on PT).

4. Positive tests for nitrites and leukocyte esterase are usually indications of a urinary tract infection (see Chapter 3, p. 72). The *risk for infection* is a high priority because the glucose in the urine increases the risk for urinary tract infection and perineal abscess. The spilling of sugar in the urine also alerts the nurse to a possible *deficient fluid volume*, although other data do not suggest that this is a problem at present, probably because Mrs. Rios is receiving intravenous fluids (see Chapter 3, p. 70, on glycosuria).

5. A normal BUN and creatinine indicate no renal dysfunction from the chemotherapeutic drugs. Also, a normal BUN is evidence that there is no clinically significant deficient fluid volume at present (see Chapter 4, p. 83, on BUN measurements).

6. The low potassium level may be due to a loss caused by vomiting or a lack of intake. Hypokalemia is also found in alkalotic states. The chlorides are slightly elevated because another negative ion is slightly low (see Chapter 5, p. 122, on the electrolyte changes in acid–base imbalances). Because of the hypokalemia, Mrs. Rios has *imbalanced nutrition*. The physician should be notified so additional potassium can be given, probably intravenously for now, and oral supplements or by means of dietary intake later.

7. By looking at the ABGs, one can see that Mrs. Rios is in respiratory alkalosis. The most likely cause for the respiratory alkalosis is hypoxia. The reason for the hypoxia is not immediately evident. The *impaired gas exchange* may be due to the pneumonia or even to metastatic disease. The hypoxia might also be due to *ineffective airway clearance* related to mucous plugs or fluid in the lungs. *Anxiety* and an elevated temperature may be contributing to the hyperventilation and thus an *ineffective breathing pattern*. Certainly, the present method of oxygen delivery is not satisfactory. A thorough respiratory and neurologic assessment must be completed to determine the best way to raise the Pao_2 (see Chapter 6, p. 146, for possible nursing diagnoses related to hypoxia). In addition to the restlessness and anxiety from hypoxia, Mrs. Rios may also have *anxiety* related to the neuromuscular irritability found in alkalotic states (see the symptoms of alkalosis on p. 134). In this case study, sedation would be appropriate given these blood gas values, but not with Case Study 3.

8. The elevated blood glucose levels, in the absence of hyperalimentation, is an indication of a lack of enough insulin to transfer glucose into the cells. The β cells in the pancreas may have been damaged by the pancreatic tumor. The physician may have to order insulin if hyperglycemia persists. Mrs. Rios may be a candidate for hyperalimentation if nutrition continues to be a problem. Continued hyperglycemia may cause a possible osmotic diuresis, which leads to a *deficient fluid volume* and increases the *risk for infection* (see Table 8–4, p. 193, on the effects of hyperglycemia).

9. The elevation of the direct bilirubin is an indication of obstructive jaundice. Direct bilirubin is the conjugated bilirubin (BC) that is increased in the blood-stream when the normal biliary pathway is blocked (see Table 11–2, p. 260, on the types of prehepatic and posthepatic jaundice). For Mrs. Rios, the obstruction is most likely due to the pressure of the pancreatic tumor on the biliary tree. The dark orange urine with a positive test for bilirubin is further evidence that BC, which is water soluble, is being eliminated by the urine rather than through the intestinal tract. (The urine would foam if shaken.) If the obstruction is complete, Mrs. Rios's feces will become clay colored. Obstruction in the biliary tract also decreases the absorption of fat-soluble vitamin K, needed for the manufacture of prothrombin and other coagulation factors. Thus, Mrs. Rios has an increased *risk for bleeding* (see Chapter 13, p. 303, on the relation of obstructive jaundice to the PT). Because of the biliary obstruction, Mrs. Rios will have *imbalanced nutrition* caused by the inability to tolerate fats in the diet. As mentioned earlier, hyperalimentation may be needed during this acute phase until the obstruction is relieved with surgical intervention. The need to improve nutritional status will be a long-term goal. Two other nursing diagnoses related to the elevated direct bilirubin may be *sensory–perceptual alterations* caused by

the pruritus from bilirubin deposits in the skin and *disturbed body image* related to the appearance of the jaundice (see Chapter 11, p. 268, for further discussion of the care of a client with obstructive jaundice).

10. The markedly elevated alkaline phosphatase and GGTP provide further evidence that Mrs. Rios has biliary obstruction (see Chapter 12, p. 275, on enzymes used to assess for biliary obstruction). Unfortunately, Mrs. Rios has many serious problems. She needs a caring, knowledgeable nurse to devise an individualized care plan. Mrs. Rios and her family are at *risk for ineffective coping* as they decide what further treatments, if any, are warranted in the case of her medical diagnosis.

SALLY JAMISON

Sally Jamison, 14 years of age, has just been admitted to the hospital because of uncontrolled diabetes mellitus. She responds to questions but is drowsy if not stimulated. Her skin is flushed and dry. Her eyeballs are soft, and she reports blurred vision.

Vital signs are as follows: BP 106/88, P 128, R 32, T 100°F (38.1°C). The physician is writing orders now. Sally's sister states that the client has been under a great deal of strain caused by a family conflict. The admission laboratory results are as follows:

1. Hct 59%; RBC 5 million/mm^3; Hgb 14 g; erythrocyte indices WNL
2. WBC 15,000 per mm^3; no shift to the left
3. Platelets normal
4. Urinalysis: SG 1.040; sugar 2%; acetone moderate
5. Serum osmolality 316 mOsm; urine osmolality 1,400 mOsm
6. BUN 40 mg/dL; serum creatinine normal at 1.0 mg/dL
7. Lytes: K 5.8 mEq/L
8. ABGs: pH 7.30; Paco$_2$ 30 mm Hg; Pao$_2$ 98 mm Hg; bicarbonate 15 mEq/L
9. Random blood sugar 450 mg/dL

Plasma ketone 4+ in 1:1 diluted sample

What Are the Priority Nursing Diagnoses for This Client?

- Anxiety?
- Imbalanced nutrition?
- Risk for injury? Infection? Bleeding?
- Altered urinary patterns?
- Deficient fluid volume? Actual or risk?
- Deficient knowledge?
- Ineffective coping? Individual or family?
- Ineffective breathing pattern?
- Activity intolerance?
- Altered cardiac output?
- Noncompliance?

Discussion of Laboratory Data for Sally Jamison

1. The elevated Hct is an indication of a *deficient fluid volume*. The increase could be due to polycythemia (see Chapter 2, p. 28), but all the other laboratory data indicate deficient fluid volume. Normal erythrocyte indices indicate no apparent abnormalities with the size or amount of Hgb content of the erythrocytes.

2. The elevated WBC count indicates that the body is responding to stress or infection. There is no shift to the left. Therefore, there may not be a bacterial infection yet (see Chapter 2, p. 48, on the meaning of the shift to the left). Sally is vulnerable because of her diabetes; therefore, *risk for infection* is a priority.

3. A normal platelet count indicates no potential problem with bleeding related to thrombocytopenia.

4. The elevated specific gravity is due to the presence of glucose in the urine and also reflects an *actual deficient fluid volume* as supported by other laboratory data. The urine osmolality is a better indicator of fluid imbalance because it is not affected by glucose. The moderate acetone level in the urine indicates that Sally's condition has progressed from hyperglycemia to ketoacidosis.

5. The elevated serum osmolality reflects the *deficient fluid volume* and the hyperglycemia that have made the serum very hypertonic. The elevated urine osmolality reflects an *actual deficient fluid volume* (see Table 4–4, p. 94, on serum and urine osmolality).

6. The elevated BUN with a normal creatinine is indicative of a *deficient fluid volume*. The ratio is 40:1 rather than the normal ratio (see Chapter 4, p. 84). The other factor that could elevate the BUN, but not the creatinine level, would be a marked increase in protein intake or gastrointestinal bleeding, but the Hct shows no evidence of blood loss.

7. The hyperkalemia is expected because of the acidotic state (see Chapter 5, p. 116). Sally is at risk for altered *cardiac output* related to the development of arrhythmias. When the acidotic state is corrected, she will become hypokalemic unless her fluid and electrolyte balance is carefully monitored (see Table 6–6, p. 132, on usual electrolyte changes with acid–base imbalances). As Sally becomes able to resume oral intake, she may have *imbalanced nutrition* related to the need for electrolyte replacement as well as other dietary modifications for her diabetes.

8. The ABGs indicate that Sally is in metabolic acidosis. The test for the plasma ketones indicates that the acidosis is ketoacidosis. She does not have an ineffective breathing pattern even though her respiratory rate is 32. These rapid and deep respirations (Kussmaul's respirations) have lowered the $Paco_2$ so that there is less carbonic acid to match the bicarbonate (see Table 6–3, p. 129, on the carbonic acid–bicarbonate ratio). The acidotic state can put Sally *at risk for injury* related to a change in her perceptual awareness and level of consciousness. Her weakness and fatigue cause *activity intolerance*.

9. The hyperglycemia is due to the uncontrolled diabetes mellitus. These levels of glucose and ketones are consistent with moderate ketoacidosis (see Table 8–5, p. 194). In addition to the nursing diagnoses identified, others will become appropriate as Sally's diabetes is controlled. Does she have *deficient knowledge* regarding the balance of food, insulin, and exercise? Or is the problem one of

noncompliance that could be due to many factors? Sally's sister noted that there is a family conflict. Is there *ineffective individual or family coping*? What kind of referrals may be needed?

JACK LEE

Jack Lee, 77 years of age, was admitted to the hospital 4 days ago because of increased difficulty in breathing. He has had several previous admissions related to his chronic obstructive lung disease. He takes 0.25 mg digoxin daily and a mild diuretic.

Vital signs are stable. Mr. Lee states that he is ready to go home today. He lives alone and has no close relatives. The most recent laboratory findings are as follows:

1. Hct 60%; Hgb 19.8 g; RBC 7.1 million/mm^3; erythrocyte indices WNL
2. WBC normal
3. Platelets 450,000 per mm^3; PTT 28 seconds (control 34 seconds)
4. Urinalysis negative except for 2+ proteinuria and consistently low urine osmolality
5. BUN 45 mg/dL; creatinine 2.9 mg/dL
6. Lytes: K 4.0 mEq/L; Cl 90 mEq/L; bicarbonate 35 mEq/L
7. ABGs: pH 7.35; Paco$_2$ 58 mm Hg; Pao$_2$ 60 mm Hg; bicarbonate 35 mEq/L
8. FBS 99 mg/dL
9. Serum digoxin 1.2 ng/mL

What Are the Priority Nursing Diagnoses for This Client?

- Activity intolerance?
- Impaired gas exchange?
- Ineffective airway clearance?
- Risk for injury? Thrombophlebitis? Infection? Bleeding?
- Altered urinary patterns?
- Anxiety?
- Impaired home management maintenance?
- Risk for deficient or excess fluid volume?
- Deficient knowledge?

Discussion of Laboratory Data for Jack Lee

1. The elevated Hct, Hgb, and RBC are expected in response to chronic hypoxia. There are no laboratory data to support a deficient fluid volume, which would be another reason for an elevated Hct, as noted in the second case study. Although Mr. Lee's erythrocytosis or polycythemia is most likely secondary to his hypoxia, he could have polycythemia vera because his platelet count is also elevated. The actual medical diagnosis is the puzzle for the physicians. From a nursing point of view, the presence of polycythemia or erythrocytosis should alert the nurse to the fact that this client is at *risk for injury* because the increased viscosity of his blood can lead to venous thrombi. Mr. Lee may have *deficient knowledge* regarding

ways to decrease the risk for deep venous thrombosis (see Chapter 2, p. 26, for appropriate nursing instructions about fluids and exercises).

2. A normal WBC count indicates that Mr. Lee is unlikely to have any current problems related to infection. However, elderly clients may not always have an increased WBC count in response to an infection; therefore, careful assessment for any other signs of infection is warranted (see Chapter 16, p. 422, on infections in the elderly).

3. Mr. Lee's elevated platelet count could be due to many factors, including polycythemia, as discussed earlier. Compared with the normal (the control), the PTT is decreased. A decreased PTT can also be caused by many factors (see Chapter 13, p. 313). The decreased PTT gives additional data to suggest that Mr. Lee is at *risk for injury* related to the formation of venous clots. There is no evidence that his platelet count showed an abnormal type of platelets; however, if abnormal platelets were present, bleeding could be a problem (see Chapter 13, p. 318).

4. The proteinuria indicates renal dysfunction as verified by the laboratory data. The consistently low urine osmolality is evidence that the kidneys have lost the ability to concentrate urine. Furthermore, a urine osmolality is much more precise than a specific gravity in evaluating renal function (see Chapter 4, p. 92).

5. Elevations of both the BUN and the serum creatinine indicate that Mr. Lee does have renal insufficiency (see Chapter 4, p. 89). Because of this limited renal reserve, there is a *risk for injury* or a worsening of renal function caused by infection, stress, deficient fluid volume, and some drugs. The use of contrast media for x-ray procedures can also be dangerous. (see Chapter 20, p. 515.)

6. Mr. Lee has no problem with hyperkalemia because his renal disease is not severe. The diuretic has not caused hypokalemia, which could be dangerous with the digoxin. The other electrolytes are consistent with compensated acid–base imbalance. The bicarbonate is elevated to balance the increased $Paco_2$, as noted in the ABGs. Because bicarbonate, a negative ion, is elevated, another negative ion, chloride, is decreased in the serum to maintain an electrical neutrality (see Chapter 5, p. 105, on electrical neutrality).

7. Mr. Lee's ABGs show that he is in *compensated* respiratory acidosis. His pH remains within the normal range even though his $Paco_2$ is quite elevated. The $Paco_2$ level increased very gradually; therefore, the kidneys have had time to retain enough bicarbonate to keep the bicarbonate–carbonic ratio at 20:1 (see Tables 6–3 and 6–4, pp. 129–130). Although Mr. Lee's condition is stable with regard to the chronic obstructive lung disease, the laboratory data suggest that Mr. Lee may develop *impaired gas exchange* if he contracts a respiratory infection or is given high doses of oxygen or opioids (see Chapter 6, p. 137, on the danger of oxygen therapy and drugs). Mr. Lee may have some *activity intolerance* and thus must learn how to conserve energy.

8. Mr. Lee does not have diabetes. This is important to know in an elderly client who already has several other problems common in the aged population. Elderly clients do have an FBS slightly higher than that of young adults (see Chapter 8, p. 184).

9. This serum digoxin level is within the usual therapeutic range for a dose of 0.25 mg/day. Because of Mr. Lee's renal insufficiency, however, he is at *risk for injury*

related to his inability to excrete drugs at a normal rate (see Chapter 17, p. 460, on digoxin toxicity). Mr. Lee may have *deficient knowledge* regarding the way to check his pulse and watch for adverse reactions related to his medications. Mr. Lee's condition is stable now, and he is eager to go home; an astute nurse would recognize that Mr. Lee may have *impaired home maintenance management* unless he is aware of his health concerns. Perhaps a nurse should conduct a follow-up home visit.

MAX GOLDSTEIN

Max Goldstein, 2.5 years of age, was brought to the emergency department an hour after he took an unknown number of his grandmother's pills. She had hydrochlorothiazide (50 mg), furosemide (40 mg), and acetylsalicylic acid (ASA) on a shelf in the bathroom. On the advice of a neighbor, Max's father gave Max 3 teaspoons of *ipecac* syrup, but no pills were noted in the emesis. Admitting vital signs included P 160 and R 54. Max was drowsy and resisted further examination. He kept putting his hands over his ears. Initial laboratory results are as follows:

1. Hct 60%; RBC 6.5 million/mm^3
2. Urinalysis positive for salicylates; SG 1.030; negative for glucose and acetone
3. BUN 35 mg/dL; creatinine 1.0 mg/dL
4. Electrolytes: Na 130 mEq/L; K 2.6 mEq/L; Cl 90 mEq/L
5. ABGs: pH 7.30; Paco$_2$ 25 mm Hg; Pao$_2$ 100 mm Hg; bicarbonate 18 mEq/L
6. Serum salicylates 45 mg/dL (toxic level in children is >30 mg/dL)

What Are the Priority Nursing Diagnoses for This Client?

- Risk for bleeding?
- Deficient fluid volume?
- Ineffective breathing pattern?
- Impaired family coping?
- Imbalanced nutrition?
- Deficient knowledge related to safety needs of toddlers?
- Altered cardiac output?
- Anxiety?

Discussion of Laboratory Data for Max Goldstein

1. As in the case of Sally Jamison (Case Study 2), the elevated Hct and RBC count are reflective of a severe *deficient fluid volume* (see Chapter 2, p. 28).
2. The urine specific gravity also supports *deficient fluid volume*. Young children cannot concentrate urine as well as adults can do (see Chapter 3, p. 66, on specific gravity). The positive salicylate is expected, given the finding in the serum.
3. The elevated BUN and the normal serum creatinine level are further evidence of *deficient fluid volume* (see Chapter 4, p. 84, on BUN–creatinine ratio).

4. The low values for electrolytes are evidence of a massive diuresis. Note that even with deficient fluid volume, the sodium and chloride levels are low, and even with acidosis, the potassium level is low (see Chapter 6, p. 132). Hypokalemia is probably the greatest concern because of the risk for *altered cardiac output* related to the development of arrhythmias. The deficient fluid volume may also lead to shock and *altered tissue perfusion* as well as *decreased cardiac output*. Medical interventions are needed to restore fluid and electrolyte balance. Later on, Max may have *imbalanced nutrition* because he may need oral electrolyte replacements.

5. The ABGs for Max indicate metabolic acidosis. The salicylates are acid products that have used up the bicarbonate in the serum. The low $Paco_2$ is most likely a compensatory mechanism for the acidotic state. ASA is a respiratory stimulant and can cause respiratory alkalosis in the first stage of poisoning, particularly in adults (see Chapter 6, p. 131, on types of acidosis). In very young children, metabolic acidosis occurs very rapidly. The *risk for injury* related to sensory–perceptual alterations and loss of consciousness should be considered. The *anxiety* levels of Max and his parents also are a high priority.

6. The effect of ASA on the acid–base balance has been discussed. Large doses of ASA may also cause gastrointestinal irritation and a decrease in clotting factors. Hence, Max should be monitored for *risk for bleeding*. As various medical interventions are used to stabilize Max, the nurse needs to keep in mind the risk for *ineffective coping by the family* related to their fear and possible guilt over the accident. After Max's condition is stabilized, attention may have to be focused on any *deficient knowledge* of the parents regarding the safety needs of toddlers. However, nurses should know that active toddlers can often outwit even the most conscientious parents.

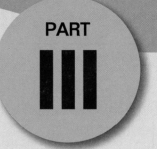

PART

III

DIAGNOSTIC PROCEDURES

CHAPTER

20 Diagnostic Radiologic Tests

- Reducing the Hazards of
  Radiation Exposure 508
- Nursing Diagnoses Related
  to Radiographic Procedures 511
- Chest Radiographs or Chest
  X-Rays 517
- Plain Radiographs of the
  Abdomen: Flat Plates,
  Three-Way Films, and KUB 519
- Bone or Skeletal Radiographs 519
- Upper GI Series and Small-
  Bowel Series 520

- Barium Enema Radiographs 521
- Cholangiograms: Intravenous,
  Operative, Transhepatic,
  and Endoscopic 523
- Intravenous Pyelograms 525
- Angiograms and Digital
  Subtraction Angiograms 526
- Hysterosalpingograms 528
- Mammograms 529
- Myelograms 531
- Arthrograms 532

OBJECTIVES

1. Describe the difference between fluoroscopy and routine radiography.
2. Explain how the four densities of air, fat, water, and bone are represented on x-ray film.
3. Identify three methods to reduce the hazards of exposure to x-rays.
4. List several important points to teach clients on how to protect themselves from unnecessary x-ray exposure.
5. Identify possible nursing diagnoses for clients undergoing radiologic studies.
6. Identify possible nursing diagnoses when clients return from undergoing radiologic studies.
7. Identify radiologic tests that require a contrast medium, and explain how the agent adds additional nursing implications.
8. Name specific nursing actions appropriate in assisting a radiographic technician using portable equipment to obtain a high-quality radiograph of a client in bed.
9. Compare the diagnostic tests described in this chapter, and identify the tests that cause pain, which often necessitates the use of analgesics.

The first part of this chapter briefly describes the three ways in which x-rays are used in diagnostic testing and how the hazards of radiation can be reduced when diagnostic radiographs are needed. The second part discusses the general nursing diagnoses to prepare a client for x-ray studies and to take care of the client after the radiographs are obtained. The last part of this chapter describes each of the common x-ray studies and the key nursing implications in caring for the client before and after each test. Although the preparation for each test is outlined in this book, the reader is advised to consult with the radiology department regarding the exact protocol to be followed at the particular institution, especially the guidelines given for pre- and posttest care. Most radiology departments have printed guidelines on the preparations needed for each test. The nurse should never hesitate to consult with members of the radiology department if a question arises about what is or is not necessary before a test. In addition, the nurse may need to consult the radiology department when several different tests are ordered for a client. For example, a radioactive iodine (RAI) test must be completed before radiographs are obtained with iodine contrast medium. Also, barium studies may make it impossible to perform other abdominal tests for 1–2 days.

Although rare, some radiology departments have a nurse as part of the staff. If a nurse is employed by the radiology department, she or he may have several roles, including (1) extended temporary floor nurse and guardian; (2) teacher; (3) consultant on how to deal with intravenous bottles, chest tubes, and other materials; (4) liaison with the clinic staff; and (5) team helper for a critical care nurse who may accompany the client to the radiology department.

How X-Rays Are Used in Diagnostic Tests

X-rays (or roentgen rays) were discovered in 1895 by the German physicist Roentgen, who received the first Nobel Prize in physics (1901) for his discovery. By 1896, the first x-ray machines were in use. Since that time, much has been learned about both the benefits and the risks of x-rays and radiographs. X-rays are electromagnetic radiation of very short wavelengths, which are commonly generated by passing a current of high voltage (from 10,000 volts up) through a Coolidge tube. X-rays can penetrate most substances, including human tissues, by strongly ionizing the tissue through which they pass. They cause some substances to fluoresce and affect photographic plates, qualities extremely useful for diagnostic tests. X-rays are, however, harmful to living tissue. X-rays can alter cells so they cannot reproduce. Consequently, radiation therapy is used to treat various types of cancer. (See Chapter 22 for further examples of diagnostic and therapeutic use of radiation in the form of radioisotopes.)

At present, there are three principal ways in which x-rays are used as diagnostic tests: (1) radiography, (2) fluoroscopy, and (3) tomography. Tests using the first two methods are discussed in this chapter, and tomography is discussed in Chapter 21.

Radiographs

Radiographs, or x-ray pictures of body structures, are like negatives of photographs. X-rays go through the body and reach the film positioned on the other side of the body. X-rays penetrate air easily; therefore, areas filled with air or gas appear very dark on the film. For example, lungs, which contain a large amount of air, appear very dark on a plain x-ray film. In contrast, bones or contrast media appear almost white on the film because the x-rays cannot penetrate these substances to reach the sensitive x-ray film. Organs and tissues appear as shades of gray because they have more mass than air but not as much as bone. For example, heart tissues contain a large amount of water, and the heart appears lighter on film than fatty tissues. From the blackest to the whitest, the four densities of substances on radiographs are as follows:

1. Air—blackish
2. Fat—dark gray
3. Water—lighter gray
4. Bone—whitish

Fluoroscopy

In fluoroscopy, the client is placed in front of an x-ray tube and a fluoroscopic screen is held over the body part to be examined. Recall that x-rays have the ability to make certain substances, such as those used to coat the screen, fluoresce, or give off light. As with radiographs, different structures of the body allow different amounts of x-ray beam to project on the fluoroscopic screen. The image remains on the monitor for continuous observation; therefore, any movements in the body can be monitored. For example, as a client swallows barium, the flow of barium can be monitored on a fluoroscopic screen. Fluoroscopy is valuable in cardiac catheter-izations to help the physician see the exact position of the catheter in the heart. (See Chapter 26 on cardiac catheterization.) Fluoroscopy is performed in the dark, so that images of the various densities are seen in sharper outline. Before fluoros-copy is performed, the physician puts on goggles with red lenses, which help the eyes adjust to the dark. Fluoroscopy prolongs the time of exposure to radiation; therefore, it is used only when it is deemed very important to observe the change in position or movement in the body. Videotapes of the fluoroscopic procedure (cine-radiography) enable the movements to be studied at later times. Cineradiography is also valuable as a teaching tool.

Tomograms and Computed Tomography

A tomogram, also called *laminagram* or *planogram*, is a special type of radiograph that is taken with both the x-ray tube and the film in motion during exposure. The camera takes pictures of several different planes of tissues. With each change in the position of the camera, a slightly different level of tissue is in focus. Computed tomography (CT) uses computers, scanners, and tomography to obtain a 3-D, cross-sectional view of any body structure. (CT scans are discussed in Chapter 21.)

REDUCING THE HAZARDS OF RADIATION EXPOSURE

Probably the most important point for the nurse to remember about radiation is that exposure to any type of radiation is cumulative. The nurse must be aware of the serious risks to clients or personnel who are repeatedly exposed to radiation. Some of the risks associated with cumulative doses of radiation are as follows: (1)

increased risk for cancer or genetic damage, (2) sterility, (3) alterations in the composition of individual cells, and (4) depression of the production of bone marrow. Leukemia and skin cancer are more common in people who use radioactive substances in their occupations. The amount of radiation in one radiograph is not enough to cause these problems, but radiation exposure must always be as limited as possible.

The effect on humans of any kind of radiation, natural or synthetic, is measured in a unit of quantity called *rem* (*roentgen equivalent for man*). A millirem is 1/1,000 of a rem. Most references estimate that the average American receives 100–200 mrem of radiation a year from the sun, cosmic rays, television sets, and diagnostic radiographs. Medical irradiation is probably between 50 and 70 mrem/person/year. For radiographs, 1 rem is equivalent to 1 rad (radiation adsorbed dose); the SI unit is the gray (1 Gy = 100 rad). X-ray exposure is designated in millirad.

The exact amount of radiation allowed for the general public cannot be expressed in millirem. The general guide of the National Council on Radiation Protection and Measurements is that all radiation exposure be held to the lowest practical level. The permissible level of radiation incurred under occupational circumstances is 5 rem or 5,000 mrem/year. The allowable amount for workers in nuclear plants or in radiology or nuclear medicine departments, however, is not a simple numerical rule. The formulas used to calculate the allowable radiation exposure for these workers take into account the lifetime exposure of workers. People who work with radiation must wear badges to monitor the exact amount of exposure to ensure that these limits are not exceeded. For example, the increased use of x-rays and fluoroscopes in the operating room increased the number of nurses who are exposed to radiation on a daily basis.

Time, distance, and shielding are three ways to offer radiation protection. For example, the time of exposure to x-rays should always be as short as possible. Fluoroscopy is not performed if a simple radiograph will suffice—exposure is shorter with a conventional radiograph. Keeping a distance from the x-ray machine is a second way to avoid radiation exposure. Thus, all personnel should leave the room when x-ray studies are being conducted. Occasionally, a nurse may be asked to help with a radiographic procedure being performed at a client's bedside. (See the discussion on portable chest radiography.) If the nurse must be involved in the procedure, shielding is important. Shielding (the third method of protection from radiation) involves the use of lead as a barrier to the x-rays (e.g., lead aprons and sometimes lead gloves). The walls of the radiography room are also shielded with lead, as are containers for radioactive materials.

It is sometimes difficult for health personnel to remember that x-rays are present, because the rays cannot be seen, heard, or felt. One type of monitor gives an audible beep when the wearer is exposed to a specified level of radiation.

Teaching Clients About X-rays

In 1984, the House of Delegates of the American Nurses Association passed a resolution that the Association educate its constituents about the new criteria for chest radiographs and the role of the consumer in reducing the number of unneeded radiographs. Clients should be encouraged to keep their own record of all x-ray exposures. This x-ray record can be carried to the physician, clinic, or hospital. The card should be filled in each time the client undergoes a radiologic examination. It should include the date, type of examination, address where the films are kept, and the name of the referring physician. Other tips for the public from the Department of Health and Human Services are the following:

1. Do not decide on your own that you need a radiograph.
2. Do not insist on a radiograph as part of a routine physical.
3. If your physician orders a radiograph, ask how it will help with the diagnosis.
4. Tell your physician about any similar radiographs you have undergone.
5. Ask if gonad shielding can be used for you and your children. (A lead apron should be routinely provided.)
6. Tell your physician if you believe you are pregnant.

Information on the safety of radiology tests and current information on all common tests including those in this chapter as well as CT (Chapter 21) and radionuclides (Chapter 22) is available at www.radiologyinfo.org. These guidelines are jointly developed by the American College of Radiology and the Radiological Society of North American (www.radiologyinfo.org).

Pregnant and Potentially Pregnant Women: The 14-Day Rule

Ideally, a woman in her childbearing years should undergo radiography only during her menses or 10–14 days after onset to avoid any exposure to a fetus. The routine use of lead aprons offers some protection to the fetus of the woman who is aware that she is pregnant.

Benefit Versus Risk, Including Costs

Over time, the public has become aware of the health risks of unnecessary radiographs. The controversy about nuclear plants caused an increased awareness by the public of the potential dangers of radiation. In addition to the health hazards from overuse of x-rays, the cost of unnecessary radiographs should be considered. As more stringent criteria are used to control insurance payments, consumers have become aware of costs. If consumers can take more responsibility for avoiding unnecessary radiography, there may be a financial gain as well as a decreased risk of illness or mutations from radiation exposure.

The point does need to be emphasized that if a client needs a radiograph for diagnostic purposes, the benefit far outweighs the risk, and cost should not be a deciding factor. It is beyond the scope of nursing practice to evaluate the usefulness and safety of specific tests ordered for a client. If the nurse encounters a client who is refusing a radiograph because of fear of radiation, it would probably be better to have the radiologist or physician explain the benefits of the test in relation to the small risk of radiation. An informed public can cooperate with health professionals to reduce the risks and increased costs of x-ray tests. When radiography is performed, the client should feel confident that the benefit of a specific test far outweighs the risk. The nurse can be instrumental in educating the public to have a healthy respect for x-rays as diagnostic tools.

Digital Radiographs

Digital radiography uses a detector that displays a digital image on a computer screen. No film is needed, so digital radiography may be called "filmless x-rays." Images are stored in a database and accessed on a computer screen. Compared to traditional radiographs, the digital radiographs offer a better quality of picture. Also, the radiologist can enlarge one section or sharpen the contrast to search for abnormalities. Nurses are able to assess digital radiographs instantly on a special high-resolution screen in the Emergency Department, operating room, or special care unit. Computer files can also be sent to other locations.

Conventional radiography is still common, but the rapid development of a picture archiving and communication system (PACS) has necessitated the need for digital imaging. See Chapter 21 for more about PACS.

NURSING DIAGNOSES RELATED TO RADIOGRAPHIC PROCEDURES

Pretest Nursing Diagnoses Related to Radiographic Procedures

Deficient Knowledge Related to Test Procedures

When radiologic tests are necessary for a client, the physician or nurse practitioner is responsible for informing the client why the tests are needed and describing the benefits and risks associated with the specific tests. If a radiograph is part of an invasive test, a special permit must be signed (see Chapter 25). Most radiology departments have printed material that gives information about how the test is carried out and what is necessary for client preparation. The role of the nurse is primarily to clarify the information the client has received and to follow up on anything that seems unclear. The nurse must understand enough about the test to be able to give simple, accurate information to the client. (Key points about specific tests are discussed later in this chapter.)

Anxiety Related to Unknown Sensations of the Procedure

Often the client may be more concerned about what the test feels like than a technical explanation of the test itself.

- Physical sensations should be described, but not evaluated.
- Clients should be told what causes the sensations (i.e., contrast medium causes flushing), so they will not conclude something has gone wrong.
- Clients should be prepared for aspects of the experience that are noticed by most clients.

Anxiety Related to Possible Findings of Test

The nurse can often relieve some of the client's anxiety by making sure that the client has received all the information he or she needs about the test, including any preparations that are needed. However, even with adequate information, many clients are anxious about x-rays.

(Continued)

Pretest Nursing Diagnoses . . . *(Continued)*

In addition to the fear of pain and discomfort from some radiographic procedures, there is often a certain amount of worry about what might be found. The nurse must not overlook the psychological needs of the client when focusing on the physical preparation. Clients may be relieved to find a nurse who not only listens but also actively encourages them to express any feelings they have about the upcoming test. Specific questions about the interpretation of the test should be referred to the physician who is diagnosing the problem. The nurse may help the client think of specific questions that should be answered.

Readiness for Enhanced Coping Related to the Procedure

Sometimes the amount of time that a client waits in the radiology department is longer than expected and may be exhausting to clients. Therefore, the nurse can alert the department personnel that the client is confused or incontinent or in a great deal of pain so that the client with a serious problem is not left unattended for a long period of time. If a very weak client must wait, a gurney should be used for transportation rather than a wheelchair. If permissible, pain medications may be given before the trip. Enemas or suppositories should be introduced early enough so that the client can rest before going to the radiology department. If possible, the nurse can promise to let the client rest once the examination is finished. For some clients, the waiting time in the radiology department causes boredom. The nurse can encourage the client to take some reading material or other activity, such as knitting, to help pass the time.

The nurse should see if the client is ready for the examination. Glasses, dentures, and hearing aids should not be removed before the examination if they are needed. X-ray personnel should be informed that a client is hard of hearing or has other communication problems. The client needs to empty his or her bladder. A robe should be worn for privacy and warmth, as should slippers if the client is to stand during the test.

These suggestions for ensuring client comfort are basic and thus often not mentioned. However, unless the nurse attends to these details, the radiography experience may be more uncomfortable than necessary. If the x-ray examination is being performed on an outpatient basis, the nurse can give the client tips on how to come prepared for the procedure. It is also important the client know the approximate duration of the test so business or home affairs do not present problems.

Risk for Deficient Fluid Volume Related to NPO Status

The nurse must make sure that the client understands when he or she is not allowed to eat or drink before a test (NPO). If feasible, having the client drink eight glasses of water for 1–2 days before the test decreases the risk for a deficient fluid volume. With some tests, a light breakfast or clear liquid may be allowed. Clients may need clarification that clear liquid means just that. Orange juice, milk, and so on are not clear liquids—one cannot see through them. Because of dehydration, especially in the very young or the elderly, the nurse must find out if the test requires strict NPO status or if clear liquids are permissible. For children, the restrictions of NPO status may be for only 3 hours rather than the usual 6–8 hours for adults.

Altered Elimination Pattern Related to Need for Intestinal Preparations

X-ray studies that involve structures in the lower abdomen may require intestinal preparation before the procedure. Table 20–1 summarizes the criteria needed to maximize intestinal

Table 20–1 Summary of Criteria Needed for Intestinal Preparation[a]
1. Restriction of diet to clear liquids (check for times)
2. Hydration of the client with adequate clear liquids (check for amounts)
3. Use of an evacuant that stimulates the small intestine (check for laxative ordered)
4. Use of an evacuant that stimulates the colon (check for laxative or suppositories ordered)
5. Use of an enema as an additional cleansing method (check for orders for tap water enemas or small medicated enemas)

[a]See text for more details on specific preparations for various procedures and the use of total intestinal irrigation.

preparation. Note that clients with ileostomies are not given enemas or laxatives as intestinal preparation. The preparation may be accomplished by cleansing enemas, cathartics, or suppositories. For example, a client may be given a bisacodyl tablet or magnesium citrate the night before the radiograph and a suppository the next morning. It is important for the nurse to assess the effectiveness of the intestinal preparation. If the method used did not cause evacuation of the intestine, other methods may be needed before the client goes to the radiology department. A poorly prepared client may mean that the radiographs have to be repeated.

An extensive intestinal preparation involves a total intestinal irrigation with a mixture of electrolytes and polyethylene glycol. The glycol prevents transfer of electrolytes into or out of the solution and also prevents production of gas in the intestine. This type of preparation is more often used for colonoscopy (Chapter 27) or surgical procedures, but it may be used for some radiographic preparations. The solution is prepared by adding tap water to a powder to make 1 L of solution. The solution tastes better if refrigerated, but for some clients, the coldness is unpleasant. The client drinks one glass of solution every 10–15 minutes or about 1.5 L an hour until the bowel return is clear or until the maximum of 4–6 L is ingested. The first bowel movement usually occurs about 1 hour after the last of the solution is ingested, and the intestine is clear in 4 hours (Deglin, Vallerand, & Sanoski, 2011).

Children and Elderly. A series of cleansing enemas or strong cathartics or repeated suppositories may be very taxing to elderly, frail clients. Also, the irrigation method with an electrolyte solution results in many trips to the bathroom. The nurse should question "standard" orders for intestinal preparation when the client is very small or frail. Smaller doses may be sufficient. Cathartics or enemas may be contraindicated if the client has had severe diarrhea or bleeding. Children younger than 1 year are usually not given any suppositories as intestinal preparation. Children 1–9 years of age may be given half a suppository. Any dose of laxative must be calculated on the basis of the weight of the child.

Teaching at Home. When intestinal preparation is to be conducted at home, the client must be taught exactly what to do if the procedure does not clean out the intestine. The client also needs to be shown exactly how to insert the suppository or how much fluid may be needed for the irrigation method. Often what is obvious to the health professional may not be to the client. Written instructions are standard, but a time for verbal interaction is often needed and may be much appreciated.

(Continued)

Pretest Nursing Diagnoses . . . *(Continued)*

Risk for Injury Related to Allergic Reactions to Contrast Medium

Many contrast media contain iodinated compounds, which can provoke allergic reactions (Table 20–2). Some newer agents contain less iodine, but they are more expensive. The radiology department should be notified if the client has any allergies. In the past, clients were asked if they are allergic to seafood as this was thought to be due to iodine content. However, this is a medical myth as allergies to seafood are due to a specific protein and not to the iodine content of the food (Huang, 2005). The exact reason for severe reactions to contrast medium is not well understood. For clients known to be at high risk for allergic reactions, pre-procedure treatment with prednisone and diphenhydramine and the use of low osmolar contrast medium reduce the risk to less than 1% (McPhee, Papadakis, & Rabow, 2011).

Before the radiologist injects the contrast medium intravenously, the client again is questioned about possible allergies. The radiologist still watches carefully for any signs of allergy, such as nausea, vomiting, palpitations, dyspnea, and dizziness. Sometimes antihistamines, such as hydroxyzine, and the H_2 blocker cimetidine are ordered at bedtime and in the morning before the procedure. Radiology departments are always equipped with drugs (epinephrine, antihistamines, corticosteroids, and nebulizers with albuterol) (Brege, 2008). The intravenous radiographic contrast material can also cause a vagal reaction marked by profound bradycardia and hypotension. Treatment of a vagal response includes intravenous atropine. Serious thromboembolic events have also been reported with contrast media, so hydration is important.

Clients need to understand that normally the contrast medium causes a flushing, warm sensation when it is injected intravenously, and may also cause a salty taste in the mouth. Nurses should be aware that contrast medium may temporarily cause false low pulse oximetry readings. Values usually stabilize within a few minutes. (See Chapter 6 on pulse oximetry.)

Table 20–2 Nursing Implications When Contrast Medium Used for X-Ray Tests

Examples of Common Radiologic Tests Using Iodine Contrast Medium

1. Intravenous cholangiograms (IVC)

2. Intravenous pyelograms (IVP)

3. Arteriograms

Pretest	**Posttest**
Assess for allergies	Assess for any allergic reactions
Instruct on sensations of contrast medium	Encourage fluids (may have intravenous)
Check what drugs should be withheld	Assess serum creatinine
(e.g., metformin)	Assess for phlebitis at injection site
Assess serum creatinine, and GFR	

Note: In addition to allergic reactions, a vasovagal reaction may occur during instillation of the contrast medium. See text for details.

Risk of Injury Related to Development of Contrast-Induced Nephropathy

Clients with preexisting renal problems are at risk for contrast-induced nephropathy (CIN). Estimation of the serum creatinine and GFR helps determine if the procedure is safe (Chapter 4). Factors that may contribute to CIN include dehydration, age over 70, diabetes or multiple myeloma with renal involvement, proteinuria, and concurrent administration of other nephrotoxic drugs. In addition to the use of a low osmolar agent, clients at high risk may be given intravenous fluids before the procedure and for 12 hours afterward (Barrett & Parfrey, 2006). Nonsteroidal antiinflammatory drugs (NSAIDS) and diuretics should be withheld for at least 24 hours before and after the procedure. Metformin, a drug used to treat diabetes, can cause lactic acidosis (Chapter 6) in clients with poor renal function, so it is also withheld before tests with contrast medium (Deglin et al., 2011). The timing for resuming medications depends on the serum creatinine level after the procedure. Because acetylcysteine has little harm and possible benefit, especially for clients with low GFR, the drug may be used. Other drugs such as sodium bicarbonate may also be used as a preventive measure (McPhee et al., 2011).

Posttest Nursing Diagnoses Related to Radiographic Procedures

The nurse or client performing self-care needs to know exactly what type of procedure was carried out, because specific implications are related to specific tests. (Care after a test is detailed in the descriptions of the tests later in this chapter.) Some hospitals may have a small recovery room for clients who need special observation, such as neurologic checks. More commonly, clients are returned to their rooms as soon as the procedures are finished. Many clients undergo radiography on an outpatient basis; therefore, the client or a significant other needs careful instruction on possible complications.

Risk for Injury Related to Use of Contrast Medium

Usually, if the client is allergic to the contrast medium, an immediate allergic reaction occurs in the radiology department, but delayed reactions are possible. Consequently, any symptoms such as urticaria, nausea, vomiting, or dyspnea should be reported immediately. Oral antihistamines or corticosteroids may be ordered for allergic reactions not acute enough to require epinephrine. Occasionally, the vein used for the contrast medium injection may become inflamed. Any local tissue reactions should be reported. Warm compresses may be used for phlebitis. Rarely, the high osmolality of the contrast medium can pull enough fluid into the intravascular space to cause pulmonary edema. Clients may need a diuretic and other treatment for respiratory distress (Geiter, 2006).

Imbalanced Fluid and Food Requirements

Contrast medium given intravenously for radiographic diagnostic tests is excreted in the urine. The contrast medium acts as an osmotic diuretic. Thus, if other conditions allow, a client who has a contrast medium injection should be given extra fluid to replace the fluid lost with excretion of the agent. Some clients may report bladder irritation or burning on urination caused by the

(Continued)

Posttest Nursing Diagnoses . . . *(Continued)*

contrast medium. As noted earlier, the contrast medium poses a risk of nephrotoxicity in clients with preexisting renal problems. The contrast medium is not visible in the urine, but it may elevate the specific gravity of the urine. (Contrast medium does not change the osmolality of the urine, so a urine osmolality test would be a valid test of fluid balance [Chapter 4].) Some of the newer contrast medium has less osmotic effect.

The contrast medium barium sulfate, used for studies of the GI tract, may cause constipation; therefore, consumption of fluids should be encouraged after these radiographic examinations. The barium is visible in the stool as white streaks.

The client may be very hungry or thirsty from being on NPO status for a long time. If allowed and tolerated, a cup of tea or some milk is appreciated until more solid food can be obtained. The liquids can help eliminate the dehydration, which may develop from the extended NPO status.

For many people, food is more than just physically satisfying. Food can be a symbol of love and care. Concern about the client's lack of food may be interpreted by the client as a sign of warmth and caring. (One of the cornerstones of professional nursing is nurturing.) It becomes routine for the nurse to withhold food and fluids because of diagnostic procedures. It is not routine for the client to go without food or fluids, and mere acknowledgment of this deprivation may be satisfying to the client.

Pain After Procedure

Waiting in the radiology department and the test procedures themselves may be exhausting. Clients should, therefore, be allowed to rest and be disturbed only for necessary procedures, such as checking vital signs and inspecting dressings for bleeding. Lying on a hard table causes a backache for some people. A backrub often is appreciated. A heating pad may also be helpful if muscles or joints hurt from the positioning during the test. (A physician's order is needed for heat applications.) Some procedures cause pain severe enough to require the use of analgesics. The nurse must assess whether the pain is the expected type for the procedure. For example, pain at the site of arterial puncture is expected, whereas pain in the foot may be a symptom of an embolus from the puncture site.

After diagnostic tests, an outpatient may need to rest before going home. (Monitoring may also be needed for a few hours.) If advisable, clients should be told in advance to have someone available to drive them home. The client should be informed about the level of pain to be expected. For example, hysterosalpingography may cause severe abdominal pain a few hours after the procedure. The client should be alerted that if the pain is not relieved with analgesics, she should notify the clinic or physician because pain can be a sign of a complication, such as a perforation. Arthrography also can cause considerable pain after the test. The manipulation of the joint entailed in the procedure can cause severe pain when the local anesthetic wears off. Instruction on the use of warm compresses or sitz baths to relax the tense, tired muscles from the painful radiographic session may be helpful. Mild analgesics may be needed.

Anxiety Related to Waiting for the Results of the Test

Interpretation of the test results is usually not available for 1–2 days. The client may be concerned about the results of the test. The nurse can act as a sounding board and help the client formulate questions to ask the physician. The nurse can also let the client express feelings about any pain or discomfort experienced during the test.

Nursing Implications for Future Care

By listening to the client's personal account of the test, the nurse not only helps the client put the experience in perspective, but also learns something that might help in preparing the next client for a radiologic test. As noted earlier, clients should be prepared for sensations experienced by most clients who undergo a diagnostic procedure. Nurses make lists of all aspects of a client's experience. Then using the list, the nurse can interview clients to learn what aspects of the experience are noticed by at least 50% of clients. The nurse also learns the words clients use most often to describe the sensations. Clients' descriptions are usually less technical and complex than the descriptions used by the nurses.

CHEST RADIOGRAPHS OR CHEST X-RAYS

Description

Chest radiographs are obtained not only in the radiology department but also at the client's bedside if the client cannot be transported to the radiology department. However, bedside, portable chest x-ray machines are not of as good a quality as those in the radiology department. In the radiology department, the client stands 6–9 feet from the x-ray machine, whereas the small, portable chest x-ray machines must be at most 3 feet from the client. In the radiology department, a conventional chest radiograph is a posteroanterior (PA) view because the client stands with the anterior part of the body next to the film. A portable chest x-ray machine provides only an anteroposterior (AP) view because the film is behind the client's back. In describing positions of the client, the first part of the term refers to the site of entry and the second to the exit of the x-ray beam, which is captured on the film. Note the basic working principle: The part that needs to be studied should be next to the film. Chest radiographs may be lateral views or oblique views as well. If there is question about the presence of free pleural fluid, the radiograph is taken with the client supine or in a lateral decubitus position, so the fluid pools. (*Decubitus* means lying down; hence, a decubitus ulcer results from a sustained lying-down position.) If the presence of air is suspected, the client is kept sitting up. For most chest radiographs, the client is asked to take a deep breath and hold it so that the lungs are fully expanded and the diaphragm is descended.

Purposes

Radiographs of the chest are used to identify abnormalities of the lungs and structures in the thorax. In addition, the size of the heart and abnormalities in the ribs or diaphragm can be determined. The normal heart shadow at its widest point is 50% or less the width of the thorax, so this cardiothoracic ratio is the simplest way to evaluate heart size. In heart failure, the heart shadow enlarges to greater than 50%. A smaller-than- normal heart shadow may be seen in chronic obstructive pulmonary disease because overexpanded lungs compress the heart. The three most common abnormalities diagnosed with chest radiographs are pneumonia, atelectasis, and pneumothorax. A chest radiograph is sufficient to help diagnose pneumonia, which is the most common cause of infectious death in the elderly. Unfortunately, in early stages of tuberculosis or asthma, the client may have a normal chest radiograph. Also in chronic obstructive pulmonary disease (COPD), the chest radiographic findings may not correlate with the clinical status. Expiration radiographs are used to detect a small pneumothorax or to demonstrate alterations in ventilation caused by emphysema or partial bronchial obstructions. Tumors of the lung can be identified with chest radiographs, but CT scans (Chapter 21) give much more detail. See Chapter 21 and the Lung Alliance (www.lungcanceralliance.org) for current use of CT screens for at-risk populations. Chest radiographs are also used to validate correct placement of central venous catheters and pacemaker leads. Peripherally inserted central catheters (PICCs), often inserted by specially trained nurses, also need the position confirmed by x-ray.

Feeding tube placements are also checked by chest radiographs. The first radiograph is taken to assess that the tube is in the esophagus and not the tracheobronchial tree. A second radiograph is done after the tube has been advanced to the proper location in the gastrointestinal tract. In some institutions, feeding tubes may be placed under fluoroscopy.

Client Preparation

A chest radiograph obtained in the radiology department requires no special preparation. The client should not wear jewelry or any metal around the neck or on the hospital gown. Most clients are very familiar with chest x-rays and realize that there is no pain or discomfort.

Nurse's Role with Portable Chest Radiography

If portable chest radiography is used at the client's bedside, the nurse may have a more active role in preparing the client than when the client goes to the radiology department. For example, chest electrodes need to be temporarily removed so the metal does not interfere with the picture. Intravenous tubing and arterial lines may cause shadows; thus, nothing should be lying on top of the client's chest. The client's back must be in even contact with the film holder. If the client is slumped in bed, the picture may be of poor quality. If it is absolutely necessary for someone to help hold the client in a position, the helper should wear a lead apron. (Lead gloves may also be used for protection.) As discussed earlier, although the radiation from one chest radiograph is minimal, the nurse must remember that radiation exposure is cumulative over a lifetime. Pregnant nurses should definitely not be exposed to any x-rays during a client's examination.

Posttest Nursing Implications Related to Chest Radiography

There are no special implications for nursing care after chest radiography. If the x-ray film shows atelectasis, the client needs vigorous pulmonary toilet for ineffective airway clearance. While the final interpretation of radiographs is the responsibility of the radiologist, nurses may view them to better understand the client's condition. Viewing chest radiographs can complement a physical assessment.

PLAIN RADIOGRAPHS OF THE ABDOMEN: FLAT PLATES, THREE-WAY FILMS, AND KUB

Description

Plain, or scout-view, radiographs, also known as "flat plates," of the abdomen may be obtained as the first step in assessing a variety of abdominal problems. They may be obtained with the client lying flat, turned to the left, and upright. These three positions are called a *three-way abdominal radiograph*. If the main focus is on the kidneys, ureters, and bladder, the radiograph is called a *KUB*.

Purposes

Abdominal radiographs can help detect loops of dilated intestine, patterns of gas, and possible obstructions. Stones and calcified areas in the pancreas, biliary system, or urinary system may be detected, but radiographs with contrast medium are needed for diagnosis. Perforations in the GI tract result in the escape of air into the peritoneal cavity, which causes an elevation of the diaphragm on the affected side. The elevated diaphragm is seen on the plain radiograph.

Client Preparation

In abdominal trauma, a flat-plate radiograph is ordered as a stat procedure. If there are questionable abdominal injuries, there will not be any attempt to clear the intestine of feces and gas. In nontraumatic conditions, however, the client may need an intestinal preparation before the radiograph is obtained. (See the introductory remarks on types of intestinal preparation that may be performed.)

> ### Nursing Implications Related to Plain Radiography of Abdomen
>
> There are no special nursing implications related to a flat-plate radiograph of the abdomen. However, the nurse should be aware that the client may be scheduled for other radiographs that involve the use of a contrast medium to identify particular structures. The nurse should also assess and record the exact nature of any abdominal pain and absence or presence of bowel sounds, which could be useful in the differential diagnosis of acute abdominal problems.

BONE OR SKELETAL RADIOGRAPHS

Description and Purpose

Skeletal radiographs are routinely used to detect fractures. They may also be used to detect tumors of the bone, but scans are more useful. Scintigraphy may also be used to detect stress fractures in clients with pain but a negative skeletal x-ray. (See Chapter 22 for the use of bone scans with radionuclides to detect tumors and stress fractures.) Simple radiographs are useful in assessing skull fractures; however, the presence or absence of a skull fracture does not correlate with the possible severity of any underlying brain damage. (CT scans, discussed in the next chapter, are extremely valuable in detecting soft-tissue injuries.) Skeletal radiographs are also used to assess arthritic conditions and to detect osteomyelitis.

Client Preparation

Skeletal radiographs require no special preparation. If the radiographs are being obtained to assess a possible fracture, the client should be treated as having a fracture until it is ruled out. The client needs careful handling and immobilization of the affected part. Pain relief may be needed before transportation. If skull radiographs are required, the client should undergo a neurologic assessment before transportation to the radiology department. If any drainage is present, a check for the presence of glucose reveals if the fluid is cerebral fluid. Glucose in cerebral fluid makes the test positive. Mucus contains no glucose. The nurse should notify the members of the radiology department of any instability in the client's vital signs, so that the radiographs can be obtained immediately and the client watched carefully.

Nursing Implications Related to Skeletal Radiographs

Exercise the precautions regarding care of potential fractures. If the client is undergoing skeletal radiography because of arthritis, the client may need an analgesic after the manipulation.

UPPER GI SERIES AND SMALL-BOWEL SERIES

Description and Purposes

Barium swallows are used for radiographs of the upper GI tract. The client drinks barium sulfate, which is a chalky radiopaque substance. Its non-water-soluble quality prevents it from being absorbed by the GI tract. Sometimes, the radiologist uses a contrast agent, meglumine diatrizoate, which is water soluble. Fluoroscopy during the barium swallow outlines the esophagus and any structural defects. Esophageal varices may also show on the radiograph.

The swallowed barium coats the stomach wall so that defects, such as tumors or ulcers, are seen as dark areas with a white background. An endoscopic examination (Chapter 27) is the definitive test for gastric and duodenal ulcers. The time it takes for the barium to empty out of the stomach is important in some cases because duodenal ulcers may cause pyloric obstruction or gastric outlet obstruction. As the barium goes through the small intestine, another series of radiographs may be taken, called a *small-bowel series*.

An upper GI series takes about 45 minutes. If a small-bowel series is performed, it may take as long as 5 hours to complete the examination. Also, a follow-up series may be performed in 24 hours. (See Chapter 27 for capsule endoscopy of the small intestine.)

Drugs may be given during an upper GI series. For example, glucagon may be given to relax the intestinal tract. Drugs may also be used to accelerate the passage of barium through the stomach and small intestine to promote better visualization of the jejunum and ileum. Metoclopramide is such a promotility agent. These drugs are given intravenously after the client reaches the radiology department.

Client Preparation

The client usually eats a light meal the evening before the radiograph is obtained and ingests nothing by mouth from midnight until the test. Food or medicine in the GI tract interferes with the barium coating the walls. Sometimes oral medications may be continued until 2 hours before the scheduled examination if gastric emptying is normal. However, any administration of medication should be authorized by the physician. Some parenteral medications, such as antibiotics, are continued; others may not be (e.g., regular insulin would be withheld, whereas a longer-acting insulin may be given). Because opioids and anticholinergic drugs, such as atropine, slow the motility of the intestinal tract, the radiologist should be notified if these drugs have been given to the client. Sometimes atropine might be ordered before an upper GI series if the client has a hyperactive intestine. The client should be told that fluoroscopy is performed in the dark and that the table is tilted to help the flow of barium. If a small-bowel series is to be performed, the client needs to know that it is a long procedure that requires two trips to the radiology department. The client should also be told that the barium has a chalky taste. Many radiology departments use flavored barium sulfate (e.g., peppermint or chocolate), but most clients still find it unpleasant to drink.

Posttest Nursing Implications Related to Upper GI Radiography

The client may need to wait for a second series of radiographs to be taken. Food and water should not be allowed until the radiologist completes the test. If the client has an ulcer, the lack of food in the stomach may aggravate abdominal pain, so food or antacids should be resumed as soon as possible. The client should be informed that his or her stool will be light colored because of the barium being excreted. For some clients, the barium may be constipating, so laxatives or enemas may be needed. Gastrografin may cause diarrhea. Barium in the intestine interferes with other abdominal tests, so the others should be scheduled first; otherwise, the client may need an enema so that other structures can be visualized with these other tests.

BARIUM ENEMA RADIOGRAPHS

Description

For examination of the lower colon, an enema of barium sulfate is given. This enema is performed in the radiology department. The client must retain the barium while a series of radiographs are obtained. After the barium is excreted, a final radiograph of the intestine is obtained. Sometimes air is put into the empty colon afterward for a double-contrast examination. The introduction of air may cause slight discomfort. A barium enema examination takes about 1–1.5 hours to complete.

Purpose

A barium enema examination is commonly used when any kind of lower intestinal problem is suspected. Tumors, strictures, polyps, and diverticula can all be well visualized with this method. Sometimes a barium enema is also therapeutic;

it may reduce an obstruction caused by intussusception or telescoping of the intestine (Hay et al., 2011).

Client Preparation

The lower colon must be prepared with the bowel preparation used in a particular setting. As noted in Table 20–1, bowel preparations may include enemas, laxatives, electrolyte irrigations, or suppositories. It is essential that there be no fecal matter in the lower colon. The client may be given a cleansing enema early in the morning of the radiograph. Some institutions do not schedule enemas the day of the radiograph. If the client has a severely inflamed intestine or active bleeding, strong cathartics or other bowel preparation is contraindicated.

A liquid diet may be ordered for the day before the examination. Clients are given a light breakfast the day of the examination because the food does not reach the large intestine by the time of the examination. However, if there is any question about complications, food may be withheld. Perforation of the colon is an unlikely complication, but it can occur if the intestine is diseased and friable. When there may be complications, it is always better that the client not have a full stomach. Adequate ingestion of liquids is important so that the client is well hydrated. An example of client instructions for use with outpatients is shown in Table 20–3.

Table 20–3 Instructions for Barium Enema	
THE SUPPOSITORY AND LAXATIVES MAY BE PURCHASED AT THE PHARMACY. (*Senokot* and *X-prep* are brand names for senna preparations: bisacodyl may also be used.)	
ON THE DAY BEFORE YOUR APPOINTMENT, EAT AND DRINK ONLY THE FOLLOWING:	
LUNCH	This meal may include clear broth, white chicken meat sandwich (no butter, lettuce, or other additive), or two hard-boiled eggs, strained fruit juices, Jello or other gelatin (without fruits or nuts), coffee or tea (without cream or milk), or carbonated beverages
3 PM	Take 2.5 oz of the prescribed laxative and drink one full glass of water
SUPPER	Limit your evening meal to liquids without milk products. This meal may include clear broth, strained fruit juices, Jello or other gelatin (without fruits or nuts), coffee or tea (without cream or milk), or carbonated beverages
10 PM	Insert one suppository into your rectum
ON THE DAY OF YOUR APPOINTMENT:	
BREAKFAST	Limit to coffee or tea (without cream or milk), strained fruit juices, and continue to drink water until 1 hour before the test
Two hours before your scheduled examination, insert one suppository into your rectum.	
PLEASE REPORT TO THE X-RAY DEPARTMENT ON _____ AT _____	
WHAT IS A BARIUM ENEMA?	
This is an x-ray examination of the large intestine. For this study, it is most important to clean the bowel of all retained fecal matter. A tube is placed into your rectum, and the barium liquid flows easily into your bowel. The radiologist studies the bowel with a fluoroscope. Several x-rays are taken.	
NOTE: If you have severe diarrhea or considerable rectal bleeding, consult your physician before taking the laxative or suppository. If you have any questions, or require a change of appointment, please call the x-ray department.	

Note: X-ray departments may modify these instructions as to whether 12-, 24-, or 48-hour prep is needed.

If a client is unable to retain the fluid of the enema, the nurse needs to inform the radiology department so a special tube can be used to instill the contrast medium. A client who can retain the enema fluid can be spared this extra discomfort. Most people can retain the amount of fluid used for a barium enema, but it is often a concern for the client.

A barium enema can be administered through a colostomy. Usual bowel preparations are completed, and the colostomy is irrigated before the procedure. Mechanical bowel cleaning differs for clients with ileostomies because enemas and laxatives are not used.

Posttest Nursing Implications Related to Barium Enema Examination

A barium enema can be exhausting physically and psychologically. It is embarrassing to many people to be given an enema in the radiology department and then to be asked to assume awkward positions in front of other people. If the client did not retain the barium well, a bath may be in order. Although most clients do expel the barium in the radiology department, some, particularly the elderly, may become constipated from barium still in the intestine. Fluids should be encouraged, 2,000 mL a day for adults, unless contraindicated. Cleansing enemas or a laxative may be given if there is a problem with defecation. If the barium was instilled via a colostomy, irrigations can rid the intestine of the residual barium. As mentioned earlier, the client's first stool will be a light color or will have white streaks.

CHOLANGIOGRAMS: INTRAVENOUS, OPERATIVE, TRANSHEPATIC, AND ENDOSCOPIC

Description and Purposes

A cholangiogram is a radiograph of the biliary tree obtained with contrast medium so the cystic, hepatic, and common bile ducts can be visualized.

Intravenous Cholangiogram

When the contrast medium is given intravenously, the liver excretes the contrast medium into the biliary tree. X-ray pictures are taken at intervals after the contrast medium is injected. The contrast medium begins to appear in the biliary tree about 10 minutes after the intravenous administration of the contrast agent. It takes about 4 hours but sometimes 8 hours for the contrast medium to be totally excreted, so the client may be in the radiology department for several hours.

T-Tube Cholangiography

Cholangiograms are also obtained during surgical procedures to check for stones in the common bile duct, which might not be seen or felt. With the operative method, the contrast medium is injected directly into a drainage catheter (T tube) placed in the common bile duct during a surgical procedure. X-ray films are taken immediately after the contrast medium is instilled. A T-tube cholangiogram may also be obtained several days postoperatively to evaluate the patency of the biliary tree. Clients who undergo exploration of the common bile duct have a T tube for bile drainage until the edema in the common bile duct is relieved.

Transhepatic Cholangiography

Transhepatic cholangiograms are obtained by means of percutaneous insertion of a needle into the common bile duct. The insertion is carried out with the aid of fluoroscopy. After the needle is in the common bile duct, contrast medium is injected.

Endoscopic Cholangiopancreatography

A fourth way to inject contrast medium into the biliary system is with the use of an endoscope passed into the GI tract through the sphincter of Oddi into the biliary tract. (See Chapter 27 for a discussion of endoscopic procedures.)

Client Preparation

Of the four procedures described, intravenous cholangiography is most commonly used. The client takes nothing by mouth for 6–8 hours before the test. A preparation is ordered to clear the intestinal tract. Intravenous cholangiography is performed in the radiology department and is not particularly uncomfortable except for the sensation of contrast medium being injected intravenously.

If cholangiograms are part of an operative procedure, the client receives the routine preoperative preparation. A percutaneous transhepatic cholangiogram is conducted in the radiology department. Because this is an invasive procedure, the physician must explain the specific risks to the client. The endoscopic procedure is also invasive and entails risks; consequently, institutions have special protocols to follow regarding permission. (See Chapter 25 for nursing implications for invasive tests.) Because obstructions in the biliary system tend to increase bleeding, the client usually has a prothrombin time (PT) performed before any type of invasive procedure on the biliary tree. GI absorption of vitamin K, a fat-soluble vitamin, is hampered when there is a biliary obstruction and thus a lack of the bile salts for fat absorption. If the PT is increased, vitamin K must be given parenterally before traumatic tests are done. Chapter 11 discusses laboratory tests used to assess for biliary obstruction and the nursing diagnoses for clients with elevation of direct bilirubin (obstructive jaundice).

Posttest Nursing Implications Related to Cholangiography

The aftercare for a client who has had contrast medium instilled for an intravenous cholangiogram would be the routine nursing diagnoses discussed at the beginning of this chapter.

See Chapter 25 for the nursing implications when a client has undergone an invasive procedure that may cause bleeding. Frequent checking of vital signs and bed rest for a specified amount of time are important. Just as in a liver biopsy, complications such as leakage of bile into the peritoneal cavity can occur when a needle is inserted into the common bile duct. Any abdominal pain, which could mean bile peritonitis, should be called to the attention of the physician. Chills and fever may be due to inflammation of the bile duct.

INTRAVENOUS PYELOGRAMS

Description

Diatrizoate sodium and diatrizoate meglumine are contrast media used for pyelograms because they are excreted by the urinary system. Another name for intravenous pyelography (IVP) is excretory urography because it demonstrates the ability of the entire urinary tract to excrete contrast medium. After the contrast medium has been injected intravenously, radiographs are obtained every minute for 5 minutes, allowing visualization of the cortex of the kidney. Approximately 15 minutes later, radiographs are obtained as the contrast medium collects in the pelvis of the kidney and is excreted via the ureters into the bladder. The contrast medium outlines the bladder in about 45 minutes. The client is asked to void, and a postvoiding radiograph is obtained to see how well the bladder empties. The entire set of radiographs takes about an hour. If the contrast medium is not well excreted, a 24-hour follow-up radiograph must be obtained.

Purposes

Structural defects or tumors can be observed when the urinary system is outlined with contrast medium. A retrograde introduction of contrast medium, through ureteral catheters, to outline the urinary system is carried out with a cystoscope. (See Chapter 27 for endoscopic procedures.) Renograms, conducted with radionuclides (Chapter 22), can be performed if clients are allergic to the contrast medium used for IVP.

Client Preparation

The client is given a light meal the evening before the test. Different radiology departments may have different instructions regarding nothing-by-mouth status. Some radiologists prefer that the client not take in any fluids so the contrast medium will not be diluted. Other radiologists want the client to be given clear liquids so that the client is not dehydrated before the examination. A lack of normal renal function may make it hazardous for a client to receive contrast medium that is excreted via the kidneys; therefore, serum creatinine and BUN levels are assessed before the test is begun (Chapter 4). The intestinal preparation for an IVP must be thorough. A cathartic agent as well as suppositories the evening before and the morning of the examination may be necessary. Enemas may be necessary if the client has undergone a barium study in the preceding 48 hours.

The client should be instructed about the sensation of the contrast medium being injected. (See the general implications about contrast medium discussed earlier in this chapter.) There may be more than one venipuncture. The only other discomfort results from lying in one position during the series of radiographs. Voiding in the radiology department may be embarrassing for clients who must use a urinal or bedpan if they cannot go to the bathroom.

> ## Posttest Nursing Implications Related to IVP
>
> See the general implications for contrast medium use, including a fluid intake of 2,000–3,000 mL. The client should be observed for any signs of urinary problems, such as difficulty voiding or bladder irritation. Note that the serum creatinine levels and creatinine clearance tests may be used to assess any loss of renal function.

ANGIOGRAMS AND DIGITAL SUBTRACTION ANGIOGRAMS

Description

Angiography is a broad term meaning visualization of blood vessels that are either arteries or veins. *Arteriography* is a more precise term designating visualization of arteries. *Digital Subtraction Angiography* (DSA) uses digital images pre- and post-contrast medium to better visualize the vessels. Use of a sophisticated imaging system with a computer allows the pre-images to be subtracted from the post-images. Other applications give a 3-D image of the vessels. The most common site of contrast medium injection for an arteriogram is the femoral artery. Arterial catheters are positioned with a guidewire that is used to advance the catheter to a specified location in the arterial tree. Because the arterial catheter is radiopaque, movement of the catheter is noted with fluoroscopy. After correct placement is obtained, contrast medium is injected into the catheter to outline a portion of the artery. In this way, the circulation in the lower extremity can be visualized. Also, the catheter can be threaded via the femoral artery into the abdominal aorta to the level of the renal arteries for renal arteriograms. The arteries of the GI tract can be visualized if the contrast medium is instilled in the celiac axis. The brachial artery can be used for upper extremity visualization. Carotid arteriography may also be performed but can disrupt atherosclerotic plaques, which can become cerebral emboli. Therefore, the carotid arteries are usually visualized with contrast medium administered through a catheter threaded through other arteries.

Purposes

Arteriograms are extremely valuable for observing the blood flow to a part of the body and to detect lesions that may be amenable to surgical treatment. The catheter used to administer the contrast agent to confirm the diagnosis of a suspected kidney or liver lesion may also become a vehicle for the selective delivery of chemotherapeutic drugs or drugs to stop bleeding. Catheters in arteries are also used to remove atherosclerotic plaques in a procedure called *percutaneous transluminal angioplasty* (PCTA). Magnetic resonance angiography (MRA) and CT angiography

(Chapter 21) have largely replaced invasive angiography to determine the location of occlusive disease in blood vessels (McPhee et al., 2011).

Client Preparation

The client must sign a special permission form. At some hospitals, it is routine to discuss the possibility of angioplasty and obtain informed consent at the time a client signs a consent form for arteriography because the therapeutic maneuver may immediately follow the diagnostic procedure. After premedication is administered, the client cannot legally consent to a procedure not cited on the original consent form. (See Chapter 25 for the nurse's role in preparing clients for invasive procedures.) Because arteriography involves intravenous administration of an iodinated contrast medium, the implications for contrast medium use should be considered. (See the discussion on contrast medium at the beginning of this chapter.) The client ingests nothing by mouth for 6–8 hours before the procedure; some institutions do allow liquids before an arteriogram. There may be an order to shave an area, but usually any preparation of the puncture site is performed in the radiology department.

Posttest Nursing Implications Related to Arteriography

The client stays supine for a minimum of 4–6 hours to decrease the possibility of bleeding from the puncture site; some institutions may instruct the client to stay supine longer. The nurse should make an observation of the puncture site as soon as the client returns from the radiology department. This serves as a baseline comparison if later there is blood on the dressing or swelling around the site. There may be more than one site if one puncture was not successful. The pressure dressing on the site should not be removed. An ice bag may also be placed on the site to decrease the possibility of bleeding or hematoma formation. Vital signs should be taken every 15 minutes for the first hour and then every 2–4 hours as ordered or deemed necessary. Frequent temperature checks are not necessary, but temperature should be recorded every 4 hours to detect beginning septicemia or a reaction to the contrast medium. Pulses distal to the arterial puncture must also be checked with the vital signs. Thrombus formation, emboli release, nerve damage, or spasms of the artery are all possible complications. Pain at the puncture site is not uncommon and may require analgesics, but pain distal to the puncture site may indicate an embolism. A false aneurysm, a cystic-like mass that communicates with the damaged arterial wall, may develop immediately after the trauma or develop weeks later.

Femoral Arteriogram. For a *femoral* arteriogram, the pedal pulses are checked. (See Chapter 23 for the use of a Doppler probe to assess arterial pulses.) The client may not have had detectable pulses before the arteriogram; this must be taken into account. The color, sensation, and warmth of the foot on the side examined should be compared with the other foot. Any pain in the foot or leg should be carefully assessed and compared with the pain before the arteriogram.

(Continued)

> **Posttest Nursing Implications . . . (*Continued*)**
>
> *Brachial Arteriogram.* If a *brachial* arteriogram is obtained, there is concern not only for spasm, embolism, or thrombus formation but also for nerve compression. Pain or numbness in the fingers or hand should always be reported immediately. Blood pressure readings should not be taken on the examined arm because they temporarily compromise arterial circulation in the lower arm.
>
> *Carotid Arteriogram.* The client should be assessed for any signs of transient ischemic attacks (TIAs), such as facial weakness, visual disturbances, or slurred speech. The client's head should be kept elevated about 30 degrees. Carotid angiograms are reserved for cases that cannot be resolved by less invasive imaging such as ultrasound (Chapter 23) and MRI (Chapter 21). Pressure on the carotid arterial site should be avoided; this can cause a vagal response that can slow the heart.
>
> *Renal Arteriogram.* If a *renal* arteriogram is performed, hypotension may result from a decrease in the formation of renin for a short time. Renal function must be closely monitored. BUN and serum creatinines may be ordered (Chapter 4).
>
> Fortunately, all these complications of arteriograms are rare, but the nurse who makes skilled assessments may detect a problem before it becomes serious.

HYSTEROSALPINGOGRAMS

Description

The client is placed in the lithotomy position, and a vaginal speculum is inserted. Contrast medium is injected through the cervix into the uterus and fallopian tubes. The client is awake during the procedure. There is likely to be some abdominal discomfort from the pressure of the contrast medium, even though only about 5–10 mL is used. Water-based contrast medium tends to cause less cramping than oil-based contrast medium; however, oil-based contrast medium has a fertility-enhancing effect (DeCherney et al., 2007). Fluoroscopy is used to monitor the progression of the contrast medium through the fallopian tubes. Ultrasonography (Chapter 23) with contrast medium may be used to establish tubal patency so that there is no exposure to radiation. The examination is scheduled within a week to 10 days after the client's menstrual period, to ensure that the client is not pregnant. The test takes about half an hour.

Purposes

The test is used to detect blocked fallopian tubes. Other abnormalities in the uterus, such as fibroid tumors, also are demonstrated on the radiograph. This is one of the tests performed as part of an infertility evaluation. (See Chapter 28 for a discussion of the five basic tests for infertility.) Occasionally, the injection of the contrast medium may also be included to evaluate the success of a tubal ligation, but laparoscopy with contrast medium instillation is the gold standard (see Chapter 27).

Client Preparation

A hysterosalpingogram is often carried out on an outpatient basis. There are no restrictions of food or fluid. The client should have finished a menstrual period within the preceding 7–10 days. The client must void immediately before the procedure. Although some institutions have the client take an enema or suppository before the examination, no special intestinal preparation is usually necessary. The client must remove her clothes from the waist down. Some clients are given a mild analgesic. (See Chapter 25 on ways nurses can help prepare clients to cope with painful procedures.)

Posttest Nursing Implications Related to Hysterosalpingography

A few hours after the procedure, the client may have severe uterine cramps that require analgesia. Warm sitz baths may be soothing. Although rare, perforation of the uterus can occur, so any severe cramping or profuse bleeding should be called to the attention of the physician or clinic. The client may have some vaginal spotting for a day or two, so she should be informed about the possible need for a vaginal pad. There is a slight chance of infection. Very rarely, a pulmonary embolism could result from the entrance of the oil-based contrast medium into the bloodstream.

MAMMOGRAMS

Description

A mammogram is a radiograph of the breast to detect the presence of tumors too small to be discovered at palpation. Mammograms may include injection of a contrast medium into the mammary ducts, but routine screening procedures do not include the use of a contrast medium. Contrast medium is useful in identifying intraductal papillomas. During the examination, the client stands or sits with breasts pushed against the film holder. An inflated rubber cushion is used to decrease the discomfort of the flattened breasts against the film holder. The procedure takes less than 30 minutes.

As discussed earlier in this chapter, digital mammograms are becoming more widely available. They do cost more than the conventional (film screen) mammogram, but radiation time is short and the quality is better in some situations. Digital mammograms have a diagnostic advantage for women less than 50 years, women with dense breasts, and premenopausal or perimenopausal women. Digital mammograms were FDA approved in 2000.

Purposes

Because breast cancer is a leading type of cancer in women, mass screening for this disease is recommended. Mammograms became popular in the early 1960s as a tool to detect early breast cancer. Studies have confirmed that both screening mammography and treatment have helped reduce the rate of breast cancer in the United States (Berry et al., 2005). In late 2009, the U.S. Preventive Services Task Force (USPSTF) (www.uspreventivetaskforce.org) recommended that women of average risk begin screening for breast cancer at age 50 instead of 40. Mammograms should then be done every other year until the age of 74. Many organizations have not accepted these recommendations. The American Cancer Society (www.cancer.org) continues to recommend mammograms annually beginning at age 40. The Susan G. Komen foundation also recommends women of average risk begin annual mammograms by age 40 and perform breast self-exams (BSE) beginning in their 20s (www.komen.org). The National Cancer Institute recommends mammograms every 1–2 years beginning at age 40 (www.cancer.gov). Women are encouraged to talk to their healthcare provider to see what screening schedule is best for them.

The goal of USPSTF is to help clinicians make informed decisions based on current research. The recommendations are not a substitute for clinical judgment.

Women with a strong history of breast cancer may begin screening earlier and be a candidate for genetic screening (see Chapter 10). MRI (Chapter 21) may be an option for high-risk women. Spots seen on a mammogram are followed up by ultrasound (Chapter 23) to differentiate cysts from solid lesions. Various types of breast biopsies are discussed in Chapter 25. Pregnant women should not have mammograms.

There are no standard guidelines regarding the use of mammograms in males, but screening may be done for men with a palpable mass or strong family history (Estala, 2006). See www.cancer.org for more information on risk factors for female and male breast cancer.

Barriers to Mammograms

Unfortunately, many women do not undergo mammography because of fear or denial, cost, accessibility, or the lack of a physician's recommendation. African American women of diverse socioeconomic status have fewer screening mammograms than Caucasians. One study found that decision making about mammograms was heavily influenced by caregiving responsibilities (Fowler, 2006). Since 1990, Medicare has paid for the examination, and insurance companies have added the tests as the focus on preventive care increased. More publicity also is being given to the high incidence of breast cancer in the United States. Nurses can be effective in educating women about the value of mammograms and the need for continued research in this area.

Client Preparation

The client should not use deodorant, perfume, or powder on the day of the test; these chemicals may interfere with the x-ray picture. The client should wear clothing that is easy to remove from the waist up. Small adhesive markers may be used to cover nipples and any large moles. The client should be prepared for some physical discomfort related to the manipulation of the tender tissue, particularly if the breasts are pendulous and much compression must be performed. The introduction of radiolucent breast cushion pad in 2001 made mammograms less uncomfortable, but not all breast imaging centers offer the option of the pad. Suggestions to reduce the pain of a mammogram include scheduling the examination during the first 2 weeks after menses, reducing caffeine intake for 3 months before the mammogram, and working with the technician to have more control with the compression of the breasts. Women who have considerable breast pain may be advised to take a mild analgesic an hour before the mammogram. Topical lidocaine has also been used to reduce pain.

The potential diagnosis of cancer may cause much anxiety; thus, attention to psychological needs also helps the woman have a more pleasant experience with mammography. A mammogram performed to place a needle or wire marker in the lump as a guide to subsequent biopsy is anxiety producing. (See Chapter 25 on breast biopsies.)

Posttest Nursing Implications Related to Mammography

Women may ask nurses about BSE, and nurses have been very involved in teaching clients about monthly exams. In 2003, the American Cancer Society no longer recommended monthly exams, but did advise healthcare providers to inform women about the benefits and limitations of BSE, so they could choose whether, and how often, to do the exam. Despite lack of definite evidence for or against BSE, some healthcare providers continue to recommend monthly BSE (Koren & Hertz, 2007; www.komen.org). A monthly breast exam may still be a useful tool so that women can recognize any changes such as skin dimpling, thickening, nipple retraction, or rashes that could be signs of a rare breast cancer called inflammatory breast cancer. This type of cancer usually does not have a distinct lump (Morris, 2010).

MYELOGRAMS

Description

A myelogram is a radiograph of the subarachnoid space of the spinal column in which air or contrast medium may be used. The contrast medium may be either an oily contrast agent or a water-soluble medium. Water-soluble contrast medium is most often used and is suitable for both inpatient and outpatient procedures. If an oil-based contrast medium is used, it is removed at the end of the procedure. The water-soluble contrast medium is not. The contrast medium or air is injected by means of lumbar puncture. The client lies on a tilted table to allow the contrast medium to flow into different parts of the spinal column.

Purposes

Radiography and fluoroscopy performed after the contrast medium is instilled can show distortions of the spinal cord caused by tumors or changes in bone structure. Herniations or protrusions of intervertebral disks can also be visualized. CT or MRI may give more detail (Chapter 21).

Client Preparation

The client should ingest nothing by mouth for 4–6 hours, and an intestinal preparation may be ordered. Intravenous fluids may be used to hydrate the client. The client should be prepared for the positioning necessary for a lumbar puncture. (See Chapter 25 on lumbar punctures.) Sedatives may be ordered. Phenothiazines are not used because they lower the seizure threshold. Consent forms are needed.

Posttest Nursing Implications Related to Myelography

If an oil-based contrast medium is used, the client should be instructed to stay flat in bed 6–8 hours after the contrast medium is removed. If water-soluble contrast medium was used, the head of the bed should be kept elevated for at least 8 hours to keep the contrast medium from irritating the cerebral meninges. The client may need analgesics if headache, pain, and stiffness in the neck occur. About 20% of clients experience headaches, nausea, and vomiting after the test. Fewer than 1 in 1,000 have a seizure. If conditions permit, fluids should be encouraged to at least 2,000 mL for adults to help with the production of adequate cerebrospinal fluid (CSF). The motor sensations of the lower extremities should be assessed to make sure that there was no nerve damage. The voiding pattern of the client should be assessed because urinary retention may be a problem in the first 24 hours.

Outpatient clients are monitored for at least 2 hours and accompanied home by a friend or family member.

ARTHROGRAMS

Description

For an arthrogram, contrast medium is injected into a joint, usually the knee and sometimes a shoulder or other joint. The procedure is performed under local anesthesia in the radiology department. After the needle is inserted into the joint space, fluid is usually aspirated for analysis. Then the contrast medium, and sometimes air, is injected. The client may be asked to run in place to spread the contrast medium around the knee joint. Also, the joint is manipulated to spread the contrast medium. (Some clients find the movement of the joint uncomfortable.) Radiographs are taken with the joint in various positions.

Purposes

Arthrograms help evaluate suspected joint damage such as tears in the cartilage of the knee. If surgical intervention is anticipated, arthroscopy may be performed in place of the arthrogram. Arthroscopy allows the physician to examine the joint directly and even perform simple repairs (Chapter 27).

Pretest Nursing Implications Related to Arthrography

Precautions related to the use of contrast medium should be noted. If the procedure is being performed on an outpatient basis, and many are, a friend or family member may have to drive the client home.

Posttest Nursing Diagnosis Related to Arthrography

Altered Comfort Related to Knee Manipulation

Mild-to-moderate discomfort may be present after the procedure. The joint should rest for about 12 hours. The knee may be wrapped in an elastic bandage for 12–24 hours. Ice bags can be used to reduce swelling, and mild analgesics may be needed. Some slight grating may be present for a day or two after the procedure. Strenuous activity, such as jogging, should not be resumed until advised by the physician. Exercises to strengthen the knee may be prescribed, depending on the results of the examination. Two possible complications after arthroscopic surgical procedures are hemorrhage and thrombophlebitis, but the incidence of either is quite low.

Questions

1. Which one of the following is *not* useful in providing radiation protection?
   a. Scheduling radiographs a few days apart so there is a time interval between exposures
   b. Shielding the client with lead aprons to protect uninvolved areas
   c. Having all personnel maintain distance when the x-ray machine is in use
   d. Making the exposure of the client as short as possible

2. Which of the following is an inappropriate action by a client?
   a. Asking for a lead apron to be used if dental x-rays are needed
   b. Carrying a card that lists all x-rays that have been performed
   c. Asking the physician to explain how x-rays will help with the diagnosis
   d. Refusing care until x-rays are obtained to validate any unexplained symptoms

3. Which of the following factors probably creates the least stress for a client undergoing a barium enema?
   a. Moving about on a hard x-ray table
   b. Being given information on the sensation of the x-ray procedure
   c. Darkness and noise during fluoroscopy
   d. Enemas or suppositories given before the test

4. General nursing implications for clients undergoing any type of radiologic test would *not* include
   a. Helping the client prepare for waiting by giving a magazine or other diversion
   b. Making sure that the client has slippers if he or she must stand during the test
   c. Instructing the client about any restrictions on foods and fluids
   d. Listing the complications that may occur

5. General nursing implications when a client returns from a radiologic test would *not* include
   a. Offering a back rub to relieve the discomfort from lying on a hard table
   b. Encouraging extra fluids (if the pathophysiologic condition allows) if contrast medium was used
   c. Finding out if the client can eat, and if so, offering food as soon as possible
   d. Instructing the client to maintain bed rest for 4–6 hours

6. The specific gravity of urine will be unchanged after a client has undergone which one of the following x-ray tests?
   a. KUB
   b. Cholangiography
   c. Arteriography
   d. IVP

7. Which of the following nursing actions should not be considered part of a routine procedure for a client who is undergoing portable chest radiography?
   a. Helping the client sit up as straight as possible before the radiograph is obtained
   b. Removing electrodes from the chest before the radiograph is obtained
   c. Helping the technician place the film holder behind the client's chest
   d. Holding the client in a fixed position while the radiograph is obtained

8. An adolescent has a history of severe epigastric pain relieved by food or milk. Which of these nursing actions is routine when she undergoes an upper GI series (barium meal)?
   a. Telling her to take nothing by mouth before the examination
   b. Telling her that when fluoroscopy is performed (as the barium is swallowed) the room will be very bright
   c. Giving an enema to her after radiography is completed
   d. Informing her that the barium sulfate often causes diarrhea

9. A client is undergoing a barium enema because of slight rectal bleeding. Which of these nursing actions is *not* routine for a client undergoing a barium enema?
   a. Administration of cathartics or suppositories the evening before the examination
   b. Informing him that he will need to hold the barium in the colon while a series of radiographs are taken
   c. Giving a light diet the evening before the examination
   d. Withholding food when he comes back from the radiology department because a second set of radiographs is obtained in 3–4 hours

10. The nurse in the Emergency Department should be aware that a routine radiograph will most likely be the primary diagnostic tool for
    a. A client, 72 years of age, who has fever and a productive cough
    b. A client, 44 years of age, who has abdominal pain that occurs after eating a large amount of fats
    c. A client, 8 years of age, who has acute pain in the right upper outer quadrant
    d. A client, 21 years of age, who has a severe head injury from a motorcycle accident

11. A client has just returned to his hospital room after a femoral arteriogram. Which nursing action would be inappropriate?
    a. Allowing him to stand if he cannot void in bed
    b. Checking vital signs every 15 minutes for the first hour, then every 2 hours if vital signs are stable
    c. Keeping an ice bag on the puncture site
    d. Checking pedal pulses and the color and warmth of the feet when vital signs are taken

12. The possible need for a mild oral analgesic for procedure-related pain is least likely for a client undergoing
    a. Mammography
    b. Arthrography
    c. Small-bowel series
    d. Hystosalpingography

References

Barrett, B. J. & Parfrey, P. (2006). Preventing nephropathy induced by contrast medium. *New England Journal of Medicine, 354*(4), 379–386.

Berry, D. A., Cronin, K. A., Plevritis, S. K., Fryback, D. G., Clarke, L., Zelen, M., et al. (2005). Effect of screening and adjuvant therapy on mortality from breast cancer. *New England Journal of Medicine, 353,* 1784–1792.

Brege, D. J. (2008). Contrast reaction. *Nursing 2008, 38*(3), 72.

DeCherney, A. H., Nathan, L., Goodwin, T. M., & Lauter, N. (Eds.). (2007). *Current diagnosis & treatment: Obstetrics & gynecology* (10th ed.). New York: Mc Graw-Hill.

Deglin, J. H., Vallerand, A. H., & Sanoski, C. A. (2011). *Davis's drug guide for nurses* (12th ed.). Philadelphia: F. A. Davis.

Estala, S. M. (2006). Proposed screening recommendations for male breast cancer. *Nurse Practitioner, 31*(2), 62–63.

Fowler, B. A. (2006). Social processes used by African American women in making decisions about mammography screening. *Journal of Nursing Scholarship, 38*(3), 247–254.

Geiter, H. (2006). Contrast-media-induced pulmonary edema. *Nursing 2006, 36*(1), 88.

Hay, W. W., Levin, M. J., Sondheimer, J. M., & Deterding, R. (Eds.). (2011). *Current diagnosis and treatment: Pediatrics* (20th ed.). New York: McGraw-Hill.

Huang, S. W. (2005). Seafood and iodine: An analysis of a medical myth. *Allergy and Asthma Proceedings, 26*(6), 468–469.

Koren, M. E. & Hertz, J. E. (2007). Older women's breast screening behaviors: What nurses need to know. *MEDSURG Nursing, 16*(2), 80–84.

McPhee, S. J., Papadakis, M. A., & Rabow, M. W. (Eds.). (2011). *Current medical diagnosis and treatment* (50th ed.). New York: McGraw-Hill.

Morris, L. (2010). Targeting the red-hot danger of inflammatory breast cancer. *Nursing 2010, 40*(9).

Website

www.cancer.gov (National Cancer Institute information on cancer screening.)
www.cancer.org (American Cancer Society guidelines and information on cancer screening.)
www.komen.org (Susan G. Komen Foundation for information on breast cancer.)

www.lungcanceralliance.com (Information on screening methods for lung cancer.)
www.radiologyinfo.org (Information on safety and details on radiological tests developed jointly by American College of Radiology and Radiological Society of North America.)
www.uspreventiveservicestaskforce.org (Recommended guidelines for mammograms.)

Answers

1. a, 2. d, 3. b, 4. d, 5. d, 6. a, 7. d, 8. a, 9. d, 10. a, 11. a, 12. c

Body Scans: CT, DXA, MRI, PET and SPECT

- Advantages and Disadvantages of Scans ... 538
- Picture Archiving Communication System ... 539
- Full Body Scans for Screening Purposes ... 540
- Computed Tomography ... 540
- Dual Energy X-Ray Absorptiometry ... 545
- Magnetic Resonance Imaging ... 547
- Positron Emission Tomography ... 552
- Single Photon Emission Computed Tomography ... 554

OBJECTIVES

1. Discuss the basic advantages and disadvantages of computed tomography (CT), magnetic resonance imaging (MRI), positron emission tomography (PET), and single photon emission computed tomography (SPECT) as body scans.

2. Compare and contrast the preparations needed for infants, children, and adults who undergo various body scans.

3. Describe the usual preparations for CT scans with and without contrast medium.

4. Explain the purpose of dual x-ray absorptiometry (DXA).

5. Describe the special precautions needed for clients undergoing MRI.

6. Describe how PET and SPECT allow clinicians to examine metabolic functions rather than structure.

7. Identify priority nursing diagnoses for clients undergoing various types of scans.

Tomography is a method of body-section radiography. A specially designed x-ray machine and film holder move around the client in an arc, focusing at various angles, each with a slightly different depth. With each change in the angle of tomography, a selected body plane becomes sharply defined while the areas above and below the focal point become slightly blurred.

CT uses the principle of tomography with the addition of detectors, computers, and a scanner, which make possible a 3-D cross-sectional view of the body. The basic principles of computerized image reconstruction of an object are common to four types of scans (CT, PET, SPECT, and MRI).

Cormack, an American physicist, and Hounsfield, an English research engineer, working independently, conducted the research that culminated in the development of CT. They shared the 1979 Nobel Prize in physiology or medicine. The Nobel

Committee acknowledged that no other method of x-ray diagnostics had led to such remarkable success in such a short time. Another type of body imaging, which uses a magnetic field and no radiation, MRI, became the success story of the 1980s. Bloch and Purcell received a Nobel Prize in 1952 for the work that led to the development of MRI, and Lauterbur and Mansfield in 2003 for their work that led to the development of the modern MRI. Like CT, MRI is now used all around the world in millions of procedures. For example, see the American College of Radiology Imaging Network (www.acrin.org) for more information on clinical trials for clients with cancer.

ADVANTAGES AND DISADVANTAGES OF SCANS

These sophisticated imaging modalities are noninvasive examinations that require a skilled technician to operate the machine. Much research is being conducted to compare the advantages and disadvantages of scans with those of invasive diagnostic procedures (Chapter 25), sonography (Chapter 23), and radionuclide scans (Chapter 22) for assessing various pathophysiologic conditions. The advantage of the scans and MRI is the exquisite detail of the images. Now computers may be used to tie together the results of MRI and CT to give incredibly detailed pictures of all parts of the body.

CT does have two disadvantages. One is the cost of the test, which must be considered if other less expensive tests can provide satisfactory results. Although CT scans are expensive, the cost may be less than the combined charges for the tests they replace. The second disadvantage of CT is the time of exposure to radiation. Although the amount of radiation is small, all radiation exposure is cumulative through life. (See Chapter 20 for a detailed discussion on the role of the nurse in relation to the radiation hazards of repeated diagnostic tests.) Fear of radiation is easily evoked, so it is important that clinicians realize that the radiation dose from high-resolution chest CT is actually less than that for conventional CT and only slightly more than that for chest radiograph. As discussed later, low-dose helical (spiral) CT used in some screening programs emits no more radiation than 1–3 standard x-rays. However, a conventional CT of the abdomen may have the equivalent radiation of 250–500 chest x-rays. Estimates of the amount of radiation from a CT procedure vary depending on the length of the procedure, the size of the client, and the type of system and operating techniques. See the discussion on faster CT scans. The newest scanners can adjust radiation for pediatric clients.

MRI does not create any radiation exposure, but it costs more than CT and is not available in all healthcare settings. As noted later, some clients must not enter the MRI area because of problems that can arise from the presence of ferromagnetic materials that can be moved by the imager. Compared with CT, MRI excels in demonstration of some pathologic conditions, such as those of the central nervous system. Artifacts of bone do not interfere with MRI as they may with CT. See Table 21–1 for comparison of CT and MRI.

PET and SPECT have the advantage of detailing metabolic function rather than structure. Both require minute amounts of radioisotopes, so radiation exposure is minimal. At present, PET is available only in large medical centers and is very expensive, but a SPECT scan is more widely available.

Table 21-1 Comparison of CT and MRI*

	CT	MRI
Radiation	Yes	No
Improved image quality	Multidetectors (MDCT)	Stronger magnets (1.5 T and 3 T scans)
Ferromagnetic items	No danger	Major danger as projectile items
Thermal burns	No danger	Possible
Claustrophobia	Not an issue	Yes, but less with open MRI
Effect of movement on image quality	Some effect, must lie still	Major effect, essential to lie very still
Noise level	Not an issue	Need earplugs
Pacemakers, other implanted devices	Usually OK	Will interfere with function
Pregnant clients	Not recommended	Useful in certain cases
Children	To use lower doses	Safe for children
Fetus	Not recommended	Useful in certain cases
Time for scans	Few seconds to minutes	20 minutes to 2 hours
Available to consumers from commercial vendors	Yes	Yes
Cost	Expensive	1/3 more than CT

*See Bucsko (2005), Harvey (2006), and also text for advantages and disadvantages of each type of scan, and see text for common uses for each type of scan.

Note: There are dangers from contrast agents from both types of scans.

If angiography with contrast medium is part of a CT scan, the risks associated with the contrast medium must be acknowledged. (See Chapter 20 on nursing precautions with contrast medium.) The type of contrast medium used with MRI does not have as great a disadvantage as that used with CT, but there are some risks, as discussed later. The radioisotopes used with PET and SPECT do not cause untoward reactions.

Fusion or Hybrid Scans

As noted earlier, technological advances made it possible to use different types of scans together with a computer. Now some companies manufacture fusion or hybrid scanners. For example, a PET/CT system detects more detailed and higher quality images in less time and with a reduction in the amount of injected tracer. The use of combination PET–CT scans has improved the diagnosis and management of clients with cancer (Ott, 2010). SPECT/CT scanners are also available.

PICTURE ARCHIVING COMMUNICATION SYSTEM

The use of digital images and computers has revolutionized radiology information services (RIS). Digital images eliminate film and problems linked to the film. Film images require processing, storage, and manual transport, which are labor intensive and time consuming. Digital imaging provides a superior quality image that can be sent to experts in any location. Many companies offer innovative systems and products that can archive all kinds of radiological images including the 4-D color and motion effects of PET/CT. This picture archiving communication system (PACS) can be shared as part of an EMR and can also be used worldwide by interactive Web access. The reader is encouraged to discover how PACS is being used in a local setting.

FULL BODY SCANS FOR SCREENING PURPOSES

The development of electron beam CT and other types of high-tech scans has made it possible to do body scans in about 15–20 minutes in a variety of settings. Because a prescription or referral is not necessary, commercial companies now offer these scans to the public. Various types of CT scans may cost around $500–$1,500 and a PET $2,000–$3,000. (Insurance companies will not pay for these scans as screening devices but will pay if follow-ups are needed.) Most healthcare organizations do not recommend body scans for people who have no symptoms or a family history of a problem because of lack of supporting data as to benefit. Other concerns are the risks related to radiation exposure and the variability in quality of the scanning techniques. Some clients may be willing to pay for screening scans in order to relieve anxiety about their health status. Ironically, these scans may produce more anxiety, as they may lead to other testing for something that turns out to be an artifact or a harmless condition.

Beinfeld, Wittenberg, and Gazelle (2005) estimated that for every 1,000 whole body scans done to rule out eight conditions—six cancers (ovarian, pancreatic, lung, liver, kidney, and colon), abdominal aortic aneurysm, and coronary artery disease—908 clients (90.8%) had at least one false positive. Follow-ups for false positive are costly for the healthcare system. The researchers also estimated that whole body scans, compared to regular health care, provided minimal gains in life expectancy (about 6 days) for those with a detected abnormality. Studies have shown that unexpected asymptomatic brain abnormalities such as brain infarcts (7.2%), cerebral aneurysms (1.8%), and benign primary tumors, mainly meningiomas (1.6%), are found in the general population (Vernooij et al., 2007); these incidental sub-clinical findings can lead to intense anxiety for the client and a dilemma for the clinician on the best clinical management for something that has not created any difficulty. For example, clients with small meningiomas who remain asymptomatic should be followed with MRIs annually to make sure the tumor does not grow.

Commercial companies also offer ultrasound scans of the carotid arteries, abdominal aorta, peripheral pulses, and a bone scan for less than $200. Unlike CT scans, cheaper ultrasound scans (Chapter 23) do not have the disadvantage of radiation exposure, but may lead to anxiety from false positives and unnecessary costs for follow-up care.

COMPUTED TOMOGRAPHY

Description

CT, CAT scan, and *EMI scan* all refer to what used to be called *computerized axial tomography*. The EMI scanner was developed by Electrical and Musical Industries, a Britain-based group of international companies. The preferred term is *computed tomography* (CT), which produces a *CT scan*.

A CT scan is obtained with an x-ray machine that rotates 180 degrees around the client's head or body. Detectors read the amount of radiation each body tissue or organ absorbs. A computer processes these readings and converts them to an image shown on a screen. The resulting pictures show a 3-D cross-section of all body parts. A CT scan divides each area of tissue being viewed into an area 3 mm square and 13 mm thick for most imaging examinations. The results are available in a few minutes. A CT scan can depict almost all types of tissue except nerves.

A CT scan, a noninvasive procedure, causes no pain. The client simply lies still while the machine goes around the body. As emphasized before, no risks are entailed, other than being exposed to a small amount of radiation. The procedure takes 15–30 minutes. If contrast medium is used, the procedure takes 30–60 minutes, and there are the usual risks associated with an iodine contrast medium.

Newer Types of CT Scans

There are now two other types of CT scans in addition to the first-generation or conventional scanner addressed earlier. The second type, *spiral or helical,* developed in the late 1980s, has a single x-ray beam that rotates continuously around the client giving better views in a shorter amount of time. For example, spiral CT scanning can obtain an image of the chest during a single breath. This scanner is very rapid, as 150 images can be done in 25 seconds. Some of these newer scanners are programmed to instruct the client when to breathe in various languages including a Mickey Mouse voice for children. The third type, multislice CT scanner, may be considered a supercharged spiral scanner. Conventional and spiral CT scans use one row of detectors to pick up the x-ray beam after it has passed through the client. The multislice scanner uses up to eight rows and acquires images two to three times faster than a spiral scanner.

Multidetector CT

The MDCT scans used to be 8 slice/sec, but new scanners have made the slices thinner and thinner. As the slice gets thinner, the image has better quality and the speed of the scan increases. MDCT scans had advanced to 64 slice/sec in 2004, and to 256 slice/sec by 2008, and today, some have 320 slice/sec. Older scanners of fewer slices are still useful for many routine CT procedures. The older one-slice scans may still be useful to evaluate some tumors for cancer clients. But a portable eight-slice CT may be used in the Emergency Department to rule out intracerebral bleeding before stroke treatment (www.neme.org). The faster scanner is most useful when scanning regions of the body that contain moving organs such as the heart and lung. (See the discussion on screening for coronary artery disease.) A typical EBCT (electron beam CT) scan can image the entire heart in 30–40 seconds, while MDCT with 32- or 64-slice scans can do that in as little as 5–10 seconds (Bucsko, 2005). A chest scan can be done in 2–5 seconds and a carotid artery and circle of Willis in 5 seconds. The 256-slice CT, available in 2008, can do a heart beat in 1–2 seconds, while the 320-slice scanner that is being promoted can produce images in less than a second. As CT scans become faster and faster, radiation time is less and there is little interference from client movement.

Purposes

Around 1972, the first CT scans were used for identifying brain abnormalities and head injuries. CT was found to be much more valuable in diagnosing problems in the brain than the older x-ray tests, such as pneumoencephalogram or cerebral arteriogram. The details available with a CT scan are remarkable. For example, a CT scan can clearly show if a brain abscess is becoming smaller after treatment with antibiotics. CT scans are also used to locate foreign objects in soft tissue, such as the eyes. For example, a piece of metal lodged in an eyeball can be precisely mapped out so the surgeon has to do much less probing. Intracranial lesions, such as neoplasms or hematomas, can be located without a craniotomy. The surgeon thus has a much better understanding of the location and extent of brain disease before performing an operation.

In clients who have strokes, a CT scan is important to rule out hemorrhaging so that thrombolytic drugs can be started. A CT scan is preferable to an MRI because it is faster and more reliable for detecting intracranial bleeding (McPhee, Papadakis, & Rabow, 2011). Sometimes, after a stroke, the client may be asked to inhale xenon gas to locate how much blood is reaching key areas. A noncontrast CT head scan may be used to detect a subdural hematoma (Vacca, 2006).

CT may be the first-line test for evaluating malignant neoplasms of solid organs as well as unexplained masses, abscess collections, and trauma. CT scans have been very useful to detect appendicitis and prevent unnecessary surgery (negative appendectomy rate). Rhea et al. (2005) noted that a greater use of CT, particularly in female pediatric clients, would lower the negative appendectomy rate. Imaging for suspected appendicitis in pediatric clients may begin with an ultrasound (Chapter 23) and then a CT for a follow-up of a negative ultrasound (Hay et al., 2011). For pregnant clients who need imaging, an ultrasound is followed up by an MRI.

CT Colonography (Virtual Colonoscopy)

Over the past few years, research suggested that CT colonography (virtual colonoscopy) might be as effective as colonoscopy (Chapter 27) for detecting colorectal polyps and colorectal cancer. Though colonoscopy is still considered the "gold standard," virtual colonoscopy may be a reasonable alternative to clients who refuse the recommended colonoscopy, sigmoidoscopy, and fecal occult blood testing (see Chapter 27).

Prep for Virtual Colonoscopy

For the CT scan the client must have clear liquids for a day, have a bowel prep (see Chapter 20), and drink a contrast agent. No sedation is needed as with the traditional colonoscopy. Air injected into the rectum may cause some discomfort. If polyps are visualized on the scan, a colonoscopy may be done right away while the bowel is still prepped. (See Chapter 27).

Use of Electron Beam for Coronary Artery Screening

Electron beam CT (EBCT), 10–20 times faster than a conventional CT, is sometimes called ultrafast CT or electron beam tomography (EBT). The client wears cardiac electrodes and is enclosed in a scanner so that images can be taken at the end of diastole just before atrial contraction. Ultrafast CT is highly sensitive in detecting calcium in coronary arteries, a possibly useful marker for the presence of coronary atherosclerosis. Healthy arteries do not show calcium deposits, but small amounts of calcification may occur with aging. A normal screening virtually rules out clinically significant atherosclerosis, particularly in young people, but false-negative results can occur. An abnormal scan does not have a specific correlation with critical coronary artery stenosis, although more calcium usually means more widespread atherosclerosis. Concerns remain about appropriate management of clients with asymptomatic coronary artery calcification. For clients with some known risk for coronary disease, the use of EBCT may help to refine the clinical risk prediction and support the use of more aggressive lowering of lipid levels (McPhee et al., 2011). EBCT may also be combined with an intravenous contrast agent so blockages can be identified. (See Chapter 20 for implications for contrast agents.)

Use of Multidetector Cat Scan for Coronary Artery Screening

Advances in MDCT have given another option for coronary artery screening. A growing number of studies have shown that coronary CT angiography is highly accurate for the exclusion of significant coronary stenosis. In addition, MDCT can detect calcified and noncalcified plaques (Hoffmann et al., 2006).

Prep for MDCT

Preparation for MDCT for coronary artery screening includes a creatinine test for renal function because a contrast agent is given intravenously. (See Chapter 20 on contrast agents and the possibility of acute renal failure.) In addition, the client may be given a beta blocker to slow the heart rate to below 60. But with faster scans the medication is not needed to slow the heart.

Use of Coronary Artery Calcium Scores

Calcium scores may be reported as the number of Hounsfield units from 0 to over 400. The units, developed by one of the inventors of the CT, measure the radio density on CT scans. Most adults have some arterial calcium as they age. Some data support the hypothesis that a coronary artery calcium score (CACS) above 300 is predictive of risk of death from coronary artery disease (Greenland et al., 2004). As with EBCT discussed earlier, the scores for MDCT calcium may be more useful when they are low, as this usually means the client does not have significant arteriosclerosis. However, a high calcium score is not easy to interpret because there is no direct proof of a causal relationship between high calcium scores and stenosis. The higher scores may mean more risk, but other factors such as the pattern of calcium and the appearance of plaque may be important variables (Bucsko, 2005). The appropriate management of clients with asymptomatic coronary calcification is unclear except to modify other known risk factors for coronary artery disease.

Use of CT to Screen for Lung Cancer

Studies using low-dose helical (spiral) CT have shown that lung cancer may be detected earlier than with conventional x-rays. In 2010, the National Cancer Institute announced that the 8-year trial of CT scanning for lung cancer in high-risk screening was effective in reducing lung cancer deaths by 20% (www.cancer.gov). This was ground-breaking news as lung cancer causes more deaths than breast, prostate, colon, and pancreatic cancers combined (www.lungcanceralliance.org). CT screening should be done following a lung cancer screening protocol such as one outlined by the International Early Lung Cancer Action Program (www.ielcap.org)

Pretest Nursing Diagnoses Related to CT

Deficient Knowledge Related to Preparation for a Head Scan

Unless contrast medium is to be used, the client can eat and drink before the examination. Wigs and any objects in the hair, such as bobby pins, are removed. The client can be assured that the procedure is not painful and is much like putting one's head in a hair dryer. Although CT is not painful, the thought of having one's head immobilized can be frightening. The person must lie still during the procedure. A two-way intercom allows communication with the radiology personnel. (See the discussion on claustrophobia in the section on MRI.)

Radiopaque contrast medium may be given intravenously to outline the cerebral vessels. If contrast medium is given, the client may need preparation. (See Chapter 20 on how to prepare for reactions to contrast medium, which include flushing and possible allergic reaction.)

Risk for Ineffective Coping of Children and Confused Adults

One suggestion is to encourage a child to play at home by lying still with head flexed toward chest. The parent can dim the lights in the room and move an arm around the child's motionless head. By humming softly, parents give children an idea of the sounds they will hear during the test. Children should be taught that they can open and close their eyes but not move their head. This preparation may work for children older than 3 years. Infants sleep during the procedure if kept awake and then fed just before the test. The greatest problem is with toddlers and confused adults: Sedation may be required. (See Chapter 27 for a discussion on adverse reactions to sedatives.)

Deficient Knowledge Related to Preparation for CT Body Scans

Scans of the thorax or pelvic region may or may not require special preparation. The nurse must ask the radiologist what specific preparations are required. A tampon may be used as a vaginal marker. The client may be required to have a full or empty bladder. A contrast medium may be given to outline various organs. There are flavored beverages designed specifically to mask the taste of oral iodinated contrast agents (www.beekley.com). Low-density barium solutions and dilute water-soluble iodinated contrast materials are used. The client must be assessed for allergies and prepared for a flushing sensation and possible nausea (Chapter 20). However, some of the newer contrast media made for CT scans contain less than 10% of the iodine found in older products.

Intestinal preparations vary in importance with the various parts of the body being scanned. Contrast medium can be given by means of an enema. Drugs may be used to decrease peristalsis during the test, including propantheline and glucagon. Synthetic cholecystokin may also be given to increase peristalsis to cause filling of the gastrointestinal (GI) tract with swallowed contrast medium. These medications are given during the procedure and require an intravenous injection. If a biopsy is planned, guided by the scan, the general nursing implications (Chapter 25) for invasive procedures should be heeded.

Posttest Nursing Implications Related to CT

There are no specific nursing implications related to the scanning procedure. If a contrast medium has been given, the nursing implications about contrast medium should be followed. (See the general nursing diagnoses discussed in Chapter 20.) The nurse must be aware of any sedatives or other drugs given as part of the procedure because untoward effects from drugs are always possible. (See the discussion of the side effects of medications used for endoscopic procedures in Chapter 27.) If invasive procedures were performed, vital signs and the other assessments described in Chapter 25 are appropriate.

DUAL ENERGY X-RAY ABSORPTIOMETRY

Description and Purpose

Various types of scans have been developed to measure bone mass or bone density, but only CT assesses bone density as a volume. (Plain x-rays do not detect early signs of osteoporosis but will show significant bone loss.) CT scans to assess bone density are still widely available, but the radiation and cost are greater than the dual energy x-ray absorptiometry (DXA), which is now the method of choice. An x-ray machine emits two photon energy beams. The radiation from DXA is minimal. (See Chapter 23 for another FDA-approved test that uses ultrasound to assess for osteoporosis.) DXA can determine the density of any bone and is quite accurate for both assessment and follow-up of clients who need treatment for osteoporosis. DXA can measure bone mineral density (BMD) and bone mineral concentration (BMC) within a few minutes. The lower spine and hip density are measured by positioning the client on a table and having an arm of the machine pass over the body parts. The machine does not touch the client.

In 2011, the U.S. Preventive Services Task Force (USPSTF) updated guidelines on the screening and treatment of osteoporosis. At the age of 65, all women should be offered screening with DXA. Younger women with known risk factors may also benefit from screening. Current evidence was insufficient to recommend for or against screening of men (www.uspreventiveservicestaskforce.org). Risk factors besides age, female sex, and being white include smoking, alcohol intake, low body mass, and familial history of osteoporosis. Glucocorticoid-induced osteoporosis is the most common type of secondary osteoporosis, but other drugs such as antiepileptics may also contribute to the development of this condition.

Client Preparation

The client needs no special preparation. The client should remove all metal from the body and be dressed in comfortable clothing. The test should be given before tests that use radionuclides.

Reporting of Results

The results may be reported in tables that show the following:

1. T scores show the number of standard deviations the client differs from the normals of a 30-year-old (based on World Health Organization Guidelines). T scores between −1 and +2.5 indicate osteopenia, and scores below −2.5 indicate osteoporosis.

2. Z scores are the number of standard deviations the client differs from age-matched normals. A Z score below −1.5 may indicate a need for interventions.

3. BMD expressed as percentage of normal.

4. More important than the score on a single bone density scan is the amount of bone loss over a period of time. Scans should be done every 2–5 years, to determine rate of bone loss.

Nursing Implications Related to DXA

Detecting low bone mass early allows the woman to implement preventive measures. Although studies suggest that as much as 80% of the risk of osteoporosis may be genetic, attention to other risk factors and promotion of a healthy lifestyle can lessen the genetic predisposition. Nurses have an important role in educating women and men all through the life span about diet and exercise and other lifestyle modifications to prevent the insidious onset of osteoporosis. See Table 21–2 on teaching points for clients at risk for osteoporosis. Pharmacologic treatment may be initiated when the BMD T score is below −2 by DXA or when it is below −1.5 if the client has one or more risk factors. A prior vertebral or hip fracture may be another reason for treatment. Two main types of medications to treat or prevent osteoporosis are bisphosphonates and selective estrogen receptor modulators (Deglin, Vallerand, & Sanoski, 2011).

Table 21–2 Methods to Decrease Risk of Osteoporosis

1. Limit caffeine beverages to 2–3 cups daily

2. Do not smoke

3. Limit alcohol to one drink daily

4. Do weight-bearing and strength-training exercises at least three times a week for 30 minutes to an hour

5. Eat a diet that contains sufficient calcium (see Chapter 7 for guidelines)

6. Use calcium supplements to reach a goal of 1,200 mg daily (age 50 and above); do not take more than 500 mg at one time

7. Take 600 IU of vitamin D as adults or 800 IU daily if over age 70 (see Chapter 7)

8. Talk to healthcare provider about timing of repeat DXA scans and criteria for beginning medications

9. Ask healthcare provider if any medications may be contributing to the development of osteoporosis

Note: See Brown (2009), Holcomb (2006), and Wrotny (2005) for more details on these teaching points and risk factors for the development of osteoporosis.

MAGNETIC RESONANCE IMAGING

Description

MRI uses a huge magnet and radio waves to produce an energy field that can be transferred to a visual image. Use of the older term, *nuclear magnetic resonance* (NMR), was discontinued in 1984. The word *nuclear* may be frightening to clients because it may conjure up a vision of the nuclear fission of the atomic bomb. Nuclear in the sense of NMR simply refers to the dense core of the atom. Not only is the test not related to atomic bombs, but it also does not involve any kind of radiation hazard. Perhaps, NMR should stand for *no more radiation*. The richness of detail of the images often without the use of contrast medium and the lack of radiation hazard are advantages of MRI over CT. MRI costs about one-third more than CT.

The huge magnet in the imager produces a magnetic field. The magnetic field causes atoms in the tissues to line up in a parallel configuration. The hydrogen ion, a single proton, is used for imaging because of its abundance in water and fat tissues. The signal from fat tissue can be suppressed so that other signals can be observed. Most diseases manifest themselves by an increase in water content. When the technician pushes a switch, radio waves are sent into the magnetic field, and the lined-up ions pick up some of this energy. When the radio wave is switched off, the atoms revert to their lined-up configuration influenced by the magnet. The change in the energy field is sensed and converted to a visual display on a computer screen.

The entire MRI machine must be enclosed in a room to protect the image from interference with outside radio signals. The magnetic field around the imager is always present and stops watches, erases credit cards, and even pulls stethoscopes out of pockets. In an emergency, the magnet can be turned off, but it is expensive to restart it. In the past, MRI disrupted some intravenous drip regulators, but others were not affected. Special routine and emergency equipment compatible with MRI have been developed but may not be generally available. Thus, a client may have to be moved out of the MRI room for resuscitation. If a ventilator-dependent client needs an MRI, an alternative to the MRI-compatible ventilator is the use of extended ventilator tubing and the presence of a critical care nurse and a respiratory therapist.

Safety Issues for Projectile Items

Many articles have been written about the potential projectile effects of numerous ferromagnetic items. (Typical ferromagnetic materials contain iron, but nickel and cobalt are also magnetic). Other metals are not magnetic, but they can conduct heat, as noted later. The death of a child undergoing MRI because of an oxygen tank that became projectile and cases of other injuries from projectiles such as mop buckets made it clear that more safety education and use of detectors might be helpful. Even sandbags may contain ferromagnetic iron shavings. One used in the MRI room was pulled into the MRI coil, damaging the system (Gallauresi, 2008). Since magnetic strengths are increasing and new products enter the market regularly, professionals need to look for items that are marked as MRI safe (Hardy, 2010). (See www.mrisafety.com for updates on safety issues.) Some MRI suites now have a free-standing detector, a safe distance from the magnet room. A handheld scanner may also be used. However, these detectors do not replace the intensive questionnaire of the client as small objects could still be missed. And education about safety is essential for all personnel including those who clean the unit.

Safety Issues for Magnet Strength and Radio Frequency Heating

The first MRI scanners in the 1980s contained a magnet measured in Telsa units as 1 T. Now most scanners operate at 1.5 T and some have advanced to 3 T. 3 T is the gold standard for neuro- and musculoskeletal imaging. The FDA-approved limit on magnetic strength for clinical use is 4 T, but research institutions have even higher-strength magnets. Safety related to mechanical forces seems essentially the same for 1.5 T and 3 T, but more powerful magnets raise questions about radio frequency heating, which could interfere with some mechanical devices such as neuro-stimulators (Harvey, 2006). Traditionally, clients with pacemakers or other cardiac devices have been excluded from MRI scans but some manufacturers are working on devices that can be used even with strong MRI scans. Clients with a pacemaker or an internal cardiac defibrillator (ICD) may be able to have an MRI if a cardiologist remains in the MRI suite and the client is continuously monitored (Lee, 2006). Tattoos and some types of permanent cosmetics may cause artifacts and possibly burns from an increased radio frequency (Armstrong & Elkins, 2005; DeBoer et al., 2008). Burns are not very likely and may be prevented by using a cooling pack on the site of the permanent tattoo (Kanal, 2006). Burns have been reported from transdermal medication patches, so these should be removed before an MRI. Even electrodes and cables approved for MRI use may cause burns if the electrodes are not in complete contact with the skin surface (Lange & Nguyen, 2006).

Problems of Noise

The client is put on a moving pallet that is pushed into the large cylinder containing the magnet. As the radio signals are switched off and on, the client hears a variety of noises. The sound has been described as initially like the slow beat of an Indian drum and then with abrupt stops and starts like a muffled jackhammer. Stronger magnets usually mean louder noises. The 3 T scanner is considerably louder than the older 1 T and 1.5 T scanners, and the 4 T scanners used for research are very loud. However, some of the newest scans have a vacuum that can significantly reduce the exam noise. In addition to earplugs, special headsets with music as an auditory distraction may be used. Goggles and a headset make it possible for the client to see a DVD while undergoing longer tests, which can also address the next problem, possible claustrophobia.

Problems with Claustrophobia: Use of Open MRI

The enclosure of the entire body in the large cylinder may cause claustrophobia. (See the nursing diagnosis section.) Also, children may be very frightened by the large closed scanner. To enhance client comfort, manufacturers have developed open scanners. The open MRI has no tunnel and no loud noises. The early ones did not give the image quality of the closed systems, and even now, the closed system may be needed to get the highest-quality image. The need to combine the scanning power of the closed system with the client comfort of an open MRI system led to the development of short bore systems, which are twice as wide and half as long as the traditional closed system. These scanners now come in 1.5 T and 3 T. Other innovations are small MRI scanners for viewing an extremity such as the wrist or elbow. These scanners give as good an image as the 1.5 T whole body scan for many orthopedic conditions and cost considerably less. Also available is a stand-up scanner that allows clients to walk in and be imaged while standing.

Adverse Effects of Gadolinium Contrast

Gadolinium-based contrast agents have been used for over 20 years with MRIs. Although it is safe and effective for almost all clients, those with impaired renal function can develop nephrogenic system fibrosis (NSF). This disease may affect internal organs and the skin (McPhee et al., 2011). Since 2006, all clients receiving any of the five gadolinium-based contrast agents need to have a serum creatinine (Chapter 4) done within 30 days of the MRI (Harvey, 2009). Research is ongoing on the safety of gadolinium contrast agents and the development of other imaging agents. (See www.fda.gov for current information on these agents.)

Purposes

Although the MRI is relatively expensive, the detailed scan may be well worth it. MRI can do some things CT cannot. For example, MRI not only clearly defines internal organ structure but also helps detect changes in tissue, such as edema or infarcts. Blood flow patterns and detailed information on blood vessel integrity can give an earlier warning than ever before of developing atherosclerotic disease. Because of the lack of bone artifacts, MRI can help identify tumors in the pituitary gland. For clients with multiple sclerosis, the MRI demonstrates the amount of plaque on the nerves. MRI reveals bone bruises (osseous contusions) that occur with traumatic injuries. Researchers are investigating if these bone bruises have predictive value for future development of posttraumatic arthritis.

Another use of MRI is to differentiate normal kidney tissue from acute tubular necrosis (ATN) and acute rejection in a transplanted kidney. Ultrafast MRI, called *cine MRI,* can produce a complete image of the heart at the rate of 30–40 images per heartbeat. Conventional MRI produces an image about every 1–2 seconds. Cine MRI, like cine CT, is really a movie of the heart. The ultrafast MRI is also useful for assessing fetal problems.

Advances in MRI hardware and software have resulted in better resolution and faster screening techniques. For example, MRI may be a sensitive imaging technique for high-resolution images of great-vessel anatomy and for mapping of blood vessel flow. The results may be very close to actual cardiac catheterization measurements. MRI is invaluable for long-term follow-up of children who have had cardiac surgery (Hay et al., 2011).

Magnetic Resonance Angiography

As discussed earlier, a special type of MRI called magnetic resonance angiography (MRA) uses signals from the blood flow in vessels that are transferred into a computer image. Other structures are subtracted by the computer so that only the signals from the blood flow are shown on the image. This technique, sometimes called digital subtraction angiography, is also done with invasive arteriograms (discussed in Chapter 20).

Use of MRI to detect breast cancer

Screening with contrast-enhanced breast MRI detects cancer earlier but is much more expensive than mammograms and results in more false positive scans (Plevritis et al., 2006). However, in 2007, based on research, the American Cancer Society began recommending that women with a family and genetic history of breast cancer be screened with MRI. MRI is used to follow up women identified as having gene mutations BRCA1 or BRCA 2. (See Chapter 10). Mammograms (which may detect calcified nodules not seen on MRI) and MRIs may be alternated every 6 months for women at high risk for breast cancer. Dedicated MRI breast scanners are available to the public.

For breast MRI, the woman lies prone and the contrast medium is given IV to highlight the concentrations of blood around the tumor. No breast compression is needed for the 15-minute scan. The woman lies face down so that her breasts fall into two holes, and hang down in the magnetic field.

MRI in Pregnancy

MRI is not used in pregnancy if ultrasound (Chapter 23) will suffice. CT is avoided because of radiation risks. MRI may be very useful to diagnose acute appendicitis in pregnant women when the appendix is not visualized by ultrasound (Pedrosa et al., 2006).

Fetal Imaging

While ultrasound (Chapter 23) is the mainstay for fetal screening, MRI can detect fetal abnormalities in greater detail. Also, MRI can give detailed images of the brain and central nervous system. The ultrafast MRI eliminates the problem of fetal movement.

MR Spectroscopy and functional MRI

MR spectroscopy (MRS) uses the same type of magnet and hardware as a conventional MRI but has specialized sequences that produce a spectrum of different biochemical compounds in biological tissues. The use of MRS can provide molecular imaging on neurological conditions such as multiple sclerosis, Alzheimer's disease, and brain tumors. More recently, researchers are using MRS to study not only the brain but also other tissues such as breast tumors. Spectroscopy adds another measure to improve the overall accuracy of tumor screening.

Functional MRI (fMRI) looks at the function of the brain by taking many pictures of the blood flow in the brain while the subject completes some sensory-motor tasks. Researcher can thus see which part of the brain is activated by different types of activity such as tapping a finger, solving a math problem, or reading. Experts predict increased use of fMRI in at least three clinical areas—mapping of critical areas in clients undergoing brain surgery, early identification of psychiatric and central nervous system disorders, and evaluation of the effectiveness of therapies for disorders of the brain (Orenstein, 2006).

Pretest Nursing Diagnoses Related to MRI

Deficient Knowledge Related to Needed Preparation

Watches, tapes, and credit cards are damaged by the magnetic field; therefore, clients must shed these items. Clients must also remove jewelry, clothing with metal fasteners, and hair clips. Objects containing ferrous metal produce artifacts. Also, the movement of the object can be detrimental to the client. For example, clients who have metal implants such as surgical clips, heart valves, or orthopedic clips cannot undergo MRI because the magnet may move the object within the body. Implantable ports made from stainless steel may produce artifacts during MRI. Titanium ports reportedly produce minimal artifacts, but this should be checked with the imaging department. Artificial joints that are not ferrous present no problems. Clients should also be asked about any injuries that could have left some metal embedded in a sensitive place such as an eye. Any movement of even a small fragment could cause permanent damage. Clients may feel odd sensations from dental work in their teeth if a filling or bridge contains ferrous material. The machine can deactivate pacemakers, so clients with pacemakers need to be evaluated prior to undergoing MRI. All institutions have a client prescan screening form that must be signed by the client or guardian and the technologist.

The nurse should check with the MRI department to determine if contrast medium is to be used because the material may affect whether the client needs to have any food or beverage restrictions. Various oral contrast agents, including barium sulfate, antacids, or supplements with multivitamins and iron, may be used to improve the contrast between the GI tract and the surrounding organs. Glucagon may be given to decrease peristalsis. Drugs such as gadoteridol and gadopentetate dimeglumine are given intravenously to increase the detectability of some lesions. Unlike the iodinated contrast media used for CT, these agents are not commonly associated with adverse reactions, but nausea and taste disturbances may occur. As noted earlier, clients with impaired renal function may develop nephrogenic systemic fibrosis (NSF) after being given contrast medium containing gadolinium. Therefore, a serum creatinine (Chapter 4) must be performed no more than 30 days before the procedure. The client also signs a consent form due to the possibility of NSF.

Many scans take as long as 45 minutes to an hour, so the client should void before entering the cylinder.

Anxiety Related to Feelings of Claustrophobia

Measures to decrease claustrophobia are visualization of peaceful scenes or other relaxation techniques. A circulatory air system may also reduce the feeling of not being able to breathe normally. Special prism glasses are available so a client can have a view outside the cylinder. Also some cylinders are now made of see-through plastic material. The use of a new MRI-compatible audio-visual reality system may not only dramatically reduce noise but also banish claustrophobia. Comfort levels may also be increased by massaging the feet as the client lies in the tube. An open MRI may be feasible for some procedures.

(Continued)

Pretest Nursing Diagnoses . . . (*Continued*)

Having the parent present helps to calm children. Parents may read or talk to the child, because there is no risk of radiation from the procedure. (Parents must be debriefed about watches, credit cards, and such, which may be damaged by the magnet.)

Because clients must lie still for a long time, young children and very anxious adults may need sedation. Drugs do not interfere with the examination. General anethesia is often required for children under 8 years of age who need a cardiac MRI (Hay et al., 2011).

Posttest Nursing Implications Related to MRI

There is no special aftercare of the client. (See the discussion in Chapter 20 on the anxiety related to waiting for results that may take 1–2 days.) Although there are no known hazards from the test, clients with tumors may be concerned about the possible effect on the tumor.

POSITRON EMISSION TOMOGRAPHY

Description

In the past, CT and MRI were used to diagnose internal problems, but they primarily looked at the structure of the body. Positron emission tomography (PET) and SPECT give additional information because they measure the functions of the body. The first PET scanner was developed at UCLA in 1973, and for many years PET was mostly used in research centers to obtain detailed mapping of brain and heart function. Now PET is also very useful in determining whether a tumor is benign or malignant. All the organ systems can be scanned in one exam to diagnose and define hidden recurrent cancer. The exam is expensive, but usually costs less than $2,000; however, the benefits may outweigh the cost. Medicare now covers the use of PET in clients with cancer and other conditions such as epilepsy, Alzheimer's, and heart disease.

PET may be combined with CT as a fusion or hybrid scan. The integrated PET/CT scanner helps improve diagnosis and treatment by providing anatomical, biochemical, and functional details. Not only does PET/CT improve the staging of cancer, but it also helps determine if a tumor is resectable (McPhee et al., 2011).

For PET studies, the client receives an injection of a biochemical substance tagged with a radionuclide, which emits positrons. When the radioactive particles combine with the negatively charged electrons normally found in the cells of tissue, they emit gamma rays that can be detected with a scanning device. The PET scanner translates the emissions into color-coded images. For example, radioactive glucose can be used to map biochemical activity in the brain. The half-life of the isotopes used is short, so there is minimal radiation dosage. The radiation is usually less than one-fourth that of a CT scan. However, the gamma rays that are the byproduct of all positron-emitting isotopes are more penetrating than the type of gamma rays emitted by other isotopes (Chapter 22), so thicker shields are used for the holders and containers.

FDG-PET

The most common radioisotope used in PET is fluorodeoxyglucose (FDG) made by adding radioactive fluorine to a glucose analog. Cells use glucose as an energy source, so the most active cells take up more of the FDG tracer. Tumor cells are rapidly dividing, so these cells take up FDG faster than other cells and show up as "hot spots" on the scan. Although FDG is an exquisite tumor-locating tracer, it is not tumor specific. Infections and inflammatory changes will cause cells to uptake more FDG, so recognition of these imaging pitfalls is crucial in diagnosis. Theoretically, any physiological substance can be tagged and traced as it is metabolized in the body, and research is ongoing to find new uses for PET such as identifying occult infections.

Purposes

PET, as a measure of brain activity, is used to study the effects of stroke, epilepsy, migraine headache, Parkinson's disease, dementia, and other disorders, such as schizophrenia. PET studies of the heart have three general uses. First, and perhaps most important, is the assessment of myocardial viability. Other uses are to measure regional myocardial perfusion and to assess cardiac metabolism. PET is sometimes used to evaluate angina, but SPECT provides acceptable images and is less expensive and more readily available (McPhee et al., 2011). Research on cardiac diseases is looking at how PET could detect early changes in vessel walls even before plaque develops.

As noted earlier, PET and PET/CT scanners have become very important in detecting occult recurrent cancer. A PET may be the follow-up for clients whose blood tests show increasing levels of tumor markers. (See Chapter 10 on tumor markers). In 2005, Centers for Medicare and Medicaid Services (CMS) approved coverage for PET exams for clients with various cancers when they are listed on an FDG-PET registry. PET is also being investigated for its ability to predict response or lack of response to treatment at an early stage. Also, PET scans used in research protocols are aimed at testing or comparing the efficacy of new medications (Juweid & Cheson, 2006). The use of PET/CT scans complement each other as CT creates anatomic images to localize and define tumor borders so that a biopsy or radiation therapy is as accurate as possible (Ott, 2010).

Pretest Nursing Implications Related to PET

Some scans require avoidance of food and fluids; others do not. Alcohol, caffeine, and nicotine should be withheld for most types of scans. Usually food is withheld because increased glucose can interfere with the results. The client may have their blood glucose measured, and if it is over 150 mg/dL, the scan may need to be rescheduled (Ott, 2010). Sedatives should not be used if the scan requires brain activity. Check with the radiology department about any medications to be used or temporarily discontinued. Two lines may be needed: one for serial arterial blood samples and one for intravenous injection of the isotope. The client should void

(Continued)

Pretest Nursing Implications . . . (*Continued*)

because the scan may require a couple of hours. The waiting period after the injection of the radioisotope may be 45 minutes and another 45 minutes for the actual scan. A Foley catheter may be inserted if the scanned area is close to the bladder.

For some types of cardiac scans, the client uses a treadmill or exercise bicycle. (See Chapter 26 for more information about stress tests.) For brain scans, blindfolds and earplugs are used to reduce external stimuli to the brain. For some PET brain scans, the client may be asked to recite passages or perform other intellectual tests to see how the brain activity changes with remembering or reasoning. Lights or other stimuli may be used to stimulate the brain.

Posttest Nursing Implications Related to PET

See Chapter 22 for the discussion of general nursing implications for intravenous radioisotopes, such as (1) observing the site for phlebitis, (2) relieving anxiety, and (3) encouraging ingestion of fluids to hasten urinary excretion of the isotope. Usually clients can drive home and resume all daily activities as before (Hoerl, 2009).

SINGLE PHOTON EMISSION COMPUTED TOMOGRAPHY

Unlike PET, which uses a radiopharmaceutical labeled with a positron-emitting isotope, SPECT (single photon emission computed tomography) uses several of the common radionuclides discussed in Chapter 22 that are commercially prepared. A brain SPECT costs about as much as a CT brain scan.

SPECT has become the scan of choice for a diagnostic evaluation for dementia and some other types of central nervous system disorders. SPECT is used to measure blood perfusion in the brain, in contrast to the neuronal uptake of glucose in PET. Some of the major uses for SPECT are to localize the foci of epilepsy, detect and grade brain tumors, and evaluate brain damage from trauma that cannot be detected by CT or MRI.

Also, SPECT imaging with Tc-99m (See Chapter 22) can improve the assessment of cardiac ischemia. Bone SPECT may be superior to FDG-PET (see earlier discussion) for detection of bone metastases in breast cancer (Uematsu et al., 2005).

Coupling SPECT with the high-powered CT scanners discussed earlier in this chapter will no doubt lead to many new uses, as research focuses on these hybrid or fusion scans. SPECT/CT costs considerably less than PET/CT and is more readily available in many settings.

Pretest and Posttest Nursing Implications Related to SPECT

Usually there are no restrictions on food or fluids. (See Chapter 22 on general nursing implications for clients receiving radionuclides.)

Questions

1. Which of the following is the main disadvantage of CT scans as compared with MRI or ultrasound procedures?
   a. The number of personnel needed to run the machine
   b. The amount of preparation required for the client
   c. The amount of radiation exposure to the client
   d. The lack of detailed images

2. The priority nursing intervention after a client is finished with a body scan is to assess
   a. Vital signs because of possible adverse effects, such as bleeding
   b. Level of anxiety related to outcome of procedure
   c. Pain level caused by the procedure
   d. Effects of radiation, such as nausea

3. Which one of the following would be *inappropriate* for a 3-year-old child who is undergoing CT head scanning that does not involve the use of any contrast medium?
   a. Nothing-by-mouth status for 3–4 hours before the examination
   b. Use of sedation 30 minutes before the test
   c. Removal of bobby pins or other items in the hair
   d. Have the child practice keeping his or her head still while a humming noise is made

4. Some types of CT scans require specific client preparations. Which of the following types of CT scan requires the most physical preparation of the client?
   a. Brain scans
   b. Pelvic scans
   c. Thoracic scans
   d. Abdominal scans

5. Nursing implications related to the use of intravenous radioisotopes are appropriate for a client undergoing
   a. MRI
   b. PET
   c. CT
   d. Tomography

6. In a client scheduled for MRI, which of the following is an essential part of pretest teaching?
   a. The area to be scanned needs to be shaved
   b. Any objects containing ferrous metal must not be taken into the MRI room
   c. Food and fluids are withheld for 4–6 hours before the test
   d. The client may turn side to side during the scan, but he or she must not sit

7. In educating a client about the sensations of MRI, the nurse would *not* need to prepare the client for the possibility of
   a. A strange feeling around tooth fillings
   b. Slight redness of the skin
   c. A variety of noises, some rather loud
   d. Claustrophobia or a closed-in feeling

References

Armstrong, M. L. & Elkins, L. (2005). Body art and MRI. *American Journal of Nursing, 105*(3), 65.

Beinfeld, M. T., Wittenberg, E., & Gazelle, G. (2005). Cost-effectiveness of whole-body CT screening. *Radiology, 234*(2), 415–422.

Brown, D. A. (2009). Osteoporosis: Not just for women. *American Nurse Today, 4*(3), 10–12.

Bucsko, J. K. (2005). Keeping score on calcium scoring. *Radiology Today, 6*(14), 8–11.

DeBoer, S., Seaver, M., Angel, E., & Armstrong, M. (2008). Myths about body piercing and tattooing. *Nursing 2008, 38*(11), 50–54.

Deglin, J. H., Vallerand, A. H., & Sanoski, C. A. (2011). *Davis's drug guide for nurses* (12th ed.). Philadelphia: F. A. Davis.

Gallauresi, B. A. & Woods, T. (2008). Danger: "Sandbag" in the MRI room. *Nursing 2008, 38*(12), 60.

Greenland, P., LaBree, L., Azen, S., Doherty, T., & Detrano, R. (2004). Coronary artery calcium score combined with Framingham score for risk prediction in asymptomatic individuals. *JAMA: Journal of American Medical Association, 291*(2), 210–215.

Hardy, K. (2010). MRI safety evolution. *Radiology Today, 11*(6), 16–19.

Harvey, D. (2006). On patrol: Ensuring implant & device safety. *Radiology Today, 7*(6), 13–16.

Harvey, D. (2009). Gadolinium contrast: An update on imaging understanding and prevention of NSF. *Radiology Today, 10*(18), 16–19.

Hay, W. W., Levin, M. J., Sondheimer, J. M., & Deterding, R. (Eds.). (2011). *Current diagnosis and treatment: Pediatrics* (20th ed.). New York: McGraw-Hill.

Hoerl, K. (2009). PET scans. *Nursing 2009, 39*(8), 30.

Hoffmann, U., Ferencik, M., Cury, R., & Pena, A. (2006). Coronary CT angiography. *Journal of Nuclear Medicine, 47*(5), 797–806.

Holcomb, S. S. (2006). Osteoporosis. *Nursing 2006, 36*(2), 48–49.

Juweid, M. E. & Cheson, B. (2006). Positron-emission tomography and assessment of cancer therapy. *New England Journal of Medicine, 354*(5), 496–507.

Kanal, E. (2006). Tattoos and MRI. *Nurseweek, 19*(15), 25.

Lange, S. & Nguyen, Q. (2006). Cables and electrodes can burn patients during MRI. *Nursing 2006, 36*(11), 18.

Lee, T. (2006). Clash of the titans: The pacemaker and the MRI can't work together—at least not yet. *Harvard Heart Letter, 16*(8), 1–2.

McPhee, S. J., Papadakis, M. A., & Rabow, M. W. (Eds.). (2011). *Current medical diagnosis & treatment* (50th ed.). New York: McGraw-Hill

Orenstein, B. W. (2006). Planning ahead—clinical uses for MRI. *Radiology Today, 7*(7), 26–29.

Ott, L. K. (2010). PET-CT scans can improve care for patients with cancer. *Nursing 2010, 40*(4), 62–63.

Pedrosa, I., Levine, D., Eyvazzadeh, A., Stewert, B., Ngo, L., & Rofsky, N. (2006). MR imaging evaluation of acute appendicitis in pregnancy. *Radiology, 238*(3), 891–899.

Plevritis, S. K., Kurian A. U., Sigal, B. M., Daniel, B. L., Ikeda, D. M., Stockdale, F. E., et al. (2006). Cost-effectiveness of screening BRCA1/2 mutation carriers with breast magnetic resonance imaging. *Journal of American Medical Association, 295*(20), 2374–2384.

Rhea, J. T., Halpern, E., Ptak, T., Lawrason, J., Sacknoff, R., & Novelline, R. (2005). The status of appendiceal CT in an urban medical center 5 years after its introduction: Experience with 753 patients. *American Journal of Roentgenology, 184*(6), 1802–1808.

Uematsu, T., Yuen, S., Yukisawa, S., Aramaki, T., Morimoto, N., Endo, M., et al. (2005). Comparison of FDG PET and SPECT for detection of bone metastases in breast cancer. *American Journal of Roentgenology, 184*, 1266–1273.

Vacca, V. M. (2006). Subdural hematoma. *Nursing 2006, 36*(3), 88.

Vernooij, M. W., Ikram, M. A., Tangher, H. L., Vincent, A. J. P. E., Hofman, A., Krestin, G. P., et al. (2007). Incidental findings on brain MRI in the general population. *The New England Journal of Medicine, 357*(18), 1821–1828.

Wrotny, C. (2005). Osteoporosis: What women want to know. *MEDSURG Nursing, 14*(6), 405–407.

Websites

www.acrin.org (American College of Radiology Imaging Network for study protocols.)
www.beekley.com (Information on medical products for imaging.)
www.cancer.gov (National Cancer Institute for updates on clinical trials.)
www.fda.gov (Information on warning about gadolinium-based contrast agents.)
www.ielcap.org (International Early Lung Cancer Action Program for updates on screening for lung cancer.)
www.lungcanceralliance.org (Information on risk factors for lung cancer.)
www.mrisafety.com (Institute for Magnetic Resonance Safety, Education and Research for updates on MRI and safety issues.)
www.neme.org (For information on portable CT scans.)
www.uspreventiveservicestaskforce.org (Guidelines for osteoporosis screening.)

Answers

1. c, 2. b, 3. a, 4. d, 5. b, 6. b, 7. b

Nuclear Scans: Diagnostic Tests with Radionuclides or Radioisotopes

- General Information on Nuclear Medicine 559
- Nursing Diagnoses Related to Radionuclide Studies 565
- Bone Scans 567
- Brain Scans 568
- Gallium Scans 568
- Indium Scans or Leukocyte Imaging 569
- Sentinel Node Scans in Breast and Other Types of Cancers 569
- Breast Scan with Somatostatin Receptor Scintigraphy 570
- Gallbladder Scans 570
- Gastrointestinal Scans 570
- Liver and Spleen Scans 571
- Lung Scans: Perfusion Images and Ventilation Studies (V/Q Scans) 571
- Cardiac Scans 572
- Renal Scans 575
- Thyroid Scans 575
- RAI Uptake Study 576
- Compatibility and Red Blood Cell Survival 577
- Blood Volume Studies 577

OBJECTIVES

1. Differentiate between the use of common radionuclides for diagnostic testing and for therapy.
2. Compare and contrast the procedures used for in vitro and in vivo testing.
3. Explain why pregnant women and children are advised not to undergo radionuclide studies if other nonradioactive tests can suffice.
4. State the general nursing implications for preparing a client for any organ scan with technetium (Tc-99m).
5. State the principal use of a bone scan performed with radionuclides.
6. Explain the purpose of a gallium scan in a client with a fever of undetermined origin.
7. Plan a teaching program for a client who is to undergo a radioactive iodine uptake study in 2 weeks.
8. Explain the purpose of administration of potassium iodine before an iodine-125 (I-125) scan for sites other than the thyroid.

The terms *radionuclide* and *radioisotope* are both used to describe the radiopharmaceuticals used for diagnostic tests in the nuclear medicine department. Often, in general practice, the older term *radioisotope* is still used. However, recent literature uses the more precise term *radionuclides*, and this term is used in this chapter. The term *radionuclide* conveys that the element has a nucleus that has been made radioactive.

In diagnostic nuclear medicine, the radionuclide is given to the client and the radiation emitted from a particular organ is measured. The basic rationale for the use of radionuclides is to observe the function—not the structure—of an organ. However, positron emission tomography (PET) and its cousin, single photon emission computed tomography (SPECT), do assess both structure and function because radionuclides and a sophisticated computer are used to record and plot the effect of the radioactive substance in the body. PET and SPECT are discussed in Chapter 21 and at www.acrin.org.

GENERAL INFORMATION ON NUCLEAR MEDICINE

Radionuclides As Radioactive Elements

Radiation occurs when there is a lack of stability in the nuclei of atoms. As the atom spontaneously disintegrates, radiation is emitted in the form of α-, β-, and γ-rays. Some of the synthetic radionuclides are purified so that only γ-rays are emitted. About 50 of the roughly 350 isotopes of all elements in nature are naturally radioactive. Isotopes of an element are slightly different molecular forms of the same chemical element. The discovery that certain natural elements were radioactive was made in 1896 by Antoine Henri Becquerel, who was working with uranium compounds. In 1903, Becquerel shared a Nobel Prize with Marie Curie and Pierre Curie, who discovered another naturally occurring radioactive substance, radium. The unit used to measure the activity of radionuclides is the curie (Ci) named in honor of the Curies. The SI unit is the becquerel (Bq; 1 Ci = 37 gigabecquerels [GBq]).

In the early part of the 20th century, scientists discovered that it was possible to make naturally nonradioactive elements radioactive by bombarding the nucleus with subatomic fragments to make it unstable. The invention of the cyclotron (atom smasher) in 1931 made it possible to make many elements radioactive. Some of these synthetic radionuclides, such as iodine-131 (I-131), have been used extensively for therapy and diagnostic testing. Therapy with I-131 for cancer of the thyroid was begun in 1943—a time when both peaceful and war uses of nuclear products were being explored. The use of I-131 for cancer of the thyroid was dubbed the "atomic cocktail" (www.snm.org). Because of the length of its half-life, I-131 is infrequently used for diagnostic tests. Newer shorter-lived substances have replaced I-131, as discussed later.

Use of Radionuclides As Therapeutic Agents

This chapter focuses on the use of radionuclides for diagnostic tests, but it should be pointed out that radionuclides are also used in therapy. One commonly used radionuclide is I-131, used to treat some cases of hyperthyroidism (Katzung, Masters, & Trevor, 2009).

Table 22–1 In Vitro Sampling Tests

Test	Example of Radionuclide Used	Timing of Test After Dosage	Special Preparation
Red blood cells (RBCs)			
Compatibility	Cr-51	1 h	Blood drawn from client, then reinjected after tagged
Survival and sequestration	Cr-51	3–4 wk	Blood samples drawn 2–3 times a week
Blood volume studies			Blood drawn from client, then reinjected after tagged
RBC plasma volume	Cr-51 Radioiodinated human serum albumin (RIHSA)		Record height and weight Must have normal hydration

Cr, chromium.

Methods of Diagnostic Testing with Radionuclides

In Vitro Testing

With in vitro testing (sample testing), the radionuclide is given intravenously or orally, and at a later date, samples are taken from the blood or urine. Blood volume studies, and red blood cell (RBC) studies, use samples not scans to measure radionuclides. Sample tests are discussed at the end of this chapter, with specific points about nursing implications. Although radioactive iodine (RAI) uptake testing may also involve the collection of urine samples, it is primarily an in vivo test because the radioactivity of the thyroid gland is measured with a counter. Table 22–1 lists in vitro sampling tests. Many other laboratory tests, such as those for antibodies (Chapter 14) and hormones (Chapter 15), are in vitro tests that use radionuclides for tagging the substance to be measured.

In Vivo Testing (Scintigraphy)

The in vivo method (organ scan or scintigram) of measuring the amount of radionuclide in the body is performed by means of organ scanning. Table 22–2 lists in vivo tests. The scan of an organ is referred to as a scintigram because a scintillation camera is used to make a scan or picture. The scintillation camera, which came into use in 1964, has made testing with radionuclides a very useful method of diagnostic testing. The client is given a radionuclide compound (radiopharmaceutical) intravenously, orally, or by inhalation, depending on the organ to be scanned. Minutes or hours later, or sometimes the following day, the scintillation camera takes a radioactivity reading from the target organ and feeds these readings into a computer. The computer translates these readings into a 2-D image or scan. A gamma camera scanner gives a 2-D planar image, and the SPECT scanner (Chapter 21) gives a 3-D image. The scintigram is printed in a gray scale so there is more variation than in a black-and-white picture. Scintigrams may also be produced in color. These varying shades of gray or color show the relative distribution of the radionuclide in the different parts of the organ. Very dark spots on the scintigram are called *hot spots* because more of the radionuclide was deposited in that spot. Parts of the tissue that do not pick up the radionuclide are seen as light-colored areas. Spots without

Table 22–2 In Vivo Testing (Organ Scans or Scintiscans)

Scan	Examples of Radionuclide Type and Route	Timing of Scan After Dosage	Special Preparation
Bone	Tc-99m tagged phosphate compounds (IV)	Immediately and 2–4 hours (takes 1 hour to scan entire body)	Push fluids 2–4 h before; Void before test Intestinal preparation
Brain			
Perfusion	Tc-99m pertechnetate (IV)	Immediately	None
Static views	Tc-99m Glucoheptenate (IV)	Immediately 15 minutes 1–4 hours	None
	Radio iodinated human serum albumin (RIHSA) (IV)	18–48 hours	None
Functional	IMP or HMPAO	Varies	None
Cardiac			
For infarction	Tc-99m pyrophosphate (IV)	90 minutes–3 hours	See text
Perfusion scan	(Th-201) (IV)	3–5 minutes; also in 3–6 hours	See discussion of dipyridamole and stress tests
Ejection-fraction studies	Albumin or red blood cells tagged with Tc-99m	Immediate with first pass analysis	See text
Gated cardiac pool imaging	Same as above	Continuous over 1–2 h	
Gastrofunctional studies	Tc-99m sulfur colloid	Varies with part of GI tract studied	Maintain nothing-by-mouth status; see text about medications
Hepatobiliary			
Liver and spleen (reticuloendo-thelial cells)	Tc-99m sulfur colloid	10–15 min	None
Gallbladder	Tc-99m with HIDA or PIPIDA (IV), Tc-99m DISIDA (IV) (Hepatolite)	Immediate and intervals to 24 h	Maintain nothing-by-mouth status for 2 h before Fat restriction during time of test
Lung	Tc-99m with albumin (IV)	15 min	None
Perfusion	Xe-133 (inhalation)	Immediate	None
Ventilation	Kr-85 (inhalation)	Immediate	None
Renal[a]			
Perfusion	Tc-99m DTPA, DSMA glucoheptanate (IV)	Immediate (20 min)	Hydrate as ordered
Static views	As above	Up to 4 h	
Functional	I-131 or I-123 tagged to orthoiodohippurate (IV)	Immediate and up to 1 h as continual scan	Hydrate as ordered Potassium iodide solution as ordered
Thyroid	Tc-99m pertechnetate (IV)	30 min	No prep
Screening	I-123 (oral)	24 h	Maintain nothing-by-mouth status 8 h before No iodine for 4 wk pretest and 2 h posttest

(*continued*)

Table 22-2 In Vivo Testing (Organ Scans or Scintiscans) *(continued)*

Scan	Examples of Radionuclide Type and Route	Timing of Scan After Dosage	Special Preparation
RAI (radioactive iodine uptake) Total body scans	I-123 or I-131 (oral)	2, 6, 24 h	As above; see text
Inflammatory lesions and neoplasms	Gallium citrate, Ga-67 (IV)	4–6 and 24–72 h or longer (up to 5 days)	Usually needs intestinal preparation
Inflammatory only	Tagged leukocytes with In-111 (IV)	4–24 h	None
Thyroid malignancy	I-131	3–7 days	See text

*a*A triple renal study uses two IV injections to obtain perfusion, static views, and excretory function of the kidneys. HMPAO, Tc-99m exametazine; IMP, I-123 iodoamphetamine; In, indium; IV, intravenous; Kr, krypton; Th, thallium; Xe, xenon. See www.radiologyinfo.org for updates on these tests

radionuclide uptake are *cold spots* or *cold nodules.* The scintigram is interpreted by a physician trained in nuclear medicine, and a written report of the scan is put in the client's chart. Some common findings on scintigrams are discussed for each scan in this chapter. In general, imaging with radionuclides is most useful when there is disturbance of function rather than a structural defect.

Types of Radionuclides Used in Diagnostic Testing

In the past, I-131 was used not only for diagnosis of and therapy for thyroid disorders but also as a radioactive tag carried to other organs. Now other forms of iodine are used as radionuclides, including I-123, which has a half-life of 13 hours compared with a half-life of 8 days for I-131. (The importance of half-life is discussed in the section on hazards.) Other radionuclides, such as gallium and thallium, are used for certain types of scanning. Sodium chromate (Cr-51) is used to tag RBCs. Although various radionuclides are useful for certain tests, Tc-99m is the most commonly used for nuclear medicine diagnostic testing. In fact, 80% of the 20 million nuclear tests done annually in the United States use Tc-99m Although the United States does the most nuclear scan testing, Tc-99m is made from molybdenum-99 (Mo-99) in reactors in other countries. When Canada had to shut down a reactor in 2009, there was a shortage of this isotope (Orenstein, 2009). (See www.snm. org for current information on legislation to promote domestic production of this isotope.)

Technetium (Tc-99m)

There are several isotopes of technetium, and all are naturally radioactive. A very unstable form of technetium, Tc-99m, has a half-life of only 6 hours. Tc-99m is combined with various compounds that carry the radionuclide to various target organs. For example, bone uses most of the phosphorus in the body, so Tc-99m combined with pyrophosphate is used for a bone scan. Tc-99m combined with albumin is used as a lung scan because the radio-tagged albumin disperses in the pulmonary precapillary arterioles. RBCs can be tagged with Tc-99m to help diagnose gastrointestinal (GI) bleeding. Other compounds can carry Tc-99m to other specific organs, such as the hepatobiliary system, thyroid, or brain. If Tc-99m is given without another compound (straight), it is excreted in the urine and in the saliva. Thus, straight Tc-99m can be used to study the parotid glands or immediate flow through the cerebral vessels. Tc-99m is always administered intravenously. The timing of the scans after the administration of the radionuclide depends on the target organ to be viewed. Some organs may take up the substance in a few hours, so scans are performed relatively soon, whereas others may not be completed for 24 hours or longer.

Somatostatin Receptor Scintigraphy and Octreotide Scans

Tumors that have somatostatin receptors can be identified by the use of radio-tagged octreotide. One of the original uses for octreotide scans was to identify and localize carcinoid tumors, a type of neuroendocrine tumor with somatostatin receptors on the cellular membrane. At present, SRS has an expanded use in oncology because other types of cancer sometimes have somatostatin receptors. When a primary tumor has this type of receptor, metastatic lesions will have them too. Tc-99m-tagged depreotide, an analog of somatostatin, is discussed under bone scans and breast scans.

Octreotide is used to treat carcinoid tumors and acromegaly (Deglin, Vallerand, & Sanoski, (2011), so the client must be off the medication before having the scan with radio-tagged octreotide or somatostatin analogs. Exams may be scheduled for 3 consecutive days with a laxative given before the final scan.

Radiation Hazards from Radionuclides

The radiation hazard from radionuclide diagnostic testing is very slight because the doses used are usually very small. Also, duration is brief because of the short half-life of the radionuclides used. It was mentioned earlier that the curie (Ci) is the unit used to measure the activity of radionuclides. The curie is based on the radioactivity of a standard gram of radium. The dosages used in therapy are in millicurie (mCi) levels (0.001 Ci). In contrast, dosage levels for the radiopharmaceuticals used for diagnostic testing are in microcurie (μCi) levels (.000001 mCi). Thus, the radiation from diagnostic testing is roughly a thousand times less than with therapy. When millicurie levels are being used for therapy, other clients and personnel should be protected from the radiation in the client. The National Council on Radiation Protection and Measurements has guidelines that the hospital *must* follow when therapy is being performed with radionuclides. The guidelines for diagnostic procedures are less complicated than those for therapeutic procedures; however, nuclear medicine personnel must take precautions in handling samples. If urine or fecal matter must be saved for sample testing, the worker should wear waterproof gloves when putting the samples in containers or in cleaning bedpans. If urine can be disposed of by means of dilution in the sewage system, no special precautions are needed. Thus, from a nursing point of view, the usual precaution with urine is not to touch the urine, and if samples must be obtained, waterproof gloves should be worn to handle the sample. (See the discussion in the section "Posttest Nursing

Diagnoses Related to Radionuclide Studies.") The ALARA rule (*as low as reasonably achievable*) is appropriate for any diagnostic test that uses radioactive material.

Waste Disposal for Diagnostic Testing Materials

The minimal radiation hazard from radionuclide diagnostic testing is brief because the half-life of most diagnostic radiopharmaceuticals is short. Half-life is the time it takes a radioactive element to lose half of its radioactivity. An unstable radioactive element continuously disintegrates, but some take much longer than others to "physically decay." I-123 has a half-life of only 13 hours compared with 8 days for I-131. Tc-99m has a half-life of only 6 hours, and disposal is not a problem. In dramatic contrast, radium has a half-life of 1,590 years. In addition to less exposure for the client, the shorter is the half-life, the less is the problem of waste disposal. For nuclear medicine diagnostic testing, the waste disposal problem is not acute because wastes can be held until physical decay occurs.

Radionuclides As Low-Level Radioactive Wastes

Because radiation from any source is cumulative, it should always be kept at a minimum for clients, personnel, and the general public. The Nuclear Regulatory Commission (www.nrc.gov) grants a license to a physician or an institution to conduct research, therapy, or diagnostic testing with radioactive material. Specific standards must be maintained, and they are the responsibility of a person designated as the Radiation Safety Officer.

Radionuclide Diagnostic Testing During Pregnancy

Radiation destroys or alters cells as they go through the dividing stages of growth. In the fetus, and to a lesser degree in the child, cell growth is rapid; thus, many cells are vulnerable to alteration by radiation. (This, of course, is why radiation is used as a therapeutic agent for cancer cells, which divide and grow at an increased rate.)

As a rule, radionuclides are not used for diagnostic testing during pregnancy if other tests suffice. Although the amount of radioactivity in diagnostic testing is small, it is prudent to protect the fetus from any radiation whenever possible. As with radiography, elective diagnostic tests with radionuclides should be performed during menses or within 10–14 days after onset of menses for women who could become pregnant. When a test cannot be postponed, pregnant women may need to sign a special consent form for radionuclide testing. If testing is conducted, the pregnant woman should empty her bladder frequently after the test is begun.

Radionuclide Tests for Infants and Children

Women who are nursing should not breast-feed the infant until the radionuclide has been eliminated. If children need scans, the dosages of the radiopharmaceuticals are calculated to provide maximum results with the minimum dose possible.

Radionuclide Tests for Elderly Clients

Radionuclide testing is noninvasive and well tolerated by elderly clients.

NURSING DIAGNOSES RELATED TO RADIONUCLIDE STUDIES

Pretest Nursing Diagnoses Related to Radionuclide Studies

Deficient Knowledge Related to Procedure

The nurse should be familiar with the particular procedure being used for the test so that the client's questions can be answered. If the client is not sure why the test is needed, the nurse can help the client obtain the correct information from his or her physician. The nurse can assure the client that the scans do not hurt. The nurse should also inform the client that he or she will have to lie still during the scan, but the positioning is usually not uncomfortable. The scans may take 30–60 minutes. The machine makes clicking noises at times. Some scanners can be brought to the client's bedside, but usually it is preferable to obtain the scan in the nuclear medicine department. A parent can accompany a child. Some clients may need a sedative or pain medication before the scan, but this is not a common practice. Sedatives do not interfere with the test. Most of the radionuclides are given intravenously, so the client should be told that a venipuncture will be performed in the nuclear medicine department. All the Tc-99m compounds used for organ scans are given intravenously. Iodine compounds may be given orally or intravenously, depending on the test. If radioactive iodine is being used for studies other than of the thyroid, potassium iodide is given before and after the scan to block uptake by the thyroid gland. For some lung studies, the radio-tagged substance is inhaled.

Anxiety Related to Timing of Scans

The length of time between the administration of the radioisotope and the scan varies depending on the type of scan (see Table 22–2). A member of the nuclear medicine department notifies the nurse of the specific time the client should return for the scan or if the client is to remain in the nuclear medicine department for the entire time of the test. Clients should know if they are to stay in the nuclear medicine department for an extended length of time so they can bring reading material or handwork. For ambulatory care, the client may be given the radiopharmaceutical and told when to return for the scan. Specific written instructions should be given.

Anxiety Related to Possible Effects of Radiation

The nurse needs to understand fully the standard procedures for diagnostic radionuclide testing in a specific setting so the client is not confused about inconsistencies. The nurse can reassure the client that the dose of radiation used for diagnostic testing is small and that all necessary precautions for safety are being taken. It may also be helpful to point out that only the radioisotope is radioactive. The scintillator acts as a detector of the radiation emitted from the client as opposed to a conventional x-ray machine, from which radiation is emitted to penetrate through the body. Thus, the long time, sometimes as much as an hour, spent in front of a scintillator does not cause any radiation effects as would long exposure to x-rays. The clicking of the scintillator reflects only measurements of radioactivity already present. (Even health workers may need education about the relative safety of procedures performed in the nuclear medicine department.)

Posttest Nursing Diagnoses Related to Radionuclide Studies

Risk for Injury Related to the Procedure

Comprehensive assessments are not needed after most scanning procedures because there is no risk for most of the procedures. If a stress test is performed as part of a thallium scan for coronary perfusion, there are specific posttest considerations. (See Chapter 26 on stress tests.) If the radionuclide is given intravenously, and almost all are, the site of the needle puncture should be assessed for inflammation. Warm packs can be used for any phlebitis that develops. The medications used for testing are unlikely to cause any side effects.

Anxiety Related to Test Results

As discussed in Chapter 20, the nurse is often able to act as a sounding board for a client who has anxiety about his or her condition. The results of the scan are not usually available for a day or two, so the nurse can help the client formulate specific questions to ask the physician. For example, if a liver scan is obtained to assess for possible metastasis, the client may be anxious while awaiting the results. The nurse can help the client express feelings and identify the main areas of concern regarding choices about treatments.

Altered Fluid Requirements Related to Need to Excrete Isotopes

As noted in the pretest preparations, most of the scans do not require any restrictions in diet, either before or after the scan. If there are no contraindications, the client should be encouraged to drink extra fluids to help expedite excretion of the radionuclide. This is particularly advised for pregnant clients.

Deficient Knowledge Related to Effects on Radiation Detectors

Radiation lingering in a client after a nuclear diagnostic test does not pose a danger to others, but it can be enough to set off a radiation detector alarm at airports or other checkpoints. This detection may occur more frequently as very sensitive detectors are installed for heightened security. If clients plan to travel soon after a nuclear diagnostic procedure, they should be given a letter that documents the date of the procedure, the name and half-life of the radioactive substance, and a person to contact if needed.

Disposing of Urine

Although the amount of diagnostic radionuclide excreted in the urine is low, urine should not be used for any laboratory tests. Clients should be told to flush the toilet three times after voiding. The nuclear medicine department must supply the information about the timing of the precautions with urine, based on the half-life of the radionuclide used.

Some hospitals have developed specific guidelines and appointed safety advisors for personnel who care for clients who must stay in bed and who are undergoing nuclear medicine diagnostic procedures. Infants also pose a problem for disposal of wastes because the nurse must handle the urine. Common guidelines may be as follows:

1. Wear disposable gloves (not sterile ones) when handling wastes. If there must be direct contact with body fluids deemed to be radioactive, two sets of gloves are recommended.
2. Flush the toilet three times after excreta is discarded.
3. Rinse reusable containers twice before general cleaning.
4. Rinse disposable containers twice before discarding in the general waste.
5. Wash hands with gloves on. Remove gloves and wash hands again.
6. For infants and incontinent clients, use disposable diapers, wear disposable gloves when changing diapers, and discard gloves and waste as described earlier.

Readers are encouraged to talk to nuclear medicine personnel in their own setting to obtain accurate up-to-date information about guidelines used for clients undergoing tests with radionuclides. The nurse should not unduly alarm clients. If urine is accidentally spilled or touched, this is not an emergency. Immediate disposal of the waste is not of the same urgency as when clients undergo therapy with radioactive substances. The nurse should act in a prudent manner so that any and all exposure to radiation is minimized. (See Chapter 20 for more discussion on radiation hazards for health workers.)

BONE SCANS

For a bone scan, Tc-99m-labeled phosphates or phosphonates are given intravenously. Scintigraphy with Tc-99m depreotide, a somatostatin analog, may be used if the primary tumor exhibits somatostatin receptors (Mena et al., 2004). In 2–4 hours, the radionuclide concentrates in the bone tissue. It takes about an hour for the scintillation camera to scan the entire body, front and back. If there is increased bone activity, the bone tissue takes up more of the radionuclide. The scan outlines areas of osteoblastic and osteolytic processes in the bones.

Purposes

A bone scan is most often performed to check for silent metastasis to the bone. A metastatic lesion in the bone shows up on a scan about 6 months earlier than on a conventional radiograph. Bone scans may be obtained on a routine basis after detection of malignant tumors of the breast or prostate, because bone metastasis is a strong possibility with these tumors. A bone scan may reveal the reason for an elevated level of alkaline phosphatase (ALP), an enzyme associated with bone activity (Chapter 12).

Bone scans may also help diagnose fatigue or stress fractures in the elderly with negative skeletal x-rays but continued pain and clinical symptoms. Also, researchers are determining if bone scans that document bone marrow edema or bruises in traumatic knee injuries may have value as a predictor of future arthritis.

Nursing Implications Related to Bone Scan

Consumption of large amounts of fluids should be encouraged for 2–4 hours before the test to ensure that the client is well hydrated and thus will quickly eliminate the radionuclide not absorbed by the bones. The client must void before a bone scan so the pelvic bones can be seen. If the client cannot void, a Foley catheter must be inserted before the client goes to the nuclear medicine department. Pain medications or a sedative may be required so the client can lie still for the prolonged scanning time.

BRAIN SCANS

Brain scans are conducted as perfusion scans and static views of the brain tissues. A cerebral perfusion scan is performed 30 seconds after intravenous injection of Tc-99m. If straight Tc-99m is used, some of it is excreted in the saliva; the client must not touch the saliva and then put his or her hands near his or her head. Tc-99m pertechnetate static scans of the brain are obtained at intervals, such as 15 minutes, 1 hour, and 24 hours. Potassium perchlorate in solution or capsule may be given 30–60 minutes before the procedure to prevent uptake by saliva and other tissues. If a lesion has damaged the blood–brain barrier, the radionuclide localizes in that area. The blood–brain barrier is a complex system of membranes and fluid spaces that keeps substances in the blood from diffusing into the brain tissue. Tumors and other lesions destroy this protective barrier; consequently, more of the radionuclide diffuses into the brain tissue. Radio-iodinated human serum albumin (RIHSA) may be used to evaluate changes in the blood–brain barrier. The advent of lipid-soluble radiopharmaceuticals that can cross the intact blood–brain barrier has made it possible to study the perfusion of the brain and to document the distribution of the tracer over several hours. These agents are a breakthrough in brain imaging compared to the older tagging agents, which are only localized in the disrupted area of the brain barrier. In addition, the use of SPECT (Chapter 21) has improved the quality of brain scans.

GALLIUM SCANS

Gallium citrate (Ga-67) is useful in diagnostic scanning because gallium localizes in inflammatory lesions and in some tumors. A gallium scan may be used to detect a hidden abscess or metastatic nodules. Ultrasonography (Chapter 23) may show the presence of a mass, but is not useful in determining if a mass is benign or malignant. A gallium scan can be a complementary procedure in studying the nature of a mass found with other diagnostic modalities. Chronic osteomyelitis may be detected with a gallium scan. (See indium scans for acute infections.) Gallium scans have become very useful for identifying the diffuse pulmonary inflammation that occurs with *Pneumocystis carinii* pneumonia. Also, gallium scans are useful in evaluating residual mediastinal tumors after treatment for Hodgkin's disease (Hay et al., 2011).

If the purpose is to identify an abscess, the client may be screened in 6 hours and then again in 24, 48, or 72 hours if needed. For malignant neoplasms, such as melanoma or lymphoma, the scans may be performed at 24, 48, and 72 hours or longer. Gallium has a half-life of 78 hours.

> ### Nursing Implications Related to Gallium Scan
>
> Enemas or laxatives are sometimes given before a gallium scan to empty the GI tract. The intestinal tract collects gallium, and confusing results may occur if there are shadows in the GI tract. Not all institutions require intestinal preparation, and the dual-isotope scanning performed with indium reduces the amount of confusing results. As noted earlier, women who are breastfeeding should not resume feedings for 2 weeks after the gallium test.

INDIUM SCANS OR LEUKOCYTE IMAGING

Indium (In-111) is used to label leukocytes, which then go to infected areas of the body. In contrast to gallium, In-111-labeled leukocytes are not taken up by neoplastic lesions. Any infected area in the body can be visualized in 4–24 hours. Indium is also used to label platelets and RBCs for other types of studies. For white blood cell (WBC) imaging, 40 mL of the client's blood is withdrawn 2 hours before the scan so the WBCs can be labeled with indium. Thus, this test may also be called *indium-labeled autologous leukocytes*. If the client's granulocyte count is less than 2,000 per mm³ (Chapter 2), WBCs from a compatible donor may be tagged and used for the test. These tagged WBCs tend to localize in acute infections that are less than 8 days old. Gallium scans are more useful for chronic infections, but sometimes both scans may be performed for a client who has a persistent fever of undetermined origin (FUO). There is no special preparation of a client for an indium scan except for the blood drawing before the test. Indium may be labeled to other substances. For example, In-111 pentetreotide (OctreoScan) is a radio-labeled analog of somatostatin. This agent is used to help locate neuroendocrine tumors that bear somatostatin receptors.

SENTINEL NODE SCANS IN BREAST AND OTHER TYPES OF CANCERS

Sentinel nodes are the first nodes that receive drainage from a tumor, so identifying these nodes so they can be biopsied lessens the need for wide-scale axillary dissection. Dyes, contrast medium, and radioactive tracers are methods used to identify these sentinel nodes. Sentinel node biopsy (SNB) was originally used when breast tumors were not larger than 1.5 cm, but based on research, all clients with breast cancer should be offered SNB at the time of their surgery (Lacovara & Yoder, 2006). In addition to breast cancer, a study has shown that SNB is also useful in the management of melanomas (Morton et al., 2006). Studies are ongoing for the use of SNB for other tumors.

Typically, the surgeon injects a small amount of a radioactive tracer into the tumor and in the skin over the tumor. Sometimes a blue dye may also be injected around the primary tumor. The dye and the radionuclide help the surgeon locate and remove the sentinel node. If the node is negative, the client is spared removal of other nodes and the possible complication of lymphedema. Clients may be allergic to the blue dye.

BREAST SCAN WITH SOMATOSTATIN RECEPTOR SCINTIGRAPHY

Usually clients with advanced breast cancer receive either hormonal treatment or chemotherapy, based on the hormone receptor status of the primary tumor (See Chapter 10). This in vitro assessment of hormone receptor status is not always accurate, so in vivo imaging by Tc-99m depreotide may offer additional information for treatment decisions. Although SRS is routinely used in diagnosis of tumors that take up somatostatin, research now focuses on using SRS to predict the effect of treatment for advanced breast cancer (Van Den Bossche et al., 2006). SRS is also used for localization of some pancreatic tumors (McPhee et al., 2011).

GALLBLADDER SCANS

The newer method of evaluating biliary function is with Tc-99m combined with chemicals, such as HIDA and PIPDA. These scans are obtained immediately, every 5 minutes for 30 minutes, and at intervals over a 24-hour period. Clients need to be NPO for 24 hours before the exam. If clients have been NPO for longer than 24 hours, they may be given a drug, sincalide (a synthetic active ingredient of cholecystokinin), to empty the gallbladder 30 minutes before the radionuclide is given. During the test, morphine may be given to differentiate between delayed visualization and nonvisualization. The morphine causes contraction of the sphincter of Oddi.

Hepatobiliary scans are obtained in conjunction with ultrasonography (Chapter 23) and x-ray studies of the gallbladder (Chapter 20) for chronic cholecystitis or for assessment of obstructive jaundice (see Chapter 11 on bilirubin).

Nursing Implications for Gallbladder Scan

The client stops consuming anything by mouth 24 hours before the test. Sometimes clear liquids are allowed. The client may eat after the initial scan, but fats are restricted during the 24-hour test period to decrease rapid emptying of the gallbladder. The client should be assessed for any allergies to morphine, because the drug may be given as part of the gallbladder scan. The use of morphine can cause posttest sedation.

GASTROINTESTINAL SCANS

Esophageal Motility Studies (Transit Time)

The measurement of the transit time through the esophagus can be measured by having the client drink a liquid tagged with Tc-99m sulfur colloid. The study takes approximately 30 minutes.

Gastroesophageal Reflux Studies

The client is given Tc-99m sulfur colloid in acidic orange juice, and images are taken with the client in a supine position. An abdominal binder is used to obtain increasing predetermined external pressure gradients.

Gastric Emptying Studies

The client is given Tc-99m sulfur colloid mixed with scrambled eggs, which is eaten with bread. Images are taken to evaluate the time for gastric emptying, which should be 70–125 minutes. A longer time indicates impaired gastric emptying, and a shortened time indicates hypermotility. If there is no gastric outlet obstruction, metoclopramide may be given to assess if the drug will help improve gastric motility.

Gastrointestinal Bleeding Studies

Radionuclide studies are more commonly used to assess active lower GI bleeding, but they also may be useful for upper GI bleeding. Two types of scans, both with Tc-99m, are used. For acute bleeding, labeled sulfur colloid is injected intravenously, and if the bleeding is rapid, the scan may be positive at the spot of blood loss. The colloid disappears within minutes after injection so it does not detect slow bleeding. To detect slow bleeding, labeled RBCs are used as markers in the circulation for 1–2 days, so they may help pinpoint the bleeding site. A positive scan indicates the need for repeat endoscopy. (See Chapter 27 on endoscopy for bleeding.) Because a client with active GI bleeding may need careful monitoring, a nurse or physician may be required to go to the nuclear medicine department with the client.

> ### Nursing Implications Related to Gastrointestinal Function Tests
>
> Consult with the nuclear medicine department to see how long the client should abstain from food and drink before a specific test. Also note that anticholinergic drugs and opioids should not be given before the test because they decrease GI motility.

LIVER AND SPLEEN SCANS

Hepatobiliary scans are used primarily to note biliary function; however, liver function is assessed, too, because the agents used to outline the biliary tree are excreted by the liver. Many different radiopharmaceuticals can be used for specific liver scans to assess the reticuloendothelial system or the structural changes in cirrhosis. A liver scan is a common procedure for clients in whom liver metastasis is suspected. Tc-99m is combined with sulfur colloid to assess for neoplasms in the liver. Liver scans may also be useful in assessing trauma to the liver or the presence of an abscess. The spleen is visualized simultaneously, if desired. The scan is obtained 10–15 minutes after the radionuclide is injected intravenously. No special preparation is needed.

LUNG SCANS: PERFUSION IMAGES (V/Q SCANS) AND VENTILATION STUDIES

Lung scans may be performed either as perfusion studies or as ventilation scans. These two scans are usually performed together as a V/Q scan. V and Q are initials used in the mathematical calculations to quantify airflow (ventilation) and blood flow (perfusion) in the lungs. Perfusion studies use macroaggregated albumin (MAA) tagged with Tc-99m, which disperses in the pulmonary precapillary arterioles. Perfusion lung scans are used to evaluate the possibility of pulmonary embolisms. Ventilation lung scans are performed with radioactive gas. The client inhales a bolus of xenon-123. The lungs are then scanned for about 5 minutes to determine how much gas enters each lobe of the lung and how long it takes the gas to be expelled. Krypton is another radioactive gas used for ventilation studies. Ventilation–perfusion studies may be performed in clients who have possible smoke inhalation injury even though a bronchoscopy appears normal. These scans may be useful in identifying pulmonary hypertension caused by recurrent emboli (McPhee et al., 2011).

> **Nursing Implications Related to Lung Scans**
>
> A current chest radiograph should be sent to the nuclear medicine department with the client. Clients need to be prepared for the sensation of the mask used for the ventilation study.

CARDIAC SCANS

Infarction Scans

A test for detecting myocardial infarction uses Tc-99m pyrophosphate (the same compound used in bone scans). If there is an infarction in the myocardium, the uptake of radionuclide is increased in this "hot" spot. The scan of the myocardium is obtained 1.5–3 hours after intravenous injection of the radionuclide. The test can be performed at the client's bedside to prevent exertion on the part of the client. The hot-spot myocardial imaging test is most helpful 1–3 days after the infarction. This test may be useful when the more traditional ways of diagnosing myocardial infarction, cardiac troponins (Chapter 12), and electrocardiographic (ECG) readings (Chapter 24) have not given enough information. However, with the availability of assays of troponins, these imaging techniques have become less important (McPhee et al., 2011).

> **Nursing Implications Related to Infarction Scans**
>
> There is no special preparation of the client. A physician or critical care nurse may be required to go with the client to the nuclear medicine department. SPECT is desirable if available (Chapter 21).

Perfusion Scans

A thallium scan is useful for evaluating coronary perfusion. Thallium is a physiologic analogue of potassium in regard to distribution in the myocardium. A thallium scan may show the site of an old infarction or demonstrate partial obstructions to coronary blood flow. Poorly perfused regions of the myocardium are depicted as low levels of thallium uptake. These "cold" spots may be seen in both acute and old infarctions. A stress test is commonly performed as part of a thallium scan because coronary perfusion may only decrease with a certain amount of exertion. Research has suggested that combining a thallium scintigram with a stress test improves the prognostic ability of the tests. (See Chapter 26 for a description of the protocol for stress tests.) The client may actually exercise, or the heart may be paced to obtain the tachycardia associated with exercise. Scans are performed a few minutes after the thallium is injected and within 3–4 hours after the exercise or pacing to see the redistribution of the thallium. If there are still areas of poor distribution, scans are performed again in 18–24 hours to differentiate ischemia from infarction. Many institutions also use SPECT (Chapter 21) in conjunction with thallium treadmill testing to obtain 3-D images of the heart.

Pharmacologic Stress Testing with Dipyridamole or Adenosine

For clients who have orthopedic, neurologic, or other limitations that preclude an exercise stress test, the dipyridamole–thallium test is a safe and reliable substitute. Clients who are on beta blockers or other negative chronotropic medications may need a pharmacologic stress test because they would not be able to reach the maximal heart rate needed for conventional treadmill stress testing. The test is conducted in a specialized cardiac laboratory where the client can be carefully monitored for both cardiac and noncardiac effects of the drug used to elicit stress on the heart. Dipyridamole is given intravenously followed by an intravenous injection of thallium-201 or Tc-99m sestamibi. Dipyridamole is a coronary vasodilator for healthy arteries. If the client has coronary artery disease, the diseased arteries do not respond to the drug, so certain areas take up less thallium. Aminophylline may be given to reverse the effect of dipyridamole. Another drug that can be used to stimulate the effect of exercise on the heart is adenosine. A positive stress test may be followed up with a cardiac catheterization (see Chapter 26).

Myocardial Imaging with Tc-99m Sestamibi

Tc-99m-labeled agents with better imaging characteristics, combined with advances in equipment, provide better imaging quality. The problems of breast artifacts with myocardial imaging is considerably lessened with these newer agents as compared with thallium-201 imaging. Another advantage of Tc-99m sestamibi is that it allows direct measurement of both myocardial perfusion and ventricular function.

Tc-99m sestamibi remains fixed in the myocardium longer than other agents. As with thallium, an area of diminished uptake reflects relative hypoperfusion. The tracer may be used with dipyridamole or adenosine, as discussed earlier, or the test may be part of an exercise-induced stress test (Chapter 26).

Pre- and Posttest Nursing Implications Related to Myocardial Imaging

Imaging scans require the client to abstain from food and drink for 4–6 hours and no caffeine for at least 12 hours before the test. Check with the cardiologist to see what medications should be withheld. For a dipyridamole–thallium scan, the client should not have had any theophylline preparations for 48 hours or dipyridamole for at least 24 hours. Clients with a history of bronchospasms should not undergo the dipyridamole test. Posttest care is usually uneventful; adverse reactions, such as nausea, headaches, and angina, tend to occur during the test. If needed, cardiac monitoring may be maintained after the test (Chapter 25). The precautions for handling urine are appropriate for a few hours after the test. If the thallium or another radionuclide is given as part of an exercise stress test, there are more specific nursing implications, which are discussed in Chapter 26. The client should be prepared for having about 10 electrodes connected to the body.

Multiple Gated Acquisition Scan: Wall Motion Studies and Ejection Fractions

A multiple gated acquisition (MUGA) scan is a sophisticated study of heart function that includes wall motion studies and ejection fraction studies. The scan is performed in conjunction with ECG monitoring of cardiac function. Signals from the ECG trigger the scintillation camera to record the flow of blood at precise times in the cardiac cycle. A computer is used to break down the time from one R wave to the next into fractions of a second called *gates*. These scans from multiple gates within the cardiac cycle can be used to assess if the motion of the ventricular walls is normal. For example, a ventricular aneurysm causes abnormal wall motion. Computer analysis of the data also determines the percentage of ejection of blood from both ventricles. A normal ejection fraction is more than 55% for the left ventricle and more than 45% for the right ventricle. Clients with severe cardiomyopathy have very low ejection fractions. Measurement of ejection fraction is now standard in clients who have had a myocardial infarction.

A MUGA scan is done in a specialized cardiology laboratory. The client is first given an intravenous injection of a nonradioactive material that binds with RBCs in the plasma. In about 30 minutes, a second intravenous injection of Tc-99m is given, and this radioactive substance binds to the material coating the RBCs. The monitoring of the first pass of the radionuclide through the heart is completed, and then scanning may be either a resting MUGA that lasts about an hour or an additional stress MUGA that requires exercise and may last up to 3 hours.

Nursing Implications Related to Wall Motion Studies or MUGA Scans

There are no special preparations other than the general ones for all clients undergoing radionuclide scans. Usually, the test is not performed less than 3 hours after a meal. The client should be told why there are two injections and that ECG monitors are used. Some parts of the study may require special approval. (See Chapter 26 for more information on preparations for the exercise part of the test.) The scan is usually performed in the nuclear medicine department, but the equilibrium studies can be performed at the bedside if the client is too ill for transportation.

RENAL SCANS

Scans of the kidneys evaluate both renal perfusion and function. Tc-99m is tagged to a compound such as dimercaptosuccinic acid (DMSA). The tagged compound is administered intravenously, and a series of scans is taken to assess the dynamic perfusion of the kidneys. Static scans are taken for 20 minutes to 4 hours to assess the structure of the kidneys. Another type of compound, orthoiodohippurate tagged with radioactive iodine, can be given as a second intravenous injection so continuous images can be obtained over approximately an hour to measure the time it takes to travel through the cortex and pelvis of each kidney. The times of uptake, transit, and excretion of the radionuclide by each kidney can be plotted on a graph called an *isotopic renogram curve*. Plotted curves are compared with normal reference curves to determine abnormalities in either kidney. The use of two intravenous injections to assess the perfusion, structure, and excretory ability of the kidneys is sometimes called a *triple renal study*. A loop diuretic, furosemide, may be used to stimulate a large urine output. Captopril, a drug that inhibits an angiotensin-converting enzyme, is used with a renal scan to assess for renal arterial stenosis. Captopril produces a transient decrease in perfusion to the kidney that has severe renal arterial stenosis. The client's blood pressure must be carefully monitored after the drug is given.

Intravenous pyelography (IVP) involves the use of a radiopaque contrast medium to evaluate the excretory ability of the renal system (see Chapter 20 for IVP). For clients allergic to the contrast medium used for IVP, renograms can be used as a substitute to assess the excretory pattern. However, CT scans if available may be more accurate (McPhee et al., 2011). Renal imaging to assess renal dysfunction is used in conjunction with various other diagnostic studies. Renal biopsies (Chapter 25) are sometimes performed in conjunction with renal scans.

Nursing Implications Related to Renal Scans

See the general nursing diagnoses in the introduction. In addition, the client should be well hydrated. If a captopril study is planned, the client should not have had any antihypertensive drugs for 24 hours and no angiotensin-converting enzyme inhibitors for at least 48 hours before the test. For aftercare, see the discussion on safety precautions for disposing of urine.

THYROID SCANS

Iodine, such as I-123, can be given either orally or intravenously. Scans of the thyroid are performed to assess nodules, which may be felt in the thyroid gland. Benign nodules appear as "warm" spots on the scan because they tend to take up the radionuclide. Conversely, malignant tumors appear as "cold" spots because they do not tend to take up the radionuclide. The actual presence of a malignant neoplasm must still be determined with a biopsy. (A special type of scanning of the thyroid called an *RAI uptake* is discussed in a separate section because the RAI uptake scan is different from organ scans in general.)

For someone with no symptoms of thyroid problems, thyroid scans can be obtained with Tc-99m because the screening can be completed faster with less radiation exposure because of the short half-life of Tc-99m. Thyroid scans are also performed on people who have no thyroid problems but do have a history of radiation to the face and neck. Until the late 1950s, x-ray therapy was used in the treatment of acne and thymus gland disorders, and this past radiation exposure may promote malignant growths in the thyroid gland. Thyroid scans with Tc-99m require no special preparation. Currently, ultrasound is usually used to screen for cancer of the thyroid gland. (See Chapter 23.)

I-131 Whole Body Imaging for Thyroid Tumor Metastasis

A whole body scan with I-131 uses a dose 100 times greater than the dose normally used for thyroid imaging. The whole body scan is used to detect metastasis from a proved malignant tumor of the thyroid. Scans are taken 3 and 7 days after the client is given the oral dose of I-131. (See Chapter 15 for more on thyroid cancer follow-up.)

> ### Nursing Implications Related to Whole Body Scans with I-131
>
> Inform women of childbearing age that a pregnancy test is performed to rule out pregnancy and that the test should be performed during the first 10 days of the menstrual cycle. Consult with the physician concerning the schedule for withdrawing all thyroid medication before the test. (See precautions for urine handling discussed at the beginning of this chapter.)

RAI UPTAKE STUDY

For an RAI uptake study, the client is given radioactive iodine either in an oral capsule or intravenously. The uptake by the thyroid gland is measured with a scanner at several time intervals, such as 2–4 hours and 24 hours. A person with hyperthyroidism has increased uptake of iodine, more than 35%. Conversely, a person with hypothyroidism has decreased uptake of iodine by the thyroid gland. The values of the RAI uptake are expressed in percentages: the amount of thyroid uptake divided by the amount of the dose given. The reference values vary depending on the locality because normal iodine consumption varies in different locales.

REFERENCE VALUES FOR RAI	
Scan (uptake)	1–13% after 2 hours
	4–19% after 4 hours
	11–30% after 24 hours

Nursing Implications Related to RAI Uptake

Because the amount of iodine consumption before the test affects the uptake of radioactive iodine, it is important that the client not have additional iodine uptake for several weeks before the test. A list of medications currently being taken by the clients should be recorded on the laboratory request. Thyroid medications and amiodarone interfere with the test.

As mentioned in Chapter 20, most contrast media used for x-ray studies have an iodine base. A client should undergo an RAI uptake study before studies that use iodine dye. Clients need to be instructed to avoid all sources of iodine. Some foods, such as kelp and enriched breakfast cereals, are high in iodine. Vitamin preparations may contain iodine, as do most cough syrups. Even suntan lotion and nail polish can be sources of exogenous iodine. Such a small amount of iodine is used for the RAI uptake scan that it does not cause any allergic problems, even in people who are allergic to iodine. (In contrast, x-ray dyes that contain iodine can cause anaphylactic shock in people with allergies to iodine.)

The client abstains from food and drink by mouth 6–8 hours before the test but can resume food 1 hour after the oral dose is taken. Scans are performed a few hours after administration of iodine and the next day. For outpatients, make sure the client knows what time to return for scans.

RAI is contraindicated in pregnancy. Women of reproductive age may need a urine pregnancy test (Chapter 18) prior to administration of the radioactive iodine.

COMPATIBILITY AND RED BLOOD CELL SURVIVAL

Sodium chromate (Cr-51) readily binds with the protein of hemoglobin (Hgb) so RBCs can be tagged to evaluate the rate of hemolysis or RBC survival in some hemolytic diseases. A sample of blood is withdrawn from the client, tagged with the radioactive Cr-51, and injected back into the client. A collection of blood samples are drawn at various time intervals. One sample may be drawn within 1 hour to measure compatibility and then two to three times a week to assess survival. No special preparation of the client is required. No blood transfusions should be given 48 hours before the study.

BLOOD VOLUME STUDIES

Cr-51 is used to tag the RBCs, and RHISA or another isotope is used to tag plasma. A measured amount of blood is withdrawn from the client, tagged with radionuclides, and injected back into the client. After 30–60 minutes, samples of blood are drawn and the amount of dilution of the original sample is calculated. The total blood volume of a client can thus be estimated.

Nursing Implications Related to Blood Volume Studies

It is important that the hydration of the client be normal before the blood studies are performed. Intravenous solutions invalidate the test, as does abstinence from food and drink. The nurse must record the height and weight of the client before the test is conducted. The client should be told that two in-line catheters will be used for injecting the two radionuclides and taking multiple blood samples.

Questions

1. Technetium (Tc-99m) is useful as an agent for diagnostic testing because this radioactive element
   a. Has a half-life of only 2 days
   b. Can be tagged to go to the brain, bone, liver, or lung
   c. Is radioactive only when it reaches the target organ
   d. Is excreted only in the urine

2. Scintigraphy involves taking the reading of radioactivity from a body organ and transforming the reading into
   a. Audible sounds (Geiger counter)
   b. Quantitative measurements
   c. A 2-D image of the organ
   d. A vertical graph

3. The radiation hazard from the radionuclide diagnostic testing is much less than when radionuclides are used for therapy because the dose used for diagnostic testing is about
   a. Half as much as used in therapy
   b. 10 times less than in therapy
   c. 100 times less than in therapy
   d. 1,000 times less than in therapy

4. Which of the following would be a reason to postpone, if possible, radionuclide diagnostic studies in a female client? She is
   a. Seven days past onset of menstrual period
   b. Pregnant in first trimester
   c. Menstruating
   d. Allergic to iodine

5. Which of the following nursing actions is appropriate in preparing a client for any organ scan with technetium (Tc-99m)?
   a. Explain to the client that all urine must be monitored after the test
   b. Make sure the client ingests nothing by mouth
   c. Explain that the test involves intravenous administration of a very small dose of a radioactive substance
   d. Shave the area that will be viewed during the scan

6. The main use of a bone scan with radionuclides is to detect
   a. Silent metastasis from the breast or prostate gland
   b. Silent metastasis from the liver or kidney
   c. Utilization of phosphorus by the body
   d. Fractures

7. A client is going to undergo a gallium scan this morning because of a fever of undetermined origin (FUO). Gallium is useful as a radionuclide for scintigraphy because gallium localizes in
   a. Inflamed tissue and some types of tumors
   b. The lungs
   c. The brain and spinal column
   d. The hepatobiliary system

8. A client is scheduled for a radioactive iodine uptake (RAI) scan in 4 weeks, so she is to have no iodine intake. Therefore, which one of the following would be allowed because it contains no iodine?
   a. Suntan lotions
   b. Vitamin preparations
   c. Contrast medium for x-ray test
   d. Soft drinks, such as colas

References

Deglin, J. H., Vallerand, A. H., & Sanoski, C. A. (2011). *Davis's drug guide for nurses* (12th ed.). Philadelphia: F. A. Davis.

Hay, W. W., Levin, M. J., Sondheimer, J. M., & Deterding, R. (Eds.). (2011). *Current diagnosis and treatment: Pediatrics* (20th ed.). New York: McGraw-Hill.

Katzung, B., Masters, S. B., & Trevor, A. J. (Eds.). (2009). *Basic and clinical pharmacology* (11th ed.). New York: McGraw-Hill.

Lacovara, J. E. & Yoder, L. (2006). Secondary lymphedema in the cancer patient. *MEDSURG Nursing, 15*(5), 302–306.

McPhee, S. J., Papadakis, M. A., & Rabow, M. W. (Eds.). (2011). *Current medical diagnosis and treatment* (50th ed.). New York: McGraw-Hill.

Mena, D., Camacho, V., Estorch, M., Fuertes, J., Flotats, A., & Carrio, I. (2004). 99mTc- depreotide scintigraphy of bone lesions in patients with lung cancer. *European Journal of Nuclear Medical Molecular Imaging, 31*(10), 1399–1404. [E-Pub]

Morton, D. L., Thompson, J. F., Cochran, A. J., Mozzillo, N., Elashoff, R., Essner, R., et al. (2006). Sentinel-node biopsy or nodal observation in melanoma. *New England Journal of Medicine, 355*(13), 1307–1317.

Orenstein, B. W. (2009). Lack of imaging isotopes may be hazardous to patients. *Radiology Today, 10*(14), 14–17.

Van Den Bossche, B., Van Belle, S., De Winter, F., Signore, A., & Van de Wiele, C. (2006). Early prediction of endocrine therapy effect in advanced breast cancer patients using 99m-Tc-depreotide scintigraphy. *Journal of Nuclear Medicine, 47*(1), 6–13.

Website

www.acrin.org (American College of Radiology Imaging Network for information on nuclear scans.)

www.nrc.gov (Nuclear Regulatory Commission guidelines for use of radioactive material.)

www.radiologyinfo.org (Information for consumers on various radiological tests including nuclear scans.)

www.snm.org (Society of Nuclear Medicine for news about nuclear tests, and a history of events important to the field.)

Answers

1. b, 2. c, 3. d, 4. b, 5. c, 6. a, 7. a, 8. d

Diagnostic Ultrasonography

- Ultrasound Principles   581
- Doppler Techniques   584
- Ankle-Brachial Index   585
- Compression Ultrasound
  of Veins   586
- Cerebral Circulation Scans   586
- Carotid Artery Scans for
  Intimal Medial Thickness   587
- Pelvic Sonograms: Ultrasound
  Scans in Pregnancy and
  Gynecologic Conditions   587
- Transvaginal Ultrasound
  Scanning   588
- Abdominal Sonograms   589
- Transrectal Ultrasound Scanning   591
- Transthoracic Echocardiograms   591
- Stress Echocardiograms   592
- Transesophageal
  Echocardiograms   592
- Echoencephalograms   594
- Thoracic Sonograms   594
- Thyroid and Parathyroid
  Sonograms   594
- Breast Sonograms   595
- Bone Sonograms   595
- Bladder Sonograms   595
- Ultrasound-Guided Peripherally
  Inserted Central Catheters   596

OBJECTIVES

1. Explain the differences between A-mode, B-mode, and real-time scans as methods of pulse–echo recordings.
2. Describe three clinical situations in which the nurse uses ultrasound for assessment.
3. Describe the preparation of the client for pelvic and abdominal sonograms.
4. Compare and contrast the pre- and posttest care of clients undergoing transthoracic and transesophageal echocardiograms.
5. Describe the responsibilities of the nurse when a child undergoes echoencephalography.
6. Explain why ultrasound examinations of the thorax are of limited usefulness.
7. Identify at least two nursing diagnoses for clients undergoing sonography.

Ultrasound, a noninvasive method of diagnostic testing, uses sound waves to detect physical changes in the client. Sound is a physical force, and thus sonograms are in no way related to radiographs (Chapter 20), CT (computed tomography) scans (Chapter 21), or radionuclide scans (Chapter 22).

Table 23–1 Ultrasound Methods Used for Assessment

Method	Example of Use
Pulse–echo methods	
1. A-mode (amplitude modulation)	Echocardiogram
2. B-mode (brightness modulation)	Sonograms of fetus, pelvic, and abdominal structures
Doppler method	
1. Doppler stethoscope	1. Monitoring fetal heart rate
2. Doppler instrument	2. Monitoring peripheral pulses
3. Pulse volume recorder	3. Assessing extent of vascular disease
4. Color flow imaging	4. Assessing direction of blood flow

Ultrasound, first used in industry to detect flaws in metal, is used as a sonar system to locate objects in the water and for depth sounding of the ocean floor. For health care, ultrasound first gained importance as a diagnostic tool in pregnancy in the 1960s. Sonograms of the heart (echocardiograms) soon followed, and later ultrasound became commonly used to view many areas of the body. Common tests using both pulse–echo recordings and Doppler methods are described in this chapter (Table 23–1). (More information on ultrasound tests is available at www.radiologyinfo.org.) The Doppler method of assessment is often used by the nurse in obstetric settings, in medical–surgical units, and in home care.

ULTRASOUND PRINCIPLES

Ultrasound As Therapy

Although this chapter focuses on the use of ultrasound as a diagnostic tool, ultrasound waves are also used in therapy. Ultrasound, in large and continuous doses, can generate heat in tissues; therefore, ultrasound treatments are used for various kinds of low back pain. Ultrasound has also been tried as a method to promote tissue regeneration and to generate heat to kill malignant growths. A procedure called *percutaneous ultrasonic lithotripsy* (PUL) has become well established as a therapeutic use of ultrasound to pulverize kidney stones and gallstones. In 2004, the FDA approved a type of focused ultrasound (FUS) to shrink uterine fibroids. Magnetic resonance imaging (MRI; Chapter 21) keeps track of the volume and temperature of the fibroids during treatment.

Description

Ultrasonics is part of the science of acoustics that deals with sound waves that are beyond the range of audible sound. The human ear can hear sounds that are of a frequency between 16,000 and 20,000 cycles/sec. The unit of frequency is hertz (Hz), which is equal to 1 cycle/sec. Thus, ultrasound waves are of a frequency higher than 20,000 Hz. Sonograms are performed with transducers, which produce sound waves of varying strength or intensity. Intensity is the measurement of the strength of a sound wave and is measured as the amount of power per cross-sectional area. However, more useful to the nurse than figures of frequencies and intensities is the comparison of dosages used in tests. Intensities used for treatment are at least 20 times the intensities used in diagnostic testing.

For diagnostic purposes, ultrasound waves are sent into the body with a small transducer pressed against the skin. Technically, the transducer is the piezoelectric crystal, which changes electric energy to sound waves and vice versa. However, the unit that houses the crystal is also called the *transducer* in general terms. A transducer changes one form of energy into another. An electric signal from the machine is converted to ultrasound waves. Air almost completely impedes the transmission of the ultrasound waves into the body; thus, the transducer must be in good contact with the skin as it is being moved. A lubricant, such as mineral oil, glycerin, or a water-based jelly, is used to ensure good contact with the skin. The lubricant is called the *coupling agent.* The transducer not only sends the sound waves into the body but also receives any returning sound waves, which are deflected back as they bounce off various structures. Some sound waves pass through the body. The transducer converts the returning sound waves into electric signals that can then be transformed with a computer into either scans or graphs (pulse–echo methods) or into audible sounds (Doppler method).

Pulse–Echo Method of Displaying Ultrasound

All the pulse–echo techniques measure the time it takes the sound waves to reach various structures and return to the transducer. There are various ways that the readout can be presented. In A-mode (amplitude modulation), the echoes are displayed in a graphic form (e.g., the graph completed for an echocardiogram). In B-mode (brightness modulation), the echoes appear as different intensities of brightness. B-mode scans use dots of brightness to show a two-dimensional cross-sectional view of the various structures. Thus, with a B-mode scan, one can actually see a "picture" of the fetus in the womb, for example. B-mode scans may be still (static scans), or motion may be added.

Real-Time Imaging

The terms *real-time* and *real-time imaging* describe scanners that are capable of scanning so rapid that motion is displayed. In other words, real-time scanning is like a movie. A fetus can be seen moving around, sucking a thumb, or performing other motions. The use of a scanner with rapid sequencing is valuable in observing heart action. For real-time imaging, there is no need for the client to suspend respiration during the scan, as was true of older static scans.

Innovations in Ultrasound

The first sonograms were black and white and two dimensional. In 1979, gray-scale imaging became possible. In a few years, computerized sonographic machines could magnify a selected area five to seven times and thus give a view as powerful as with low-power microscopic techniques. Color-coded sonography became available in the 1980s. In the 1990s, the first contrast agent for ultrasound became available, as did three-dimensional viewing techniques. Techniques such as intravascular ultrasound have been used to follow up calcified spots seen on other scans (van der Hoeven et al., 2006). Computer-aided detection (CAD) software, first developed to help differentiate between benign and malignant breast lesions, is being developed for other diseases also. Larger cart-based machines have been refashioned into smaller formats that include laptop devices that are wireless. These hand-carried units have made it possible to do point-of-care testing with ultrasound anywhere (Harvey, 2006). Now an even smaller device, a "pocket" ultrasound, weighs only 1.6 pounds and easily fits in a lab coat pocket. The small device is intended to complement initial diagnostic care and triage. For more information see www.pocketultrasound.com.

Volumetric 3-D and 4-D Scans

Traditional 2-D ultrasound takes 20–40 minutes to get a complete scan as the sonographer moves the transducer over the area to take many images. The final 2-D scan shows cross-sections. Inadequate scans must be repeated. A volumetric ultrasound scanner uses newer technology to create a 3-D image. This volumetric or 3-D scanner is done with the probe just placed over the body part and not moved over the surface as with the traditional scanner. All the needed views are captured in a few seconds and then manipulated to create the 3-D image. The client does not need to have the scan repeated as the images are very detailed and accurate.

Time is the "fourth dimension" added to 3-D technology. At the present time, 2-D ultrasound is the standard and 3-D/4-D technology is used when clinicians need additional information or if the diagnosis is uncertain. This new technology is considerably less expensive than CT and MRI scans and does not have their disadvantages, as discussed in Chapter 21.

Elastography

Elastography is a technique used with ultrasound to determine the firmness by measuring the stiffness or the physical elasticity of a tumor when pressure is applied. The resulting image is called an elastogram. Images are compared to the ones before pressure was applied. Malignant tumors tend to be firm and dense and are stiffer than the surrounding tissue.

Possible Risks from Ultrasound

There are two known effects of ultrasound in tissue: the production of heat and cavitation. Cavitation is the appearance of gas-filled bubbles in a sound field. Ultrasound waves greater than 100,000 Hz cause formation of gas bubbles in bacterial cells, killing the bacteria. As far as is known, the low-intensity dose of ultrasound used for sonograms is harmless to humans; there is no heat formation or cavitation in the tissues. The sound waves are delivered intermittently for sonograms and not continuously as with therapy.

Sonograms have been used in pregnancy since the mid-1960s, and there have not been reports of damage to either the woman or the fetus. In the past, some authorities questioned the risks of ultrasound to the developing fetus. The Doppler devices used in fetal monitoring are of low enough dosages to be free of adverse heating effects or cavitation in tissues. However, the Doppler instrument used in arterial studies does use intensities of sound that produce some heat in tissues; consequently, arterial Doppler monitors are not considered suitable for fetal investigation. As far as is known, routine Doppler monitoring and other uses of ultrasound in pregnancy have no adverse effects on the fetus (DeCherney et al., 2007).

Cost Versus Benefits of Routine Screening

Although routine ultrasound screening is often conducted during pregnancy to detect fetal abnormalities and to estimate gestational age, it is not certain if ultrasound screening is useful for pregnant women who are at low risk for perinatal morbidity or mortality. Although research has not supported the use of ultrasound as routine screening in healthy pregnant women, women want the screening, and insurance does cover the cost. This leads to interesting philosophical and ethical questions about the proper use of technology.

Fetal Portraits with Moving 3-D/4-D Images

The newer technology of 3-D/4-D has become very popular for commercial fetal portraits and is advertised as "live-motion" 3-D ultrasound. Although the FDA views fetal keepsake portraits as an unapproved use for ultrasound, several commercial companies offer 3-D/4-D ultrasounds to pregnant women not as a medical device but as keepsake portraits, videos, and DVDs. Most of the companies require that customers have a prior medical ultrasound. In addition to discussing the issue with a healthcare provider, consumers need to know how to choose a reputable outlet that has certified sonographers and properly maintained equipment so that scans can be obtained within the recommended time limit (McClintock, 2005). Several states are attempting legislation to limit the sale of ultrasound equipment to anyone but licensed healthcare facilities.

Commercial Mobile Ultrasound Units for Adult Screening

Consumers may pay to have ultrasound screening to detect certain conditions. The four tests most often offered as a package (for about $140.00) are screening for carotid artery plaques, abdominal aneurysm, peripheral arterial disease, and osteoporosis. A board-certified physician reviews and confirms all results before the report is sent to the customer. If something is abnormal, the customer is referred to his or her personal physician. Although these tests may not be needed for low-risk customers, the tests are not harmful and may give peace of mind to the "worried well." Nurses need to realize a false positive can be anxiety producing and costly. See the discussion on other types of body scans in Chapter 21.

DOPPLER TECHNIQUES

With the Doppler method, returning sound waves are transformed into audible sounds, which can be heard with earphones. Not only are sound waves produced by moving objects, but also sound waves that are bounced off different moving objects have slightly different frequencies. The sound produced by an artery is pulsatile and multiphasic, whereas the sound from a vein is intermittent and varies with respiration. Doppler ultrasound is used to assess the movement of the opening and closing of the heart valves and the flow of blood. This technique is used for bedside assessments and as a laboratory diagnostic aid. A Doppler stethoscope can detect the presence of fetal heartbeats, even when the heartbeat is inaudible with a conventional stethoscope. Doppler ultrasound can be used for fetal monitoring during labor and delivery. It is also used to monitor the fetus during an oxytocin challenge test (OCT) or a nonstress test, which may be performed during the last trimester of pregnancy (Chapter 28).

In suspected cases of intrauterine growth inhibition, umbilical artery flow can be assessed by Doppler. Low flow correlates with fetal acidosis and hypoxia. However, Doppler ultrasound of the umbilical artery has not been shown to have value as a screening test in all pregnant women.

In addition to using a Doppler stethoscope or monitoring to evaluate fetal status, the nurse may also use a Doppler instrument to monitor blood flow in clients who have altered arterial circulation. A portable Doppler instrument is about the size of a tissue box. A small flat transducer is placed over the vessel to be assessed, and when the unit is turned on, transmitted sound waves bounce off the moving blood, producing a pulse heard with earphones. The portable Doppler unit, useful in the first few days after an arterial graft to assess the continued patency of the graft, may also be used in a clinic to assess chronic perfusion problems. Another type of Doppler unit is sometimes used to monitor blood pressure in shock when the blood pressure is barely audible. Pulses can be detected with a Doppler unit when they are too faint to be felt with the fingertips. A Doppler unit with blood pressure cuffs also can be used to measure the pulse volume of both arteries and veins and obtain a pressure index by means of comparison of leg and arm pressure readings.

ANKLE-BRACHIAL INDEX

The ankle-brachial index (ABI), a ratio of the pressure in the arms and legs, is one of the simplest and most useful tests to assess for peripheral arterial disease (PAD). The client rests in the supine position while the brachial blood pressure is measured in both arms by a Doppler blood pressure cuff. Then both the dorsalis pedis (DP) and posterior tibial (PT) pressures in the ankles are measured with a handheld Doppler. Results are calculated by dividing the highest pressure of each ankle by the higher systolic pressure. For example, if the systolic pressure is 120 and the right ankle pressure is 60, the index is equal to 0.5. If the systolic pressure is 120 and the left ankle pressure is 120, the index will be 1.0.

REFERENCE VALUES FOR ABI	
0.40 or less	Severe PAD
0.41–0.90	Moderate to mild disease
0.91–0.99	Borderline
1.00–1.29	Normal

Nurses may perform this noninvasive exam so they need to know the risk factors and symptoms of PAD (Moye, 2011). Risk factor modification is the first line of treatment and includes smoking cessation, exercise, and dietary changes (Johnson, 2010). The peripheral arterial disease coalition offers up-to-date information about PAD (www.PADCoalition.org) as does www.vascularweb.org.

Color Flow Imaging

Doppler flow imaging is sometimes called *color flow imaging* or *mapping* because the color is used primarily to detect the direction of blood flow and to assist in determining whether the flow is laminar or turbulent. For example, valvular regurgitation can be displayed in vivid colors that dramatically emphasize the areas of turbulence. Color flow imaging is also useful in documenting the shunts seen in some congenital heart defects. Color flow imaging technique also can help differentiate the true and false lumens in aortic dissection.

Duplex Scanning

Duplex scanning uses both real-time imaging and Doppler flow imaging to obtain information about many vascular problems, such as plaques in arteries or the presence of aneurysms. The real-time imaging shows how the veins and arteries function. The Doppler technique shows flow as well as the velocity within the vessels. Duplex scanning may also be used to scan renal transplants for rejection. A duplex scan may be performed in a specialized vascular laboratory or in the radiology department. The procedure usually lasts less than an hour. If an abdominal scan is obtained, the client may need to fast for 12 hours.

COMPRESSION ULTRASOUND OF VEINS

The approach to diagnosis of deep vein thrombosis (DVT) now includes physical assessment, the D-dimer test, and possible ultrasound imaging of the veins in the legs. Recent evidence suggests that a negative D-dimer test (Chapter 13) may eliminate the need to do ultrasound imaging (Scarvelis & Wells, 2006). If the D-dimer is positive, ultrasound imaging is done as the next step. The imaging is called compression ultrasound (CUS) because the goal is to see if the vein can be compressed. If a segment of the vein cannot be compressed, the test is positive for DVT. There is no special preparation of the client.

CEREBRAL CIRCULATION SCANS

Transcranial Doppler ultrasound can measure blood flow in the middle cerebral artery, distal internal carotid, anterior and posterior cerebral artery, and the basilar artery. These cerebral scans identify children with sickle cell anemia who are at high risk for stroke. (See Chapter 18.) Peak velocity blood flow of the middle cerebral artery is useful to monitor the fetal well-being of the Rh negative mother who may have antibodies against the red blood cells of her fetus. (See Chapter 11 on bilirubin levels and fetal anemia.)

Definitive studies of the cerebral arteries may include the invasive arteriogram, as discussed in Chapter 20, or the noninvasive magnetic resonance arteriography, discussed in Chapter 21. Another noninvasive way to study the cerebral circulation is the duplex ultrasound discussed earlier. This method is considered by some the method of choice for symptomatic clients. McPhee, Papadakis, and Rabow (2011) note that the results are so reliable that symptomatic clients may proceed directly to surgery for carotid endarectomy or other procedures.

CAROTID ARTERY SCANS FOR INTIMAL MEDIAL THICKNESS

Ultrasound has also been used to screen asymptomatic clients because the thickness of carotid arteries has been found to predict stroke and heart attack risk. Researchers found that the risk for cerebral and cardiac vascular disease increases in direct proportion to the thickness of the carotid lining, as this thickness represents atherosclerotic plaque. The National Institutes of Health noted that this test has great potential for preventing myocardial infarctions and strokes by early identification of high-risk clients.

Several commercial companies have marketed a 4-minute ultrasound of carotid arteries as a stroke screening. Clients who have a positive test are referred for testing with more sophisticated equipment. Opponents of commercial use of this test contend that overuse of the test by poorly prepared technicians will lead to unnecessary further testing. Others feel that the test can be beneficial for screening, particularly if coupled with blood pressure and cholesterol checks for more in-depth assessment. As stroke screening evolves, healthcare providers must determine how to use the information for asymptomatic clients. Teaching about lifestyle modifications for diet, exercise, and stress (Chapter 9) may be needed.

PELVIC SONOGRAMS: ULTRASOUND SCANS IN PREGNANCY AND GYNECOLOGIC CONDITIONS

Sonograms were originally used for evaluating the position of the placenta and the status of the fetus. Before amniocentesis (Chapter 28) is performed, the position of the placenta is determined with ultrasound. The fetal growth rate can also be determined by measurements of the images obtained with ultrasound. At about 18 weeks' gestation, detailed measurements can be obtained. Ectopic pregnancies, hydatidiform moles, or structural abnormalities in the fetus can be detected with ultrasound, as can death of the fetus. For ectopic pregnancies, ultrasound scans are easier to interpret after 6 weeks' gestation. Ultrasounds confirm a ruptured ectopic pregnancy, one of the leading causes of maternal death in the first trimester (Young, 2010). The presence of twins can almost always be detected. It is possible, however, for one twin to "hide" behind the other, so the two-dimensional scan may not show the second fetus.

For some situations, a Level II ultrasound scan may be ordered. This type of scan takes longer and is more expensive than a conventional scan, but the quality of resolution is better. For example, a Level II scan is performed if a pregnant woman has a positive α-fetoprotein (AFP) test (Chapter 18). A Level II sonogram is sometimes called a "targeted" or "anatomical ultrasound" because it allows the healthcare provider to visualize more details such as the chambers of the heart. Also discussed in Chapter 18 is the use of fetal ultrasound to screen for Down syndrome in the first trimester by using a measurement of the amount of fluid in the nape of the neck (nuchal translucency). A sonogram is also an important component of assessing the status of the fetus in the last trimester. The biophysical profile (Chapter 18) combines the finding of a stress test with four observations made by ultrasound of amniotic fluid volume, fetal breathing, fetal body movements, and fetal tone.

Ultrasound scans may also be obtained after delivery to check for any retained placenta. Pelvic sonograms are also used to evaluate pelvic inflammatory disease and abscess formation. Pelvic masses can also be detected with ultrasound.

Pretest Nursing Diagnoses Related to Pelvic Sonograms

Anxiety Related to Well-Being of Fetus

The movement of the transducer over the abdomen is not painful. The client can see the scan on the monitor. Most pregnant women are thrilled to be able to see an image of the fetus on the monitoring screen. The technician can point out the head, feet, and other features as the fetus moves about. The heartbeat is seen as a blip of light. It is also understood, however, that watching the monitor can be an unbelievable, chilling moment for a woman whose fetus is dead or if the scan is being performed to assess malformations.

Pain Related to Full Bladder and Positioning

Besides the anxiety of finding possible abnormalities with the sonogram, two other factors may make a sonogram uncomfortable. One factor may be the need to have a full bladder during the procedure. A full bladder is an acoustical window so that other structures can be seen in relation to the bladder. Sound waves travel well through liquid. Pregnant women do not need a full bladder for a pelvic ultrasound if the fetus is more than 26 weeks' gestation. But they must lie flat for 20 minutes or so during the procedure. Some pregnant women experience hypotension due to the pressure on the vena cava. It may be necessary for the woman to turn on her left side to relieve this pressure. For pregnant women beyond 25 weeks' gestation, a small hip roll may be used to prevent this supine hypotensive syndrome.

Deficient Knowledge Related to Physical Preparation

There is no need to restrict medications or alter the client's diet before the test. If it is essential that the client's bladder be full during the sonogram, the client must drink about 750 mL of water before the test. A full bladder is an acoustical window. If the client has an intravenous infusion going, the nurse needs to check to see how much the rate of infusion should be increased. If the client has a Foley catheter, it must be clamped so that the bladder is full for the pelvic sonogram (Table 23–2).

TRANSVAGINAL ULTRASOUND SCANNING

Vaginal ultrasonography uses a probe placed inside the vagina to pinpoint ovulation, diagnose tubal pregnancies, or evaluate other gynecologic problems, such as endometriosis. Transvaginal ultrasonography may be particularly useful in differentiating acute appendicitis from pelvic inflammatory disease. Transvaginal ultrasonography combined with transfundal pressure has been used to detect an incompetent cervix in pregnant women at risk for this condition. Clients with gynecological symptoms may have a sonogram to assess the thickness of the endometrium. An abnormal thickness may require an endometrial biopsy (Chapter 25). Women who are at risk for ovarian cancer will need periodic vaginal ultrasounds and a CA 125 (Chapter 10).

Table 23-2 Preparation of Client for Sonography

Test	Nothing by Mouth?	Intestinal Preparation	Other Tips
Cerebral	Maybe	No	See if contrast used
Bone	No	No	See on bone density
Breast	No	No	Assess area if biopsy done
Pelvic sonogram	No	No	May need full bladder
Abdominal sonogram	Usually but not always	Varies	See text for medication and other preparation
Echocardiogram	No	No	None
Echoencephalogram	No	No	Sedation for children
Thoracic sonogram	No	No	None
Transesophageal	Yes	No	Invasive procedure—see text
Transrectal sonogram	No	No	None
Vaginal sonogram	No	No	None
Bladder sonogram	No	No	Done by nurse—see text

Pretest Nursing Implications for Transvaginal Sonograms

The woman needs to be told that the transvaginal approach is only minimally uncomfortable. A lubricant is used for the probe. Clients need to be asked about latex allergy so that a non-latex cover can be used for the probe, if needed. For this approach, the woman may not need to have a full bladder, an appreciated advantage for a client who may undergo ultrasonography for 10 days in a row to assess ovulation (see Chapter 28 on infertility tests). For other exams, a full bladder may be needed.

Posttest Nursing Implications Related to Pelvic and Transvaginal Sonograms

There are no special nursing implications after the client has undergone pelvic or transvaginal sonography. If the sonogram was obtained to assess for fetal abnormalities or fetal death, the nurse must be sensitive to helping the woman find support to cope with the distressing news. (See Chapter 28 for a discussion on the role of the nurse in helping couples deal with loss.) Other abnormal findings may create anxiety because of the need for further testing.

ABDOMINAL SONOGRAMS

Sonography of the abdomen is being used more and more as the equipment becomes more sophisticated and clinicians become more adept at identifying abdominal problems with a sonogram. A sonogram of the abdomen may mean the client does not undergo exposure to radiation or invasive procedures to diagnose a problem. Bedside ultrasound is very useful in critical care units. In the Emergency Department, focused assessment with sonography for trauma (FAST) is very useful in detecting free fluid in the abdomen or thorax. Intraperitoneal hemorrhage or pericardial tamponade can be detected by a rapid (3-minute) scan. The small scan can be used while other procedures are being done on an unstable client.

For some abdominal conditions, ultrasonography may be the first examination performed. For example, ultrasonography has been a first test for conditions such as appendicitis and cholelithiasis. But CT may be preferred to diagnose appendicitis (McPhee et al., 2011). Abdominal sonography is also the diagnostic study of choice for aneurysms of the aorta and for identifying cysts and tumors in organs such as the liver. The U.S. Preventive Services Task Force (2005) recommends routine screening for abdominal aortic aneurysm (AAA) in men aged 65–75 who have ever smoked. The evidence for screening for women is less certain, so other risk factors must be assessed. As discussed earlier, AAA screening is available commercially. Ultrasound confirms the presence of ascites and is used to help guide needles for paracentesis. In other clinical conditions, abdominal sonograms are complementary to other examinations, such as radionuclide studies (Chapter 22), x-ray studies (Chapter 20), or CT and MRI (Chapter 21). In addition to no radiation hazard, sonography has the advantage of being less expensive than CT or MRI and is readily available in most healthcare settings.

Pretest Nursing Diagnoses Related to Abdominal Sonograms

Deficient Knowledge Related to Preparation

The actual procedure for an abdominal sonogram is similar to that for a pelvic sonogram. However, the client does not need to have a full bladder for an abdominal sonogram as for a pelvic sonogram. The client may be instructed to abstain from food and drink or may be allowed only liquids, depending on the exact nature of the abdominal sonogram. For example, if the gallbladder is the focus, the client must take nothing by mouth for 12 hours and may have a fat-free meal the evening before the examination. If the client eats before a sonogram of the gallbladder, the gallbladder is not full and thus is not easily visualized. For other scans, the purpose of allowing only liquids is to reduce gas formation in the colon, because gas does interfere with the scan. Another way to reduce gas in the gastrointestinal (GI) tract is by administering medications that contain simethicone. Smoking and gum chewing are prohibited because they increase gas formation. Sometimes an enema is needed to clear the intestine. Barium used for other tests interferes with a sonogram. (See Chapter 20 for principles of intestinal preparation.) Abdominal scars and obesity make it difficult to obtain a good abdominal sonogram. Abdominal dressings must be removed before a sonogram. Contrast medium may be given.

Risk for Ineffective Coping of Child

Children should be accompanied by a parent if possible. Even young children can cooperate if they are not overly anxious. A parent may lie down with the child to calm him as there is no radiation risk. Also, the transducer can be first placed on a doll and the child allowed to see the shadows on the screen. (See Chapter 25 on preparing children for diagnostic procedures.)

> ### Posttest Nursing Implications Related to Abdominal Sonograms
>
> The client may be ill from the pathophysiologic condition that necessitated the sonogram, but there is no concern over the direct effects of a sonogram. Occasionally, a sonogram may be only a preliminary test to an invasive procedure, such as liver or renal biopsy. If so, the invasive procedure has some nursing implications (Chapter 25).

TRANSRECTAL ULTRASOUND SCANNING

Transrectal ultrasound scanning produces a clear image of the prostate gland so tumors can be detected at an early stage. Clinicians use the digital rectal examination (DRE) and the prostate-specific antigen (PSA) test (Chapter 10) to screen for prostate cancer. Transrectal ultrasound is not usually used as the first-line screening tool. If a malignancy is suspected, an ultrasound-guided biopsy can be done under local anesthesia. Clients may be given prophylactic antibiotics because the procedure runs a risk of causing sepsis. Ultrasound may also be used to help with implantation of radiation seeds for treatment.

> ### Pretest Nursing Implications Related to Transrectal Screening
>
> The client needs to be told that the rectal probe will be well lubricated and will cause only minimal discomfort. Clients need to be asked about latex allergy so that a non-latex cover can be used for the probe, if needed. A small enema may be given before the exam.

TRANSTHORACIC ECHOCARDIOGRAMS

Ultrasound has become a well-established diagnostic tool for valvular defects. Ultrasound was first used to detect abnormalities in the mitral valve and has become the standard method for diagnosing mitral valve prolapse. Modern echocardiograms are so sensitive that many clients show some leakage of the mitral and tricuspid valves. These findings may not be clinically significant. In contrast, the aortic valve does not normally leak. An echocardiogram is also used to measure the diameters of the cardiac chambers and evaluate other structural abnormalities of the heart such as atrial septal defect and patent ductus arteriosus. Pleural effusion and cardiac tamponade are other abnormalities identified with ultrasound. An electrocardiogram (ECG) is often run simultaneously; therefore, echographic findings can be correlated with the cardiac cycle. Earlier echocardiograms used the M-mode (motion) to conduct time–motion studies of the heart. Newer types can also produce cross-sectional scans, which can be used to detect some changes in coronary vessels. Echocardiograms also use the color flow imaging discussed earlier. The color is useful in detecting the direction of blood flow and whether the flow is laminar or turbulent. Contrast agents, such as perflutren, given as a bolus or continuous infusion during the scan, enhance visualization of the left ventricular chamber for difficult-to-image clients. (Ejection fraction for the left ventricle should be 55–75% of the blood it holds, when full.)

A transthoracic echocardiogram (TTE) may have to be followed up with a transesophageal echocardiogram (TEE), which gives more detail because there is no impedance by the lungs and chest-wall structures. Unlike a TTE, a TEE is invasive.

Pretest Nursing Implications Related to Transthoracic Echocardiograms

The client needs no special preparation. The echocardiography technician directs the transducer at specific points on the client's chest to obtain images of the mitral valve and other structures. During the test, the client may be asked to perform the Valsalva maneuver. Also, the client may be given a vasodilator, such as amyl nitrite, which can have the side effect of tachycardia. If a contrast agent is used, the client should be informed that sometimes headaches, flushing, or nausea occur. Allergic reactions or other severe effects are rare compared to the contrast agent used for radiology. If an ECG is performed, the client needs instruction about the procedure (Chapter 24).

Posttest Nursing Implications Related to Transthoracic Echocardiograms

There is no special care of the client after a TTE because it is a noninvasive procedure.

STRESS ECHOCARDIOGRAMS

A stress echocardiogram may be used as an alternative to the nuclear medicine stress test using thallium or technetium (Chapter 22). Advantages of the stress echocardiogram are faster results (1 hour rather than 4 hours), no radiation, and less cost. Echocardiograms may be done during or after exercise to see the effect on heart wall motion. Some medication, such as dipyridamole and dobutamine, may be used to stress the heart. Depression of wall motion suggests ischemia. In experienced laboratories, the ultrasound test is as accurate as a nuclear medicine scan (McPhee et al., 2011).

TRANSESOPHAGEAL ECHOCARDIOGRAMS

The introduction of the transesophageal approach to echocardiography has given clinicians a new "window on the heart," because this approach is unimpeded by chest-wall structures and lung interference. A TEE can be safely performed on critically ill clients at the bedside and demonstrates abnormalities that are missed with TTE. For example, a TEE allows clear visualization of posterior structures of the heart, such as the left atrium and the aortic root, which are needed to evaluate prosthetic heart valves. Other clinical uses of TEE are for the diagnosis of infective endocarditis;

the diagnosis of aortic abnormalities, such as aortic dissection; the assessment of a cardiac source of an embolus; monitoring of atrial fibrillation; and the evaluation of clients who have had a myocardial infarction. A TTE with color flow Doppler is the test of choice to identify mitral regurgitation (Ziegler & Quillen, 2005).

A TEE is obtained with a transducer mounted on the end of a gastroscope. The physician inserts the scope and has the client swallow as the scope goes down the esophagus. Over the next 5–20 minutes, the probe is manipulated and then gently withdrawn to provide various views of the heart. A video camera records the findings. Special contrast medium may be given intravenously.

Although a TEE is clearly superior to a TTE in detecting many potential cardiac abnormalities, it carries a small risk related to esophageal intubation and the use of medications. Complications that may occur are bleeding, aspiration, vocal cord paralysis, and arrhythmias. Pain in the esophageal or abdominal area could indicate perforation. Therefore, a harmless and painless TTE may be used as a screening test with a follow-up TEE if deemed necessary. A TTE is not reliable in detecting the presence of left atria thrombi, the origin of most cardiogenic emboli. Therefore, TEE has become an important tool for detecting left atrial thrombi and managing treatment protocols.

Pretest Nursing Implications Related to Transesophageal Echocardiograms

The client needs to fast for 4–6 hours before the examination. If the client has a prosthetic valve, antibiotics are given prophylactically before and after the procedure. An informed consent should be obtained and eyeglasses and dentures removed before the procedure begins. If present, a nasogastric tube is usually removed to prevent entanglement with the endoscopic probe. If the client has an endotracheal tube, a special latex cover may be used to protect the probe. The client is usually sent to a specialized room, but bedside units are available for critically ill clients.

The client needs to know that before the scope is inserted, a local anesthetic is used to numb the throat and the gag reflex. The client is asked to lie on the left side during the procedure, which usually takes 5–20 minutes. Clients may also be given small intravenous doses of opioids or antianxiety agents to reduce the discomfort of the procedure. Occasionally, glycopyrrolate may be used to reduce respiratory secretions. A bite block in the client's mouth protects the patient's teeth if he or she does not have removable dentures. Oxygen saturation is monitored, and oxygen may be administered. (See Chapter 6 on pulse oximetry.) Cardiac rhythm is monitored. (See Chapter 24 on cardiac monitoring.)

Posttest Nursing Implications Related to Transesophageal Echocardiograms

After the probe is removed, the client may need to cough to clear secretions. Nothing is taken by mouth until the gag reflex returns. Throat lozenges or saline rinses may be used to soothe the sore throat. Observations of vital signs, cardiac rhythm, and oxygenation may continue for 45 minutes after the probe is removed. (See Chapter 27 for more on monitoring for unwanted effects of medications.) Outpatients should have someone drive them home.

ECHOENCEPHALOGRAMS

Ultrasonic visualization of the head may be used to evaluate some head injuries, but the adult brain cannot be well imaged because ultrasound cannot penetrate bone. CT and MRI are more valuable in identifying masses and tumors because these studies give a 3-D cross-section of the entire brain (Chapter 21). Echoencephalograms are effective in monitoring certain cerebral abnormalities that cause shifts of cerebral midline structures. For example, ultrasound has been useful in monitoring the state of hydrocephalus in young infants. The size of the ventricles and the functions of the shunts are monitored with echoencephalograms or echoventriculograms. Because the newborn's skull is not completely fused into a solid bony structure, ultrasound is a useful tool for detecting intracranial hemorrhage.

Pretest Nursing Implications Related to Echoencephalograms

As with most other ultrasound procedures, there is no pain or risk for the client. The head is placed on a foam sponge. If the echoencephalogram is performed on a small child, the nurse may need to hold the child's head. Then, a water-soluble gel is applied to the skull. Thick hair may make it difficult to obtain a sonogram, but any cutting of the hair must be completed according to hospital procedure. During the sonogram, the client must remain motionless. If the client cannot lie still during the examination, the physician may order a sedative. Medications, food, and fluids can be taken normally. Portable ultrasound units may be wheeled to neurologic units or newborn nurseries to avoid transporting critically ill clients.

Posttest Nursing Implications Related to Echoencephalograms

There is no special aftercare, but the nurse should be aware of the underlying pathophysiologic problem, which may indicate a need for frequent neurologic assessment. The nurse should assess if the gel has been washed off the scalp or is matted in the hair.

THORACIC SONOGRAMS

Because ultrasound does not penetrate air, sonograms are not as useful for thoracic disease as for abdominal disease. For a lesion to be identified with ultrasound, there must be no air-filled lung between the chest wall and the lesion. Sonograms of the chest may be useful in identifying pleural fluid, abscess formation, or malposition of the diaphragm.

THYROID AND PARATHYROID SONOGRAMS

Ultrasound of the neck is the preferred imaging for the initial assessment of thyroid nodules (McPhee et al., 2011). A fine needle aspiration (FNA) biopsy is performed for suspected cancer. After surgery for a malignancy, surveillance may include ultrasound and RAI (Chapter 22), PET scanning (Chapter 21) can detect metastases that are not visible on RAI scans. Parathyroid scans are performed if clients present with unexplained elevated serum calcium levels (Chapter 7).

BREAST SONOGRAMS

Ultrasound of the breast is often done as a follow-up to mammograms to differentiate between cysts and solid lesions. Documentation of cysts that are often filled with fluid eliminates the need for a biopsy. Ultrasound may also improve cancer detection in women with dense breasts, as both glandular tissue and cancer show up as white areas on a mammogram. On an ultrasound, the cancer appears black and thus may be easier to detect on a predominantly white background. Ultrasound has also been useful during diagnosis of and treatment for breast cancer during pregnancy (Yang et al., 2006). A routine breast ultrasound requires no special preparation.

Ultrasound may also be used in conjunction with a breast biopsy. Percutaneous breast biopsy can be done using real-time ultrasound guidance and a probe that extracts tissue by a vacuum. Postbiopsy ultrasound determines the amount of tissue biopsied and verifies that no hematoma has occurred. A sterile stainless steel clip may also be placed to mark the site for a more extensive surgical excision. (See Chapter 25 for the care of a client before and after a breast biopsy.)

BONE SONOGRAMS

In the late 1990s, the FDA approved a portable device that can diagnose osteoporosis by ultrasound. The sonometer sends high-frequency sound waves into the heel. Healthy bone sends back the sound faster than does a bone with osteoporosis. The nondominant heel is used for the test. This painless, noninvasive, and nonradioactive test takes about 5 minutes to complete. Clients may obtain testing at health fairs or in other locations, as no prescription is needed. A low reading requires a referral to a health professional for further testing. Early detection can prevent later fractures. (See the discussion on dual energy x-ray absorptiometry [DXA] in Chapter 21 for the nursing role in helping prevent and detect osteoporosis.)

Another example of the use of ultrasound is for assessment of newborns for dysplasia of the hip (dislocated hip). Although physical findings may make the diagnosis, an ultrasound can confirm doubtful findings. The use of ultrasound has virtually replaced the use of conventional x-rays for this disorder. Ultrasound is most useful after a newborn is at least 4 weeks of age (Hay et al., 2011).

BLADDER SONOGRAMS

In the past few years, a diagnostic unit using ultrasound has been designed for use by nurses to assess the amount of urine in the bladder. The scan must be programmed for male or female by pushing a button. If the woman has had a hysterectomy, the male button is pushed. The client should be in the supine position. A generous amount of gel is placed on the abdomen and the scan head placed firmly on the skin 1.5 inches above the pubic bone. The transducer is moved until the image of the bladder fits within the marked area on the screen. A calculated urine volume is displayed. Measuring the volume of urine in the bladder can prevent unnecessary catheterizations. Integrating bladder ultrasound into a urinary tract infection-reduction project has given evidence that this addition is a "best clinical practice" approach (Altschuler & Diaz, 2006; Baumann, Rogers, & Newbury, 2010). Now handheld units are available.

ULTRASOUND-GUIDED PERIPHERALLY INSERTED CENTRAL CATHETERS

Nurses began using ultrasound to insert peripherally inserted central catheter (PICC) lines, in the 1990s. A handheld transducer (probe) positioned on the skin can give longitudinal (sagittal) and cross-sectional (transversal) views of veins to help the nurse select a vein. Then the ultrasound image is used to guide the entry of the catheter and to check the position. The nurse doing the procedure uses a sterile probe cover and sterile gel. A 2-hour training session for nurses improved placement success rate, but some nurses found it difficult to master the technique quickly (Blaivas, 2005).

Questions

1. Sonograms or ultrasound scans are performed with ultrasound waves, which are
   a. Waves of energy closely related to the γ-rays of radiographs
   b. High-frequency sound waves, which are beyond the range of audible sound
   c. Sound waves of very low frequency that are undetectable by the human ear
   d. Part of a still undefined physical force

2. The type of ultrasound scan that demonstrates motion, such as the movement of a fetus, is
   a. A-mode scan
   b. B-mode scan
   c. Real-time scan
   d. Doppler scan

3. The nurse is least likely to use Doppler ultrasound to assess which of these clients?
   a. A client who is in the first stage of labor
   b. A client who has had an aortofemoral bypass
   c. A client who had a pacemaker inserted yesterday
   d. A client who is undergoing an oxytocin challenge test (OCT)

4. The nurse should be aware that abdominal sonography is particularly useful as first-line testing for
   a. Cholelithiasis and appendicitis
   b. Gastrointestinal bleeding
   c. Metastasis to the liver or other abdominal organs
   d. Renal arterial stenosis

5. Which of the following is necessary before a pelvic sonogram? The client must
   a. Maintain nothing-by-mouth status
   b. Be given an enema or suppository

    c. Not take any medication

    d. Have a full bladder

6. Which of the following preparations is necessary when a client is undergoing an abdominal sonogram?

    a. Reinforcing abdominal dressings

    b. No smoking or gum chewing for several hours before the examination

    c. Using medications for sedation

    d. Having the client drink two to three glasses of water before the examination

7. An elderly man underwent a transthoracic echocardiogram (TTE) yesterday and is now scheduled for a transesophageal echocardiogram (TEE). The nurse preparing him for the TEE should emphasize that

    a. A TEE is much the same as a TTE

    b. The radiation exposure is minimal

    c. Food and fluids do not need to be withheld

    d. Dentures need to be removed before the procedure

8. An infant is undergoing an echoencephalogram to monitor a ventricular shunt that was inserted for hydrocephalus. The responsibilities of the nurse who accompanies the baby to the ultrasound department may include

    a. Explaining the results of the sonogram to the parents

    b. Reassuring the mother that anesthesia is used

    c. Giving an ordered contrast medium before the examination

    d. Holding the baby's head while the sonogram is being done

9. The use of ultrasound in the thorax is difficult because

    a. The transducer cannot be moved evenly on the chest wall

    b. Ultrasound does not penetrate air

    c. Thoracic tumors are solid masses

    d. The movement of the heart interferes with the sound waves

References

Altschuler, V. & Diaz, L. (2006). Bladder ultrasound. *MEDSURG Nursing, 15*(5), 317–318.

Baumann, B. M., Rogers, C. J., & Newbury, K. (2010). Nurses using volumetric bladder ultrasound in the pediatric ED: A painless method to guide the timing of catheterization. *American Journal of Nursing, 108*(4), 73–76.

Blaivas, M. (2005). Ultrasound-guided peripheral IV insertion in the ED. *American Journal of Nursing, 105*(10), 54–57.

DeCherney, A. H., Nathan, L., Goodwin, T. M., & Lauter, N. (Eds.). (2007). *Current diagnosis & treatment: Obstetrics & gynecology* (10th ed.). New York: McGraw-Hill.

Harvey, D. (2006). The incredible shrinking modality. *Radiology Today, 7*(5), 18–24.

Hay, W. W., Levin, M. J., Sondheimer, J. M., & Deterding, R. (Eds.). (2011). *Current diagnosis and treatment: Pediatrics* (20th ed.). New York: McGraw-Hill.

Johnson, C. (2010). Peril on the periphery. *American Nurse Today, 4*(6), 28–30.

McClintock, R. (2005). Should three-dimensional fetal imaging be used for nondiagnostic portraits? *MCN: American Journal of Maternal Child Nursing, 30*(1), 8–9.

McPhee, S. J., Papadakis, M. A., & Rabow, M. W. (Eds.). (2011). *Current medical diagnosis and treatment* (50th ed.). New York: McGraw-Hill.

Moye, M. (2011). Understanding the ankle-brachial index, *Nursing 2011, 41*(1), 68.

Scarvelis, D. & Wells, P. (2006). Diagnosis and treatment of deep-vein thrombosis. *Canadian Medical Association Journal, 175*(9), 1087–1092.

U.S. Preventive Services Task Force. (2005). Screening for abdominal aortic aneurysm: Recommendation statement. *Annals of Internal Medicine, 142*(3), 198–202.

van der Hoeven, B. L., Liem, S. S., Oemrawsingh, P. V., Dijkstrra, J., Jukema, J. w., Putter, H., et al. (2006). Role of calcified spots detected by intravascular ultrasound in patients with ST-segment elevation acute myocardial infarction. *American Journal of Cardiology, 98*(3), 309–313.

Yang, W. T., Dryden, M., Gwyn, K., Whitman, G., & Theriault, R. (2006). Imaging of breast cancer diagnosed and treated with chemotherapy during pregnancy. *Radiology, 239*, 52–60.

Young, D. (2010). Ruptured ectopic pregnancy. *Nursing 2010, 40*(6), 72.

Ziegler, K. & Quillen, T. (2005). Mitral valve regurgitation after myocardial infarction. *Nursing 2005, 35*(11), 88.

Website

www.PADCoalition.org (Current information on diagnosis and treatment of peripheral arterial disease.)

www.pocketultrasound.com (Information on pocket ultrasound.)

www.radiologyinfo.org (Information on types of ultrasound tests.)

www.vascularweb.org (Society for vascular surgery for diagnostic testing for peripheral arterial disease.)

Answers

1. b, 2. c, 3. c, 4. a, 5. d, 6. b, 7. d, 8. d, 9. b

Common Noninvasive Diagnostic Tests

- Electrocardiography 601
- Electrocardiographic Imaging 605
- Telemetry and Cardiac Monitoring 608
- Ambulatory Electrocardiography 609
- Electroencephalography 610
- Quantitative Electroencephalograms or Brain Mapping 611
- Electromyelography 612
- Pulmonary Function Tests: Spirometry 613
- Peak Flow Meters 617
- Nitric Oxide Breath Test 617
- Urea Breath Test for *Helicobacter pylori* 618

OBJECTIVES

1. Identify two general nursing diagnoses useful in preparing clients for noninvasive diagnostic testing.
2. Describe five basic characteristics of a normal sinus rhythm on a lead II electrocardiogram (ECG) strip and how common arrhythmias change these characteristics.
3. Given an ECG of a normal sinus rhythm, calculate the heart rate of the client.
4. State what nursing assessments are useful in monitoring the mechanical events of the heart when the client has an abnormal ECG or is undergoing telemetry.
5. State four important nursing functions to help prepare a client for an electroencephalogram (EEG).
6. Describe what a nurse should teach a client about an electromyelogram (EMG).
7. Explain how the pulmonary function tests (forced vital capacity [FVC], forced expiratory volume [FEV], maximum voluntary ventilation [MVV], and forced expiratory flow [FEF]) are used in assessing lung ventilation defects that are obstructive or restrictive.
8. Describe the importance of peak flow meters in promoting self-care for clients with asthma.
9. Explain the rationale for the urea breath test in clients with peptic ulcer disease.

Table 24–1 Noninvasive Diagnostic Procedures Using Various Types of Measurements

Tissue	Electricity	Ultrasound	Magnetic Field	Air Flow	X-rays
Heart	ECG Telemetry Holter monitors	Echocardiogram	Magnetic resonance imaging (MRI)		Chest radiographs Cine computed tomographic (CT) scan
Brain	EEG	Echoencepha-logram	MRI		Skull radiographs CT scan
Muscles	EMG				
Lungs		Thoracic sonogram	MRI	Pulmonary function tests	Chest radiographs CT scan
Tumors or inflam-mation		Abdominal and pelvic sonograms	MRI		Flat plates of abdomen CT scan

Note: See this chapter for nursing diagnoses for most noninvasive tests, Chapter 20 for radiographs, Chapter 21 for CT and MRI, and Chapter 23 for sonograms.

The preceding four chapters describe noninvasive procedures that use x-rays (Chapters 22 and 21), radionuclides (Chapter 22), and ultrasound (Chapter 23). This chapter discusses several types of noninvasive tests, including measuring such diverse things as electric events (ECG, EEG, and EMG) and air flow (pulmonary function tests) (Table 24–1). The unifying theme throughout all these tests is that because they are noninvasive, there is little or no risk to the client. These tests give an indirect assessment of an organ and its structure or function. Most are fairly easy to perform (usually completed by a skilled technician) and are relatively inexpensive.

Invasive diagnostic tests are those that use methods that invade the body, such as cardiac catheterization (Chapter 26) or an endoscopic procedure (Chapter 27). Other common invasive procedures are the subject of Chapter 25. The nurse must realize that this division of invasive and noninvasive tests is strictly from the professional's view. For the client, *any* test is an invasion of his or her personal space and privacy. Although health professionals consider an ECG noninvasive (because the body is not entered), the client may (because of the use of electrodes on the body) perceive it as being invasive.

General Nursing Diagnoses Related to Noninvasive Tests

Deficient Knowledge Related to Test Procedures and Preparation

It is the nurse's responsibility to see that the client is both physically and psychologically ready for the test. Preparation of the client should include reassurance that the test is neither painful nor harmful. Special consent forms are not needed because there is no anticipation of any complications from the test itself. There are specific physical preparations for several of the tests, such as a shampoo before an EEG. Some medications affect the results of several of these tests; thus, the nurse must be aware of the information required on laboratory requests. Also, the nurse must make sure the client understands any restrictions on medications, food, or liquids. Preparation for a child must take into account children's concepts of illness (Hay et al., 2011). School-aged children are usually very receptive to teaching. (See Chapter 25 for more on children's reactions to procedures.)

Anxiety Related to Outcome of Test

The focus of nursing care after a noninvasive test is to let the client rest once an assessment has been performed. It is important for the nurse to validate that the client is physically stable and not psychologically upset by the test performed. The results of the test may not be known immediately, and this may be a source of anxiety for the client. (See the discussion in Chapter 20 on posttest anxiety.) With few exceptions, there are no specific nursing implications after noninvasive testing. Although these tests are relatively simple to perform and there is practically no risk to the client, the client may be quite ill from the basic pathologic problem. The aftercare of the client is therefore geared to the underlying problems.

ELECTROCARDIOGRAPHY

Description

An electrocardiogram (ECG) comprises the electrical impulses generated by the heart during its depolarization and repolarization. The impulses are picked up by electrodes and displayed on a strip of graph paper. The electrodes are fastened to all four extremities of the client by means of rubber straps. A jelly or paste is used under each electrode to help conduction of the electrical impulse. The electrodes on both arms and the left leg are used to record impulses. The electrode on the right leg is a ground. A suction bulb is moved across the client's chest to obtain recordings for six different areas of the heart (precordial leads).

A common lead used for monitoring (and the one usually displayed in nursing textbooks) is lead II, which records the electrical activity of the heart with the negative electrode on the right arm and the positive electrode on the left leg. As the electrical current moves through the heart, the current moving toward the positive electrode shows as a positive deflection on the graph (above the baseline). If the electrical current moves away from the positive electrode, the graph shows a negative deflection (below the baseline). In lead II, as the electrical current goes through the atrium and the ventricles, there are two positive deflections: the P wave and QRS complex. In other leads, such as the augmented leads, the P wave and the QRS complex are seen as negative deflections because of the placement of the electrodes. Lead I uses both arm electrodes and lead III uses the left arm and left leg electrodes. In addition to these three leads (I, II, and III) and the six precordial leads (V_1–V_6), there are also three augmented unipolar leads (VR, VL, and VF), which make up the standard 12-lead ECG. Six-inch recordings of each lead are taken. With all 12 leads of the ECG, a clinician can gain a great deal of knowledge about the total electrical activity of the heart. Evidence-based guidelines recommend using two specific leads (leads 11 and V_1) for continuous monitoring of arrhythmias with the capability of performing a 12-lead ECG in an emergency (Hamilton, 2010).

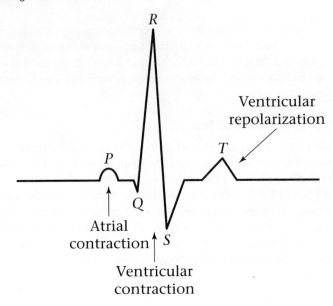

Figure 24–1 Basic components of an ECG tracing. (Note that atrial repolarization is hidden in the QRS complex.) See text for definition of P wave, PR interval, QRS complex, T wave, QT intervals, and ST segment.

Purposes

The ECG is a diagnostic tool used very frequently for clients with chest pain or other cardiac symptoms. Toxicity to certain medications, such as tricyclic antide-pressants, can be monitored with ECGs (Deglin, Vallerand, & Sanoski, 2011). The ECG is the definitive way to diagnose the various arrhythmias. It is also very helpful in differentiating myocardial infarction from myocardial ischemia. A cardiologist interprets the ECG and writes a formal summary of the findings. This summary is put in the client's chart with samples from the various leads of the ECG. Although a 12-lead ECG can tax the skill of even an experienced cardiologist, nurses in expanded roles may conduct an initial analysis.

Characteristics of a Normal Sinus Rhythm

All nurses need to have a basic understanding of what a normal sinus rhythm looks like (Figure 24–1), so arrhythmias can be detected on a rhythm strip. Electrolyte imbalances of potassium, calcium, and magnesium cause characteristic changes in rhythm, so nurses need to be able to identify these changes. The characteristics of a normal ECG are as follows:

1. The heart rate is 60–100 beats per minute in an adult (two ways to calculate rates are discussed later).
2. The rhythm is regular.
3. A P wave precedes each QRS complex.
4. The PR interval is 0.12–0.20 second (shorter in children).

5. The QRS complex is normal and less than 0.12 second.
6. The T wave is normal.

Describing Arrhythmias

In describing arrhythmias, a normal sinus rhythm means that the heart rate is under the control of the sinoatrial (SA) node. A *sinus* tachycardia means that the rate is faster than 100 beats per minute in an adult, but the SA node is still controlling the rate. *Atrial* tachycardia means the atrium is controlling the heart rate, whereas *ventricular* tachycardia means the ventricle is controlling the heart rate. In *nodal* or junctional arrhythmias, the atrioventricular (AV) node is controlling the rate. Thus, by simply reading the name of the arrhythmia from the ECG report, the nurse can assess something about the origin of the arrhythmia.

Ectopic or Premature Beats

A premature ventricular contraction (PVC) occurs when the ventricle originates a beat before the normal conduction of the impulse from the SA node. In rhythms with an occasional premature beat, the cardiac rate is still being controlled by the SA node. Another name for premature beat is *ectopic beat. Ectopic* means *displaced* or *malpositioned.* (An ectopic pregnancy occurs outside the uterus.) Ectopic or premature contractions can arise from the atrial tissue (premature atrial contraction [PAC]), ventricular tissue (PVC), or AV junctional tissue.

P Wave

The P wave occurs at the beginning of each contraction of the atria (depolarization). The rounded P wave is the impulse that spreads through muscle, not through conductive tissue in a straight line. (In contrast, the QRS complex is a straight line with a peak because the impulse travels straight through conductive tissue.)

Abnormal P Wave

In a PAC, the P wave does not demonstrate the usual sequence seen with normal sinus rhythm. In arrhythmias, such as atrial fibrillation, the P waves cannot be distinguished on the ECG because the atria are quivering or fibrillating. In atrial enlargement, the P wave looks different from normal because the impulse travels through more tissue.

PR Interval

The PR interval is the time it takes the impulse to travel from the atrium to the ventricle through the AV node and the bundle of His. Normally, the PR interval is 0.12–0.20 second. (One large square on the ECG paper measures 0.20 second.)

A PR interval longer than 0.20 second indicates a slowing of the impulse through the AV node and bundle of His. Medications, such as digoxin, can cause a widening PR interval or first-degree heart block. Other types of medications may also prolong the PR interval. In one type of second-degree heart block, the PR interval becomes longer and longer until the ventricular beat is dropped. In complete heart block, the PR interval cannot be measured because the ventricles are originating beats that are totally independent of the SA impulses, which generate the atrial beats. Thus, in complete heart block, the P waves may be normal, but no QRS complex follows. The P waves and QRS complexes are totally independent of each other.

QRS Complex

The QRS complex reflects the contraction (depolarization) of the ventricles. Normally, the QRS complex is less than 0.12 second.

A PVC causes a distorted and widened QRS complex. It usually looks very different from the other QRS complexes in the strip. Often, the QRS complex is a negative deflection rather than the positive deflection seen in lead II. All these changes in the QRS complex are due to an impulse that originated in ventricular tissue and traveled through the ventricle differently from the normal impulse, which comes from the SA node.

In myocardial infarction, the appearance of the QRS complex is one part of the ECG that is changed. Abnormal Q waves are characteristic of some types of myocardial infarction.

In ventricular tachycardia, the ventricles have taken control of the heart rate, and the ECG shows only spikes of QRS complexes, which are wide and rather bizarre looking.

ECG Documentation of the Type of Cardiac Arrest

In ventricular fibrillation, there are only wavy lines on the ECG with nothing that resembles a P wave or QRS complex. Ventricular fibrillation causes cardiac arrest—when the ventricles are fibrillating (quivering), there is no cardiac output—and the ECG shows chaotic electrical activity. For the other type of cardiac arrest, cardiac standstill or asystole, the ECG shows a straight line—even the quivering or fibrillation of the ventricle has stopped. Only the ECG can be used to differentiate whether a cardiac arrest is due to asystole or fibrillation.

T Wave

The T wave occurs as the ventricles recover from the contraction period. This period of electrical recovery is called *repolarization*. (The repolarization of the atrium is not seen on the ECG graph because it is hidden in the larger electrical event of the QRS complex.)

Myocardial damage may cause inversion of the T waves. High levels of serum potassium (hyperkalemia) cause tall, peaked T waves. An ECG on an oscilloscope is sometimes used to monitor potassium replacement in severe cases of hypokalemia. Low levels of potassium (hypokalemia) cause inverted T waves. A flattened T wave means the ventricle is not able to repolarize normally. (See Chapter 5 for a discussion on the effects of potassium on cardiac function.)

QT Interval

The QT interval covers the period of both ventricular depolarization and repolarization. Its normal duration is 0.36–0.44 second.

The QT interval is useful in evaluating the effects on the heart of medications such as quinidine. Ischemia or electrolyte changes may prolong or shorten the QT interval.

ST Segment

The ST segment is the time between completion of depolarization and the beginning of repolarization of the ventricles. One often interprets only a nonspecific ST abnormality on an ECG.

A decidedly depressed or downward slope of the ST segment is somewhat characteristic of myocardial ischemia. Digoxin depresses the ST segment. (See the stress test in Chapter 26 for more explanation about ST changes from exertion and other factors.) Conversely, an elevated ST segment is one of the characteristics of a myocardial infarction. As with all other changes in the ECG, the meaning of the changes may be open to several interpretations, depending on other clinical data.

ELECTROCARDIOGRAPHIC IMAGING

At present, there is no easy way to identify the exact location of cardiac arrhythmias. Standard ECGs determine the origin of the arrhythmia (e.g., atrial or ventricular). Electrophysiology studies (Chapter 26) are invasive and expensive ways to map the exact location of the arrhythmia in the atrium or ventricle. A new noninvasive way to map arrhythmias uses a multielectrode vest that records 224 body-surface ECGs. These ECGs are then reconstructed on the heart's surface by using a CT scan and a mathematical algorithm. The first clinical application of ECG imaging (ECGi) identified the exact location of PVC in a young athlete (Intini et al., 2005). See Chapter 26 for another new test called microvolt T-wave alternans (MTWA).

Determining Heart Rate with an ECG

Because the ECG paper is horizontally marked for time, heart rate can be determined by looking at an ECG strip. (The vertical deflections reflect the amplitude of the voltage, but this is not of great use to a nurse who is just beginning to learn about ECGs.) As seen in Figure 24–2, each tiny square of ECG strip measures 0.04 seconds, and each larger square (which consists of five tiny ones) is 0.20 seconds. By remembering that each large square signifies 0.20 second, one can calculate the heart rate by means of several different formulas. Two simple methods that a nurse can use to time a heart rate by scanning an ECG strip are described in the following sections. Both methods assume a steady rate of impulses.

Method A: Counting the Squares Between the Beats

The squares between each QRS complex can be counted to determine the time between each beat. For example, if there are three large squares between each beat (QRS complex), this implies a time interval of 0.6 second (3 squares × 0.2 second) between each beat. Thus, in 60 seconds, there would be 100 beats (60 seconds ÷ 0.6). If there were five large squares between each beat, this would mean 1 second (5 squares × 0.20 second) between each beat. In 60 seconds, there would be 60 beats

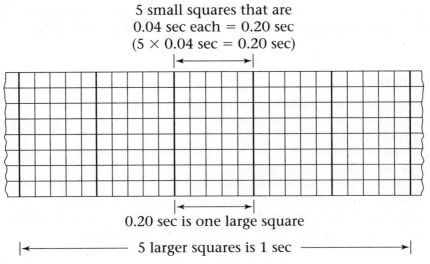

5 small squares that are
0.04 sec each = 0.20 sec
(5 × 0.04 sec = 0.20 sec)

0.20 sec is one large square

5 larger squares is 1 sec

Method A: Count the number of large squares that occur between each QRS complex.

$$\textit{Formula: } \frac{60\ sec}{Number\ of\ squares\ between\ beats \times 0.2\ sec} = \text{Beats per min}$$

Method B: Count the number of beats in 30 large squares.
Formula: Number of beats in 30 squares × 10 = Beats per min

Figure 24–2 Two methods to determine heart rate from an ECG tracing. See text for examples of use.

(60 seconds ÷ 1 second per beat). Thus, when a client has a normal rhythm on an ECG strip, which has no fewer than three squares and no more than five squares between beats, the rate is within the normal adult range of 60–100 beats per minute. The formula for calculating heart rate by this method is

$$\frac{60\ sec/min}{Number\ of\ squares\ between\ beats \times 0.20\ sec} = \text{Beats per min}$$

EXAMPLE

$$\frac{60}{3\ (\text{squares between beats}) \times 0.20} = \frac{60}{0.6} = 100$$

Method B: Counting the Beats in 30 Squares

Another way to calculate heart rate from an ECG strip is to count the number of QRS complexes in a certain number of squares. Recall that the large square measures 0.20 second. By counting the beats in 30 large squares, one has counted the number of beats occurring in 6 seconds because 30 squares times 0.20 second equals 6 seconds. The number obtained for 6 seconds is multiplied by 10 to obtain the number of beats per minute. The time markings on the ECG strip designate 3-second intervals and can also be used to determine 6-second segments. For example, if the total number of beats in 30 squares is 5, the heart rate is 50 beats per minute (5 beats in 0.6 second × 10). The formula for this method of calculating heart rate is

Number of beats in 30 squares (or 0.6 sec) × 10 = Number of beats per min

EXAMPLE:

5 beats (in 30 squares) × 10 = 50 beats per min

Pretest Nursing Diagnoses Related to ECG

Deficient Knowledge Related to Preparation for ECG

It is not necessary for a client to discontinue medications or abstain from food and drink before an ECG. The client should not wear metal jewelry. Clothing must be loose so the electrodes can be fastened on the arms and legs and the suction bulb moved across the chest. Women need to remove hose because the electrode paste must be applied directly to the skin. The jelly or paste used with the electrodes is nonallergenic, but it may feel messy to the client. Clients may be skeptical about "being strapped to an electrical box," as a client once said. Therefore, the client may need reassurance that the machine detects only electrical signals *from* the client, not to the client. Because many medications, such as quinidine or digoxin, affect certain aspects of the ECG, it is important that the cardiologist who interprets the test be aware of any cardiac medications the client has received. ECG requests have a place to note the cardiac medications that the client has received.

Risk for Injury Related to Malfunctioning Equipment

From a safety point of view, any electrical equipment does present an electrical hazard if the machine is defective and not properly grounded. As a rule, all electrically operated appliances should be plugged into the same wall outlet so there is no difference in grounding points. Improperly grounded or defective equipment can cause a current leakage through the client if the two pieces of equipment are plugged into outlets more than 12 feet (3.6 m) apart. The ECG technician has the responsibility of checking the machine to make sure that there are no frayed cords or other problems and that the machine is properly grounded. With a changing economic climate, nurses may find that running a 12-lead ECG becomes a nursing task. The nurse needs to keep in mind that for very ill clients, such as those with electrodes placed into the ventricle, all electrical equipment must be checked and grounded properly, including ECG machines. The nurse should consult with the hospital's electrical engineer about any problems that occur and how to perform safety checks of routine equipment.

Posttest Nursing Diagnosis Related to ECG

Risk for Altered Cardiac Output Related to Underlying Pathophysiologic Condition

The ECG technician or nurse helps the client wipe off the electrode paste or jelly. Aside from this, there is no other special client care related directly to the test. However, if the ECG was

(Continued)

> ## Posttest Nursing Diagnosis . . . (Continued)
>
> done to evaluate a possible myocardial infarction, cardiac precautions should be continued until other diagnostic tests, such as cardiac markers (Chapter 12), are interpreted by the client's physician. If the ECG was performed to evaluate an arrhythmia, the nurse may need to inquire about any changes in medication orders. Usually, the ECG technician scans the graph for blatant abnormalities and calls this to the attention of the physician. An experienced nurse can often differentiate between benign supraventricular abnormalities and potentially dangerous ectopic beats arising from the ventricle. Sometimes the ECG strip is kept with the client's chart; thus, the client's personal physician can immediately evaluate the strip. Otherwise, the ECG is interpreted by a cardiologist, and a typed summary appears on the client's chart.
>
> Heart rate, rhythm, and the presence or absence of a pulse deficit should be routinely monitored by the nurse if there is any question of arrhythmias. The nurse must remember that the ECG measures only the electrical events in the heart and not cardiac output. The quality of peripheral pulses, capillary filling time, and color of the client are all signs of adequacy or inadequacy of cardiac output. Dyspnea, angina, abnormal heart or breath sounds, and a decrease in urine output are all detected by the nurse—not from an ECG reading. Therefore, even when a monitor is used to show the ECG pattern, the nurse must still collect information to obtain a complete idea of the efficiency of the heart.

TELEMETRY AND CARDIAC MONITORING

Telemetry is taking measurements at a distance from the client by the use of radio signals. It has been extensively used in physiologic assessments during space travels. In the hospital setting, telemetry is used to monitor the ECG of a client without the client having to be hooked up to a monitor. The telemetry nurse monitors the monitor.

Small electrode disks are applied to the client's chest to obtain a good reading on the monitor. Disposable prelubricated disks can be kept on the client for several days unless skin irritation is noted. The wires from the electrodes are connected to a portable transmitter. A newer device called "wireless ECG" has replaced the lead wires with radio signals. The portable transmitter is about the size of a small tissue box and can be left lying in bed by the client or can be strapped to an ambulatory client's waist. Current ECG monitors can assess heart rate, cardiac arrhythmias, and myocardial ischemia by ST-segment monitoring (Pelter, 2008), but the nurse is still needed to assess the mechanical events (i.e., cardiac output) in the client.

Telemetry with Telephone and Facsimile

Telephone recordings of ECGs originated in 1971. A special instrument is used with the telephone. The graphic representation of heart rhythm is fed into a computer and a duplicate is made for analysis by a cardiologist. The response time for emergency requests is 10–15 minutes for a complete reading. Clients with pacemakers may have phone checks completed every 3 months or so to supplement office visits. Clients may use cordless phones with some devices. The telephone transmitter is supplied through the physician or pacemaker clinic.

Facsimile technology made it possible to send complete ECGs to a cardiologist on call, making a well-organized 24-hour system for ECG interpretation available in even small community hospitals or clinics.

AMBULATORY ELECTROCARDIOGRAPHY

In outpatient settings, clients may be given a portable recorder (sometimes referred to as a Holter monitor) to wear, which records the ECG on magnetic tapes. When the tapes are returned to the cardiology laboratory, a computer scans the tapes to identify points of interest. This method is expensive, but it can be helpful in pinpointing the type of arrhythmia causing the client's symptoms. Also, the ambulatory ECG can be used to evaluate the effects of some treatments. The usual duration of Holter monitoring is 24 hours. However, some arrhythmias, such as those associated with syncope, may not be detected in the first 24 hours, so a longer time may be required. Holter monitoring may be as useful as the more expensive electrophysiologic studies (Chapter 26) to predict the efficacy of antiarrhythmic medications for ventricular tachyarrhythmias.

New types of monitors for ambulatory ECGs, called arrhythmia event recorders, allow the client to record an ECG during a symptomatic episode with a small device that is capable of transtelephonic transmission. Some units look like a wristwatch; one electrode forms the back of the monitor worn around the wrist. When symptoms occur, the client activates the record button and rests a hand on top of the other electrode. A high-quality ECG strip is recorded. This stored ECG can be sent by phone anywhere in the world. Readers should consult current literature on the various items available, since technologic advances continue at a fast pace. See Chapter 26 on implantable loop recorders.

Nursing Diagnosis Related to Ambulatory ECG

Deficient Knowledge Related to the Procedure for Monitoring

Clients need to clip or shave hairy areas so the electrodes make good contact and are less painful to remove. The skin should be washed with soap and water to rid the skin of oil and debris. (In the hospital an alcohol prep pad may be used). Good skin preparation means better ECG tracings. The leads are attached to the event recorder, which may be carried in a pouch. It is important that the button to record symptoms be quickly accessible so the event can be recorded as it occurs. For bathing, the cables can be removed and the electrodes left in place, but they should not get wet. Electrodes may be changed every 2 days or as directed by the information supplied by the manufacturer. The client must not have any radiographs taken while the monitor is being used—radiographs erase the tape. Metal detectors, remote control TV, CB radios, microwave ovens, and even electric blankets may interfere with the readings. The client should be instructed to keep a diary of any events that cause symptoms such as shortness of breath, dizziness, or angina. The client should also keep a record of such activities as sleeping time, exercise, eating, bowel movements, cigarette smoking, sexual activity, and emotional stress, which may be related to the cardiac symptoms.

(Continued)

Nursing Diagnosis Related . . . (Continued)

It has been observed that clients are often unaware that symptoms, such as dizziness, are due to an arrhythmia. In addition to the usual cardiac symptoms, symptoms such as headache, indigestion, or weakness may be linked to the specific time of an arrhythmia. Thus, a 24-hour strip may elucidate the cause of vague client symptoms so that the symptoms can be treated.

ELECTROENCEPHALOGRAPHY

Description

An electroencephalogram (EEG) is a recording of the electrical activity of the brain. The EEG primarily records activity of the superficial layers of the cerebral cortex. Approximately 20 surface electrodes are applied to the client's scalp. A jelly may be used to help conduction of the electrical signals. The electrode wires are attached to the EEG machine that records the electrical signals on a piece of graph paper.

If the client is comatose, the EEG can be performed at bedside. However, for routine diagnostic studies, the client is taken to the EEG laboratory, where the environment can be better controlled. The recording takes an hour or two and may include a nap. The first part of the recording is obtained with the client as relaxed as possible, to obtain a baseline reading. The client is then asked to hyperventilate for several minutes, to see how this changes the patterns of the brain. The client may become light headed from hyperventilating. Evoked potential (EP) studies evaluate changes in the brain in response to various stimuli such as flickering light and auditory signals. In addition, somatosensory signals may be generated by skin electrodes. Sleep may evoke abnormal patterns that are not present when the brain is more active, so sleeping patterns may also be obtained.

Purposes

Although the EEG is nonspecific, it can help identify a focus of disturbance in the brain. Most clients with cerebral seizures have abnormal EEGs, but a normal EEG does not rule out a seizure disorder. Normal EEGs are seen in about 20% of children and 10% of adults who have epilepsy. However, these percentages are reduced when serial tracings are obtained (Hay et al., 2011). Classification of the type of seizure disorder is important for determining the most appropriate antiepileptic medication. Imaging is important to rule out a neoplasm in persons over 20 years who present with a new onset of seizures (McPhee, Papadakis, & Rabow, 2011). Disadvantages of an EEG to confirm brain death are interferences from the surroundings and the possibility of false positives. However, the EEG is a standard confirmatory test used in many hospital facilities (Hills, 2010).

When the brain is dead, the electrical activity of the brain is absent, and the EEG is usually flat. EEGs may be performed to evaluate narcolepsy, sleeping patterns, and sleep apnea. These types of studies are conducted in a specially equipped sleep laboratory. Concurrent measurement of the client's oxygen level can be monitored with a pulse oximeter (Chapter 6). EEGs to evaluate sleep disturbances are called *somnograms*. To evaluate abnormal EEG waves, clients may also be connected to an ambulatory EEG system. As with the Holter monitors used for ambulatory ECGs, clients keep a journal of their activities and any symptoms that occur during the 24-hour monitoring period.

QUANTITATIVE ELECTROENCEPHALOGRAMS OR BRAIN MAPPING

A quantitative EEG adds a computer and statistical analysis to the traditional EEG so that brain waves can be measured and compared to other patterns. The procedure is sometimes called brain electrical activity mapping (BEAM) or just brain mapping. The client has a resting EEG and an EP when the brain is stimulated. From the client's perspective, the procedure is much like the traditional EEG except for the use of more electrodes. The computer compares the results to a database of brain electrical activity to study location of seizures, unexplained neurological disorders, learning disabilities, and mental decline. For example, researches have found differences in brain function between relapsing and abstaining alcohol-dependent clients (Saletu-Zyhlarz et al., 2004)

Nursing Diagnosis Related to EEG

Deficient Knowledge Related to Preparation

For routine EEG testing, the client should have no medicines for 24–48 hours before the test, except medicines particularly ordered by the physician. Tranquilizers, stimulants (including coffee, tea, colas, and cigarettes), and alcohol all cause changes in brain patterns. The client should have normal meals because hypoglycemia can cause changes in brain patterns. The client's hair should be shampooed the day before the test, and no oils, sprays, or lotions should be applied to the hair. It may be desirable that the client not have much sleep before the EEG recording because sleep deprivation may evoke abnormal brain patterns. The last part of the EEG recording may be conducted with the client asleep, and the client may have trouble falling asleep if he or she has just slept. Therefore, the adult client may be instructed to go to bed late the night before the test and to awake early. Children and infants should not be allowed to nap before the scheduled test. For ambulatory EEG monitoring, the client needs instructions on how to keep the electrodes in place. A journal of activities is needed for this type of monitoring.

If an EEG is being performed to evaluate the possibility of brain death, it is important that artifacts be kept to a minimum. Artifacts can be caused by manipulation of the electrodes or by electrical interference. The nurse should follow the specific guidelines of the institution when EEGs are performed at the client's bedside. (The electrical hazards for ECG also apply to EEG, in which several electrical appliances may be in use at once.)

> ## Posttest Nursing Diagnosis Related to EEG
>
> ### Risk for Injury
>
> The only specific care after an EEG is a shampoo to remove electrode gel from the hair. If seizure activity is a possibility, seizure precautions should be noted.

ELECTROMYELOGRAPHY

Description

An electromyelogram (EMG) measures the electrical activity of muscles. Needle electrodes are inserted into selected skeletal muscles. (Although in one sense the test is somewhat invasive, it is discussed here because of the similarities between ECGs and EMGs.) This procedure does cause some pain. The skin is cleaned with alcohol or iodine, but no local anesthetic is used. The muscle activity is recorded at rest, during voluntary activity, and with electrical stimuli. The findings from the EMG are recorded and usually summarized in narrative form for use on the client's chart. Informed consent is needed for this test.

Purposes

In nerve atrophy, there may be characteristic fibrillation, even in the resting muscle. Usually, a resting muscle has no electrical activity. The test can be useful in determining the extent of peripheral nerve injuries and differentiating paralysis of psychological origin.

EMG cannot be used to diagnose specific neuromuscular diseases, but it can differentiate between neuropathy and myopathy. All neuromuscular abnormalities are classified into two categories:

1. *Myopathy* is a disease or disturbance of striated muscle fibers or cell membranes. Myasthenia gravis and primary muscular dystrophy are examples of myopathies that produce abnormal EMGs.
2. *Neuropathy* is a disease or disorder of the lower motor neuron. Toxic effects of medications, hypothyroidism, polio, and diabetes can all cause neuropathy.

> ## Nursing Diagnoses Related to EMG
>
> ### Deficient Knowledge Related to Procedure for EMG
>
> No special physical preparation of the client is required before or after the test. Premedications for sedation or pain relief are avoided to assess a normal neuromuscular pattern. Muscle aches after the procedure may be relieved with mild analgesics. The procedure may take 1–2 hours if extensive testing is performed. The nurse should prepare the client for the discomfort and sounds of an EMG. The client may feel pain on insertion of the needle electrodes and hears audio amplification that sounds like firecrackers. If nerve conduction studies are carried out, the feelings may be similar to static electricity.

Risk for Impaired Mobility

Before and after an EMG, the nurse can be very useful in evaluating the functional capacity of the client with an unknown neuromuscular problem. Thus, the gait of the client, ability to perform range-of-motion (ROM) exercises, and any motor–power–sensory deficits should be recorded. Clinical data are always used as part of the base for interpreting EMG reports.

PULMONARY FUNCTION TESTS: SPIROMETRY

Description

Pulmonary function tests (PFTs) can be classified as (1) ventilation tests and (2) specialized PFTs of gaseous diffusion and distribution. PFTs, performed in a pulmonary function laboratory, cover the entire range of respiratory volume and capabilities. On the other hand, PFTs performed on the unit or in ambulatory care settings are modified to ventilation tests of forced expiratory volume (FEV), vital capacity (VC), and maximum voluntary ventilation (MVV). This section focuses only on the more common ventilation studies. Chapter 22 includes information about lung perfusion scans. The clinical significance of blood gas analysis, an important aspect of most pulmonary studies, is discussed in Chapter 6.

For ventilation studies of lung volume and capacity, the client breathes into a machine called a *spirometer*. A spirometry system consisting of a plug in a spirometric module connected to a computer graphic, such as blowing out birthday candles, is used to test pulmonary function. The computer analyzes the results and prints a report. Reports are stored so that comparisons of tests can be made over time. (The nurse sometimes uses a portable spirometer, the Wright spirometer, for clinical assessment of the client's ventilation status.)

Purpose

PFTs for lung volume and capacity help identify whether the client has an obstructive defect, a restrictive defect, or a combination of both. When there is an increase in airway resistance, the defect in ventilation is called an *obstructive defect*. Asthma, bronchitis, and emphysema cause obstructive defects in ventilation. (See Chapter 10 on alpha-1-antitrypsin deficiency as an inherited cause of obstructive pulmonary disease.) When the defect in ventilation is due to a limitation on chest expansion, the defect is called a *restrictive defect*. Pathologic conditions that limit chest expansion include fibrosis of the lungs, muscle dystrophy, obesity, and abnormal curvature of the spine. Conditions such as pulmonary congestion may cause both obstruction and restriction of ventilation. The ventilation tests help delineate the type of defect present and whether the defects are reversible with therapy such as bronchodilation. Ventilation tests are may be often ordered before a client undergoes an operation, so any respiratory problems can be anticipated and better treated or prevented. Nurses in ambulatory settings may be actively involved in conducting ventilation tests as part of a nursing assessment. Nurse-directed clinics for clients with chronic lung disease have routinely measured FEV, FEV_1-to-VC ratios, and MVV for many years. PFTs are an important tool in neonatal intensive care and may be performed by nurses skilled in this area. Home testing can even be conducted by clients with inexpensive peak flow monitors that can be used by people with asthma to assess a worsening of their status. More expensive handheld spirometers can also be purchased by clients to measure FVC, FEV, and MVV.

Pretest Nursing Diagnosis Related to Pulmonary Function Tests

Deficient Knowledge Related to Procedure

The clinician conducting a PFT gives the client specific instructions for each step of the test. The client must breathe only through his or her mouth. A noseclip is used on the nose. The client needs to rest before the test so that he or she can perform as well as possible. The client should not take any bronchodilators or opioids before the test because they can change breathing capabilities. Because the various breathing maneuvers require the maximal cooperation of the client, the test is not reliable in young children or confused adults. Food and fluids may be consumed, but not a heavy meal. Clients should not smoke for at least 4 hours before the test.

Posttest Nursing Diagnosis Related to Pulmonary Function Tests

Risk for Ineffective Breathing Patterns

The client may be discouraged if the tests showed less-than-optimal lung functioning. Poor test results may be an incentive for the client to stop smoking to prevent further damage. Also, the test results can help guide the clinician in determining what breathing exercises may be beneficial for the client and whether medications such as bronchodilators are effective. Clients with restrictive defects may need help to maximize respiration. Clients with obstructive defects need to learn how to get more air out by using techniques such as pursed-lip breathing. Nurses skilled in teaching breathing techniques may foster positive changes in the client.

Summary of Findings from Ventilation Studies

VC and FVC

The VC is the maximum amount of air that can be expired after a normal inspiration. The VC when the breathing is forced is the forced vital capacity (FVC).

Reference Values for VC and FVC

Must be determined with charts, which are specific for sex, age, and height. A value less than 75–80% means the predicted value is abnormal.

Clinical Significance

For most clients, the results of VC and FVC are similar. The VC increases with physical fitness. In fact, the FVC may be a good indicator of overall good health. In restrictive diseases, the VC or FVC is decreased—this test is the best assessment of restrictive defects. In obstructive defects, the VC may not be appreciably decreased. However, the more severe the obstruction, the more likely it is that the air trapping will reduce the VC.

FEV

The FEV is the percentage of VC that can be expressed in 1, 2, or 3 seconds. The figures are expressed as FEV_1, FEV_2, and FEV_3. The test is useful to evaluate the severity of airway obstruction and to evaluate the effectiveness of bronchodilators. For the client with obstructive diseases, an increase in FEV_1 of at least 12% is considered a positive response to a bronchodilator.

Reference Values for FEV_1

Normally 65–85% of the vital capacity can be expressed in the first second and up to 95–97% by 3 seconds. For FEV_1, less than 75% of the predicted value is considered abnormal.

Clinical Significance

In obstructive disease, FEV_1 is decreased. In restrictive disease, FEV_1 is normal or can be decreased. In some restrictive diseases in which there is an increase of elastic resistance, the FEV_1 may be normal or elevated.

Reference Values for FEV_1 Compared with FVC

Younger people can expel 75–85% of the VC in 1 second. Older people can normally expel about 65–75% in the first second. This is the only PFT in which age is an important determinant and in which increases as well as decreases may be abnormal.

Clinical Significance

The ratio of the total FVC to FEV_1 is decreased with obstructive disease and increased, normal, or sometimes decreased with restrictive disease. The amount of disability from obstructive disease may be rated by the ratio of FEV_1 to VC. In chronic obstructive disease, the FEV_1-to-FVC ratio will be below 70%. An FEV_1 of 80% or above indicates mild obstruction, noted usually by a chronic cough and excess sputum. An FEV_1 of 50–79% indicates moderate obstruction with noticeable shortness of breath on exertion and progression of symptoms. An FEV_1 below 50% indicates severe obstruction and below 30% may be life threatening. This is the staging system used by the Global Initiative for Chronic Obstructive Lung Disease (www.goldcopd.com). Clients with any degree of lung disability need to know how to prevent further damage. Preventing further decline in FEV_1 requires elimination of any noxious substances that damage lungs, such as air pollutants and smoking. Vaccines for flu and pneumonia may prevent further injury (Bauldoff, 2009). Symptomatic relief includes the use of bronchodilators. For the inherited type of emphysema, alpha-1-antitrypsin deficiency may be treated with augmentation therapy of alpha-1-antitrypsin. (See Chapter 10 on tests for alpha-1-antitrypsin.)

VE, MVV, or MBC

These tests measure the volume exhaled (VE) in 1 minute. The volume exhaled per minute at rest is VE. The VE in 1 minute when the person breathes as deeply and rapidly as possible is called the maximal voluntary ventilation (MVV) or the maximal breathing capacity (MBC). Usually, the minute volume is 15–20 times the one-time volume of the FVC.

Reference Values for VE, MVV, or MBC

Values are matched on a chart for age and weight. Less than 80% of predicted value is considered abnormally low.

Clinical Significance

Clients with obstructive defects have volumes less than 80% of the predicted values. In restrictive disease, the values usually are normal. Severe ventilation defects may show less than 35% of the predicted value.

FEF

Forced expiratory flow (FEF) measures how fast a person can exhale a specified amount of air. This test is useful in screening clients for subclinical obstructive disease. The person breathes in as deeply as possible and then times how many seconds it takes to exhale through an open mouth. The test is performed three times, and the fastest time is recorded. Most people can expel all the air in 2–5 seconds. If clients perform a simple version of this test at home, they should contact a doctor if it takes longer than 5 seconds to expel the air.

Reference Values for FEF

Values are matched on a chart for age and weight. Less than 75% of the predicted value is abnormally low.

Clinical Significance

A long-time smoker may have no symptoms of respiratory problems, but the FEF is less than 75% of the predicted value.

In summary, the test used most often for restrictive defects is FVC. The tests used for obstructive defects are the FEV, FEV_1-to-FVC ratio, MVV, and FEF for subclinical disease. For mixed types of defects, all these tests are helpful. Repeat testing by a specialist is recommended (McPhee et al., 2011).

PEAK FLOW METERS

In the past several years, small easy-to-use devices called *peak flow meters* have become available for home monitoring of clients with asthma. To test peak flow, the client sets the flow tab at the predetermined normal rate and then takes a deep breath and exhales into the tube-shaped monitor as hard and as fast as possible. A whistle blows if the flow rate achieves the predetermined set rate of flow. Some meters have more sophisticated gauges than others. Electronic peak flow meters are also available. Prices vary considerably depending on the design and whether the device is made from cardboard or plastic. The less expensive meters are reliable, but they may not last long. Most come with a carrying case and daily record charts.

If these meters are used on a regular basis, the client can detect the beginning reduction in air flow that warns of an impending asthma attack. The reductions in air flow may precede an asthma attack by hours or even a day, so the client has ample time to consult the health-care provider and make needed adjustments in medication. Or the client may be instructed to go to the emergency department if the peak flow drops below a certain point. For example, a goal for a client with asthma may be to maintain peak expiratory flow rate (PEFR) greater than 80% of the personal best and with less than 20% variation during a 24-hour period.

Nursing Implications Related to Use of Peak Flow Monitors

The sooner an asthma attack is treated, the easier it is to stop, so detailed instructions on how to use the monitor are warranted. The client should stand to perform the test, then take as deep a breath as possible, and blow out as hard and as fast as he or she can. The highest reading out of three times should be recorded. Nurses should remind their clients to bring their peak flow meters to clinic visits for repeat performances (Corbridge & Corbridge, 2010). Encouraging the use of a peak flow meter helps clients and parents of young children with asthma become partners with the health-care team in managing a frightening and unpredictable disease. This approach makes the client much more in control of the problem with more self-assurance in leading a normal life. One brochure for a peak flow meter notes that children enjoy making the whistling sound and give it their all, including following physicians' orders, so they can keep a normal peak flow rate. In the emergency department, the triage nurse must classify the severity of the asthmatic attack. Peak flow monitoring can be used to help assess children over the age of 6 years, but it may not be possible if the child is not familiar with the technique (Volpe, 2011).

NITRIC OXIDE BREATH TEST

In 2003, the FDA approved a new device for measuring exhaled nitric oxide. Nitric oxide plays an important role in the physiology of the respiratory system, and clients with bronchial inflammation have elevated levels. But some clients with asthma, especially those with non-allergic asthma, may not have elevated levels.

However, for those who do have elevated levels, the use of inhaled steroids will reduce the level in a couple of weeks. If the nitric oxide level in an exhaled breath does not decrease after steroid treatment, the client may need higher doses or other medications. (Also, the client may not be taking the prescribed medications.)

The test equipment has a mouthpiece and a breathing tube connected to a computer that analyzes the amount of nitric oxide in an exhaled breath. The test is a noninvasive, simple, and reproducible procedure that should be more widely used in practice (Zietkowski et al., 2006).

UREA BREATH TEST FOR *HELICOBACTER PYLORI*

Since the identification of urease-producing *Helicobacter pylori* in gastric secretions, a major change has occurred in the treatment of ulcers because many studies have demonstrated a causal relationship between this organism and chronic active gastritis and peptic ulcers. Eradication of *H. pylori* reduces symptoms and prevents reoccurrence of peptic ulcers. Current treatment includes anti-infectives such as amoxicillin, clarithromycin, or others combined with antiulcer agents that decrease gastric acidity (Deglin et al., 2011).

A noninvasive way to detect the presence of *H. pylori* in the gastrointestinal tract is the use of the urea breath test. After a 4-hour fast, the client is given a pudding to eat that contains a certain amount of nutrients. (The pudding acts to delay gastric emptying during the test.) A baseline breath test is obtained. The client then drinks a solution that contains synthetic urea. *H. pylori* secretes an enzyme, urease, that breaks down the urea-creating carbon dioxide (CO_2), which is absorbed in the blood and expelled in the breath. Thirty minutes later, a second breath sample is obtained and the amount of CO_2 is compared to the baseline sample. Clients need to know that antibiotics and bismuth may be restricted for 30 days and sucralfate and proton inhibitors for 14 days prior to the test. Clients may be able to continue with antacids and H_2 blockers. Specific written instructions should be obtained from the department conducting the test.

Other types of testing for *H. pylori* include direct sampling taken during esophagogastroduodenoscopy (Chapter 27). This procedure is invasive and more costly than the breath test. Several serological tests that detect serum antibodies to *H. pylori* are available (Chapter 14), but they cannot distinguish between current and past infections. The urea test and a fecal antigen immunoassay for *H. pylori* have excellent sensitivity and specificity and are not invasive (McPhee et al., 2011).

Questions

1. Special consent forms for noninvasive diagnostic tests are
   a. Usually required and are obtained by the physician in charge
   b. Always required if the client has not undergone the test before
   c. Not usually required because there is no risk to the client
   d. Completed if the client is fearful of the procedure

2. The repolarization of the ventricle is shown on the ECG as the
   a. QRS complex
   b. QT interval
   c. ST segment
   d. T wave

3. A characteristic of a normal ECG for an adult is
   a. A PR interval less than 0.10 seconds
   b. A heart rate between 70 and 80 beats per minute
   c. A positive deflection of the QRS complex on lead II
   d. A P wave after each QRS complex

4. Premature heartbeats change the appearance of the ECG. Which of the following is a characteristic of a premature ventricular contraction?
   a. A P wave precedes the QRS complex
   b. A T wave is absent after the QRS complex
   c. The QRS complex is wider than normal
   d. The QRS complex is absent

5. A client has just undergone an ECG. The nurse has noted that the rhythm is regular and that there are 8 QRS complexes in 30 large squares of the ECG graph. Therefore, the client's heart rate is
   a. 50
   b. 60
   c. 70
   d. 80

6. Another way to figure a client's pulse rate on the ECG graph would be to count the large squares between each QRS complex. If there were four large squares between each QRS complex, the rate would be
   a. 55
   b. 65
   c. 75
   d. 85

7. A client with a history of angina had some nonspecific changes on an ECG performed today. He is now undergoing telemetry. Which of the following measures of cardiac activity could be eliminated by the nurse because telemetry is being used? (Assume the telemetry equipment has been checked and is functioning properly.)
   a. Counting the apical rate and noting the rhythm
   b. Noting any dyspnea, angina, or abnormal breath sounds
   c. Checking the quality of peripheral pulses
   d. Noting the amount of urinary output

8. Which of the following nursing actions is *inappropriate* when a client is to undergo an EEG?
   a. Allowing a child to nap before the procedure
   b. Seeing that the client has a shampoo
   c. Allowing regular meals but no coffee, tea, or colas
   d. Checking to see if tranquilizers and sedatives should be withheld

9. A female client is to have an EMG to assess a weakness in her left leg. Which of the following statements is correct to tell the client when she asks about the test?
   a. There is no pain or discomfort during an EMG
   b. The test can specifically determine the type of muscular disorder present

    c. The client must remain on bed rest for a while after the test

    d. The test can help the physician determine whether the muscular problem is due to nerve or muscle dysfunction

10. Which one of the following pulmonary function tests is most useful for detecting subclinical cases of obstructive defects in ventilation?

    a. FVC (forced vital capacity)

    b. FEV_1 (forced expiratory volume in 1 second)

    c. MVV (maximum voluntary ventilation)

    d. FEF (forced expiratory flow)

11. Education about the use of a peak flow meter would be of the greatest benefit for a client

    a. Who is to undergo an exploratory thoracotomy

    b. Who is a heavy smoker

    c. Who took an overdose of an opioid and had respiratory depression for a few hours

    d. Who has a history of severe asthma attacks

References

Bauldoff, G. F. (2009). When breathing is a burden: How to help patients with COPD. *American Nurse Today, 4*(9), 17–21.

Corbridge, S., & Corbridge, T. C. (2010). Asthma in adolescents and adults: Guideline base diagnosis and management. *American Journal of Nursing, 110*(5), 28–39.

Deglin, J. H., Vallerand, A. H., & Sanoski, C. A. (2011). *Davis's drug guide for nurses* (12th ed.). Philadelphia: F. A. Davis.

Hamilton, P. (2010). Detecting cardiac injury with telemetry. *American Nurse Today, 5*(9), 64.

Hay, W. W., Levin, M. J., Sondheimer, J. M., & Deterding, R. (Eds.). (2011). *Current diagnosis and treatment: Pediatrics* (20th ed.). New York: McGraw-Hill.

Hills, T. E. (2010). Determining brain death: A review of evidence-based guidelines. *Nursing 2010, 40*(12), 35–40.

Intini, A., Goldstein, R., Jia, P., Ramanathan, C., Ryu, K., Giannattasio, B., et al. (2005). Electrocardiographic imaging (ECGi), a novel diagnostic modality used for mapping of focal left ventricular tachycardia in a young athlete. *Heart Rhythm, 2*(11), 1250–1252.

McPhee, S. J., Papadakis, M. A., & Rabow, M. W. (Eds.). (2011). *Current medical diagnosis and treatment* (50th ed.). New York: McGraw-Hill.

Pelter, M. M. (2008). Electrocardiographic monitoring in the medical-surgical setting: Clinical implications, basis, lead configurations, and nursing implications. *MEDSURG Nursing, 17*(6), 421–428.

Saletu-Zyhlarz, G. M., Arnold, O., Anderer, P., Oberndorfer, S., Walter, H., Lesch, O. M., et al. (2004). Differences in brain function between relapsing and abstaining alcohol-dependent patients, evaluated by EEG mapping. *Alcohol and Alcoholism Advances, 39*(3), 223–240.

Volpe, D. (2011). Managing pediatric asthma exacerbations in the ED. *American Journal of Nursing, 111*(2), 48–53.

Zietkowski, Z., Bodzenta-Lukaszyk, A., Tomasiak, M., Skiepko, R., & Szmitkowski, M. (2006). Comparison of exhaled nitric oxide measurements in steroid-naïve asthma patients. *Journal of Investigative Allergology and Clinical Immunology, 16*(4), 239–246.

Websites

www.goldcopd.com (Information on staging for COPD by the Global Initiative for Chronic Obstructive Lung Disease.)

Answers

1. c, 2. d, 3. c, 4. c, 5. d, 6. c, 7. a, 8. a, 9. d, 10. d, 11. d

CHAPTER 25

Common Invasive Tests

- Nurse's Role for Invasive Tests   623
- Lumbar Puncture   629
- Bone Marrow Aspiration or Biopsy   633
- Thoracentesis (Pleural Tap)   634
- Paracentesis (Abdominal Tap)   636
- Papanicolaou Smears or Exfoliative Cytologic Studies   638
- Cervical Cytology   638
- Human Papillomavirus Testing   639
- Colposcopy, Cervical Biopsy, and Endometrial Biopsy   640
- Breast Biopsy and Needle Aspiration   641
- Liver Biopsy   642
- Renal Biopsy   644

OBJECTIVES

1. Identify nursing diagnoses related to preparing adults and children for invasive diagnostic procedures performed at their bedsides, in a treatment room, or in the outpatient department.
2. Identify the key nursing implications for clients undergoing bone marrow aspirations.
3. Describe the usual procedure for the collection of spinal fluid and the normal characteristics of cerebrospinal fluid (CSF) as demonstrated in routine laboratory analysis.
4. Compare and contrast the pre- and postcare of clients undergoing thoracentesis or paracentesis.
5. Identify the key nursing diagnoses for clients undergoing breast and cervical biopsies for suspected malignant tumors.
6. Compare and contrast the pre- and postcare of clients undergoing renal and liver biopsies.
7. Identify what is important in informing consumers about the Papanicolaou smear as a cancer detection tool.

As discussed in Chapter 24, the division of diagnostic tests into invasive and non-invasive is somewhat artificial because all testing may be considered as an invasion to the person to some degree. The term *invasive* is usually used to describe diagnostic tests that entail the use of needles or instruments inserted inside the body to directly record or assess the structure and function of an organ. Some invasive diagnostic procedures are performed at the client's bedside, such as a thoracentesis or pleural tap. Others are performed in specially equipped treatment rooms, in radiology suites, or even in a specialized laboratory, such as a cardiac catheterization laboratory. Invasive tests require specialized equipment and highly skilled clinicians. When invasive procedures are performed by experienced, skilled clinicians, the incidence of serious side effects is low. But there is always the possibility of complications when the body is invaded with needles and other types of probes. The possibility of complications ranges from simple problems to severe injury and even death. After the clinician explains the possible risks to the client and the expected benefits of the test, the client or guardian must sign a consent form specific to the test. *The policy of informed consent is essential for all invasive tests.* A general form used at admission is not acceptable.

One of the goals of the Joint Commission is to improve the accuracy of client identification by conducting, prior to any surgical or invasive procedure, a final verification called a "time-out." This time-out phase is to double-check for the right client, the right procedure, as well as the right site, and to confirm that documented consent has been obtained. A review of laboratory data is an additional appropriate safety consideration, as a very low platelet count could lead to bleeding. Also, a policy should be in place for what medications, such as Acetylsalicylic acid, should be withheld before invasive procedures.

The invasive tests covered in this chapter are those that are usually performed in the hospital unit or in an outpatient clinic. A nurse is often present during these procedures and actively assists the physician and supports the client. These tests include needle aspirations or taps and various kinds of biopsies performed with the aid of local anesthesia. Nurse practitioners may actually perform some procedures on clients whose condition is stable.

The second broad type of invasive procedures are those performed in a special laboratory or specially equipped procedure room, such as endoscopic procedures or cardiac catheterizations. The role of the staff nurse for these procedures is to prepare the client for the test and to care for the client afterward. If a nurse wants to assist with endoscopic procedures or cardiac catheterization, special clinical training is required. Cardiac catheterizations and electrophysiologic studies are discussed in Chapter 26 and endoscopic procedures in Chapter 27.

NURSE'S ROLE FOR INVASIVE TESTS

General Pretest Nursing Diagnoses

Risk for Injury

The nurse needs to assess if the client is on any medications that can contribute to bleeding and if the client has an allergy to latex products or other medications. As mentioned earlier, the client or guardian must sign a specific consent form for any invasive procedure. The usual risks are mentioned on the form. The nurse coordinates the collection of any samples needed for laboratory analysis such as hematocrit (Hct) and urinalysis. The nurse also assesses the physical and mental status of the client before the test; these are baseline assessments, which

(Continued)

Pretest Nursing Diagnoses . . . (*Continued*)

are referred to after the test. One of the most critical baseline assessments is the client's normal blood pressure and heart rate. For some of these tests, the blood pressure cuff is left on the client's arm during the procedure so the nurse can take readings throughout the procedure.

Anxiety Related to Pain of Procedure and Fear of Unknown

All invasive procedures are to some degree uncomfortable for the client, and most cause some pain. At the very least, the pain is confined to the prick accompanying the injection of the local anesthetic. Some procedures also cause momentary pain or unpleasantness during the test. If the nurse is with the client during the procedure, he or she can be valuable in assisting the client in dealing with any expected momentary pain. For example, various breathing techniques or pain distractors can be taught to the client. Sometimes simply squeezing the nurse's hand helps the client cope. Depending on the interest of the client and the skill of the nurse, the client may be taught techniques, such as imaging or other methods, to divert his or her attention from the present situation. For example, if the client has learned the Lamaze breathing technique to reduce discomfort during labor, this technique could be used to lessen the discomfort during a painful procedure. The nurse should find out what the client believes will help ease discomfort. For some clients, sedatives may be needed, but accurate information about the test may alleviate anxiety and make sedatives unnecessary. The key points to emphasize are that (1) the duration of pain is brief and (2) local anesthesia is used. Pretest information should include what the client will see, smell, taste, or feel to lessen the dread of the unknown. Some clients may want a lot of technical information. Others may want to know only how much it will hurt. Research studies have suggested that adult clients who receive information about the sensations of a procedure appear to have less anxiety than clients who receive no information or only procedural information.

Sometimes intravenous drugs are needed to control the anxiety and pain of invasive procedures. For example, fentanyl and midazolam may be given before the procedure is started. Sedation occurs within 3–5 minutes after an intravenous slow push and usually lasts only for about 30 minutes. Clients remain awake after receiving midazolam but are relaxed and often have nearly total amnesia of the procedure (Deglin, Vallerand, & Sanoski, 2011). If many tests are performed and some need to be repeated, such as bone marrow aspirations and lumbar punctures (LPs) for leukemia, some amnesia may be desirable.

Anxiety and Fear in Children

Preparing children for invasive tests means preparing the parents, too. The use of a booklet designed for children is helpful. It is sometimes better to let the parents explain the procedure to the child, but it may be better to speak to adolescents when they are alone. The nurse's assessment of the child's growth and developmental stage is essential for appropriate health teaching. For example, school-aged children are usually receptive to teaching. Encouraging a child to play with some of the equipment may help alleviate anxiety. Research studies have suggested that, as with adults, telling children about the sensations they will feel may lower distress. Adolescents may be particularly interested in seeing what equipment will be used during the test. Children, as well as adults, need to know how they can help during the test. Young children may have to be restrained; thus, they deserve explanations. By the age of 3 years, children may be able to undergo procedures without the use of restraint if (1) the parent holds the child, (2) the child is allowed to participate, and (3) acceptable behavior is rewarded. Keeping a security blanket or favorite toy nearby may also help relieve the child's anxiety. Distraction, such as with the use of a kaleidoscope, has ameliorated children's perceptions of pain during needle sticks. In fact, many studies support the use of distraction to help children cope during medical procedures (McCarthy et al., 2010)

Deficient Knowledge Related to Test Procedure

Some of the tests require the client to maintain nothing-by-mouth status, whereas others do not. Medications may or may not be withheld; specific medications may be part of the test. The client should be physically comfortable; thus, he or she should be given a chance to void before the procedure begins. (For some of the procedures, such as paracentesis, an empty bladder is essential.) Physical preparation is described in the discussions of each test. (Table 25–1 lists key points about the tests.) The nurse also needs to explain what aftercare will be needed. Thus, children and parents will not be concerned because the child is being carefully watched after the test. By the same token, the adolescent or adult needs to be told before the test that his or her blood pressure will be taken, approximately every 15 minutes, so that there is no misconception that something is amiss.

Table 25–1 Common Invasive Tests: Summary of Key Points for Nursing Care[a]

Test	Nothing by Mouth Before Test	Local Anesthetic Used	Restricted Activity After Test	Assess for Complications
Lumbar puncture	No	Yes	Varies, usually several hours	Spinal headache; nerve damage to legs (very rare)
Bone marrow biopsy	No	Yes	No	None likely; infection possible
Thoracentesis	No	Yes	1 hr on unaffected side	Pneumothorax; subcutaneous emphysema
Paracentesis	No	Yes	No	Hypovolemia; peritonitis
Papanicolaou smears of uterus	No	No	No	None likely
Cervical biopsy–endometrial biopsy	No	Sometimes	No	Bleeding from biopsy site
Breast biopsy	No	Yes	No	None likely; infection at site or bleeding possible[b]
Liver biopsy	Yes	Yes	Up to 24 hr	Internal bleeding; bile peritonitis
Renal biopsy	Yes	Yes	Up to 24 hr	Hematuria and internal bleeding; urinary tract infection

[a]See text for detailed discussions about all preparations before and after each test and for possible nursing diagnoses.

[b]If breast biopsy is performed under general anesthesia, the client needs routine postanesthesia assessments.

Preparation of Equipment

For all these procedures, special trays are used. For example, the basic equipment for an LP is sterilized on one tray. A check must be completed to see if the necessary slides, chemistry tubes, culture tubes, and other equipment are included on a special procedure tray.

In some institutions, the nurse may be responsible for setting up equipment for a procedure. In other settings, the person who performs the procedure is responsible for acquiring all needed equipment. Many procedure trays are now packaged commercially with all disposable items. The nurse must check with the particular institutions to see exactly what procedures are followed in that setting. Most prepared trays contain packets of skin antiseptics, such as povidone–iodine, which has broad-spectrum microbicidal action.

Injectable Local Anesthetics

The two most common injectable local anesthetics used for invasive diagnostic testing are procaine and lidocaine. Procaine, which is shorter acting, lasts about 3/4–1½ hours; lidocaine lasts for 1½–2 hours. Sometimes a very small amount of epinephrine is combined with lidocaine (in a premixed vial) to promote local vasoconstriction. Two reasons why some local vasoconstriction may be desirable are as follows: (1) the vasoconstriction slows the absorption of the drug to lengthen its duration and (2) the vasoconstriction may cause decreased bleeding at the injection site. Epinephrine is not used in areas of the body supplied by end arteries, such as fingers, toes, penis, or nose. Epinephrine is never used with a local anesthetic if tissue circulation is compromised. Also, epinephrine is not used if a client is taking β-blockers.

The syringes and needles used for the local anesthetic are included on the various trays. These routine types of needles on a procedure tray are (1) 25-gauge 5/8-inch needles for local skin infiltration, (2) 22-gauge 1½-inch needles for deeper structures, and (3) spinal needles, which are various gauges and extra long (3 inches) for very deep injections. (Trays such as a bone marrow or paracentesis tray include cutting needles or trocars for different test procedures.) Sterile towels are also on prepared procedure trays. Usually the vial of anesthetic is not included on the equipment tray and must be added.

Adverse Reactions to Local Anesthetics

Systemic effects can arise from local injections that contain epinephrine. Nurses should assess for any skin flush or increased pulse when epinephrine is used. Anaphylaxis can occur from procaine if the client is allergic to local anesthetics, but this is rare, and an allergy to lidocaine is even rarer (Katzung, Masters, & Trevor, 2009).

Local Anesthetic Cream

EMLA, a *e*utectic *m*ixture of *l*ocal *a*nesthetics, has decreased the use of needles for local anesthesia. *Eutectic* means to melt well at a low temperature. Although lidocaine and prilocaine are crystalline solids as individual components, a mixture of these two local anesthetics in equal amounts fuses as a liquid at room temperature.

The cream, actually very small droplets, penetrates the skin and blocks neuronal transmission of pain.

This anesthetic cream, introduced in 1993, is effective for both adults and children who must undergo painful procedures, such as LPs or bone marrow taps. Modifying the pain experience has been especially helpful for clients who must undergo repeated painful procedures.

The cream is not rubbed in, but an occlusive dressing is placed over the area to promote penetration. After the designated application time, which is usually 1 hour for minor dermal procedures and 2 hours for a major dermal procedure, the cream is wiped off and the area prepared for the procedure (Deglin et al., 2011).

A newer form of EMLA contains the emulsion in a patch surrounded by an adhesive ring. The patch may not adhere as well as the occlusive dressing, but it is equally effective with no substantial differences in side effects. Parents and nurses should be aware that young children may remove dressings or patches, so use of a secure extra covering may be prudent.

Common side effects of EMLA are erythema, blanching, or slight edema in the area. Allergic reactions are very rare with this type of local anesthetic, but clients must be assessed for any possible allergic reactions, including contact dermatitis. Metabolites of prilocaine can cause methemoglobinemia in newborns and in older infants receiving other methemoglobin-inducing agents, such as sulfonamides and acetaminophen. Nurses have a role in helping patients cope with painful procedures. EMLA combined with the caring attitude of a skilled nurse is a winning combination.

Arranging Environment for the Test

The nurse or clinician performing the procedure must check the lighting in the area. Most hospitals or clinics have a treatment room, which ensures adequate lighting and privacy. If the procedure is performed at the client's bedside, a treatment light should be brought to the room. A good light is needed, so doors should not be open—closed doors ensure privacy for the client. In a multiple-bed unit, it is better to take the client to a treatment room; otherwise, the bed should be screened, and perhaps the other client can go to a waiting room, if possible. Clients should not be exposed to another client's invasive procedure. Emergency equipment and drugs should be readily available. For example, atropine may be needed for the bradycardia that can occur from a vasovagal reaction.

Nurse's Role During the Procedure

The nurse may remain with the client to offer support. It has already been emphasized that the nurse can help prepare the client for the procedure by exploring, with the client, the best way to cope with any pain or discomfort. The nurse can explain that the antiseptic feels cold to the skin and the injection of the local anesthetic causes a stinging sensation. The nurse can offer to hold the client's hand or let the client squeeze his or her hand. Hand holding also helps remind the client not to put his or her hands on the sterile field. For a child, special restraining procedures may be required to ensure the safety of the child and the sterility of the procedure. The parent may help hold the child. If the parent is not present, the nurse can hold the child. The nurse may be essential in helping the client maintain a certain position, such as with an LP. The nurse also assists the physician or the clinician who performs the procedure. This may require pouring an antiseptic into a basin, opening extra gauze packages, or holding collection tubes. The nurse must make sure all collected samples are clearly marked in the order collected. Also, the nurse is needed to observe any untoward effects of the procedure (e.g., check the blood pressure several times during a procedure).

Nurse practitioners perform bone marrow aspirations and other invasive procedures. However, the focus of this chapter is for nurses in general practice, who usually assist during invasive diagnostic procedures.

General Posttest Nursing Diagnoses

Risk for Injury Related to Adverse Reactions

One of the nursing implications for any invasive test is to carefully check vital signs before, during, and after the procedure. Routines may vary for different procedures, depending on the policy of the institution and the procedure performed. Regardless of the stability of the vital signs, they should be taken at regular intervals as long as there is any possibility of the client bleeding or having other complications. Vital signs after an invasive test include blood pressure, pulse, and respiration. (The client's temperature is *not* taken every 15 minutes. The client's temperature may become more important later if there is any possibility that the procedure has caused an infection.) If there is any indication of a possible febrile reaction, temperature should be checked routinely every 4 hours. All vital signs must be documented on the client's record and should be graphed so that trends (e.g., decreasing blood pressure and increasing pulse rate) are readily apparent. Blood for an Hct may be drawn a few hours after the procedure. (See Chapter 2 for an explanation of why Hct is only accurate several hours after any bleeding has occurred.)

The time at which the procedure was performed and the name of the clinician who performed it should be recorded. The amount of any fluid withdrawn and its color and characteristics (e.g., cloudy or bloody) should be documented. The number of specimens sent to the laboratory also should be documented.

In addition to the specific items, such as the vital signs and other items discussed later, the nurse should record the general condition of the client after the test. For example, if there were no untoward reactions, this should be recorded as "client tolerated procedure well with no complications noted at present." Specific assessments of the client's condition depend on the test. These are emphasized in the discussion about each test.

Risk for Activity Intolerance Related to Need for Bed Rest and Medications

The positioning of the client after the procedure may be important. If the client is to remain in a certain position or maintain bed rest for a specified amount of time, the client needs to know this information. Also a sign can be placed at the foot of the bed. For example, the sign may say "Flat in bed until 7 PM." Clients may be dizzy when first allowed to walk. Ambulatory care clients often need someone to drive them home.

Pain Related to Complications

The nurse must know what type of pain is usual after a procedure, so ordered analgesics (without aspirin) can be used for relief without masking what could be a symptom of a complication. There may be a need for medical follow-up if pain persists after the use of mild analgesics.

There are pain scales such as (faces) used with young children and (numeric scales) used for older children and adults. In the case of a very young child or infant, a "FLACC" pain assessment is used and evaluates the following criteria: face, legs, activity, cry, and consolability (Hay et al., 2011).

Risk for Infection

The dressing over the site of an invasive procedure should remain sterile. The nurse must use sterile technique if the dressing becomes wet and must be changed. Some procedures may require a pressure dressing, whereas others only require a small adhesive dressing.

Imbalanced Fluid or Nutritional Requirements

Any limitations on eating after the procedure are discussed for the specific tests. For some tests, encouraging fluids is beneficial.

LUMBAR PUNCTURE

Description

Positioning of the client for an LP is very important. Clients are turned on their sides and told to curl up into a ball with head and feet as close to each other as possible (fetal position). This position allows for the maximum separation of the vertebrae. For very small infants, the position is a sitting one with the head flexed. The usual preparation of the skin with antiseptic and local anesthetic is completed. The clinician inserts a spinal needle into a lumbar space, which is below the end of the spinal cord. The spinal cord usually terminates at the second lumbar vertebra. Thus, the spinal cord is not touched with the needle. Sometimes the needle does graze a spinal root, causing a sharp pain, which radiates down the client's leg. If the client has pain in one of the legs, the clinician needs to know which leg, so that the needle position can be slightly readjusted. Once the needle is positioned in the subarachnoid space, a pressure reading is taken with a three-way stopcock and a manometer (standard equipment on an LP tray). The client must relax and straighten out his or her legs before the opening pressure is performed because intra-abdominal pressure increases CSF pressure. After a baseline pressure has been obtained, the physician may want the client to strain slightly (Valsalva maneuver) to see if the increased abdominal pressure causes an increase in CSF pressure. If there is a blockage in the spinal canal, the CSF pressure may not change. The Queckenstedt test is also used to see if there is a block in the flow of CSF. The physician may ask an assistant to apply finger pressure to both internal jugular veins of the client. Obstruction of these veins causes a rise in CSF pressure, unless there is a block somewhere in the spinal column. The Queckenstedt test can be dangerous if too much pressure is put on the carotid receptors. The assistant must know exactly how and where to apply the pressure. After the pressure readings are completed, a few milliliters of CSF are obtained in tubes for (1) chemistry, (2) cell counts, and (3) microbiologic examination. A closing pressure may be obtained. The CSF pressure drops 5–10 mm of water pressure for each milliliter of fluid removed. Usually only about 10 mL is removed, but this can reduce pressure by 50–100 mm. The needle is withdrawn, and a dry sterile dressing is placed over the site.

Purposes

An LP or spinal tap measures CSF pressure and is used to obtain CSF for laboratory examination. For example, an LP is imperative when meningitis is suspected. An LP is also performed to inject dye into the spinal column (see myelograms, Chapter 20). An LP performed for a spinal tap is similar to that performed for spinal anesthesia.

Spinal fluid is formed in the lateral ventricles of the brain. The fluid bathes the brain and spinal cord and protects the central nervous system (CNS) from injury. Besides infections, measurement of different CSF components helps in the diagnosis of various conditions of the CNS. A special summary about the clinical significance of CSF changes is discussed at the end of this section.

Contraindications to LP

Measurement of CSF pressure helps detect any obstruction in the normal flow of CSF. However, if increased intracranial pressure is suspected, an LP is *not* attempted because a quick reduction in the pressure in the spinal column can cause a herniation of the brain stem into the foramen magnum. This downward shift of the brain can put lethal pressure on the vital centers in the medulla. A CT scan (Chapter 21) may be done before the LP (McPhee, Papadakis, & Rabow, 2011).

Pretest Nursing Implications Related to Lumbar Puncture

Note the general nursing diagnoses for all invasive testing (e.g., consent forms and other policies). (See the earlier discussion of EMLA as a local anesthetic.) A doll and pictures may be used to demonstrate LP to a child and thus reduce anxiety and perceptions of pain. The client does not need to maintain nothing-by-mouth status for LP. Sedation is usually not used but may be necessary for children or confused adults. A blood glucose sample must be drawn about 1/2–1 hour before the test to be used as a comparison with the CSF glucose level.

Posttest Nursing Diagnoses Related to Lumbar Puncture

Risk for Disturbed Sensory Perceptions

See the general guidelines about vital signs and assessing for pain. Special attention should be paid to any change in the level of consciousness, particularly if increased intracranial pressure is suspected.

Risk for Pain Related to Changes in CSF Volume

The exact reason for a spinal headache is not known, but it is assumed to be related to the loss of CSF. The use of a large needle or other trauma during the procedure may cause more loss of spinal fluid, and thus, there is less fluid to bathe the meninges of the brain. If a headache does begin, the client maintains bed rest and uses an ice cap and mild analgesics as ordered. If these conservative measures do not relieve the headache, interventions such as an epidural blood patch may be tried. Some clinicians may still advocate bed rest for a few hours after an LP, but no evidence exists that bed rest is effective in preventing headaches after LP.

Risk for Deficient Fluid Volume

After an LP, the client can eat and drink as soon as he or she desires. Unless otherwise contraindicated, drinking plenty of fluids should be encouraged because this helps the body replace any lost CSF. Extra fluids may decrease the risk for headache.

Possible Risk for Infections to Others

Clients with meningococcal meningitis should be admitted to a private room and placed on droplet precautions for a minimal of 24 hours after beginning antibiotics. Because meningococcal meningitis is highly contagious, individuals that have been in close contact with the client will also need to receive prophylactic antibiotic therapy (Heavey, 2010).

REFERENCE VALUES FOR CSF

Bilirubin	Negative
Cell count	0–5 lymphocytes—newborns up to 30
Glucose	50–75 mg/dL—compare with serum glucose, should be about 60% of serum level; newborns have higher levels

Protein
  Albumin
  IgG
  Oligoclonal bands
	15–45 mg/dL—higher in newborns
	29.5 mg/dL
	4.3 mg/dL
	Absent

Pressure	70–180 mm H_2O Infants and young children, 50–160 mm H_2O
Lactate	3 mmol/L—higher in newborns
Lactic dehydrogenase	About 10% of serum level

Note: Specific rapid tests for enzymes, neurotransmitters, and PCR testing for organisms may also be done (Hay et al., 2011).

General Significance of Abnormal Findings in CSF

Blood in the Fluid

Normal fluid is clear. Bleeding from the tap itself usually does not make all the tubes bloody. The collection of samples should be marked #1, #2, and #3, so it is possible to see if the blood is less in the last tube than in the first tube. Grossly bloody CSF is a sign of hemorrhage somewhere in the CNS. It may not be possible to perform any other tests on the CSF when a great deal of blood is present. Sometimes the fluid can be spun down to clear RBCs.

Bilirubin

Bilirubin (the indirect portion) can cross the blood–brain barrier in infants. Bilirubin in the spinal fluid of a newborn (kernicterus) can cause brain damage (Chapter 11).

Cell Counts

Normally there are fewer than five cells per milliliter in CSF; all are lymphocytes. In bacterial infections, there may be enough neutrophils to make the CSF cloudy. In tuberculosis and some viral diseases, lymphocytes may be increased. Tumor cells can also be identified with a Papanicolaou smear.

Glucose

The glucose level is lowered in bacterial infections because the bacteria use sugar. Viral infections do not cause a lowered CSF sugar. The blood glucose sample is needed for comparison. Ideally the blood glucose sample is drawn about 30 minutes before the LP because it takes glucose about 30 minutes to an hour to diffuse into the CSF.

Proteins

Degenerative diseases and brain tumors tend to cause increased protein in the CSF. Structural lesions that interrupt the blood–brain barrier cause increased total protein in the CSF because there is increased diffusion from the blood to the brain tissue. In general, an increase in the total protein of the CSF is a sign of a serious neurologic disorder. Because various diseases cause elevations in only some types of proteins, much research is directed toward identifying exactly what types of proteins are elevated in various diseases of the CNS. Demyelinating diseases of the CNS are those in which the myelin sheath covering the neurons is lost. During active demyelination, a basic protein is present in the serum and the CSF. Immunoelectrophoresis can be performed on CSF. IgG and an abnormal type of protein band called oligoclonal bands are often present in multiple sclerosis. IgG also increases in various CNS infections.

Gram Stains and Cultures

Cultures are performed to identify any organisms found in the CSF. If a preliminary Gram stain identifies any organisms, the physician is notified immediately so treatment can begin at once (see Chapter 16 on culture and sensitivity tests.)

Rapid Tests for Infections

A test using molecular biology can assist in distinquishing the difference in viral and bacterial meningitis within a few hours, compared to several days for a culture. See the Food and Drug Administration (www.fda.gov) for more information on these rapid tests on CSF.

Serologic Tests

The laboratory may perform various types of serologic tests to detect the presence of neurosyphilis. (See Chapter 14 for examples of serologic tests for syphilis.)

Lactic Dehydrogenase

An elevated lactic dehydrogenase (LDH) level is usually associated with inflammatory processes and bacterial meningitis. The LDH is usually 5–10% of the blood level.

BONE MARROW ASPIRATION OR BIOPSY

Description

Common sites used for bone marrow aspiration or biopsy in adults are the posterior iliac crest, anterior iliac crest, and sternum. The tibia may be used in small children. If a biopsy, rather than aspiration alone, is planned, the iliac crest is used. The area is prepared, and a local anesthetic is administered. Hair may have to be shaved from the site. The physician or nurse practitioner inserts the needle through the bone until the marrow is reached. For aspiration, the plunger of the syringe is pulled back to withdraw a small amount of marrow into the syringe. When the plunger is pulled back, the client often feels sharp pain. The client should be prepared for this momentary pain. Also, the client may hear a crunching sound and feel a "pop" as the needle penetrates the bone (Rushing, 2006). Normal bone marrow is soft and semifluid, and thus, a sample can often be obtained by means of aspiration with a syringe. Otherwise, a bone marrow biopsy can be performed with a large needle that has a cutting blade. The specimen obtained must be carefully placed in the correct container. A smear may be microscopically examined immediately to make sure tiny bone particles, called *spicules*, are present. Six or more slides may be prepared. A culture tube may also be necessary. Usually only a small adhesive dressing is placed over the site because there is minimal bleeding or drainage. A small pressure dressing is used if a biopsy was performed.

Purposes

Bone marrow studies are performed when there are abnormal types of cells on a peripheral blood smear. They are used to confirm the presence of metastatic tumors or diseases such as leukemia or various types of anemia. Bone marrow studies may be performed periodically to evaluate the response to treatment. A complete blood count with a differential and a reticulocyte count (Chapter 2) should be ordered on the day of the biopsy.

Pretest Nursing Diagnosis Related to Bone Marrow Aspiration or Biopsy

Deficient Knowledge Related to Procedure Requirements

The client is usually not given sedation, but if sedation is deemed necessary, it does not interfere with the test. The client can eat and drink before the test. The procedure, including the momentary pain, should be explained to the client. For some clients, the momentary pain is quite intense. The client is positioned with pillows under the thoracic spine if the sternum is used. When the iliac crest is used, the client is in a side-lying position or on his or her abdomen. The nurse helps the client get into as comfortable a position as possible, so the client can remain still during the procedure.

> ## Posttest Nursing Implications Related to Bone Marrow Aspiration or Biopsy
>
> Vital signs and other routines are performed as for other invasive tests, although the risk of bleeding is slight. The client may stay in bed for an hour or so to rest but then can resume normal daily activities. There may be a slight ache or pain, which requires the use of a mild analgesic without aspirin. Chapter 2 discusses nursing diagnoses related to decreased red blood cell (RBC) counts and abnormal white blood cells (WBCs), which are often present when a bone marrow aspiration or biopsy is required.

THORACENTESIS (PLEURAL TAP)

Description

The site usually used for a thoracentesis (pleural tap) is the seventh or eighth intercostal space. The clinician determines the exact site at which to insert the needle by studying the client's chest radiograph and by means of percussion and auscultation of the chest. To avoid large vessels, Doppler ultrasonography (Chapter 23) may be performed just before the tap. The client is usually sitting so that fluid pools at the base of the pleural space. If the client cannot sit, he or she may be turned toward the affected side and placed in a high Fowler position. The area is prepared and anesthetized. After the needle is positioned in the pleural space, fluid is withdrawn with a syringe and a three-way stopcock. The fluid for laboratory analysis, collected in a 50-mL syringe with 1 mL of heparin to assure accurate cell counts and pH reading, is then transferred to the appropriate containers (e.g., complete blood count [CBC] blood tube, chemistry blood tube, culture and sensitivity tube, and cytology jar). A catheter may be connected to the three-way stopcock to drain off a large amount of fluid. No more than 1,000–1,500 mL of fluid should be removed at one time. Vital signs should be monitored if large amounts of fluid are withdrawn. Atropine should always be immediately available for possible bradycardia due to a vasovagal effect. A pulse oximeter (Chapter 6) can be used to monitor for hypoxemia, and supplemental oxygen may be needed to relieve dyspnea. The client may feel some pain as the pleural space is entered, but the withdrawal of fluid is not uncomfortable. Once the fluid is withdrawn, a small bandage is placed over the site. Some clinicians may spray the site with a collodian seal. Thoracentesis is usually performed at the client's bedside or in the procedure room on the unit. Thoracentesis can also be performed in an office or clinic setting.

Purposes

A thoracentesis may be needed for aspiration of air, pleural fluid, or blood from the pleural cavity. It is often performed for therapy as well as for diagnosis. Inflammatory diseases of the lungs and neoplasms are common reasons for a large collection of pleural fluid. Blood in the pleural space (hemothorax) is usually from a traumatic injury.

Laboratory Examination of Pleural Fluid

For analysis of pleural fluid, the most cost-effective approach may be to first establish whether an exudate or transudate is present. Exudates have elevated LDH and protein levels, whereas transudates do not (McPhee et al., 2011). Transudates occur when changes in hydrostatic or oncotic pressure allow fluid to leave the circulatory system. Examples of transudates are the pleural effusion that can occur with congestive heart failure, cirrhosis, and the nephrotic syndrome. Exudates are caused by inflammation, infections, malignant neoplasms, or other abnormalities that alter or injure the pleural surface and promote fluid collection. Further examination of exudates, besides protein and LDH, includes cell counts; pH, which becomes acidic with inflammation; and various chemistries, such as glucose or amylase, if indicated. Tumor cells can be identified and organisms cultured.

Pretest Nursing Implications Related to Thoracentesis

The general pretest nursing diagnoses for bedside examinations are considered. An extra bedside table may be necessary to help position the client in a comfortable sitting position. The client can lean over the table with his or her feet on a chair for support. Chest radiographs are needed. The nurse should listen to the client's breath sounds to be used as a baseline for a posttest assessment. The nurse should also note any breathing difficulty and the color of the client's skin before the test is begun. Sedation, although not usually used, does not interfere with the procedure if needed. Food, fluids, and medicines need not be withheld.

Posttest Nursing Diagnoses Related to Thoracentesis

Risk for Injury Related to Procedure

The client is usually turned on the *unaffected* side for 1 hour to allow the pleural puncture to seal. Vital signs are recorded as per routine. The amount of fluid withdrawn for diagnosis, if more than a few milliliters, should be recorded as part of the intake and output record, and the client should be assessed for hypovolemia. There is no restriction on food or fluids after the procedure. If the client has no respiratory or other problems within an hour after the test, all normal activity can be resumed.

Clients with pleural effusion caused by malignant tumors or infection may have cytotoxic or antibiotic drugs injected into the pleural space after the fluid is withdrawn. The nurse must be aware of possible reactions to the drug injected into the pleural space.

Risk for Ineffective Breathing Patterns

Careful note should be made of the respiratory rate and the character of the respirations. The nurse should listen for any diminished breath sounds, which could be a sign of a pneumothorax. Any dyspnea or shortness of breath should be carefully compared with the respiratory status before the test. If a large amount of fluid is withdrawn as therapy, the client should be able to breathe with less effort. A chest radiograph is obtained to evaluate the amount of fluid removed and to check for any pneumothorax.

PARACENTESIS (ABDOMINAL TAP)

Description

The word *paracentesis* actually means puncture of any cavity for the aspiration of fluid. An abdominal paracentesis is used for the removal of fluid from the peritoneal cavity. In general practice, abdominal paracentesis is usually simply called paracentesis because withdrawals of fluids from other cavities have specific names (i.e., thoracentesis, amniocentesis).

Paracentesis is performed at the client's bedside or in an outpatient setting. The client must sit with the feet supported. A bedside table may be used to support the arms in a comfortable position. The physician inserts a large-gauge needle or trocar through the abdominal wall. (It is essential that the bladder be empty so there is no accidental puncture of the bladder.) Doppler ultrasound (Chapter 23) can be used to avoid puncture of the large abdominal collateral vessels. Once the needle is in the peritoneal cavity, the fluid is withdrawn with a syringe if a small amount is needed for diagnosis. If the tap is also needed to relieve pressure from ascites, the needle may be connected to tubing, and a large collection bottle is used, which is much like the setup used to withdraw blood. As much as 1,000 mL of fluid may be withdrawn at one time. Another technique is to perform slow, continuous drainage of ascites. The concern when a large amount of fluid is removed is that there may be a shift of fluid from the vascular space to the now-empty peritoneal cavity. Intravenous fluid or albumin may be used to prevent hypotension when large amounts of fluid are withdrawn. Once the needle or trocar is withdrawn, a small sterile dressing is placed over the site. If the client has a great deal of ascites and only a small amount of fluid is removed, the pressure of the remaining fluid may cause a continued leakage from the puncture site. The dressing may have to be changed frequently, and extra fluff gauze is used to absorb the leakage. The use of Montgomery straps eliminates the need to change the tape every time the dressing is changed.

Purposes

Paracentesis may be performed to assess for peritonitis. If the client has undergone peritoneal dialysis, the specimen may be aspirated from the peritoneal catheter. The nurse may collect this specimen by withdrawing a small amount of fluid with a syringe and using sterile technique.

An abnormal collection of fluid in the peritoneal cavity is called *ascites*. Ascites is most often seen in clients with advanced cirrhosis or widespread malignant disease in the abdomen. For these conditions, a paracentesis is performed for therapeutic rather than diagnostic reasons. The disadvantage of paracentesis for therapeutic reasons is that ascitic fluid contains a large amount of protein. Because paracentesis causes a loss of protein, other measures, such as diuretics, are used before paracentesis is performed for therapy.

In addition to diagnostic aids or therapeutic relief in cirrhosis and malignant disease, paracentesis is also performed as a diagnostic procedure for traumatic injuries to the abdomen. A peritoneal tap or a peritoneal lavage with warmed Ringer's lactate solution or normal saline solution is performed to see if there is any bleeding into the peritoneal cavity.

Laboratory Examinations of Peritoneal Fluid

Laboratory examination of the peritoneal fluid may include RBC count, WBC count, cultures, fecal content, bilirubin, and amylase (if pancreatitis is suspected). Normal peritoneal fluid is clear and yellowish. Blood in the fluid is abnormal. If the blood is intraperitoneal blood, it does not clot, but venous blood, which may be accidentally withdrawn from a vessel, clots. The amount of protein in the fluid helps differentiate a transudate from an exudate. Exudates, which usually result from inflammation, contain more protein and LDH than transudates, which are caused by pressure changes from mechanical factors.

Pretest Nursing Implications Related to Paracentesis

In addition to the general nursing actions for invasive testing, the client should be weighed before and after the procedure to assess the fluid loss. (Recall that 1 L of fluid weighs 1 kg [2.2 lb].) The client *must have* an empty bladder so it is not pricked by the needle. If the client cannot void, a catheter may be necessary. The client needs to be in a comfortable sitting position with the feet supported on a bedside stool or chair.

Posttest Nursing Diagnoses Related to Paracentesis

Risk for Deficient Fluid Volume and Electrolyte Imbalance

When a large amount of fluid is being withdrawn, the client's blood pressure must be taken several times during the procedure. Equipment for an intravenous infusion should be readily available in case of hypotension from shifts of fluid out of the vascular space. Intravenous albumin is sometimes given immediately after the procedure. (See Chapter 10 on albumin levels.) Vital signs are checked after the paracentesis is completed, and other routine after-care for invasive procedures is carried out. The client's pre- and posttest weights should be compared. The amount, color, and character of the removed fluid should be recorded on the nurse's notes and as part of the intake and output (I&O) record. The client should record I&O for 24 hours. Depending on the causes of ascites, the client may follow a restricted fluid or sodium diet. Electrolytes must be closely monitored (Chapter 5).

Risk for Infection and Injury from Other Complications

If any excess fluid is left in the peritoneal cavity, there may be a problem with leakage from the site. The dressing may have to be changed frequently. Sterile technique must be used. The client's temperature should be taken every 4 hours for 24 hours. The nurse should carefully observe the client for other signs or symptoms of peritonitis, such as abdominal pain and tense, rigid abdominal muscles. For a client with cirrhosis, paracentesis may precipitate hepatic coma. (See Chapter 10 on ammonia levels.)

PAPANICOLAOU SMEARS OR EXFOLIATIVE CYTOLOGIC STUDIES

The Pap smear is named after Dr. George Papanicolaou, who in the 1940s developed a technique for identifying malignant cells in body secretions. The Papanicolaou (Pap) smear usually refers to a test for malignant cells in the uterus, but the test can also be performed on many other body secretions. In women, routine Pap smears have been instrumental in decreasing the incidence of cervical cancer. In gay and bisexual men, routine Pap smears of the anus are thought to be beneficial in detecting early stages of anal and rectal cancer, since the prevalence of anal cancer has dramatically increased in gay and bisexual men compared to the general population (Palefsky et al., 2007).

Malignant cells slough off (exfoliate) more readily than do normal cells. The field that involves Pap smears is sometimes called *exfoliative cytology*. In addition to uterine or cervical secretions, exfoliative cytologic studies are conducted on sputum, pleural fluid, bronchial washings from a bronchoscope, gastric contents, bladder excretions, peritoneal fluid, and even secretions from the mammary glands. The collection of a sample for exfoliative cytologic examination is often part of an invasive study. The laboratory tells the nurse exactly how the specimen should be prepared. It must be remembered that all reports of exfoliative cytologic findings are used for screening, not for a final diagnosis. Thus, the presence of a malignant neoplasm is always confirmed with a biopsy.

CERVICAL CYTOLOGY

Reporting of Cervical Cytology and Follow-up

General interpretations for cytology fall into two main categories. The first category is *negative for intraepithelial lesions or malignancy*. Non-neoplastic cellular changes and organisms may be reported under this section. The second category is *epithelial abnormalities*, which may involve squamous or glandular cells. Dysplasia in a cervical specimen may be classified as cervical intraepithelial neoplasia (CIN) 1, 2, or 3. A CIN 1 lesion is characterized as the least abnormal, and infections in this category tend to spontaneously resolve. However, a large proportion (greater than 40%) of CIN 2 lesions advance to dysplasia and require more aggressive treatment. In the case of CIN 3 lesions, many (greater than 12%) progress to squamous cell carcinoma (Schiech, 2010). Another technique used to report dysplasia is by low-grade or high-grade squamous intraepithelial lesions (SIL). This method is referred to as "Bethesda System" (McPhee et al., 2011). One of the most common types of abnormal Pap smear is an inconclusive result referred to as atypical squamous cells of undetermined significance (ASCUS). In the past, women with ASCUS would have a colposcopy and a biopsy or several Pap smears over a period of time. Now, testing for human papillomavirus (HPV) helps decide how much follow-up is needed. A woman who tests negative for HPV is unlikely to have cervical cancer. Those who test positive need further evaluation.

HUMAN PAPILLOMAVIRUS TESTING

At least 70 genetically distinct types of HPV have been identified, and several types definitely cause benign squamous papillomas (warts) in humans. HPV has also been implicated as a causative factor for squamous cell carcinoma of the cervix and ano-genital region. Men who have sex with men may develop anal cancer. Women who have chronic HPV infection are at risk for the development of cervical cancer, but other cofactors probably must be present to cause the cell malignancy. Numerous sexual partners with the risk of more sexually transmitted infectious diseases, hormonal changes, diet, smoking, or other unknown factors may be cofactors. Specimens can be screened for the presence of HPV by DNA probe (Chapter 1). Certain types of HPV are associated with cervical neoplasia. The utility of HPV typing continues to be studied, as not all HPV-infected clients develop cervical cancer, even when they harbor those types identified as oncogene types.

Vaccines for HPV

There are two vaccines for HPV. The first is Gardasil, which was approved in 2006 and acts against 2 strains of HPV that cause about 75% of cervical cancers, and 2 other strains that are responsible for approximately 90% of all the genital warts. A second vaccine named Cervarix was approved in 2009, and acts against the same two strains of HPV that are responsible for cervical cancer (Aschenbrenner, 2010). Gardasil is approved for both females and males, ages 9–26 years, whereas Cervarix is approved for females only. The 2008 Women in Government Report on Cervical Cancer Prevention reported that most states are making progress in reducing the incidence and mortality of cervical cancer. However, the availability of the HPV test and the use of the vaccine vary from state to state (Wells, 2008). Nurses can help educate the public about these new technologies, since parents are often uncomfortable in discussing their child's sexuality. The nurse should initiate the discussion because parental consent is needed in order for minors to receive the vaccine (Heavey, 2008). A vaccine is not effective if the client is already exposed to HPV, so the vaccine needs to be given before the client becomes sexually active. Unresolved issues include the most critical groups to vaccinate. See the American Cancer Society website (www.cancer.org) for current information. Another issue is when the cost of the vaccine will be low enough for use in the developing world, where 80% of cervical cancer occurs (Lowy & Schiller, 2006). Women who have the HPV vaccine will still need Pap tests because the vaccine does not protect them from all types of HPV. Men who have anal intercourse may need Pap smears as well.

Papanicolaou Smears of the Uterus

Description

A small amount of secretion is obtained from the cervix by swabbing the exterior of the cervix with an applicator. A cytobrush may be used to obtain cells from the endometrium. Most sources suggest that two smears be taken to increase the chance of obtaining any atypical cells that may be present. The smears are placed on dry slides and immediately sprayed with a fixative or in a liquid preservative. It is important that the cells not dry before they are fixed on the slide. Research supports the ability of nurse practitioners to collect technically adequate specimens and arrange for appropriate follow-up care for women with abnormal findings.

Current guidelines recommend that cervical cancer screening should begin for females at the age of 21 years and continue every 2 years until the age of 29 years. The interval may be extended to every 3 years by age 30 years. If the woman has three negative Pap smears, HPV testing is added at age 30 years. Women over the age of 65 or 70 years who have had three or more negative results in the last 10 years may discontinue screening. See the American Cancer Society website (www. cancer.org) for updates on all types of cancer screenings.

Purposes

Cytologic examination of cells from the cervix can detect premalignant epithelial abnormalities that may be present 5–10 years before invasive carcinoma develops. The cause of dysplasia is not known, but it may be associated with some vaginal infections and condyloma (genital warts) caused by the HPV. Although most cervical cancers are associated with HPV, many women with chronic HPV do not develop a malignancy. See the discussion above on HPV testing.

Pretest Nursing Implications Related to Pap Smears

A Pap smear is usually performed 5–6 days after the menses. The client should not have intercourse or douche for 24 hours before the smear. If the client has used antibiotic vaginal creams, the examination should be delayed 1 month. The use of any medications, particularly oral contraceptives, should be recorded on the request slip. For some women, a pelvic examination is an unpleasant and embarrassing procedure, and the nurse must be sensitive to the need to respect the privacy of the client with actions such as draping.

Posttest Nursing Implications Related to Pap Smears

There are no client restrictions after a Pap smear. Some women may fear abnormal results of a Pap smear, whereas others may discount any risk because they have no symptoms. The news of an abnormal Pap smear and the need for follow-up may be particularly anxiety producing for younger women and those with concurrent stressors. Therefore, nurses are often crucial in contacting women who fail to return for follow-up appointments and treatment.

COLPOSCOPY, CERVICAL BIOPSY, AND ENDOMETRIAL BIOPSY

Description and Purposes

A colposcope, or colpomicroscope, is a binocular microscope with a magnifying glass and a high-intensity light source. It is used to examine the vagina and cervix and to collect a biopsy specimen if necessary. Nurses, as primary care practitioners, perform colposcopic examinations. The biopsy is planned for about 1 week after the client's menses because the cervix is more vascular before and after menses.

The biopsy is performed after the menstrual period, so there is no possibility of pregnancy. The client is prepared for a pelvic examination as described earlier. The client is not given any local anesthetic because the cervix is sensitive to pressure but not to burning or cutting, as is the skin. The momentary pressure is somewhat uncomfortable for some clients. The biopsy site may be sealed with a silver nitrate stick or cauterized. Packing will probably be put in the vagina.

With the colposcope, the clinician can identify areas of the cervix that appear atypical and thus perform direct punch biopsies. It takes about 10 minutes to view the cervical epithelium and note suspicious areas. Normally, the cervix is pink. During pregnancy, the cervix becomes dusky in color. After menopause, the cervix is light pink. Any secretions should be odorless and clear. The stickiness of the secretions is related to ovulation time. If abnormal areas are seen in the cervix or if there are abnormal secretions, a cervical biopsy or an endocervical curettage should be performed. Endometrial biopsies may be performed as part of an infertility evaluation (Chapter 28). An endometrial biopsy is performed with a special instrument inserted through the cervix. The pain is momentary, but sharp. This procedure is quite a bit more uncomfortable than a cervical biopsy. A local anesthetic may be used, or the client may be given medication such as ibuprofen 30 minutes before the procedure. Some bleeding may be expected, so a tampon or pad is needed.

Pretest Nursing Implications Related to Colposcopy

Women undergoing colposcopy for the first time may have many unanswered questions about the procedure as well as underlying concerns about cancer and the causes of ASCUS. Preparatory information, including a review of female anatomy, the meaning of Pap results, and procedural and sensory information about colposcopy, should be made available to women before the scheduled appointment. Many institutions have written information, but the nurse should still be available to answer questions.

Preparation for colposcopy is similar to that for a Pap smear. The client should be told that the biopsy causes momentary discomfort. (If a cone biopsy is needed, the client needs anesthesia.)

Posttest Nursing Implications Related to Colposcopy

Vaginal packing or a tampon may be left in place for several hours. Any unusual bleeding or abdominal pain should be reported, but some spotting is expected for a few days. Intercourse can resume after 24 hours unless treatment was administered for the dysplasia. If cryotherapy or laser treatments were performed, the woman should abstain from intercourse for 2 weeks.

BREAST BIOPSY AND NEEDLE ASPIRATION

Description and Purposes

A breast biopsy or needle aspiration as a diagnostic procedure for malignant tumors is usually performed in an outpatient setting. For a breast biopsy, the skin is prepared and anesthetized in the usual manner. A small amount of tissue is incised. Either a biopsy or a needle aspiration takes only a few minutes to complete. A probe may be placed when a mammogram is obtained (Chapter 20) to identify the exact site for the biopsy. At the present time, breast biopsies are of five types: (1) an open incision that takes place in the operating room, (2) fine-needle aspiration, (3) core needle biopsy, (4) a newer minimally invasive technique that uses ultrasound imaging and a single probe insertion that removes tissue by vacuum, and (5) an advanced breast biopsy instrument (ABBI) that is less invasive than a surgical biopsy (Carroll, 2006). The ABBI unit has a special table in which the woman lies on her abdomen and the breast protrudes through an opening. (See Chapter 23 on the use of ultrasound for breast examinations [for cysts] and to guide biopsy.)

Pretest Nursing Implications Related to Breast Biopsy

The setup for the procedure is similar to that for any other local biopsy—sterile drapes and local anesthetic. The physical discomfort is minimal, but the anxiety level of the client is likely to be high. Although most breast lumps are not malignant, there is always the possibility that this one may be. Roughly 80% of breast lumps are benign. (See Chapter 23 on ultrasounds of the breast and Chapter 21 on CT and MRI scans.)

Posttest Nursing Diagnosis Related to Breast Biopsy

Deficient Knowledge Related to Health Maintenance

For an open biopsy, the woman should wear a supportive bra 24 hours a day until healing is complete. The newer technique that uses a vacuum makes only a tiny wound and leaves no scar. After any procedure except fine-needle aspiration, the client needs to limit physical activity until the incision heals.

Since there is a lack of strong evidence that breast self-exam (BSE) improves survival, the American Cancer Society no longer recommends monthly BSE. However, women should discuss BSE with their health care provider who can show them the proper technique if they wish to perform self-exams in between the recommended exams by their health care provider. Clients should also be informed about symptoms to report and the schedule for mammograms, which may detect a mass before it can be palpated.

LIVER BIOPSY

Description

A liver biopsy is performed under ultrasound or CT guidance (Chapter 21). The skin is prepared and anesthetized. Before the biopsy needle is inserted into the liver, the client is asked to take a deep breath and then hold the breath after an expiration. Not breathing keeps the diaphragm motionless. Also, holding the breath after expiration leaves the diaphragm farther up in the thoracic cavity than after inspiration. An uncooperative client usually makes the procedure unsafe. The actual insertion of the needle and collection of tissue takes only 1–2 minutes. The entire procedure can be performed in 10–15 minutes. When the needle is withdrawn, a pressure dressing is applied to the area. A transjugular route may be used in clients with bleeding problems or ascites (McPhee et al., 2011).

Purposes

A liver biopsy may be useful in determining the exact nature of pathologic conditions in the liver, such as tumors, cysts, cirrhosis, or chronic hepatitis. (See Chapter 14 on HCV.) Liver biopsies are also used to evaluate for rejection of a transplanted liver.

Pretest Nursing Implications Related to Liver Biopsy

The client must undergo coagulation tests (prothrombin time [PT], partial thromboplastin time [PTT], and platelet counts) before the liver biopsy. An Hct also is measured as a baseline assessment. For a liver biopsy, the rule is that the PT should not be more than 3 seconds over the control time. The platelets should be greater than 100,000/mm³. Because a diseased liver may be unable to manufacture prothrombin in normal amounts, vitamin K may be ordered in an attempt to raise the PT percentage and decrease the time in seconds. (See Chapter 13 for a discussion of laboratory tests for prothrombin and the relation between prothrombin and liver disease and vitamin K.)

The client usually takes nothing by mouth for about 6 hours before the test. Fasting makes the liver less congested and the biliary ducts less turgid. Fasting also prevents any vomiting if complications occur. The client is usually not given any sedation, but some sedation may be needed by selected patients. Baseline vital signs are taken, and the client is given a chance to practice holding the breath after an expiration.

Posttest Nursing Diagnoses Related to Liver Biopsy

Risk for Injury Related to Internal Bleeding

The client is turned on his or her right side for 1–4 hours. Ambulatory clients may go home within 6 hours if there are no complications. It is important to check the dressing for any bleeding, but a pressure dressing should not be removed to look for bleeding. Usually, serious bleeding is internal, and thus, it is not detected at visual inspection. Clients can bleed to death after a liver biopsy; therefore, vital signs are checked frequently, as with any invasive procedure. Food may be withheld until it is certain that the client is not having any immediate complications. For clients in the hospital, an 8-hour posttest Hct may be performed to assess for any blood loss. Even a slight drop in Hct should be called to the physician's attention immediately.

Risk for Injury from Other Complications

In addition to hemorrhage and shock, other complications that can occur from a liver biopsy include bile peritonitis, pneumothorax, or perforation of an abdominal organ (e.g., the colon).

(Continued)

Any pain in the abdomen or any dyspnea calls for a thorough physical assessment of the thorax and abdomen. Slight pain at the biopsy site and right shoulder pain can be expected as the local anesthetic wears off. The client may be instructed to maintain bed rest for an entire 24 hours or longer if there are any complications. The client should be cautioned not to cough or strain because this can increase intra-abdominal pressure. The day after the biopsy, the client can resume most activities but should not attempt strenuous activities or heavy lifting for a week or two.

RENAL BIOPSY

Description

A renal biopsy is usually performed in a treatment room close to the ultrasound or radiology department because the insertion of the needle is monitored by means of fluoroscopy or scanning. Renal biopsies can also be performed with a cystoscope, through which a brush is inserted up into the ureter to obtain a fragment of renal tissue. The brush technique with a cystoscope requires general anesthesia and, therefore, is carried out in the operating room, as is an open biopsy when a wedge of renal tissue is obtained. A renal biopsy, under local anesthesia, is rendered through a skin puncture or through a small skin incision. The skin is prepared and anesthetized as usual. The client is usually not given any sedation, but the use of drugs does not interfere with the procedure. The client is asked to take a breath and hold it while the needle is being inserted to obtain the biopsy specimen. Only a very small piece of tissue is obtained. When the needle is withdrawn, a pressure dressing is applied to the area, and the client is transported back to the nursing unit.

Purposes

Renal biopsies are most helpful in the diagnosis of diseases that alter the structure of the glomeruli. Biopsies are performed only on the cortex, not the medulla. In acute renal failure, a biopsy may be performed if inflammatory nephritis is suspected. Renal biopsies may also help determine the exact nature of a mass, which could be a tumor, clot, or stone. Renal biopsies may be performed periodically to evaluate and monitor the course of chronic renal disease, such as the nephrotic syndrome.

Pretest Nursing Implications Related to Renal Biopsy

Preparation is similar to that for a liver biopsy in that coagulation studies (PT, PTT, and platelet count) must be conducted, vital signs taken for a baseline, and blood drawn for an Hct. In addition, the client should undergo urinalysis and an intravenous pyelogram (IVP) performed (Chapter 20) to determine that there are two functioning kidneys. Food and fluids are withheld before the procedure. Sedation does not affect the test and might be needed if the client is anxious even after optimal preparation. The client should be told approximately how long he or she will be in the radiology or ultrasound department and what the aftercare will be.

Posttest Nursing Diagnoses Related to Renal Biopsy

Risk for Injury Related to Bleeding

The client is usually instructed to remain motionless for 4 hours. Bed rest may be continued for 24 hours. If a piece of artery is discovered in the biopsy tissue, the bed rest may be prolonged. Vital signs are obtained and dressing-check routines are followed. An Hct is usually ordered 8 hours after the procedure. During the first 24 hours, urine is collected in separate cups and left in the bathroom so hematuria can be monitored. The time at which each specimen is produced should be marked on the cup. Some urine may also be sent to the laboratory for microscopic examination. Microscopic hematuria occurs in nearly all clients, but fewer than 10% will have macroscopic hematuria (McPhee et al., 2011). There are dipsticks for detecting occult hematuria, but these are not as sensitive as a microscopic examination. (See Chapter 13 on guaiac tests and Chapter 2 on urinalysis.) Any severe jolt to the retroperitoneal area can cause bleeding, even several days after the biopsy. The client should be instructed to avoid strenuous activities or heavy lifting for several days. The client should also be told to report any flank pain, gross hematuria, or signs of dizziness or weakness.

Risk for Infection

Clients should have a large intake of fluids, if permissible. Infection can occur after a biopsy, so the client's temperature should be routinely checked for a few days after the biopsy. The client should report any burning on urination or frequency.

Questions

1. Which of the following nursing interventions is usually the *least useful* in alleviating the client's anxiety before a painful diagnostic procedure?
   a. Emphasizing the technical details of the procedure
   b. Preparing the client on ways to cope with painful sensations
   c. Explaining the purposes of any pretest preparations
   d. Providing privacy to maintain self-esteem

2. Epinephrine may be added to a local anesthetic, such as lidocaine, to
   a. Increase the duration of local anesthesia and decrease bleeding
   b. Decrease the allergic effects of the anesthetic agent
   c. Maintain the blood pressure
   d. Cause vasodilation and better blood flow

3. A young boy, 7 years of age, must undergo bone marrow aspiration. Which of the following actions by the nurse would probably be *least helpful* in preparing him for this invasive procedure?
   a. Letting him play with replicas of some of the equipment
   b. Telling him how he can help during the procedure
   c. Explaining the reason for the procedure
   d. Telling briefly about how the procedure will feel (i.e., some pain)

4. A client has just undergone a lumbar puncture. Which of these factors seems to be the most important in preventing a spinal headache?
   a. Asking him to stay flat in bed for 24 hours after the procedure
   b. Maintaining nothing-by-mouth status for 2–3 hours before and after the procedure
   c. Encouraging fluids after the lumbar puncture
   d. Using prophylactic analgesics after the procedure

5. Which of the following nursing actions is *least* appropriate for the client, who just underwent thoracentesis? Four hundred milliliters of clear fluid were obtained from the right pleural space.
   a. Encouraging extra fluids to rehydrate her
   b. Assessing the thorax for diminished breath sounds
   c. Positioning her on her left side for 1 hour after the thoracentesis
   d. Reporting any symptoms of blood in the sputum (hemoptysis) or shortness of breath (dyspnea)

6. A client is to undergo abdominal paracentesis this morning. Which of the following nursing actions is not routine for this diagnostic procedure?
   a. Making sure that the client's bladder is empty
   b. Using sterile equipment for the procedure
   c. Helping the client assume a comfortable side-lying position for the procedure
   d. Letting the client eat as tolerated

7. A client is to undergo a liver biopsy today. Which of the following nursing actions is appropriate in preparing him for the liver biopsy?
   a. Have him practice holding his breath after inspiration
   b. Encourage fluids to keep him well hydrated
   c. Explain that a local anesthetic will be used to eliminate the pain
   d. Explain that he can resume normal activities as soon as the biopsy is finished and his vital signs are stable

8. A client has just returned from the radiology department, where she underwent a closed renal biopsy with local anesthesia. Which of the nursing actions is most appropriate?
   a. Have her stay as motionless as possible in bed for 30 minutes to 1 hour
   b. Save all urine in one container for a 24-hour urine sample
   c. Administer the ordered analgesic for pain at the biopsy site
   d. Restrict fluid intake to no more than 1,000 mL/day

References

Aschenbrenner, D. S. (2010). New indication and new vaccine for HPV. *American Journal of Nursing, 110*(2), 59.

Carroll, C. M. (2006). Sorting out breast biopsy options. *Nursing 2006, 36*(3), 70–71.

Deglin, J. H., Vallerand, A. H., & Sanoski, C. A. (2011). *Davis's drug guide for nurses* (12th ed.). Philadelphia: F. A. Davis.

Hay, W. W., Levin, M. J., Sondheimer, J. M., & Deterding, R. (Eds.). (2011). *Current diagnosis and treatment: Pediatrics* (20th ed.). New York: McGraw-Hill.

Heavey, E. (2008). Start early to prevent genital HPV infection and cervical cancer. *Nursing 2008, 38*(5), 62–63.

Heavey, E. (2010). An update on meningococcal meningitis. *Nursing 2010, 40*(10), 61–62.

Katzung, B., Masters, S. B., & Trevor, A. J. (Eds.). (2009). *Basic and clinical pharmacology* (11th ed.). New York: McGraw-Hill.

Lowy, D. R., & Schiller, J. (2006). Prophylactic human papillomavirus vaccines. *Journal of Clinical Investigation, 116*(5), 1167–1173.

McCarthy, A. M., Kleiber, C., Hanrahan, K., Zimmerman, M. B.,Westhus, N., & Allen, S. (2010). Factors explaining children's responses to intravenous needle insertions. *Nursing Research, 59*(6), 407–416.

McPhee, S. J., Papadakis, M. A., & Rabow, M. W. (Eds.). (2011). *Current medical diagnosis and treatment* (50th ed.). New York: McGraw-Hill.

Palefsky, J., Hecht, J., Riggs, J., & Scarce, M. (2007). Needed: Routine HPV and pap smears for gay and bisexual men. Retrieved April 27, 2011, from http://articles.sfgate.com/2007-04-24/opinion/17239060_1_cervical-cancer-precancerous-cells-pap-smear

Rushing, J. (2006). Assisting with bone marrow aspiration and biopsy. *Nursing 2006, 36*(3), 68.

Schiech, L. (2010). Cancer: An equal opportunity danger. *Nursing 2010, 40*(10), 23–28.

Wells, S. F. (2008). Cervical cancer: An overview with suggested practice and policy goals. *MEDSURG Nursing, 17*(8), 43–51.

Websites

www.cancer.org (American Cancer Society for information on cancer screening.)
www.fda.gov (Information on rapid diagnostic tests for cerebral spinal fluid.)

Answers

1. a, 2. a, 3. c, 4. c, 5. a, 6. c, 7. c, 8. c

- Stress Tests: ECG Treadmill Test
  and Exercise Tolerance Test   649
- Microvolt T-Wave Alternans   654
- Cardiac Catheterization   654

- Electrophysiologic Studies   660
- Tilt Table Testing   661
- Implantable Event Recorders   662

OBJECTIVES

1. Describe the general purposes of stress testing (exercise treadmill electrocardiograms [ECGs]) for healthy people and for those with heart disease.
2. Explain what nurses should teach clients about stress testing.
3. Describe appropriate nursing interventions before and after stress tests.
4. Explain how stress test results are used to plan activity levels.
5. Compare the purposes and procedures of right-sided and left-sided cardiac catheterizations and electrophysiologic studies (EPSs).
6. Describe appropriate nursing interventions before and after cardiac catheterization and EPS.
7. Identify expected effects of medications used before and during the cardiac tests discussed in this chapter.
8. Compare the tests used to investigate unexplained syncope.

Chapters 24 and 25 give basic information about noninvasive and invasive testing. This chapter discusses stress testing, a noninvasive test, which, unlike other noninvasive tests, is not risk free. Although stress testing is fairly common, it is not always well understood by nurses or the general community. Even if nurses are not involved in stress-testing procedures, they should be able to explain the test and the needed precautions to clients and their families. Stress tests can be very dangerous if not conducted properly. Nurses help prepare clients for the tests, sometimes help administer the test, and are more often involved in follow-up programs for cardiac rehabilitation.

Some other tests discussed in this chapter, cardiac catheterization, EPS, and implantable event recorders are sophisticated, invasive cardiac procedures.

The cardiac catheterization laboratory or the EPS laboratory not only requires elaborate equipment but also requires a team of highly skilled clinicians. A cardiologist trained to perform cardiac catheterization heads a team of technicians who are highly skilled in using the laboratory's monitoring equipment. In addition to

Table 26-1 Examples of Cardiovascular Diagnostic Procedures

Name of Exam	Key Points	Discussed in
Basic stress test	Client on a treadmill to assess angina and arrhythmias	Chap. 26
Echocardiograms	Ultrasound to assess structure of valves, chest wall movement, and ejection fraction. Stress testing with exercise or medications	Chap. 23
Radionuclide scans	Show perfusion of myocardium. Stress testing with exercise or medications	Chap. 22
ECG	Basic test—see new variations	Chap. 24
MTWA	Microvolt T-wave alternans test predicts risk of sudden cardiac death	Chap. 26
Event recorders	Holter monitors, implantable event recorders. Used to detect hard-to-diagnose arrhythmias	Chaps. 24 & 26
EPS	Electrophysiology studies of conduction system of heart to identify arrhythmias and assess effect of treatment	Chap. 26
Tilt table testing	Helpful in assessing syncope	Chap. 26
Cardiac catheterization	Coronary angiograms have been gold standard for diagnosing coronary artery disease (CAD) and other cardiac problems. Is invasive	Chap. 26
CT scans	Ultrafast scans using electron beam (EBCT) and 64 multi-slice detectors (MDCT) for CAD called noninvasive cardiac catheterization. Can also do coronary calcium scoring	Chap. 21
MRI	Very detailed images for a noninvasive cardiac catheterization. Cannot do calcium scores	Chap. 21
PET scans	Show functional information-fusion scan combined with CT to show structures	Chap. 21
SPECT scans	Cheaper than PET to show cardiac functioning. Fusion scan combined with CT to show function	Chap. 21
Vascular screening	Ultrasound scans to detect risk for stroke, abdominal aneurysm, and peripheral vascular disease	Chap. 23

being an assistant during the procedure, the nurse may also help prepare the client for the procedure and conduct follow-up assessment. Tilt table testing is also conducted in a special laboratory. Highly sophisticated, noninvasive CT and/or MRI scans may lessen the need for invasive procedures such as cardiac catheterization and EPS. Currently CT or MRI may be part of a cardiac catheterization laboratory. See Table 26–1 for a quick summary of key points about many cardiovascular diagnostic procedures discussed in this chapter and elsewhere in this book.

STRESS TESTS: ECG TREADMILL TEST AND EXERCISE TOLERANCE TEST

Description. The forerunner of the modern heart stress test was the Master's two-step test, which involved stepping up and down on a 20-cm platform 30 times a minute while an ECG recorded the effect of the stress on the heart. The modern stress

Table 26–2 Determining Target Heart Rate for Men		
Formula	Subtract current age from 220 and multiply results by 65% and by 85%.[a]	
Example	$220 - 56 = 164$ $\qquad$ $164 \times 65\% = 106$ $\qquad$ $164 \times 85\% = 139$	
Target rate	This client, who is 56 years of age, needs to sustain a heart rate of 106–139 beats per minute for an aerobic workout. He is asked to exercise up to 139 beats per minute in a stress test.	

test is performed in a cardiology laboratory, which is set up to monitor blood pressure, ECG, and sometimes oxygen consumption, while the client exercises by walking on a treadmill. The treadmill is accelerated at intervals, and the pitch is changed to determine the exercise tolerance of the person. The test is continued until a predetermined end point has been obtained or the client shows signs of undue fatigue. A stationary exercise bicycle called a bicycle ergometer, which is portable and less expensive than a treadmill, can be used. However, it is not so easy to standardize the results because many clients develop thigh muscle fatigue before they reach their maximum heart rate. The bicycle ergometer is more common in Europe.

When exercise tolerance is assessed in clients with cardiac disease, a physician must be present so the test can be stopped if symptoms or dangerous arrhythmias develop. For a healthy client undergoing exercise tolerance testing, a physician or qualified delegate can observe the client's response while the client is using the treadmill. Examination for stress exercise testing is given by the American College of Sports Medicine (www.acsm.org). Nurses must realize that stress testing can be dangerous if not conducted properly. Only qualified personnel should conduct the tests. The American Heart Association has excellent information on quality control for operation of an exercise tolerance laboratory.

Before beginning the test, the client must be told exactly what to expect and that he or she can stop the test at any time, but the test is of greater value if the exercise is continued until a predetermined level is obtained. The predetermined levels are based on the client's age and expected response to a certain level of exercise. The target heart rate to be achieved is up to 85% of the maximal heart rate for a certain age. There are different formulas based not only on age but also for gender (Gulati et al., 2010). See Table 26–2 for the formula for men and Table 26–3 for the formula for women.

Table 26–3 Determining Target Heart Rate for Women		
Formula	Multiply current age $\times$ 0.88 and subtract the results from 206. Multiply those results by 65% and by 85% to get target heart rate.	
Example	$56\,(0.88) = 49$ $\qquad$ $206 - 49 = 157$ $157\,(.65) = 102$ $\qquad$ $157(.85) = 133$	
Target rate	This woman, who is 56 years of age, needs to sustain a heart rate of 102–133 per minute for an aerobic workout. For a stress test, she should exercise up to 133 beats per minute.	

See Gulati et al. (2010) for evidence of differences in heart rate response to exercise stress testing in women.

Table 26–4 Example of Stages for Exercise Treadmill Testing (Bruce Protocol)

Stage	mph	km/hr	Grade (%)
1	1.7	2.7	10
2	2.5	4.0	12
3	3.4	5.4	14
4	4.2	6.7	16
5	5.0	8.0	18
6	5.5	8.8	20
7	6.0	9.6	22

Note: The grade and miles per hour (mph) are increased every 3 minutes until the target rate is achieved as discussed in the text. Some institutions have modified the Bruce protocol, which was first published in 1963.

The client is connected to the apparatus necessary to monitor ECG and blood pressure. If oxygen consumption is measured, a mouthpiece is used. Baseline measurements are taken in advance, and the physician performs a brief physical examination to clear the client for the test.

The characteristic sign of myocardial ischemia is a depressed ST segment. However, some clients have a drop in the ST segment when hyperventilating, so before the treadmill is started, an ECG is obtained while the patient is standing still and hyperventilating. After the client has a chance to practice walking on the treadmill, the test is begun with the increases in grade and miles per hour shown in Table 26–4. The ECG, blood pressure, and pulse are constantly monitored and fed into a computer for analysis. The development of a computer-aided method of analyzing treadmill exercise tests eliminates some of the false positives that were common before computers were used. In addition to the concern for false-positive results, false-negative results also occur.

During the test, clinicians assess for symptoms, such as vertigo, extreme dyspnea, pallor, or signs of exhaustion. Depending on the ECG reading and other circumstances, the client may be allowed to continue with mild or moderate angina, but severe angina necessitates an abrupt end to the test. Leg fatigue or severe pain in the calves (claudication) may also necessitate cessation of the test.

Other reasons to stop the test are:

1. Decrease in systolic blood pressure of 22 mm Hg
2. Marked ST-segment depression
3. Ventricular tachycardia (VT)
4. Heart block, second or third degree
5. Atrial fibrillation (AF)
6. Paroxysmal atrial tachycardia (PAT)

Some clients do have occasional ectopic beats with exercise, so a few premature atrial contractions (PACs) or even premature ventricular contractions (PVCs) are not indications to stop the test if there is no clinical evidence of a change in cardiac output. (See Chapter 24 for a detailed discussion on common types of arrhythmias and clinical assessment for changes in cardiac output.)

Nuclear Cardiology Stress Tests and Echocardiography Stress Tests

A stress echocardiogram can provide additional information. The client exercises on a treadmill and then undergoes an ultrasound scan. A dobutamine echocardiogram may be done if the client cannot exercise (Chapter 23). Also radionuclide studies with thallium-201 and Tc-99m sestamibi may be used to highlight the difference in coronary perfusion at rest and exercise. If clients cannot exercise, they may be given adenosine or dipyridamole as explained in Chapter 22. But these drugs can cause bronchospasms in clients with reactive airway disease (Fenimore, 2010). See Table 26–1 for a comparison of the types of stress tests.

Assessing Exercise Tolerance

In the planning of exercise programs, stress tests are administered to evaluate the exercise tolerance of the client. The information from a stress test is useful in planning a graduated exercise program. The exercise tolerance of clients with known heart disease also is evaluated. For example, a client with an uncomplicated myocardial infarction most likely undergoes an exercise test before discharge from the hospital. A long-term follow-up study of clients who underwent exercise screening tests after a myocardial infarction demonstrated that three findings were strong, independent predictors of cardiovascular mortality. These three predictors, after control for clinical variables, were (1) a hypotensive blood pressure response, (2) ST-segment depression, and (3) ST-segment elevation. Clients who have these findings on a stress test may benefit from close surveillance in the years after an infarction.

Pretest Nursing Implications Related to Stress Tests

Obtaining Informed Consent. Although a stress test can yield valuable information, it is not risk free, even when clients have been carefully screened. The exercise, which is equal in stress to walking briskly or running up a steep hill, can cause severe arrhythmias, a myocardial infarction, or a stroke in susceptible clients. Most authorities quote a mortality of about 0.01%, or one death in every 10,000 clients who undergo the test. Because of the morbidity and mortality, the client must sign an informed consent after the physician explains the benefits in relation to the risks. The nurse can reassure the client that trained personnel and emergency equipment are available in the laboratory to deal with any complications that may occur.

Clients need written information about stress tests, including the risks and benefits of the test. Clients should be given time to digest verbal and written information and then make an informed decision. (See Chapter 25 for more about the role of the nurse as the advocate for the client who is undergoing invasive tests or tests that can cause complications.)

Limiting Food and Fluid Intake. The client should eat a light meal 2 hours before the test. Some clinicians prefer that the client have no beverages containing caffeine, whereas others allow 1 cup of coffee or tea before the test. Milk or other foods that may cause nausea during exercise should be avoided. The client should be adequately hydrated before the test. Some procedures, particularly those with radionuclides, require the client to take nothing by mouth for 4 hours before the test.

Administering Medications. If the client is taking diuretics, assessment of the serum potassium level is completed before the exercise test. Hypokalemia, often a side effect of diuretics, predisposes the client to arrhythmias. Nitroglycerin or other vasodilators are not given before the test, unless the test is being given to evaluate the efficacy of the medications. The nurse must confer with the physician to see what medications are permissible before the test. For example, β-blockers make the test useless because they decrease the response to exercise. Clients need clear instructions on which routine medications are to be continued and which are to be withheld.

Clothing Needs. Comfortable walking shoes are a must for the test. Bedroom slippers, sandals, or high-heeled shoes are unsatisfactory. Rubber-soled shoes provide the best grip on the treadmill.

Men wear no clothes on the upper body, so electrodes can be applied to the chest. Women can wear a bra and a hospital gown or blouse that opens in the front. A bra may interfere with imaging if a nuclear stress test is performed. Breast markers may be needed to avoid breast artifacts. Pants, skirts, or trousers should be loose and comfortable because electrodes are placed on the extremities. Constricting clothing and nylon fabrics are to be avoided. Hair should be arranged off the face, and any bothersome jewelry should be removed.

Resting Before the Test. A good night's sleep before the test is essential so that undue fatigue is not a factor in the results. Relaxation exercises before the test may be beneficial. The client performs warming-up exercises and cooling-down exercises in the laboratory.

Posttest Nursing Implications Related to Stress Tests

Assessing Vital Signs. The client remains in the cardiology laboratory until vital signs are normal. To ensure that levels have returned to baseline, ECG tracings are taken at various intervals. Rarely, the client may need to be monitored for several hours because of arrhythmias or other complications.

Resuming Activities After Radionuclide Testing. If nuclear scanning has been performed as part of the stress test, more testing is done in 2–4 hours. Clients may be allowed a light meal, but this should be verified with the nuclear medicine department. (See Chapter 22 for precautions about urine after radionuclide testing.)

Follow-up Plans. An individualized exercise program is planned on the basis of the results of the stress test. An ideal exercise plan is one that helps the client achieve target heart rate for 20 minutes three times a week. Target heart rates are usually 65–85% of the client's maximum heart rate. A target rate of 65% of the maximal heart rate strengthens the lungs, heart, and circulatory system while the upper limit of 85% of the maximal heart rate builds endurance. See Table 26–2 for the formula for men and Table 26–3 for the formula for women. The American Heart Association (www.heart.org) has detailed guidelines for exercise prescriptions. Whatever the length and type of exercise prescribed by the physician, it is important that the client also understand the importance of warm-up and cool-down exercises.

(Continued)

Posttest Nursing Implications . . . (Continued)

If the stress test is given to evaluate angina and coronary ischemia, more diagnostic tests may be ordered by the physician. For example, the client may need instructions about cardiac catheterizations discussed later in this chapter.

MICROVOLT T-WAVE ALTERNANS

In most clients, the T wave on an ECG (Chapter 24) has the same size and shape, but sometimes the T wave varies with every other beat. The change is too small to be seen on a regular ECG but can be detected with an equipment that filters and processes the signals from the heart. This test that detects microvolt T-wave alternans (MTWA) was originally developed to check astronauts for early warning of arrhythmias. People who have T-wave alternans are at increased risk for developing ventricular tachycardia and ventricular fibrillation. The T wave reflects subtle changes in how cardiac cells handle calcium.

Accurate reflection by MTWA helps identify those who would benefit from an implantable cardioverter defibrillator (ICD) (Haghjoo, Arva, & Sadr-Ameli, 2006). Medicare pays for the test ($300–400) for clients who are at risk for sudden cardiac death.

Description of Test

The test is similar to the exercise stress test discussed earlier in this chapter. (See the nursing implications for the exercise part.) Fourteen electrodes are connected to the chest by small suction cups. Recordings are made while the client is seated, on a treadmill, and resting after the exercise. The total time is about 30 minutes.

Clinical Significance

A positive test may indicate the need for an ICD, whereas a negative test usually indicates that the ICD is not necessary.

CARDIAC CATHETERIZATION

Description

A cardiac catheterization is performed under local anesthesia because the client needs to cooperate by performing deep breathing and coughing maneuvers. (Coughing helps clear the contrast agent from the coronary arteries.) The client may also be asked to perform bicycle-type leg exercises to see the effect of stress on cardiac function and coronary blood flow. (Small children undergo catheterization under general anesthesia.) Depending on the information needed, a catheter may be inserted into a vein for a study of the right side of the heart or into an artery (usually the femoral artery, but the radial artery may also be used) for a study of the left side of the heart. The catheter for cardiac catheterization is a flexible, hollow tube 100 cm (40 inches) long. For a left-sided catheterization, an artery is punctured with a short stubby needle and a guide wire is inserted. The catheter slides over the guide wire into the artery. The guide wire makes it possible to guide the catheter through the left atrium into the left ventricle.

Fluoroscopy is used to view the catheter; the room must be darkened. (See Chapter 20 for a discussion on fluoroscopy.) For a right-sided catheterization, a vein is used, and the catheter is threaded through the vena cava into the right atrium and right ventricle.

A transseptal technique uses a small needle inserted in the right side of the heart. The needle is gently maneuvered through the septum to obtain pressure readings and blood samples from the left side of the heart. In some cases of aortic stenosis, the heart valve cannot be crossed in the usual manner, and a transseptal technique is needed.

After the pressure readings and blood samples are obtained, a catheter is threaded into the coronary artery, and a radiopaque contrast agent is inserted to outline the coronary arteries. This contrast agent contains iodine. (See Chapter 20 for the precautions when a contrast agent with iodine is used for a diagnostic procedure.) During the passage of the contrast agent, the room is darkened so that the motion can be observed on the fluoroscope screen. Movies (cineography) may also be taken of the flow of the contrast agent. The table is tilted to help with contrast agent flow. Ultrasound may also be used (Chapter 23).

The entire procedure of a left-sided and right-sided cardiac catheterization takes about 1–2 hours, depending on the findings. However, clients may not need all the different aspects performed. For example, an adolescent with a valve defect may not undergo studies of the coronary arteries.

Because cardiac catheterization is an elaborate procedure that requires a specialized laboratory setup, it is not performed in small hospitals or clinics. The University of California, San Francisco (UCSF) was the first imaging suite to combine MRI with a cardiac catheterization laboratory. The new system allows the placement of stents or other devices by using a combination of x-ray and MRI (XMR) guidance.

Purposes

As mentioned earlier in this chapter, a stress test may be a preliminary test before cardiac catheterization. Cardiac catheterization is used when noninvasive forms of cardiac diagnostic tests—such as ECGs (Chapter 24), computed tomography (CT) or magnetic resonance imaging (MRI) (Chapter 21), and radionuclide scans (Chapter 22)—have not provided enough diagnostic information. As with any invasive procedure, there is some risk to the client. If less complicated, less risky, and less costly procedures will suffice, they are preferred.

Cardiac catheterization is often needed to confirm the patency of coronary arteries. For example, the need for a coronary bypass procedure is assessed with cardiac catheterization, which demonstrates the lack of coronary perfusion. Since 1979, when percutaneous transluminal angioplasty (PCTA) was introduced, many other types of percutaneous coronary interventions (PCIs) have been developed to improve coronary perfusion. These various interventions may be done immediately following a cardiac catheterization. Cardiac catheterization also defines the nature of other cardiac problems, especially congenital heart defects (Hay et al., 2011). Cardiac catheterization can also help determine the severity of heart disease and evaluate the progress of the client after medical or surgical intervention.

Conventional cardiac catheterization measures the pressures and calculates the flows in the various chambers of the heart and great vessels. Blood samples are obtained to measure dilutions of contrast agent and oxygen and carbon dioxide values. Radiopaque contrast agent is used in radiography and fluoroscopy of the heart and vessels.

Pretest Nursing Implications Related to Cardiac Catheterization

Checking the Chart. The client's chart should contain the results of other diagnostic tests, such as coagulation studies and hematocrit (Hct). In addition, vital signs and other baseline data are charted as for other invasive procedures (Chapter 25). The precatheterization physical stability of the client must be assessed and documented. For example, strokes do occur as a complication of cardiac catheterization, so a careful neurologic evaluation before the procedure makes evaluation afterward more reliable.

Although the risks of serious complications, such as a myocardial infarction or cerebrovascular accident, are slight, they sometimes occur with a catheterization. Thus, the client must sign a consent form that lists the possible complications, including such things as the possibility of a loss of a limb or cardiac arrest. The client's physician must explain the possibility of such risks in relation to the potential greater benefits of the procedure.

Physical Preparation of Client. Clients may fast 3–8 hours before the procedure. Peripheral pulses should be assessed and the skin over the pulse points marked with ink to assist with posttest assessment. The client's groin, used for the femoral puncture, should have the hair clipped. If needed, shaving may be performed on the unit or in the laboratory. The client should void and empty his or her bowels, if possible, because the procedure is a long one. The client is transported to the laboratory on a gurney. A hospital gown is worn. Glasses can be worn, as can a watch, because the client is awake. Dentures are left in place because they may be needed if the client is to perform any breathing exercises with a mouthpiece. Hearing aids should be worn if needed. The client's chart should document the presence of a hearing difficulty or any communication problems.

Use of Medications Before and During the Procedure. Routine medications are usually not withheld, but this should be checked with the cardiologist. Some drugs, such as long-term anticoagulants, are usually contraindicated before the procedure because of the risk of bleeding. Thus, if a client has been taking warfarin, this must be evaluated by the physician. Heparin is used during the procedure. The premedications differ from institution to institution. Some cardiologists prefer no sedation for clients. Others routinely order a sedative. Antihistamines or a cortisone preparation may be ordered for clients who are allergy prone. Some institutions have a policy to give cortisone or antihistamine drugs 1–2 days before cardiac catheterization. Test doses of the contrast medium also may be given. During the procedure, the client may be given vasodilators, such as nitroglycerin, to promote arterial dilation or ergonovine to constrict the arteries. Pain medications, other than a local anesthetic, are not routine before or during the procedure. More than one intravenous infusion may be started in the laboratory. Protamine is given at the end of the procedure to neutralize the effect of heparin. Clients who take NPH insulin may have antibodies to protamine and thus have an allergic reaction (Deglin, Vallerand, & Sanoski, 2011). Emergency drugs should be readily available. Manipulation of the catheter can stimulate the vagus nerve and cause bradycardia, so atropine should be one of the emergency drugs. In the past, when catheters were larger, atropine was used routinely before catheterization.

Some research supports the use of N-acetylcysteine to prevent contrast-induced nephropathy (CIN) in clients having an angioplasty (Marenzi et al., 2006) Intravenous doses may be given before the intervention and oral doses or 48 hours after the intervention. See Chapter 20 for more information on CIN.

Pretest Nursing Diagnoses Related to Cardiac Catheterization

Anxiety Related to Lack of Knowledge About Procedure

A nurse from the cardiac catheterization laboratory or from the general unit should reinforce the explanation of the cardiac catheterization procedure. Most cardiac catheterization laboratories have client information booklets that describe the procedure and answer common questions that clients may have about the preparation for the test. Some institutions use audiovisual material to explain the cardiac catheterization procedure. This can be accomplished the morning of the examination. Past studies have not shown whether it is more or less effective to have clients visit the cardiac laboratory before the procedure. Without adequate preparation, viewing the "cath lab" may be anxiety producing.

Now that most cardiac catheterizations are done on an outpatient basis, the primary caregiver at home needs education and support, too. Caring for clients must remain the focus of nurses, even though technology seems to make procedures easier and faster.

Risk for Pain and Discomfort from Cardiac Catheterization

Some clients experience much discomfort during a cardiac catheterization, whereas others do not. The anxiety level of the client seems to be an important factor. Sedatives may be given intravenously during the procedure. Certainly, the idea of a catheter entering one's heart is a frightening idea. The nurse should explain to the client that he or she may experience a small amount of discomfort so that he or she does not imagine the worst. Because the positioning of the catheter may cause a rapid or irregular pulse, the client may feel his or her heart "flip-flop" or race. Therefore, it may be comforting for the client to know that arrhythmias are common during the threading of the catheter and usually disappear without treatment. The client should be told that there will be constant monitoring for serious arrhythmias and that emergency equipment and drugs are present for immediate use. Clients should also be aware that a vigorous cough may suddenly be needed if they have an arrhythmia. This cough cardiopulmonary resuscitation (CPR) can help convert a potentially lethal ventricular arrhythmia to a normal sinus rhythm. The cough closes the epiglottis and increases intrathoracic pressure, which increases blood flow through the heart; hence coronary ischemia may be decreased.

Another discomfort is a venous or, even more so, an arterial puncture. A local anesthetic is used before an arterial puncture, but there is usually some pain associated with the procedure. Needles in general are very unpleasant for some clients. (See Chapter 25 on ways nurses can help prepare clients for momentary pain.) The injection of the contrast agent may be a source of pain or discomfort for some clients, because of a metallic taste, a warm feeling, or a more intense rush from the contrast agent. (The symptoms of an allergic reaction can occur, but this is not common; see Chapter 20.) Another discomfort may be the length of time the client must lie relatively still on the table—this may be very taxing for some clients.

Posttest Nursing Diagnoses Related to Cardiac Catheterization

Risk for Altered Cardiac Output

Vital signs are checked the same as for other invasive procedures. Arrhythmias usually occur during the procedure, not afterward, but an apical pulse should be part of the assessment each time the client's vital signs are taken. If there is any arrhythmia, the client may need to be monitored for a time. (See Chapter 24 on monitoring.) An intravenous line is kept open (k/o rate) if arrhythmias have persisted. (See Chapter 20 on anaphylactic reactions from contrast medium, which could also cause altered cardiac output.)

Risk for Altered Tissue Perfusion

Because more than one entry site may be used, the nurse needs to check for more than one bandaged area after catheterization. Occasionally, a surgical cutdown may be performed to find the vessel for the catheter. If so, the client has skin sutures at the cutdown site.

The outside of the pressure dressing should be checked for any bleeding or hematoma formation. The pulse distal to the arterial puncture site should be checked and compared with the uninvolved site for a thrombus in the artery. Spasms of the artery can also cause diminished arterial flow. The venous site is less likely to have any serious complications. Phlebitis (inflammation of the vein) can develop later and may be relieved with warm compresses.

Nurses caring for clients after cardiac catheterization and PCI procedures must understand the difference in the three methods of arterial closure after the procedure, as this helps determine restrictions on activity. The three methods are (1) pull, (2) plug, and (3) close. In the first method, the catheter is pulled, and manual compression or some type of pressure device is applied for 20–60 minutes. The client remains immobile with the leg extended for 3–6 hours. For the second method, collagen is applied on the external surface of the femoral artery followed by 5 minutes of compression. The client may ambulate after an hour. If the device fails to seal properly, abdominal distention can occur due to retroperitoneal bleeding. The last method involves local anesthetic and sutures to close the arterial puncture. Clients may sit up soon after the procedure and be ambulatory after 2 hours. Another type of closure device uses polyethylene glycol, which is applied over the puncture site when the catheter is removed. This sealant absorbs blood and other fluids and expands to three to four times its original size to close the arterial puncture site. The sealant dissolves within 30 days (www.accessclosure.com). Nurses outside the cardiac catheterization laboratory may be responsible for removing femoral sheaths, so each facility must develop protocols for client management. Protocols should include desired parameters for laboratory values and how to manage adverse reactions such as bleeding (Dressler & Dressler, 2006; Huber, 2009).

Risk for Deficient Fluid Volume

The client can eat and drink as soon as he or she desires. An adequate intake of fluids is needed to help with excretion of the contrast agent. The contrast agent, a hypertonic solution, can produce a fluid volume deficit.

Pain Related to Complications

Back pain from the positioning is common, and a backrub may be helpful. Mild analgesics may be needed for pain at the puncture site. Pain distal to the puncture site is not expected and could mean an embolus to the extremity.

Clients undergoing catheterization usually exhibit some of the following symptoms: fatigue, dyspnea on exertion, edema, paroxysmal nocturnal dyspnea (PND), or angina. Nurses need to know what symptoms were present before catheterization so that new symptoms can be identified and called to the physician's attention. New symptoms should not be masked by pain medication. Clients can have delayed allergic reactions to the iodine contrast agent, so the nurse must keep this in mind when assessing any pain or discomfort. (See Chapter 20 on radiopaque contrast agents.)

Risk for Injury Related to Cardiac Tamponade and Other Complications

In addition to arrhythmias, emboli, and infarctions, cardiac tamponade can occur after cardiac catheterization. Bleeding into the pericardial sac causes reduced cardiac output, because the heart is compressed in the pericardial sac. Symptoms of cardiac tamponade include anxiety, tachypnea, distended neck veins (when the client sits forward), muffled heart sounds, narrowing pulse pressure, and a paradoxical pulse. To detect a paradoxical pulse, the nurse must take the systolic blood pressure during inspiration and expiration, noting if the systolic pressure is less during inspiration. A difference of more than 10 mm Hg in the two is evidence of a paradoxical pulse. Any questionable symptoms or marked change in vital signs should be immediately called to the attention of the physician. Ultrasound (Chapter 23) is used to assess pericardial bleeding. Although cardiac tamponade and other complications are unlikely after cardiac catheterization, they can occur, and a prudent nurse is always alert for adverse reactions after all invasive tests.

Deficient Knowledge Related to Home Care

In the past, clients were admitted to the hospital for cardiac catheterization. Now catheterizations are performed as both inpatient and outpatient procedures. Even clients with PCI may be discharged within a day, so they must know how to recognize adverse reactions and low to take extra care of the groin site, which may have bruising and a small bump (Dressler & Dressler, 2006). Institutions provide written discharge instructions that include the information discussed earlier and specific guidelines for activities and care of the insertion site. For example, no bending or squatting or unnecessary activity should be performed the evening after the catheterization. A reclining position may be better than sitting. If the client feels or notices any bleeding, direct hand pressure should be applied to the site and the physician called for instructions.

The next day, the client can gradually resume some activity with no heavy lifting or exercise. The dressing can be removed during a shower and replaced with a small dry dressing, which is then changed daily until healing occurs. Clients should avoid baths or swimming until the site is healed. If stitches were used, they should be removed in about 1 week. The physician should also state when the client can return to work and how much exercise is allowed the first week.

ELECTROPHYSIOLOGIC STUDIES

EPSs are performed under laboratory conditions similar to those for cardiac catheterization. Electrodes that can both pace and stimulate the rhythm of the heart are connected to catheters that are inserted through the femoral, brachial, or basilic vein to the right side of the heart. Arterial catheters are used if there is a need to stimulate the left ventricle. A typical study may require three to six of these intracardiac pacing catheters. The intracardiac ECG is reported simultaneously with the regular or surface ECG (Chapter 24). This very sophisticated monitoring can give a detailed evaluation of the entire conduction system with mapping of both normal and abnormal (aberrant) pathways. EPSs are also useful to evaluate if dangerous arrhythmias can be induced. An arrhythmia may be artificially induced in a drug-free state to try to assess what has caused syncope or a previous cardiac arrest. Induction of an arrhythmia is also attempted after the client has reached a steady state with an antiarrhythmic drug to see if the drug does prevent the arrhythmia. If the drug fails the test (i.e., the arrhythmia can be elicited with an EPS), another antiarrhythmic drug is tried, and the EPS is performed again when the drug produces a steady state.

In the past few years, nonpharmacological control of arrhythmias by the ablation of abnormal cardiac pathways and the use of ICDs has lessened the need for long-term use of antiarrhythmics for serious arrhythmias (Katzung, Masters, & Trevor, 2009). EPS is used as part of the procedure for assessing the effects of catheter ablation procedures or antitachycardia devices (McPhee, Papadakis, & Rabow, 2011).

In the past, clients needed to have EPS and be refractory to medications before being considered for an ICD. Now the use of this device without intensive EPS is becoming standard practice. (See the earlier discussion on MTWA.) An ICD can be placed using a transvenous approach. The newer models can be programmed to override various arrhythmias before they progress to ventricular fibrillation. Thus the client may be spared the painful shocks needed to stop ventricular fibrillation (Sossong, 2006). The ICD is considered very effective in more than 89% of cases for preventing a sudden cardiac death (SCD) from a lethal arrhythmia (Moorman, 2010). In addition to the implantable device, an automatic wearable cardioverter defibrillator (WCD), available since 1992, may be a lifesaver for some clients, because early defibrillation is one of the most important interventions in saving a client from SCD (Morrison & Smith, 2009).

Recent progress in ICD technology includes ICD monitoring by telephone. Research supports that follow-up care by nurses continues to be important to address fears and concerns about the effects of ICD monitoring on lifestyle (Flanagan, Carroll, & Hamilton, 2010).

Pretest Nursing Implications Related to Electrophysiologic Studies

Although the physical and psychological preparation for an EPS is similar to that for a cardiac catheterization, the risk for anxiety may be even greater. During an EPS, arrhythmias are purposely induced, and the client may experience a life-threatening arrhythmia that requires emergency drug therapy or defibrillation. Also, some clients have to undergo several EPSs to find and evaluate an effective drug for their particular type of arrhythmia. EPSs are performed in large medical centers where specialists in cardiovascular nursing are available to help clients understand the purpose of repeated EPSs and to deal with the fear that an EPS can generate.

Posttest Nursing Implications Related to Electrophysiologic Studies

The nursing implications for care after cardiac catheterization also apply to an EPS. Sometimes a catheter may be left in place because of the need to repeat a study. The client may stay flat for 4 hours and then be propped up with pillows. The leg should be kept straight with no bending at the groin. A small bedpan creates less need to bend the leg than does a conventional bedpan. The client should be turned toward the side of the puncture. If using a bedpan seems to put strain on the groin site, the client may need to have a Foley catheter inserted. Lines left in place for repeat EPSs require specific orders for the care and flushing of the catheter.

TILT TABLE TESTING

For testing of the autonomic system's reaction to a rapid change of position, clients may be taken to the laboratory for a tilt table test. The test may help rule out a cardiac origin for the syncope. The client is placed on a tilt table, and blood pressure and pulse are monitored in the supine position for a period of time. Then the tilt table is elevated, head up to at least 70°, to see if the client has a significant drop in blood pressure, pulse, and symptoms of syncope. Syncope may occur due to hypotension, bradycardia, or tachycardia. Drugs such as isoproterenol may be infused as part of the test, or sublingual nitroglycerin may be used (McPhee et al., 2011).

In general when a client moves to a standing position, the autonomic nervous system achieves orthostatic stability in 60 seconds or less. The heart rate may increase 10–20 beats per minute with a simultaneous increase in diastolic blood pressure by 5–10 mm Hg. However, there is only a slight change in systolic blood pressure. One variation of orthostatic intolerance is referred to as postural orthostatic tachycardia syndrome (POTS). In this condition, the pulse increases 30 beats or more usually without a decrease in blood pressure (Grossman & McGowan, 2008). When a client has an abnormal tilt test, further testing is required to determine the cause of the imbalance. Clients who are prone to dizziness when standing should be taught to rise slowly from a lying position. Dangling at the side of the bed; contracting the abdominal muscles, buttocks, and legs; and flexing the feet may help. Clients should also avoid prolonged hot showers or standing for long periods of time while their conditions are being evaluated.

IMPLANTABLE EVENT RECORDERS

Sometimes it is very difficult to determine if syncope is due to neurological or cardiac conditions. The usual approach to assess clients with unexplained syncope involves the use of ambulatory ECG (Chapter 24), tilt table testing, and electrophysiological testing, both discussed earlier. A newer technology, the implantable event recorder (ILR) may have merit as a strategy for clients with unexplained syncope. The device, inserted under the skin like a pacemaker, may be in place for a year. When syncope or other symptoms occur, the client or another person uses an activator to save an ECG record for a time before, during, and after the episode. If the client is unconscious or not able to activate the device, it will go to auto-activation mode when the pulse falls above or below programmed limits. A health care provider accesses the stored information later.

Questions

1. A client asks the nurse why the physician has ordered a nuclear cardiology stress test rather than a conventional stress test. The nurse should base an answer on the fact that radionuclides are used with an exercise stress test for
   a. Assessing the location of partially obstructed coronary arteries
   b. Evaluating exercise tolerance after a myocardial infarction
   c. Evaluating myocardial perfusion during exercise
   d. Assessing the relation between arrhythmias and stress level

2. A client, 48 years of age, is scheduled for a stress test tomorrow because she has had some heart palpitations while exercising. She asks the clinic nurse about the procedure. The nurse would be correct in informing her that
   a. Blood pressure cuff and electrocardiogram leads are used during the test
   b. A treadmill is adjusted to decreasing and increasing speeds during the test
   c. If she has any angina, the test will be stopped
   d. Clients must be admitted to the hospital in preparation for the test

3. A client has been scheduled for a stress test in the cardiology laboratory tomorrow morning. He had an uncomplicated myocardial infarction a week ago. Which of the following nursing interventions is most appropriate in preparing him for the test?
   a. Reassuring him that there are no risks from the test
   b. Instructing him to consume nothing by mouth for 12 hours before the test
   c. Giving him nitroglycerin tablets, if needed, before the test
   d. Asking his family to bring his walking shoes for the test

4. A client, 16 years of age, is to undergo cardiac catheterization, right-sided and left-sided, this morning. She takes digitalis and consumes a no-added-salt (NAS) diet. Which of the following is not an appropriate nursing action in preparing her for the cardiac catheterization?
   a. Checking to see if all ordered laboratory reports are on the chart, such as PT, PTT, and Hct
   b. Allowing liquids but withholding all oral medicines
   c. Explaining that she will be awake and that she will be asked to do such maneuvers as coughing and deep breathing during the procedure
   d. Allowing her to wear her glasses and a watch to the cardiac catheterization laboratory

5. A client was given atropine sulfate during the cardiac catheterization procedure. The desired effect of atropine in relation to cardiac catheterization is to
   a. Promote sedation
   b. Decrease respiratory secretions
   c. Prevent bradycardia
   d. Eliminate gastrointestinal spasms

6. A client has just returned from the cardiac catheterization laboratory. She underwent a right-sided and left-sided (left femoral artery was used) catheterization with no complications, except a minor arrhythmia during the procedure. Her vital signs are stable. Which nursing action is unnecessary for the first hour that she is back on the unit?
   a. Keeping the left leg immobilized
   b. Offering her something to drink and telling her fluids help eliminate the contrast agent
   c. Checking the pulses distal to the left femoral artery and comparing these with the pulses in the right foot
   d. Taking her temperature every 15 minutes three times

References

Deglin, J. H., Vallerand, A. H., & Sanoski, C. A. (2011). *Davis's drug guide for nurses* (12th ed.). Philadelphia: F. A. Davis.

Dressler, D. K., & Dressler, K. (2006). Caring for patients with femoral sheaths. *American Journal of Nursing, 106*(5), 64A–64H.

Fenimore, G. S. (2010). Evaluating CAD with a pharmacological stress test. *Nursing 2010, 40*(5), 51–52.

Flanagan, J. M., Carroll, D. L., & Hamilton, G. A. (2010). The long-term lived experience of patients with implantable cardioverter defibrillators. *MEDSURG Nursing, 19*(2), 113–119.

Grossman, V. G. A., & McGowan, B. A. (2008). Postural orthostatic tachycardia syndrome. *American Journal of Nursing, 108*(8), 58–60.

Gulati, M., Shaw, L., Thisted, R. A., Black, H. R., Merz, C. N. B., & Arnsdorf, M. F. (2010). Exercise physiology: Heart rate response to exercise stress testing in asymptomatic women. *Circulation, 122*(2), 130–137.

Haghjoo, M., Arva, A., & Sadr-Ameli, M. (2006). Value of microvolt T-wave alternans for predicting patients who would benefit from implantable cardioverter-defibrillator therapy. *Cardiology Review, 14*(4), 173–179.

Hay, W. W., Levin, M. J., Sondheimer, J. M., & Deterding, R. (Eds.). (2011). *Current diagnosis and treatment: Pediatrics* (20th ed.). New York: McGraw-Hill.

Huber, C. (2009). Safety after cardiac catheterization: Minimizing vascular complications. *American Journal of Nursing, 109*(8), 57–58.

Katzung, B., Masters, S. B., & Trevor, A. J. (Eds.). (2009). *Basic and clinical pharmacology* (11th ed.). New York: McGraw-Hill.

Marenzi, G., Assanelli, E., Marana, I., Lauri, G., Campodonico, J., Grazi, M., et al. (2006). N-acetylcysteine and contrast-induced nephropathy in primary angioplasty. *New England Journal of Medicine, 354*(26), 2773–2782.

McPhee, S. J., Papadakis, M. A., & Rabow, M. W. (Eds.). (2011). *Current medical diagnosis and treatment* (50th ed.). New York: McGraw-Hill.

Moorman, L. P. (2010). Implantable cardioverter-defibrillator: Just another device. *American Nurse Today, 5*(1), 12–14.

Morrison, D., & Smith, J. (2009). Taking a vested interest in a wearable. *Nursing 2009, 39*(6), 30–32.

Sossong, A. (2006). About implantable cardioverter defibrillators. *Nursing 2006, 36*(11), 66.

Websites

www.accessclosure.com (Information on a sealant used to close arterial puncture sites.)
www.acsm.org (American College of Sports Medicine for updates and information on exercise tests.)
www.heart.org (American Heart Association for updates and information on cardiac tests.)

Answers

1. c, 2. a, 3. d, 4. b, 5. c, 6. d

Endoscopic Procedures

- Nursing Diagnoses Related to Endoscopy   668
- Bronchoscopy   669
- Gastroscopy   670
- Esophagogastroduodenoscopy   671
- Endoscopic Retrograde Cholangiopancreatography   672
- Endoscopic Ultrasound of the Gastrointestinal Tract   672
- Capsule Endoscopy   673
- Sigmoidoscopy and Proctoscopy   673
- Colonoscopy   675
- Cystoscopy and Ureteroscopy   676
- Laparoscopy   678
- Arthroscopy   678

OBJECTIVES

1. Describe nursing assessments for seven possible complications that may occur after endoscopic procedures.
2. Identify at least five general nursing diagnoses for clients undergoing endoscopic procedures.
3. Compare and contrast the nursing interventions before and after bronchoscopy, gastroscopy, or other endoscopic procedures involving the upper airway.
4. Identify areas for client teaching about sigmoidoscopy and other endoscopic procedures of the gastrointestinal (GI) tract.
5. Identify endoscopic procedures that may require conscious sedation (procedural sedation).
6. Describe nursing interventions for a client who has undergone cystoscopy under local anesthesia.

Endoscopes are used for direct visualization of hollow organs or body cavities. Specifically designed endoscopes are named for the cavity that is being viewed, such as a gastroscope, bronchoscope, or sigmoidoscope. Table 27–1 presents examples of endoscopic procedures. The scopes contain lights so that the interior cavity of the organ can be seen. The scopes are hollow instruments with suction tips, biopsy forceps, and other accessories for obtaining tissue samples. Stains (called chromoendoscopy) help to visualize abnormal cellular patterns. Electrodes for cauterization may also be an accessory. Photocoagulation can be used to control GI bleeding, and gallstones can be removed with a special adaptor. Cameras can

Table 27-1 Areas Visualized with Endoscopic Procedures

Name of Procedure	Area Visualized[a]
Arthroscopy	Knee or other joints
Bronchoscopy	Bronchial tree
Capsule endoscopy	Small intestine
Colonoscopy	Colon
Colposcopy	Vagina and cervix (Chapter 25)
Culdoscopy	Female pelvic organs
Cystoscopy	Urinary bladder
Endoscopic retrograde cholangiopancreatography (ERCP or ECPG)	Common bile duct and pancreatic duct
Esophagoscopy	Esophagus
Esophagogastroduodenoscopy (EGD)	Esophagus to small intestine
Gastroscopy	Stomach
Laparoscopy	Abdominal cavity
Proctoscopy	Anus and rectum
Sigmoidoscopy	Sigmoid colon
Flexible sigmoidoscopy	Sigmoid *and* descending colon
Ureteroscopy	Ureters

[a]Preparation discussed in this chapter unless noted.

be used to record the findings for later reference. Ultrasound (Chapter 23) may be combined with endoscopes.

Earlier scopes were all rigid instruments, but newer models are flexible nylon tubes, which can more easily be advanced into a body cavity, such as the intestinal tract. Fiberscopes or fiber-optic scopes are made of strands of glass fibers that reflect light and actually make it possible to see around corners. A flexible fiberscope can be threaded from the mouth into the duodenum (duodenoscopy) or from the rectum through the ileocecal valve into the small intestine (enteroscopy). The first fiberscopes were used in the early 1960s. Industry also uses fiber-optic instruments to peer into cavities, such as automobile engines, so that the engine does not have to be dismantled.

Possible Complications of Endoscopic Procedures

Although endoscopic procedures cause some pain and discomfort, topical anesthetics or conscious sedation makes the procedure tolerable for most clients. An endoscopic procedure may save the client the risk and expense of a surgical procedure under general anesthesia. Specific complications for the different types of endoscopic procedures are discussed later, but there are at least seven possible risks of any type of endoscopic procedure. These risks are

1. The possibility of perforation of the organ or cavity being examined.
2. Aspiration of saliva or gastric contents when the upper airway or esophagus is being examined.

3. Untoward reactions to the drugs used, which include the opioids, fentanyl or less often meperidine, and the benzodiazepines, diazepam and midazolam. These drugs produce conscious sedation that is also referred to as "procedural sedation." Written protocols need to be in place for the administration of these drugs intravenously and the monitoring of the client. The worst unwanted effects of these drugs are respiratory depression and hypotension. Naloxone, a specific antagonist for the opiods, and other emergency drugs should be available. As mentioned later, other drugs may be used during some endoscopy procedures and these, too, may cause unwanted effects.

   Flumazenil, a specific benzodiazepine antagonist, may be used to reverse the effects of a benzodiazepine used during an endoscopic procedure. The drug eliminates sedation rapidly, so at the end of the procedure, the client is awake, oriented to the surroundings, and cooperative. The client will have little recall of the endoscopic procedure. However, clients still need assessment for respiratory depression because the drug may not reverse hypoventilation. Also, resedation may occur, so a second dose of the antagonist may be needed (Deglin, Vallerand, & Sanoski, 2011).

   Propofol, a popular intravenous anesthetic is also used in smaller amounts for conscious sedation for diagnostic procedures and for clients in critical care units. Propofol can cause respiratory depression and hypotension (Katzung, Masters, & Trevor, 2009). Currently, there is no antidote or antagonist for propofol.

4. Cardiovascular problems, such as arrhythmias and even myocardial infarction, due to the psychological and physical stress of the procedure. A vasovagal effect can be stimulated. The vagus can cause bradycardia because the effect of the vagus nerve is to slow the heart. Atropine should be available to treat the bradycardia.

5. Hemorrhage, particularly if a biopsy has been performed as part of the diagnostic procedure. Clients should be informed a week before the procedure to avoid acetylsalicylic acid (ASA), ibuprofen, nonsteroidal anti-inflammatory drugs (NSAIDs), and herbal products such as echinacea, ginko, and ginseng, which may all increase the chance of bleeding.

6. Infections and transient bacteremia. The danger of bacteremia is explored in the section on cystoscopy. In addition to transient bacteremia from slight tissue injury, infection may occur from contaminated equipment.

7. Hypersensitivity to contrast medium is low compared to intravenous delivery, but allergies can occur. When locally instilled dye reaches peak serum levels after endoscopy is completed, clients should be monitored for delayed reactions. (See Chapter 20 on contrast media.)

The risks of these complications are low, and the exact rates of occurrence depend on the skill of the clinician performing the procedure, the physical status of the client, and the type of instrumentation used. Because of the possible risks mentioned, the physician has the client sign a special consent form. (See Chapter 25 on consent forms.) This form should be in the client's chart before any sedative medications are given. Baseline studies, hematocrit (Hct), and urinalysis are routine in most clinic and inpatient settings. Coagulation studies (i.e., partial thromboplastin time [PTT] and platelet studies) are needed if bleeding is a potential problem. If the client has undergone any other diagnostic tests before endoscopy, those results should be available on the chart.

NURSING DIAGNOSES RELATED TO ENDOSCOPY

General Pretest Nursing Diagnoses Related to Endoscopy

Anxiety Related to Unknowns About Procedure

Because the client is usually awake during the procedure, he or she should understand the general procedure. As emphasized in Chapter 25, most clients particularly want to know how the procedure feels. Some clients may want a detailed explanation of the technical aspects; others do not. Clients should also be told what causes the sensations—if they know what to expect, they are less likely to misinterpret the experience. Physical sensations should be described but not evaluated by the nurse because this may cause more anxiety.

Because endoscopy is performed in a specialized procedure room or operating room, the nurse is usually not present during the procedure. Thus, the nurse performs his or her anxiety-relieving function well before the client goes for the examination. As with other diagnostic tests, the nurse can reinforce the information given by the physician and try to find out answers to those questions that continue to bother the client about the test. Nurses who work in the procedure rooms have specific functions during the test but can also focus on helping clients deal with anxious feelings.

Deficient Knowledge Related to Physical Preparation

With the exception of sigmoidoscopy, all the endoscopic procedures discussed in this chapter require that the client maintain nothing-by-mouth status. Vital signs must be taken for baseline data, and a notation should be made of the client's general physical status before the examination (e.g., a client may have abdominal cramps before the examination or shortness of breath). Any signs and symptoms present before the procedure should be documented. The client should void before the procedure so he or she does not have to urinate during the procedure. If general anesthesia is planned, the client should be instructed on deep breathing and coughing exercises and other postoperative care. The nurse must protect the client from injury by instructing the client to stay in bed, with side rails up, after any premedications are given. The client should be informed that the drugs used before or during the procedure may cause drowsiness, euphoria, or a feeling of "not self," and that monitoring may include pulse oximetry (Chapter 6) and other devices for monitoring vital signs.

General Posttest Nursing Diagnoses Related to Endoscopy

Risk for Injury Related to Adverse Reactions or Complications

The frequency with which to record the client's vital signs is determined by the routine practices discussed for other invasive procedures in Chapter 25. The client may want to rest because the procedures are somewhat of an ordeal. The nurse should check for specific complications each time vital signs are taken. The nurse should particularly assess for bleeding if a biopsy was part of the procedure. The nurse needs to know what medicines were used both before and during the test so that untoward reactions can be identified. (See the earlier discussion of seven possible complications.)

Risk for Pain Related to Procedure

Mild analgesics may be needed when local anesthesia wears off. Because severe pain can be caused by a perforation, any severe or persistent pain should be carefully assessed.

Risk for Ineffective Airway Clearance Related to Use of Local Anesthesia

When a scope is inserted via the throat, the gag reflex can be abolished by administration of a topical anesthetic. The nurse must check to see if a local anesthetic was used. Even though the client can swallow, he or she may still not have a gag reflex. The return of the gag reflex can be checked by gently touching a tongue blade to the back of the throat. Once the gag reflex returns, the client is allowed to resume whatever diet is tolerated.

Deficient Knowledge Related to Home Care

Any specific instructions for follow-up care, such as sitz baths or warm gargles, should be explained to the client. If the client is going home after the diagnostic procedure, he or she needs explicit instructions on symptoms that should be reported immediately to the physician or clinic. The client should be accompanied to the procedure by a friend or family member who, in addition to driving the client home, can also be taught what to look for because the drugs used during the procedure can produce some amnesia in the client.

BRONCHOSCOPY

Description and Purposes

For bronchoscopy, a lighted bronchoscope is passed into the bronchial tree. A local anesthetic may be sprayed or swabbed on the throat. The client lies on his or her back with the head hyperextended. The bronchoscope is inserted via the nose or mouth into the trachea and main stem bronchi. The client must breathe around the tube. This can cause a fear of suffocation. It is important that the client be relaxed and not fight the tube. Oxygen may be administered to maintain Pao_2. Visualization of the mucosa of the bronchi shows the surgeon the area on which to perform a biopsy when cancer is suspected. Bronchial washings or brush biopsy specimens can be obtained for culturing fungi; acid-fast bacilli; *Pneumocystis carinii,* now called *P. jiroveci* and *Legionella pneumophila.* (Immune-deficit clients are prone to parasitic infections as with *P. jiroveci,* and simple sputum cultures do not identify the organism.) Bronchoscopy is also used therapeutically to remove foreign objects or for deep suctioning. Flexible bronchoscopes are easier to insert, but a rigid bronchoscope may be needed for removal of foreign objects in children and adults (Hay et al., 2011). In adults, flexible bronchoscopy can usually be performed with local anesthesia and low-dose conscious sedation. Rigid bronchoscopy, needed for massive bleeding or extraction of large foreign objects, usually requires general anesthesia (McPhee, Papadakis, & Rabow, 2011).

Pretest Nursing Implications Related to Bronchoscopy

Completing Routine Preoperative Care. Most institutions have a routine preoperative checklist that is completed before bronchoscopy. The consent form must be signed. Hct and urinalysis may be performed. The client consumes nothing by mouth for about 6–8 hours before the procedure. Good mouth care is important before the procedure so that less bacteria are present in the mouth. Dentures must be removed, and the physician must be warned about any loose teeth.

Patient Teaching. During the procedure, the client breathes through the nose with the mouth open. The client may need time to practice. The client is not able to talk while the bronchoscope is in his or her throat; therefore, the nurse should explain that the client must communicate with hand signals.

Posttest Nursing Diagnoses Related to Bronchoscopy

Risk for Ineffective Airway Clearance Related to Increased Secretions

The client is kept in a semi-Fowler position but may be turned to either side. The client should not smoke. Tissues and a paper bag are needed for expectorations. An emesis basin, lined with tissue, may be useful for copious secretions. (Lining the basin makes it easier to empty.) Once the gag reflex has returned, encouraging fluids to keep the client well hydrated makes secretions less viscous and easier to expectorate. Vigorous coughing after a biopsy can loosen a clot. A suction machine should be available. Some institutions have routine orders for oxygen for 4 hours after bronchoscopy. Pulse oximeters (Chapter 6) are used to assess persistent hypoxemia. Because severe respiratory embarrassment can occur, a tracheostomy set should be nearby. An absence of breath sounds may indicate pneumothorax. Subcutaneous emphysema (a collection of air in tissues) can occur if there is a leak in the pleural space. (See the discussion on thoracentesis or pleural taps in Chapter 25.) Some pink-tinged mucus or small amounts of blood in the sputum are not unusual after bronchoscopy, but hemoptysis can signal hemorrhage from a biopsy site.

Pain Related to Procedure

The client should not do much talking. A pad and pencil or a picture communication board can be used for communication, so the client can point out needs. Fluids, particularly warm fluids that are soothing, are encouraged once the gag reflex has returned. A gargle with warm saline solution may help relieve throat discomfort. Throat lozenges may be used. A soft diet may be better tolerated if swallowing is painful. The client may be very anxious to hear the results of the biopsy because this test is often the determinant of whether a malignant tumor of the lung is operable.

GASTROSCOPY

Description and Purposes

Gastroscopy may include viewing the esophagus (esophagoscopy) as well as the interior of the stomach. The presence of ulcers can be verified and a biopsy taken. If a client has GI bleeding, it may be possible to control the bleeding with photocoagulation, so early endoscopic treatment may be advisable. With a gastroscopy, a percutaneous endoscopic gastrostomy (PEG) tube can be easily inserted or removed at the bedside or in an outpatient setting. See the American Society for Gastrointestinal Endoscopy website (www.asge.org) for information and videos about GI endoscopy procedures.

ESOPHAGOGASTRODUODENOSCOPY

Description and Purposes

All endoscopic procedures on the upper GI tract are performed with the client in the left lateral recumbent position. Appropriate intravenous medications and local anesthetics are given to make the procedure tolerable. In addition to drugs for sedation, the client may receive atropine or glucagon to slow peristalsis. A plastic mouthpiece is used to help relax the jaw and protect the endoscope. The client may be asked to swallow once or twice while the scope is advanced down the esophagus. After that, the client should not swallow—secretions can drain from the side of the mouth or be suctioned out. The client may feel a sensation of pressure as air is instilled to help with visualization of the GI tract. This is more uncomfortable with duodenoscopy. Most of the air is removed at the end of the procedure. Burping is common. With active esophageal bleeding, endotracheal intubation may be necessary to prevent aspiration both during and after the procedure.

Esophagogastroscopy may include viewing the esophagus to detect lesions or varices. Tumors and ulcers can also be viewed and biopsies performed. Color instant photographs of the ulcerations may be placed in the client's chart. Diagnosis of a gastric infection with *Helicobacter pylori*, a gram-negative bacterium, can be made by means of biopsy of gastric mucosal samples, although noninvasive testing for the bacteria may include serologic testing or the urea breath test. (See Chapter 14 on serological tests and Chapter 25 on the urea breath test for *H. pylori* and follow-up treatment.)

If the client has GI bleeding, it may be possible to view the bleeding site and initiate treatment. Esophageal varices may be ligated with bands or less often with sclerotherapy (McPhee et al., 2011).

Pretest Nursing Implications Related to Upper GI Endoscopy

A general preoperative preparation is completed, including consent forms and laboratory work. As with bronchoscopy, it is important that dentures be removed and the client checked for any loose teeth. The client consumes nothing by mouth for 8–12 hours before the procedure.

Posttest Nursing Implications Related to Upper GI Endoscopy

The client may be kept in a semi-Fowler position or turned to the side to help expectorate any fluids. The standard vital sign routine is followed, as is careful evaluation for any signs of gastric bleeding. If a local anesthetic was used, no liquids are allowed until the gag reflex returns (see bronchoscopy care). Warm saline gargles may be used to relieve a sore throat, or throat lozenges can be used. As with other procedures, the use of drugs may cause specific posttest reactions.

ENDOSCOPIC RETROGRADE CHOLANGIOPANCREATOGRAPHY

Description and Purposes

Endoscopic retrograde cholangiopancreatography (ERCP or ECPG) involves the passage of a flexible fiberscope through the mouth, into the stomach, and finally into the duodenum, as for esophagogastroduodenoscopy (EGD), discussed in the previous section. As in EGD, the procedure starts with the client placed on the left side. However, after the scope is in the mouth, the client is turned to a supine position with the head turned to the right. When the endoscope reaches the ampulla of Vater, a contrast agent is injected to outline the common bile duct and the pancreatic ducts. Radiographs are taken of the biliary tree (cholangiogram). ERCP is an important diagnostic tool for clients with cholestatic jaundice. The usual precautions before and after esophagoscopy or gastroscopy are applicable to ERCP. The additional concerns related to the injection of a contrast agent into the biliary system are discussed in the section on cholangiograms (Chapter 20). Current guidelines recommend that the client is informed about five possible complications for ERCP: pancreatitis, hemorrhage, infection, adverse cardiopulmonary reactions, and perforations (Bruesehoff, 2010). Serum amylase and lipase levels are useful in assessing for pancreatitis (Chapter 12). ERCP can be combined with a surgical procedure (sphincterotomy) to remove a gallstone from the common bile duct. Transient pancreatitis after sphincterotomy is considered normal, and the client has an elevated amylase level for a few days. Other types of therapeutic procedures also may be performed with ERCP, including insertion of stents or catheters. Antibiotics may be prescribed for suspected biliary obstruction, known pancreatic pseudocysts, or ductal leaks. After complicated procedures, such as removal of stones or insertion of stents, the client may consume nothing by mouth or only clear liquids until the next morning. Assessment of pain, abdominal distention, and bowel sounds is important, and the findings should be documented.

Another type of endoscopy, laparoscopy, revolutionized the treatment of gallstones. General anesthesia is needed for this approach, as discussed in the section on laparoscopy.

ENDOSCOPIC ULTRASOUND OF THE GASTROINTESTINAL TRACT

For the past few years, endoscopic ultrasound (EUS) has become an important diagnostic method for evaluating and staging cancers in the GI tract. For example, an EUS measures the diameter and depth of cancer penetration in the esophageal wall to help determine treatment. A fine-needle aspiration (FNA) can be done of an abnormal mass or lymph node. EUS can also exclude common duct bile stones before surgery and avoid the need for an ERCP. It has evolved from a purely diagnostic modality to one that can be therapeutic, such as draining cysts or fine-needle injection therapy for cancer (Prasad, Wittmann, & Pereira, 2006). From the client's perspective, the procedure is much like the regular endoscopy but usually longer.

CAPSULE ENDOSCOPY

Description and Purposes

An advance technology in gastroenterology is the wireless capsule endoscope designed to gather images of the small intestine. The mechanism for video imaging is contained within a capsule that the client swallows. The capsule, about the length of a quarter, contains a camera, light source, radio transmitter, and batteries. As the capsule passes through the intestinal tract, the camera visualizes the mucosa and takes 2 pictures per second for about 8 hours. The client has a receiving antenna attached to the abdomen via a patch that resembles an ECG electrode. The electrode is connected to a receiver that the client wears around the waist. After the client returns the receiver, the data is downloaded to a computer. The capsule is eliminated in the feces later. If a client is suspected of having small bowel stenosis, he may need a barium enema before the test, or a trial capsule without the video may be tried first.

The capsule has proven very useful in identifying obscure bleeding not detected by conventional endoscopy. Other uses of CE are to detect small bowel polyps and tumors, evaluate inflammatory small bowel changes in Crohn's disease, and help diagnose malabsorption conditions. A limitation in the pediatric age group is the size of the capsule, but for older children the capsule can be "front loaded" on the end of a gastroscope (Seidman & Dirks, 2006).

Nursing Implications Related to Capsule Endoscopy

Laxatives are usually not needed before the test because the procedure involves only the small intestine, not the large. The client should start a liquid diet the day before the exam and have nothing to eat or drink, including water, for 10 hours before the exam. After the monitoring equipment has been applied, the client holds the capsule under the tongue for one minute to verify that the light source is operating. The client may leave the endoscopy department once he or she is shown how to check the data recorder on the belt to ensure recording is occurring. Usually the client can drink liquids after 2 hours and have a light snack after 4 hours. During the 8 hours of recording, the client should avoid strenuous activity or exposure to electromagnetic fields (e.g., MRI).

Esophageal pH Monitoring

Esophageal pH monitoring can be done by placing a sensor in the esophageal mucosa during outpatient endoscopy. The client wears a receiver that collects and stores radio signals from the pH sensor. After a few days, the sensor is expelled in the feces and can be flushed in the toilet (Lawrence & Taylor, 2007). Correlating the pH reading with the client's symptoms (recorded in a journal for 48 hours) helps determine if gastroesophageal reflux disease (GERD) is present. This type of monitoring is a safe and more comfortable alternative to the traditional monitoring by a transnasal catheter (www.asge.org).

SIGMOIDOSCOPY AND PROCTOSCOPY

Description and Purposes

Sigmoidoscopes are used to view the lower, or sigmoid, colon, and proctoscopes are used to view the anus and rectum. When the scope is put through the rectal sphincter, the client has a strong sensation of a need to defecate. This is only a sensation because the client undergoes intestinal preparation before the examination. The flexible scope is advanced about 60 cm into the colon. This lengthy scope provides direct visualization of the proximal sigmoid and descending colon. Air, inserted to help with visualization of the colon, may cause an uncomfortable sensation of pressure and cramps. The procedure lasts 10–15 minutes and is well tolerated by most clients. However, for some clients, the procedure may cause considerable discomfort, and the scope cannot be advanced as far as needed to produce the best view. Having the client relax and take deep breaths may help, as may removing some air. Scopes are equipped with visual monitors that may be viewed by the client as the scopes are advanced. This may or may not be an appropriate diversion for the client.

Research has shown that being female and advancing age are independently associated with the risk of inadequate sigmoidoscopy (Walter, de Garmo, & Covinsky, 2004). Women are more likely to experience pain because they have longer colons in a smaller abdominal cavity. Older clients tend to have poor bowel preparation and more coexisting problems such as prior abdominal surgeries or diverticular disease.

Pretest Nursing Implications Related to Sigmoidoscopy

Clients should continue to take all their routine medications except iron pills, bismuth subsalicylate, or bulk-forming laxatives, all of which should be discontinued for 3 days or longer. Only clear liquids are taken the day of the examination, and a laxative such as magnesium citrate may be taken the afternoon before the examination or early the day of the examination. Two sodium phosphate/biophosphate enemas are given 2 hours before the examination. Because this procedure is performed on an outpatient basis, the client needs to be clear on how to obtain and administer the ready-to-use enema sets and laxatives that are ordered. No sedation is used, so the client needs to be prepared on how to relax during the procedure. Deep breathing may help.

Posttest Nursing Implications Related to Sigmoidoscopy

Clients may drive home after this procedure. The client may have some mild abdominal cramping because of the air instilled for the test, and air will continue to be expelled for several hours.

Endoscopy of the lower colon is used to detect and perform biopsies on polyps and tumors. The clinician can sometimes see the site of bleeding or the extent of an inflammatory process. Because most cancer of the large intestine occurs in the lower colon, sigmoidoscopy is a useful detection tool for cancer.

A flexible sigmoidoscopy is recommended as one of the ways to screen for colorectal cancer. The United States Preventive Services Task Force (USPSTF) (www.uspreventiveservicestaskforce.org) recommends several methods for screening for colorectal cancer from age 50–75 years. The client or health care provider may choose any of these three methods:

A sigmoidoscopy every 5 years combined with a fecal blood test every 3 years.

A colonoscopy every 10 years as discussed next

A fecal blood test every year (Chapter 13)

These tests may be discontinued after age 75 years depending on known risk for each individual client. The USPSTF concludes that the evidence is insufficient to recommend CT colonoscopy, sometimes called a "virtual colonoscopy" (Chapter 21) or fecal DNA testing (Chapter 13) as routine screening methods.

COLONOSCOPY

Description and Purposes

For colonoscopy, a scope inserted through the rectum provides access to the lower GI tract. Colonoscopy may last from 20 minutes to more than 1 hour depending on the tortuosity of the intestine and the procedures performed. The client lies on the left side as the scope is inserted in the rectum but later may need to lie prone with the right knee flexed. Introduction of air into the colon, to help distend the intestine and aid visualization, causes some pressure and cramping. The discomfort tends to be more intense as the coloscope is maneuvered through the curves in the colon. Conscious sedation makes the procedure tolerable and usually provides complete amnesia of the event. Atropine or glucagon may be given to decrease peristalsis. Atropine may also be used for the bradycardia that may occur from the vagal effect of stimulating the colon.

Colonoscopy is useful for diagnosing inflammatory bowel disease. Older clients, who present with microcytic hypochromic anemia (Chapter 2) are always assessed for occult blood loss that could be from colorectal cancer. In women, signs of chronic blood loss may be uterine bleeding as well as occult GI loss. Polyps can be removed and biopsies performed.

A colonoscopy is recommended as one method to screen for colorectal cancer. Based on current evidence, a colonoscopy should be done every 10 years after age 50 years if this is the method chosen for screening by average-risk clients as noted previously. Medicare added coverage for colonoscopy in 2001, but there are still concerns about the cost, risk, and availability for all clients between age 50 and 75 years. See the earlier discussion on sigmoidoscopy as an alternative screening test and fecal occult blood test (FOBT) in Chapter 13.

Also see Chapter 21 on a CT colonoscopy called a "virtual" colonoscopy, which may be used in certain clients, but is not a primary screening procedure.

Pretest Nursing Implications Related to Colonoscopy

In addition to the general nursing implications for endoscopic procedures, attention must be given to ensuring a thorough cleansing of the intestine so that fecal matter does not obscure viewing. In the past, intestinal preparation included 2 days of clear liquids, in combination

(Continued)

Pretest Nursing Implications . . . (Continued)

with cathartics and enemas. Now intestinal preparation is usually completed with a balanced electrolyte solution in a polyethylene glycol base. Because electrolyte lavage is expensive and some clients may not adhere with taking the large volumes needed, oral sodium phosphate may be better tolerated and as effective. Whatever the type of intestinal preparation, the nurse needs to make sure the client understands the importance of a thorough intestinal cleaning. (See Chapter 20 for more detailed discussion of intestinal preparation and the procedure for GI irrigation.) The endoscopic colon must be free of solid stool and explosive gases before electrocautery can be used to remove polyps. The client will have an intravenous (IV) as a vehicle for receiving medication for conscious sedation. For some clients the IV will also be used to restore hydration after an intensive bowel prep.

Posttest Nursing Diagnosis Related to Colonoscopy

Pain Related to Flatus

The client has abdominal cramps after the procedure because of the air injected during the examination. Changing positions or walking, if permissible, can relieve gas pains. (See the beginning of this chapter for other concerns, such as bleeding or perforation.)

CYSTOSCOPY AND URETEROSCOPY

Description and Purposes

A cystoscope is passed through the urethra into the bladder so that the interior of the bladder can be examined for inflammation, tumors, stones, or structural abnormalities. For some diagnostic studies, such as for interstitial cystitis, it is necessary that the bladder be distended during examination to assess for changes in the mucosal lining of the bladder (McPhee et al., 2011). Small stones may be removed with the scope. Ureteral catheters may be passed into each ureter to obtain samples of urine from the pelvis of each kidney. A contrast agent (Chapter 20) may be injected for a retrograde pyelogram. Cystoscopy can be performed with topical anesthesia, but more extensive procedures require the use of general or spinal anesthesia. The topical anesthetic is in jelly form and is put into the urethra. Ureteroscopy may be used in conjunction with ultrasound (Chapter 23) to remove stones.

Pretest Nursing Implications Related to Cystoscopy

Routine preparations are performed in relation to procedures such as consent forms, vital sign checks, and laboratory work. If the client is to undergo general anesthesia, he or she should be instructed on routine deep breathing and other routines for recovery from general anesthesia. The client is allowed a full liquid diet if the procedure is to be performed with local anesthesia. Administration of prophylactic antibacterial agents may be started.

Posttest Nursing Diagnoses Related to Cystoscopy

Risk for Injury Related to Bleeding

The standard vital sign routine is followed. Some hematuria is not uncommon, but the client should be carefully watched for hemorrhage if a biopsy was performed. The client may maintain bed rest for up to 4 hours. If the procedure was performed in a urology clinic, the client and the client's family should be instructed on these routine assessments and other pertinent aftercare.

Risk for Urinary Retention

The client's intake and output should be monitored for at least 24 hours. Adult clients should have an intake of 2,500–3,000 mL, unless contraindicated. If the client does not have a Foley catheter, the nurse must check for the possibility of urinary retention with overflow. Small amounts of urine, 50–100 mL frequently, may be a sign of urinary retention with overflow. Cholinergic drugs, such as bethanechol chloride, may be needed to stimulate bladder contraction. If the client has a Foley catheter, the catheter must remain connected to a sterile drainage system.

The client may have a ureteral catheter. These catheters are very tiny and are usually fastened on a splint. It is important that there not be any tension on the catheter or any kinking. Nurses do not routinely irrigate ureteral catheters. If the catheter is to be irrigated, only a few cubic centimeters of sterile normal saline solution are used because the renal pelvis holds only about 5 mL of urine. Because the renal pelvis does not have room for much collection of urine, it is important that the physician be notified if a ureteral catheter is not draining properly.

Risk for Infection

Clients are sometimes given antibacterial agents after cystoscopy because of the high risk for urinary tract infections from the instrumentation. Any break in the tissue of the bladder may let bacteria into the bloodstream; consequently, the client may have chills and fever from transient bacteremia. This transient bacteremia may be dangerous for clients with valve abnormalities because bacterial endocarditis can occur. The client should be instructed about the signs of urinary tract infection, such as burning on urination or cloudy, foul-smelling urine. Some burning after urination is expected the first day after instrumentation. A urinalysis is usually performed as a posttest procedure. (See Chapter 3 for interpretation of routine urinalysis and Chapter 16 for culture and sensitivity tests.)

Pain Related to Bladder Spasms

The client may have some pain when urinating (dysuria) and bladder spasms. Sometimes antispasmodic drugs, such as oxybutynin, are given for bladder spasms. Urinary tract analgesics may also be needed, such as phenazopyridine (Deglin et al., 2011). If permitted, warm tub baths may be soothing. Clients with interstitial cystitis may need instructions on foods and drugs that irritate the bladder wall.

LAPAROSCOPY

Description and Purposes

An instrument can be used to inspect the abdominal viscera. If the instrument is inserted into the abdomen through a small incision in the lower abdominal wall, the procedure is called *laparoscopy*. Carbon dioxide is instilled into the peritoneal cavity to distend the abdomen so that visualization is easier. A laparoscopic examination is sometimes performed to help diagnose infertility (Chapter 28). The diagnosis of endometriosis is usually based on laparoscopic findings (DeCherney et al., 2007). Operations performed with a laparoscope are sometimes called "Band-Aid" operations because the incision, only 1–2 cm long, requires only a small dressing. In England, the term is "keyhole" surgery. In 1987, the use of laparoscopy to remove a gallbladder was a major event, and for many years the entry site has been the abdominal wall. Today, the entry site for a laparoscope can be the mouth, rectum, or vagina. This eliminates the need to cut through the abdominal muscles, which is a major source of postprocedure pain. See the National Orifice Surgery Consortium for Assessment Research website (www.noscar.org) for updates on laproscopic procedures.

Most laparoscopic procedures are performed with the aid of general anesthesia, but some procedures on selected clients can be performed with local anesthesia combined with intravenous conscious sedation. When local anesthesia is used, the client may be discharged 1–2 hours after the procedure.

Nursing Implications Related to Laparoscopy

If a laparoscopy is performed under light general anesthesia, the client needs routine preoperative preparation. A Foley catheter is inserted to keep the bladder deflated. Aftercare is the standard care discussed at the beginning of this chapter.

Gas injected into the abdominal cavity during laparoscopy can irritate the diaphragm and cause referred pain in the shoulder area. Clients can be assured the pain disappears in 1–2 days. Mild analgesics may be needed.

ARTHROSCOPY

Description and Purposes

An arthroscope is a fiber-optic endoscope used to examine the interior of joints. Although other joints can be visualized, the most common arthroscopic procedure involves the knee joint. An examination of joint fluid provides a quick and easy diagnosis of gout (see Chapter 4 on uric acid), calcium pyrophosphate deposition disease, and infectious arthritis. The synovial white cell count (WBC) helps discriminate between noninflammatory (<2,000 WBC), inflammatory (2,000–75,000 WBC), and purulent (>100,000 WBC) conditions (McPhee et al., 2011). Arthroscopy of the interior of the knee joint can reveal injuries to the meniscus as well as other abnormalities. Normal saline solution is used to flush the knee and to remove loose objects and allow easier scope management. Surgical repairs can be performed

with the use of an arthroscope. General anesthesia is used if surgical repair is anticipated or if the client has a great deal of pain. Arthroscopy is another "Band-Aid"
operation made possible with fiber-optic endoscopes and microscopic surgical
instruments.

Nursing Implications Related to Arthroscopy

Pre- and postprocedure care depends on whether the client undergoes local or general anesthesia. Nursing diagnoses discussed at the beginning of this chapter are pertinent. In addition, the nurse should assess for any possible infection, which can be serious in a joint. Some
clients may be given prophylactic antibiotics when joints are entered to prevent osteomyelitis.
Ice bags may be used to reduce postprocedure swelling. Any limitations on weight bearing
are related to the procedure performed. (See Chapter 20 on arthrograms, which may be
obtained with an arthroscope.)

Questions

1. Which of the following is *not* a potential complication for clients undergoing endoscopic
   procedures?
   a. Shock caused by perforation of a body organ
   b. Hemorrhage caused by bleeding from a biopsy site
   c. Oversedation related to the use of sedatives before or during the procedure
   d. Burns from the light on the end of the instrument

2. Which of the following nursing actions is more important in preparing a client for bronchoscopy than for other types of endoscopic procedures?
   a. Obtaining informed consent
   b. Emphasizing oral hygiene
   c. Preparing the client for discomfort and the effects of conscious sedation
   d. Demonstrating the use of a nose clip to ensure mouth breathing

3. When a client has had an anesthetic sprayed on the throat, the assessment that determines the
   client can have fluids is
   a. Ability to swallow without discomfort
   b. Presence of gag reflex when a tongue blade touches the back of throat
   c. Absence of nausea or abdominal distention
   d. Presence of active bowel sounds

4. Clients should be taught that the usual recommendation for routine colonoscopies for adults
   without symptoms is
   a. Annually for all people older than 40 years
   b. Annually for all people older than 50 years
   c. Every 3–5 years after 40 years of age
   d. Every 10 years after 50 years of age

5. An *inappropriate* nursing intervention after a client has undergone cystoscopy under local anesthesia is
   a. Recording input and output for at least 24 hours
   b. Checking for urinary retention with overflow
   c. Keeping the client on nothing-by-mouth status for 4–6 hours after the procedure
   d. Assessing for bladder spasms and giving ordered analgesics as needed

References

Bruesehoff, M. P. (2010). ERCP: Update your knowledge about the diagnostic and therapeutic uses for endoscopic retrograde chalangipancreatograpy. *Nursing 2010, 40*(10), 46–50.

DeCherney, A. H., Nathan, L., Goodwin, T. M., & Lauter, N. (Eds.). (2007). *Current diagnosis & treatment: Obstetrics & gynecology* (10th ed.). New York: McGraw-Hill.

Deglin, J. H., Vallerand, A. H., & Sanoski, C. A. (2011). *Davis's drug guide for nurses* (12th ed.). Philadelphia: F. A. Davis.

Hay, W. W., Levin, M. J., Sondheimer, J. M., & Deterding, R. (Eds.). (2011). *Current diagnosis and treatment: Pediatrics* (20th ed.). New York: McGraw-Hill.

Katzung, B., Masters, S. B., & Trevor, A. J. (Eds.). (2009). *Basic and clinical pharmacology* (11th ed.). New York: McGraw-Hill.

Lawrence, B. L., & Taylor, D. (2007). Esophageal pH monitoring goes wireless. *Nursing 2007, 10*(37), 26–27.

McPhee, S. J., Papadakis, M. A., & Rabow, M. W. (Eds.). (2011). *Current medical diagnosis and treatment* (50th ed.). New York: McGraw-Hill.

Prasad, P., Wittmann, J., & Pereira, S. (2006). Endoscopic ultrasound of the upper gastrointestinal tract and mediastinum: Diagnosis and therapy. *Cardio Vascular Interventional Radiology, 29*(6), 947–957.

Seidman, E. G., & Dirks, M. (2006). Capsule endoscopy in the pediatric patient. *Current Treatment Options in Gastroenterology, 9*(5), 416–422.

Walter, L. C., de Garmo, P., & Covinsky, K. (2004). Association of older age and female sex with inadequate reach of screening flexible sigmoidoscopy. *American Journal of Medicine, 116*(3), 174–178.

Websites

www.asge.org (American Society for Gastrointestinal Endoscopy for information on tests including videos.)

www.noscar.org (Information on Natural Orifice Surgery Consortium for Assessment and Research.)

www.uspreventiveservicestaskforce.org (Evidence-based recommendations for screening for colorectal cancer.)

Answers

1. d, 2. b, 3. b, 4. d, 5. c

Diagnostic Procedures Related to Childbearing Years

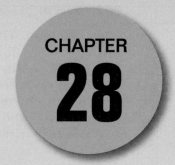

- Basal Body Temperature — 683
- Ovulation Tests for LH — 684
- Saliva Ferning Tests to Detect Ovulation (Home Tests) — 685
- Home Fertility Tests — 685
- Semen Analysis — 685
- Postcoital Examination: Sims–Huhner Test — 686
- Hysterosalpingogram — 687
- Measurement of Hormones — 687
- Other Fertility Tests and Treatment Options — 687
- Amniocentesis — 689
- Tests for Assessing Fetal Maturity (S/A Ratio and PG) — 693
- Chorionic Villus Sampling — 695
- Fetal Monitoring Nonstress Test — 695
- Biophysical Profile — 696
- Nitrazine and Fern Tests for Ruptured Membranes — 696

OBJECTIVES

1. Identify appropriate nursing diagnoses for clients undergoing tests related to reproduction.
2. Explain client instruction needed for each of the five basic fertility tests.
3. Describe basic facts about amniocentesis and chorionic villus sampling (CVS) biopsy that are helpful in planning nursing care for a couple in which the woman is to undergo a procedure for prenatal genetic diagnosis.
4. Name some common genetic diseases that are detected with three types of tests of amniotic fluid or CVS.
5. Explain the types of testing for the isoimmune disease (Rh factor).
6. Explain the clinical significance of determining surfactant-to-albumin ratio (S/A ratio) in amniotic fluid.
7. Describe the routine preparation, including client teaching, for a client who is to undergo amniocentesis in the last trimester.
8. Compare and contrast the nonstress test and biophysical profile (BPP) for antepartum monitoring.

Even a nurse who is not a specialist in maternal–child health nursing may at times be called on to assist with diagnostic procedures commonly performed during the childbearing years. The intent of this chapter is to give the reader an overview of the diagnostic procedures used to assess the ability to conceive or to carry a fetus to term. The chapter begins with the basic tests of fertility because the inability to become pregnant is a common problem. The technique of CVS for prenatal diagnosis is discussed and compared with early amniocentesis. Amniocentesis is discussed in regard to tests for chromosome defects, inborn errors of metabolism, and neural tube defects. Two other uses of amniocentesis, evaluation of the severity of hemolysis from the Rh factor and assessment of fetal maturity, are explained. Basic information about fetal monitoring is presented at the end of this chapter.

General Nursing Diagnoses Related to Fertility and Prenatal Testing

Readiness for Enhanced Coping

During the childbearing years, many couples suffer disappointments because of the inability to have the longed-for "perfect" child. For many years, nurses have been involved in helping families deal with unexpected or crisis situations. Nurses who contract with couples for follow-up visits after a family crisis can help strengthen the adaptive capability of a family. The key point is for the nurse to focus on the family as a unit. Whether it is the crisis of infertility, an unhappy report from amniocentesis, or the stress of fetal monitoring, a professional nurse can be instrumental in helping the family cope and even grow from the experience.

Anxiety Related to Test Procedures and Effect on Self-Concept

The nurse's sensitivity to the needs of clients undergoing diagnostic tests is important for short-term care as well as for follow-up care. For example, when clients are connected to monitors or undergoing technical procedures, they may begin to feel depersonalized if nurses focus first on monitors. As more and more diagnostic procedures are used to assess the natural events of childbearing, the nurse can continue to supply the essential human element of caring. (See Chapter 25 for discussion of relieving anxiety about diagnostic procedures.)

Fertility Testing

A growing number of couples in the United States seek medical help for infertility. Three possible reasons for an increased focus on infertility tests are (1) the diminished number of children available for adoption because of legalized abortion; (2) a rising incidence of sexually transmitted diseases, which can cause pelvic inflammatory disease (PID) and sterility; and (3) the fact that more women are opting to delay pregnancy until after 35 years of age, when reproduction may not be as easy.

Infertility is defined as the inability of a couple to achieve pregnancy after 1 year of unprotected intercourse. Estimates suggest that as many as one in 10 couples may be infertile. For some couples, such circumstances as past PID, suspected hormone imbalances, or other physical problems, indicate sterility may be a problem. If there are no obvious reasons why a couple should not be able to conceive, fertility tests are not advocated until after a year of unprotected intercourse. For women older than 35 years, tests may be conducted sooner than a year. A nurse can reassure a couple who seems healthy that not becoming pregnant after only a few months is not an indication to seek medical help too quickly.

For couples who have tried for much longer than 1 year to conceive, the decision to begin fertility testing may be difficult. The tests may be expensive. They are an invasion into an area that is usually very private, and beginning the tests is, in a way, an acknowledgment of failure to do something that is thought of as being natural. Clients may discuss with nurses the frustration in not being able to become pregnant. The nurse can emphasize that infertility may be caused by a problem with the man, woman, or both; therefore, both people need to be tested once the couple has decided they need help. Usually the male is tested first because the tests are noninvasive and less expensive (www.americanpregnancy.org). As noted later, several tests can be done in the privacy of the home before seeking medical attention. Some basic tests for fertility are summarized in Table 28–1.

BASAL BODY TEMPERATURE

The term *basal* refers to the lowest possible level of a physiologic measurement (i.e., baseline). The basal body temperature (BBT) is taken early in the morning before the woman gets out of bed. Because this test requires only a thermometer and a graphic chart, women may perform this test before they seek medical advice. There are special BBT or ovulation thermometers that are measured in tenths of degrees rather than the two-tenths on conventional thermometers. An electronic thermometer linked to a microcomputer can also be purchased.

In women who have a normal menstrual cycle, BBT is usually less than 98°F (36.7°C) in the preovulatory phase. Before ovulation occurs, an increasing production of estrogen may cause a slight downward trend in BBT. Then with ovulation, progesterone is secreted by the corpus luteum. Progesterone affects the hypothalamus, so there is up to a 1°F (0.37°C) rise in BBT. The increase in temperature at ovulation usually makes the woman's basal temperature greater than 98°F (36.7°C). If the woman keeps an accurate graphic recording for a few months, a physician can interpret the charts and determine if there is presumptive evidence that ovulation is occurring. The client needs to record on the chart any colds or infections, which would disrupt the normal temperature pattern.

The BBT, as a method to confirm ovulatory cycles, has limited use because it is difficult to interpret. Also, research does not support BBT as a method to achieve pregnancy because identification of the fertile period before ovulation, such as tests of cervical mucus, are more reliable for timing intercourse (Barron & Fehring, 2005).

Preparation of Client for BBT Recordings

Each morning as soon as she awakens, the client should take and record her temperature. She should be instructed to take the temperature before she goes to the bathroom or performs any physical activity, including sex. Oral temperatures are usually sufficient. The client is given a special chart to record the temperatures, which is brought back to the physician's office or infertility clinic for analysis. The newer electronic thermometers keep a daily record.

Table 28-1 Examples of Basic Tests for Infertility

Test	Purpose
Basal body temperature recordings and LH ovulation test kits	Presumptive evidence of ovulation
Semen analysis	Assessment of number and characteristics of sperm in one ejaculation
Hormone analysis	Assessment of hormonal imbalances, which may be primary or secondary hypofunction (Chap. 15). Some physicians use endometrial biopsy (Chap. 25)
Postcoital examination (Sims–Huhner)	Assessment of mobility and number of sperm in cervical mucus after intercourse and of characteristics of mucus at time of ovulation
Hysterosalpingogram	Assessment of tubal patency and any structural defects in uterus or tubes (Rubin's test tests only tubal patency). (See Chap. 20 on hysterosalpingogram.)

Note: See text for explanation of these and other tests and client teaching.

LH, luteinizing hormone.

OVULATION TESTS FOR LH

A dozen or more simple home ovulation test kits are available for over-the-counter purchase. These self-test kits measure the surge of luteinizing hormone (LH) that appears in the urine 12–36 hours *before* ovulation. The ovulation tests are useful as a beginning assessment for infertility in women. (See Chapter 15 on LH levels.) For a woman who wishes to avoid pregnancy, self-observation of cervical mucus after teaching by a qualified natural family planner may be as helpful as using and less expensive than the commercial kits. However, the kits can be used to avoid intercourse during the time of ovulation or to plan intercourse to enhance fertility. These tests, based on monoclonal technology, are quite specific and sensitive.

Preparation of Client and Collection of Sample

The various commercial test kits for LH in the urine contain written information on how to conduct the test and all the needed equipment. Some tests require droppers or vials, and some require only a stick that can be held in the stream of urine. Toll-free numbers are included with most of the test kits if the client needs more information.

Clients can begin a daily test a few days after the end of the menses. Some kits contain enough supplies to test the urine for up to 10 days each month. The first voided urine specimen in the morning is ideal because the urine is concentrated. When the surge of LH appears in the urine, a positive test results in a sharp color change.

Urine samples may be brought to a clinical laboratory for measurement of pregnanediol, a urinary metabolite of progesterone (Chapter 15). Sonograms may be obtained daily to validate ovulation (Chapter 23). A substantial number of women do not demonstrate sonographic evidence of ovulation until the second morning after detection of the urine LH surge.

SALIVA FERNING TESTS TO DETECT OVULATION (HOME TESTS)

In 2002, the FDA approved the first saline ferning test for home use. The test has been used in Italy since 1994. The test kits contain a mini-microscope that allows the woman to examine a dried saliva sample. These tests are based on the fact that estrogen levels increase before ovulation and cause a distinct fernlike pattern in dried saliva that looks like frost on a windowpane. (This same ferning pattern is present in cervical mucus as discussed later.) Fern structuring starts 3–4 days before ovulation and ceases 2–3 days after ovulation. Thus, this ferning pattern approximates the fertile period, which is about 3–5 days before ovulation and the day of ovulation. Sperm may live for 3–5 days in estrogenic cervical mucus, and an egg may live for 12–24 hours after ovulation. The test may be used to plan sexual intercourse in either fertile or non-fertile periods depending on the goal of achieving or preventing a pregnancy. (See www.americanpregnacy.org for more information on ovulation home tests.)

HOME FERTILITY TESTS

Clients may obtain a kit (Fertell at www.fertell.com) without a prescription to do preliminary tests for male and female fertility. The female test measures the level of follicle-stimulating hormone (FSH) present in the first morning urine on day 3 of menses. The male test measures the concentration of motile sperm in a semen sample. If either client's test results are outside the expected ranges, the couple can consult a physician for further testing.

SEMEN ANALYSIS

An investigation of semen is the most important initial diagnostic study for infertility in men. If the analysis seems normal, more intensive investigation of the woman's fertility is in order. In the laboratory, a sperm count is performed, as is an examination of the form of the sperm, its mobility, and the amount and characteristics of the semen. If any abnormalities are detected, or if the count is low, a second specimen is examined because there are variations with each ejaculation. Semen analysis is performed after a vasectomy to determine that the operation has been successful.

Preparation of Client and Collection of Sample

Semen is collected after 2 or more days of sexual abstinence. The client may be given privacy in a bathroom to collect the specimen in a jar by means of masturbation. This procedure is a highly intimate matter and may cause tension and anxiety in the man. Some men, for psychological or religious reasons, prefer to collect semen at home by using a condom during intercourse. The condom should not contain lubricants or substances that may interfere with the analysis. The client may be given a plastic sheath to use as the condom. (Religious practices may necessitate a small puncture in the sheath.) All the semen is put into a clean jar and kept at room temperature. It must be sent to the laboratory within 1 hour after ejaculation.

REFERENCE VALUES FOR SEMEN ANALYSIS

Color	Grayish white
pH	7.2–7.8
Volume	2.0 mL or more
Sperm count	20 million/mL or more
Motility	≥50%
Normal morphology	≥30%
Viscosity	Can be poured from a pipette in droplets rather than a thick strand

Reference for semen analysis is from DeCherney et al. (2007). Note that sperm measurements that discriminate between infertility and fertility are not well defined.

POSTCOITAL EXAMINATION: SIMS–HUHNER TEST

The Sims–Huhner test is an examination of the number and motility of the sperm found in the cervical mucus of a woman after intercourse. The test is performed 1–2 days before expected ovulation because an increased secretion of estrogen causes characteristic changes in the mucus. Estrogen increases the elasticity and sodium content of the cervical mucus. The elasticity of the mucus is called *spinnbarkeit*. Normally, these mucous changes enhance sperm survival. (Learning the mucous changes for ovulation is the basis for a form of contraception. *Ferning* refers to the pattern produced when cervical mucus dries under the influence of estrogen. Postcoital examination of the mucus and the sperm can help determine if an immunologic or hormonal problem is contributing to the infertility.

Preparation of Client and Collection of Sample

The test is planned for 1–2 days before the woman's expected time of ovulation. The couple has intercourse, and the woman then goes to the clinic or office for a pelvic examination. The woman may be told to stay in bed for about half an hour after intercourse. The sample of cervical mucus must be obtained 2–4 hours after intercourse. The couple should not use any lubricants, and the woman should not douche.

REFERENCE VALUES FOR SIMS–HUHNER TEST

The microscopic examination shows the quality of the mucus, including the pattern it makes on a slide. Patterns such as ferning are considered normal. The number and the motility of the sperm are observed. Ten or more sperm per high-power field is considered a normal count.

HYSTEROSALPINGOGRAM

The tubes can be insufflated with contrast medium (hysterosalpingogram) to see if the tubes are patent. A hysterosalpingogram is useful for identifying any structural defects in the uterus or tubes. A hysterosalpingogram is obtained in the radiology department. (See Chapter 20 for the discussion of nursing implications related to a hysterosalpingogram.)

A hysterosalpingogram may have a therapeutic effect because it breaks up adhesions in a tube or removes debris that may have been blocking the tube.

MEASUREMENT OF HORMONES

The levels of FSH and LH, as well as testosterone, progesterone, and estrogen, may be assessed with laboratory tests to determine normal hormonal balance in both the man and the woman. (See Chapter 15 for detailed information.) Some physicians prefer an endometrial biopsy to determine the quantity of progesterone rather than serum levels of the hormone. Others consider an endometrial biopsy part of a second phase. An endometrial biopsy can be performed as part of a cervical examination (Chapter 25).

OTHER FERTILITY TESTS AND TREATMENT OPTIONS

Unexplained infertility is now recognized to be due often to specific immunoglobulin factors and antibodies. Tests, such as the antinuclear antibodies (ANA) as well as antithyroglobulin and antimicrosomal antibodies (Chapter 14), may serve as indirect markers of autoimmune infertility.

Also, some couples may have chromosomal rearrangements or inversions that can contribute to infertility. For example, changes in one or both copies of the cystic fibrosis gene (see Chapter 18) can cause infertility, as can changes in the Y chromosome in men. Some women may carry a fragile X permutation that can contribute to infertility. For women who have had recurrent pregnancy losses, tests may be done for clotting disorders such as factor V Leiden (Chapter 13).

Laboratory tests may or may not be sufficient to identify the cause of infertility. Depending on the results of the basic tests, the physician may order other procedures, such as laparoscopy, to examine the female reproductive organs in more detail (Chapter 27). Surgical reconstruction may be needed. For women who are not ovulating, medications may be prescribed.

Since the first "test-tube" baby in 1978, many other options have become possible, including implantation of ova from other women into women who are postmenopausal. A survey of clients' perceptions of infertility treatment indicated that although technologic advances have allowed for more definitive diagnoses and increased chances for conception, the rigorous and sometimes experimental treatment, the long duration and expense of treatment, and the need to make complex decisions about termination of treatment are all stressful. Professional competency, sensitivity, and environmental comfort can mediate the stress.

A review of the literature related to parenting after assisted reproductive technology (ART) indicates that parents face many challenges and nurses need to have an understanding of how to intervene (McGrath et al., 2010).

Nursing Diagnoses Related to Fertility Tests

Risk for Ineffective Coping Related to Inability to Conceive

Although treatment can help many infertile clients, the success rate for all infertile clients, irrespective of the cause of infertility, is approximately 50% at most centers. The final pronouncement that it is highly unlikely that a couple can have a child by the usual biologic means is difficult for many couples to accept. Adoption may or may not be the answer for a couple. Couples may benefit from talking to other couples who have been unable to conceive. There are various support groups for infertile couples. The National Infertility Association (www.resolve.org) serves the needs of the infertile population. A person who has an infertility problem may feel guilt over the perceived inadequacy. If the couple does not remain a couple, the person may have problems explaining the infertility to a new partner.

Anticipatory Grieving Related to Loss of a Desired Goal

The loss of a child, either real or desired, does cause a period of grieving. Interventions used to help resolve grief may be applied to several situations discussed in this chapter, including infertility, the birth of a child with a defect, or the termination of a pregnancy. Interventions to help relieve grief can include (1) preparing the couple for anticipating *normal* feelings of emptiness, loneliness, and failure; (2) helping the couple reevaluate their roles in a childless family (or in a family that does not have the perfect or longed-for child); (3) encouraging the couple to explore fulfilling activities that use their special talents and abilities; and (4) supporting the couple by helping them communicate with each other and with family members who have been affected by the lack of a child. For example, potential grandparents can feel hurt by the lack of a grandchild, so they need help to express their feelings of loss.

Anxiety Related to Future Pregnancies

Women who have experienced a perinatal loss may be able to conceive again. Research has suggested that mothers with a history of prior perinatal loss may want more medically unnecessary laboratory tests and ultrasound in a subsequent pregnancy. Therefore, appropriate education and support from nurses and, if needed, referrals to mental health care providers may be a better use of health care resources (Hutti, Armstrong, & Myers, 2011).

Screening Tests Performed Preimplantation

Prospective parents who know they carry defective genes that could be passed on to their offspring may opt to a preimplantation genetic diagnosis. For example, if a parent carries the gene for Huntington disease (HD), a fertilized egg from in vitro fertilization can be tested by taking a single cell from the developing blastocyte. Only blastocytes without the HD gene mutation would be implanted (Skirton, 2005). See Chapter 18 for more information on genetic tests.

Screening Tests Performed During Pregnancy

The use of amniocentesis and CVS has increased the probability of healthy normal babies for what used to be called *elderly* (older than 35 years) *primigravidas*. These two screening techniques have made it possible for couples who may be at risk for genetic defects to undergo a pregnancy, knowing that some defects can be detected with laboratory testing. Nurses need to be aware of some of the basic tests genetic counseling can offer prospective parents because people often ask nurses for referrals and information on new trends in health care. Genetic counseling is recommended (1) for women older than 35 years of age, (2) for couples who already have one child with a genetic defect, (3) for couples with a family history of genetic defects, (4) as a follow-up for a positive serum-marker test for neural tube defects and for Down syndrome (see Chapter 18 for α-fetoprotein [AFP], serum estriol, HCG dimeric inhibin A, and PAPP-A), and (5) for women taking anticonvulsant medication (Chapter 17). To avoid arbitrariness and discrimination on the basis of maternal age, clinicians explain the risks and benefits of amniocentesis to pregnant women of all ages.

AMNIOCENTESIS

Purposes

Amniocentesis is the removal of some amniotic fluid for diagnostic purposes. The three most important reasons for amniocentesis for diagnostic purposes are (1) prenatal detection of genetic disorders, (2) follow-up and possible treatment of isoimmune disease due to the Rh factor, and (3) assessment of fetal maturity. Table 28–2 provides a summary of the different purposes of amniocentesis.

Amniocentesis for Prenatal Diagnosis of Genetic Defects: Three Assessments

Karyotyping for Chromosome Study

A variety of diseases can be detected through a study of the cells and chemicals in the amniotic fluid. Identification of the chromosomes is called *karyotyping*. A karyotype of chromosomes is a pattern of the 22 pairs of autosomal chromosomes and one pair of sex chromosomes: XX of the woman or XY of the man. All the severe chromosomal abnormalities can be detected with fetal karyotyping. Trisomy of chromosome 21 (Down syndrome) is the most common abnormality found and the most common genetic birth defect. Maternal age has a strong influence on the incidence of trisomy 21.

If there is a possibility of a sex-linked defect such as hemophilia, the sex of the fetus may be important. Some diseases, such as hemophilia, are linked to the X chromosome; therefore, if the fetus is a girl, there is little, if any, possibility of the disease. The hemophilia trait is transmitted by women and occurs in males. A woman must have two defective X chromosomes, which is a rare possibility. Although the sex of the fetus is always identified with a chromosomal study, the parents may prefer to not know the results unless there is a possibility of a sex-linked disease. Centers inform the prospective parents that they can learn the sex if they so desire.

Table 28–2 Three Purposes of Amniocentesis

Purposes	Timing	Results	Usual Follow-up
1. Assessment of genetic defects a. Karyotyping of chromosomes	15th–20th wk of gestation (some centers may perform test earlier)[a]	Can identify Down syndrome and other chromosomal abnormalities	Takes 10–14 days to obtain all results Couple may opt for abortion if serious genetic defect found
b. Biochemical defects		Hundreds of defects can be identified	
c. α-Fetoprotein levels		May indicate improper closure of neural tube	
2. Assessment of isoimmune[b] disease (Rh factor)	After 24–25 wk of gestation	Level of bilirubin in amniotic fluid indicates severity of hemolysis	Increasing levels of bilirubin may indicate need for intrauterine transfusions or induced labor
3. Assessment of fetal maturity	Near end of gestation		Labor may be induced if tests indicate mature fetus
a. Surfactant-to-albumin ratio (S/A ratio)		>55 mg/g alb = maturity	
b. Phosphatidyl glycerol (PG)		Present = maturity	

[a]See text on advantages of early (before 15 weeks) amniocentesis.

[b]Rarely done because ultrasound can monitor fetal anemia by velocity of flow through the middle cerebral artery.

Note: See text for discussion on CVS, which is also performed to assess for genetic defects but does not detect neural tube defects.

Biochemical Defects

Numerous enzymes or biochemical abnormalities can be detected with amniocentesis, as research finds more and more gene markers for diseases such as HD and muscular dystrophy. Some of the metabolic diseases tested for are galactosemia, maple syrup urine disease, Gaucher disease, and Tay–Sachs disease. Some of these diseases are tested for only if it is known that both parents are carriers. For example, Tay–Sachs disease can be detected in the carrier state in parents, and because the disease is caused by a recessive gene, both parents must be carriers for the fetus to be at risk. (See Chapter 18 for laboratory tests of carrier states for biochemical defects and the impact of mass screening.)

α-Fetoprotein Levels to Detect Neural Tube Defects

α-Fetoprotein (AFP) is manufactured by the fetal liver. Normally, there is a low level of this protein in the amniotic fluid, but if the neural tube does not close properly, large amounts of AFP leak into the amniotic fluid. If the neural tube does not close at the top, a normal brain does not develop (anencephaly). If the defect in the neural tube is lower, the fetus has spina bifida. A meningocele or myelomeningocele may be associated with spina bifida. The more involvement of the spinal cord, the more severe the handicap. The child may be paralyzed from the waist down and lack bowel and bladder control, or the damage may be slight and amenable to therapy. Severe omphalocele (protrusion of intestines) or congenital nephrosis can also cause increased levels of AFP. If the amniotic fluid is contaminated with fetal blood, the AFP level may be falsely high because the protein level is normally high in the blood. Thus, a test of fetal hemoglobin (Hgb) can be performed to rule out this artifact.

High levels of AFP in pregnant women do not always indicate a problem with neural tube defects because there may be an incorrect estimation of fetal age, twins, or other reasons for an increase, which are not well understood. Still, even with these disadvantages, AFP blood screening must by law be offered to pregnant women in most states in the United States (Chapter 18). If the AFP blood-screening level is elevated, a repeat test is performed. If the test is positive on a second blood sample, the woman undergoes ultrasonography (Chapter 23) and amniocentesis. (See Chapter 2 for the role of folic acid in decreasing the risk of neural tube defects. See Chapter 18 for a discussion of the use of serum AFP with other tests for screening for Down syndrome, such as the triple screen test.)

Counseling Before Amniocentesis for Prenatal Diagnosis. Although the technical preparation of the client for amniocentesis is simple, the psychological care of the client may be complex. If amniocentesis is being performed for genetic counseling, the ultimate question is "What action will be taken if an abnormality is found?" Counseling is initiated before amniocentesis to help the couple fully understand the ramifications of the test so that they can make an informed decision.

Although amniocentesis is considered to have little risk for the mother and less than 1% risk for the fetus, the couple must be aware of the possibility of damage to or death of the fetus. The physician in a particular center or a genetic counselor, who may be a nurse or other health professional, can explain the statistics of a particular center.

Although a couple may not want to terminate a pregnancy if the results show a defect, they may desire the amniocentesis to better plan for the birth of a child with a defect. The nurse who works in a setting where amniocentesis is performed must be aware of the difficult decisions couples must make about whether the findings from an amniocentesis are the reason for an abortion. Pressures from family and friends, and society in general, may make it difficult for the couple to choose what is right for them.

A genetic counselor can be invaluable in supplying the couple with correct data to help them make their decision. Several bioethical issues are raised when prenatal diagnosis is conducted, but nurses have historically been involved in helping clients work through the overwhelming emotions surrounding prenatal diagnosis. Nurses need to stay involved in the ethical concerns of prenatal testing as technology advances.

Timing of Early and Conventional Amniocentesis. Since the late 1960s, the standard time for amniocentesis to ensure adequacy of the amniotic fluid analysis has been between 15 and 20 weeks' gestation. Testing takes 10 days to more than 2 weeks, so results are not available until well into the second trimester, when abortions are complicated. In the early 1980s, CVS became available as a first-trimester test. (CVS is discussed later in this chapter.) In the late 1980s, early amniocentesis was introduced. At present, all three tests are useful in certain situations. Conventional amniocentesis is still needed for definite diagnosis of neural tube defects and as a follow-up examination for ambiguous results with the earlier tests.

Nursing Diagnosis Related to Amniocentesis

Anxiety Related to Waiting for Results After Conventional Amniocentesis

The waiting period after amniocentesis is a time of extreme anxiety for most couples. The woman may be trying to conceal the pregnancy until she knows the fetus is all right. (A pregnancy of 14 or more weeks may be difficult to conceal.) The couple tends to have ambivalent feelings about the fetus because it is possible that it may be aborted. Crying and indecision about the pregnancy are common. If the results indicate a serious defect and the decision is made to abort the fetus, the abortion must be carried out by induction because the client is in the second trimester. Fortunately, the most common result of amniocentesis is a prediction of normality. It is important that couples understand not all possible defects can be detected with amniocentesis, and there is always a possibility of error. It is emphasized that no test can guarantee a healthy baby. But for a couple with reason to fear one of the defects that can be identified with amniocentesis, a report of no defect is joyous news. A woman who does not have the support of the father of the child may have an even more difficult time awaiting the report of the amniocentesis than a woman who has emotional support.

Amniocentesis in Isoimmune Disease (Rh Factor)

If the mother has a rising titer of Rh antibodies, amniocentesis may be performed during the pregnancy to monitor the welfare of the fetus. (A rising bilirubin level in the amniotic fluid indicates hemolysis of fetal red blood cells.) Elevated or rising Rh antibody titers in the mother indicate that the fetus may have hemolytic disease of the newborn (HDN). This disease, formerly called *erythroblastosis fetalis,* was even more common before the introduction of immunoglobulins of Rh antibodies (RhoGam), which can be given to prevent an Rh-negative mother from making antibodies against the Rh factor of the fetal cells. Other isoimmunifactors, such as ABO incompatibility, can cause some hemolytic reactions, but it is the Rh factor that causes the severe increase in bilirubin due to massive hemolysis of the red blood cells of the fetus. (See Chapter 14 for a discussion on Rh testing.)

Amniocentesis may no longer be needed to check for anemia, as a fetal blood sample can be obtained by cordocentesis (DeCherney et al., 2007). Checking for anemia in the fetus can also be assessed by ultrasound as discussed in Chapters 11 and 23. Doppler measurement of the peak velocity of systolic blood flow in the middle cerebral artery of the fetus to detect anemia is a safe alternative to invasive testing (Oepkes et al., 2006).

REFERENCE VALUE FOR BILIRUBIN IN AMNIOTIC FLUID

The amount of bilirubin in the amniotic fluid is measured by how it changes patterns of light at a certain wave length (spectrophotometry). Charts are available to compare the concentration of bile pigments at different gestational ages.

Clinical Significance

If there is an abnormal amount of bilirubin for the gestational age, the obstetrician must decide whether to perform intrauterine transfusions of the fetus or to induce labor. One of the considerations for inducing labor is the maturity of the fetus. (See S/A ratio and PG discussed next.)

TESTS FOR ASSESSING FETAL MATURITY (S/A RATIO AND PG)

Surfactant-to-Albumin Ratio (S/A Ratio)

This test that measures the ratio of surfactant to albumin as an index of fetal lung maturity is the standard test for fetal maturity. Values above 55 mg/g albumin are indicative of fetal lung maturity. A positive predictive value of a mature result is 96–100% (DeCherney et al., 2007).

Phosphatidylglycerol (PG)

If the S/A ratio is in the transitional range, a test can be done for phosphatidylglycerol (PG). PG, a component of surfactant, is reported as being present (lungs mature) or absent (lungs immature). The predictive value of a mature result is nearly 95–100%. Other tests for fetal maturity may also be performed with different reference values.

Pretest Nursing Diagnoses Related to Amniocentesis

Anxiety Related to Unknowns About Procedure

The physical preparation of the client for amniocentesis is the same whether the collection of fluid is for prenatal diagnosis of a genetic defect, to assess isoimmune disease, or to determine if the fetus is mature enough for induced labor. As noted earlier, detailed counseling is important if amniocentesis is being performed because of possible genetic defects. Even at the time of the procedure, a couple may need last-minute reassurance. Clients undergoing prenatal amniocentesis identified (1) ongoing explanation, (2) use of relaxation techniques, and (3) presence of a trusted support person, be it husband, mother, or nurse. If the amniocentesis is being performed to determine if transfusions are needed or if labor should be induced, the client needs immediate reassurance about the purpose of the test and how the physician uses the results to make a decision about care. The client needs to sign a special consent form that indicates that she understands the purposes of the procedure and the complications that can occur. (See Chapter 25 on consent for invasive tests.)

Risk for Injury to Fetus

The nurse should take baseline vital signs. If amniocentesis is being performed in late pregnancy, the fetal heart rate should be monitored for a baseline reading. No premedication is given. Depending on the timing of the procedure, the client may or may not need a full bladder for visualization with ultrasound. (See Chapter 23 for a detailed explanation of the use of ultrasound in pregnancy.) Ultrasound is used to visualize the placenta and the position of the fetus to avoid injury.

Procedure

The client lies in a recumbent position throughout the sonogram and withdrawal of the fluid. The skin of the abdomen is prepared with an iodine solution (Betadine or Iodophor). Because only one needle puncture is used to remove the fluid, the physician does not usually use a local anesthetic. (Chapter 25 describes the medications that are used for local anesthesia.) The physician inserts a long needle through the abdominal wall into the amniotic sac and withdraws amniotic fluid. The client feels the stick, but the aspiration is not painful. The fluid sample is placed in clearly marked test tubes. If the specimen is to be tested for bilirubin, the fluid should be collected in a dark tube and protected from the light because light changes the composition of indirect bilirubin. (Light is actually used as a therapy for high indirect bilirubin in the newborn. See Chapter 11 on phototherapy.) After the needle is withdrawn, a small adhesive bandage is placed over the puncture site on the abdomen.

Posttest Nursing Diagnosis Related to Amniocentesis

Deficient Knowledge Related to Follow-up Care

If amniocentesis is performed in early pregnancy for prenatal diagnosis, the client can go home after the test. The woman may be told to avoid strenuous exercise, douching, or sexual activity for at least 24 hours. The client is told she may have some mild cramps for a short time and is given instructions to notify the physician or clinic if severe cramps develop or if bleeding occurs. The genetic counselor has already impressed on the couple that the results of the test are not available for 10–14 days, but the couple should be reminded again that they will be called as soon as the results are known. (See the earlier discussion of the anxiety of waiting for results.) Amniocentesis carries a risk for sensitizing susceptible Rh-negative pregnant women, so an injection of Rh IgG antibodies may be ordered for these women (Deglin, Vallerand, & Sanoski, 2011). (See Chapter 14 for a discussion on the importance of prenatal Rh testing and the use of immunoglobulins.)

If the amniocentesis is done in late pregnancy to assess the status of the fetus, the client may or may not be hospitalized. The fetal heart rate is monitored for 30 minutes after the test to assess for any difficulty. The pregnant woman's vital signs also are assessed.

Anticipatory Grieving

Prenatal diagnosis introduces options for management of a genetic disorder by (1) termination of the pregnancy, (2) preparation for specialized prenatal care, or (3) possibly fetal therapy in some situations (Hay et al., 2011). The decision to terminate a pregnancy may have a profound effect on a couple and so does the decision to continue a pregnancy when a severe genetic defect has been detected. Capitulo (2005) noted that throughout the last century, research on the special needs of bereaved parents has changed the context of professional intervention from protective to supportive in recognizing that grief takes many forms. Nurses can help parents by encouraging them to articulate what the loss means to them and support whatever rituals are needed. Nurses can also determine if a support group might be appropriate. Nurses caring for families can be very helpful in perinatal bereavement by establishing standards of care based on research (Limbo & Kobler, 2010). More research is now being performed to support the efficacy of current practices with various ethnic groups (Sun et al., 2011; Whitaker, Kananaugh, & Klima, 2010).

CHORIONIC VILLUS SAMPLING

This test of a chorionic sample is a test of cells similar to those of the fetus. The physician inserts a small catheter through the vagina and cervix into the uterus. Suction is applied to obtain some cells. As an alternative method, CVS may be performed with needle insertion through the abdominal wall. As with amniocentesis, ultrasound is used to guide the needle. The preparation of the client is similar to that for amniocentesis. The great advantage of CVS over amniocentesis is that it can be performed earlier in pregnancy. (See the discussion of the timing of CVS in the section on amniocentesis.) CVS cannot be used to detect neural tube defects. Ambiguous results of CVS may necessitate amniocentesis at a later date, and inability to obtain a sample at CVS may also necessitate amniocentesis.

Pre- and Posttest Nursing Implications Related to CVS

See the pre- and posttest implications for amniocentesis. Minor complications within 24 hours after CVS are cramping, spotting, soreness, and fluid leak. Clients need to be informed when results will be available, as discussed for amniocentesis.

FETAL MONITORING NONSTRESS TEST

Fetal monitoring, a noninvasive technique to evaluate the status of the fetus, is called the nonstress test (NST) to differentiate it from the contraction stress test, which does put stress on the fetus. The client is attached to a fetal monitor and the fetal heart rate (FHR) is recorded. The specific patterns of FHR acceleration may be termed reactive, nonreactive, or equivocal. An NST is considered reactive when two or more FHR accelerations occur in a 20-minute period. These accelerations must be at least 15 beats per minute above the baseline and must last at least 15 seconds. If only one acceleration occurs or if the accelerations do not meet the foregoing criteria, the test results may be called *equivocal*. If no accelerations occur the test is *nonreactive*. A second 20-minute period may be recorded.

Nursing Implications Related to Nonstress Tests

An NST may be performed in a clinic, in an office, or in a quiet room in an obstetric unit. The client is put in a recliner chair or a comfortable bed. A semi-sitting position with a slight left tilt helps avoid supine hypotension from pressure on the vena cava. The client should void before the procedure to remain comfortable. It is also advisable for the client to eat before the test because the active bowel sounds of an empty stomach may interfere with the test. Also, the fetus is more active after a meal. The nurse should take a baseline blood pressure measurement. The monitors are applied per hospital routine. Fetal movements associated with an acceleration of the fetal heart rate gives evidence that the fetus is not acidotic or neurologically

Nursing Implications Related . . . (Continued)

depressed. There should be 2 or more accelerations within a 20-minute period. The accelerations should be at least 15 beats above the baseline and last approximately 15 seconds (DeCherney et al., 2007). Vibroacoustic stimulation may be used to shorten the testing time.

Experienced obstetric nurses may perform the entire monitoring procedure, including interpretation of the findings. Consultation and follow-up readings of the strip may require the services of a physician or nurse expert. Strips are sent to a regional center to be analyzed. Home care nurses visit the client at least weekly, and a nurse is on call at all times.

Although the nonstress method of antepartum monitoring does not cause any pain or physical discomfort for the woman, most women are highly anxious about the results. Fetal monitoring is performed when there is a probability of fetal jeopardy, as when a client has diabetes or hypertension or other risk factors. The nurse should allow the woman to express her concerns and anxieties. The nurse can get answers for any questions the woman may have about her prenatal care or the process of labor and delivery. The nurse can also help the client use some of the relaxation techniques she may be learning in childbirth classes.

BIOPHYSICAL PROFILE

When the NST is nonreactive, additional testing is necessary. Most clinicians use a biophysical profile (BBP). A BPP consists of an NST combined with four observations made by ultrasound (Chapter 23). The four observations are fetal breathing movements, fetal movement, fetal muscle tone, and a determination of amniotic fluid volume. Each of the components is given a score. Some clinicians may do a modified BPP, which combines the NST with the amniotic fluid volume index.

NITRAZINE AND FERN TESTS FOR RUPTURED MEMBRANES

Nitrazine Test for Ruptured Membranes

A paper impregnated with phenaphthazine (Nitrazine) is used to detect the presence of small amounts of amniotic fluid in vaginal secretions. Vaginal secretions usually have a pH of 3.8–4.2, while amniotic fluid has a pH of 7.0–7.5. False positives may occur due to alkaline urine, blood, cervical mucus, semen, soap, or some types of vaginitis (see Chapter 16). False-negative results may be obtained if the amount of fluid is small or if the rupture occurred more than 24 hours ago.

Use of Panty Liner

Research has shown that a panty liner embedded with a pH/ammonia indicator worn by women at home can effectively differentiate amniotic fluid leakage from urine (Bornstein et al., 2009).

Fern Test for Ruptured Membranes

If the Nitrazine test is not confirmatory for ruptured membranes, a swab from the posterior fornix of the vagina should be smeared on a slide, allowed to dry, and observed under a microscope for a ferning pattern that is characteristic of amniotic fluid. In some institutions, nurses are trained to use sterile speculums to obtain samples. Another method is to use a glove and an applicator. A sterile speculum exam, pH assessment, and ferning slide preparation may be basic skills for intrapartum nurses.

Questions

1. A young couple, both 27 years of age, have been married a little more than 2 years. Although they have used no form of birth control for the past 16 months, pregnancy has not occurred. The couple desires a child, so they have asked a nurse in a clinic about fertility testing. Which statement contains appropriate information?
   a. Infertility is most likely not a problem because they have only been having unprotected intercourse for a little more than a year
   b. Infertility is usually due to female problems, so the woman needs to be tested first
   c. Most infertility problems can be treated with drugs or a simple surgical procedure
   d. Basic infertility tests include semen analysis, ovulation tests, and tubal patency tests, such as a hysterosalpingogram

2. As part of an infertility evaluation, the woman is to keep a record of her basal body temperature on a daily basis. The nurse is assessing to see if she can accurately read the thermometer. In addition, the nurse should emphasize
   a. The temperature should be taken before she gets out of bed in the morning
   b. An increase in temperature is expected before ovulation occurs
   c. Rectal temperatures are the only way to obtain a basal reading
   d. A 1-month graph of temperatures is usually sufficient

3. Which of the following statements about amniocentesis is important when planning care for a client who is to undergo amniocentesis for prenatal diagnosis of genetic defects?
   a. The amniocentesis must be performed as early as possible, usually before the eighth week of gestation
   b. The test is a guarantee of a healthy baby
   c. The results take 10–14 days, so this is a period of great anxiety for a couple who may decide to terminate the pregnancy
   d. There is a risk of 5–10% for the fetus

4. A 39-year-old primigravida has elected to undergo chorionic villi sampling for prenatal diagnosis. The advantage of CVS over a traditional amniocentesis is that CVS is
   a. Less hazardous to the fetus
   b. Less expensive
   c. Able to detect neural tube defects
   d. Performed earlier in pregnancy

5. One of the tests performed on amniotic fluid is a test for α-fetoprotein because an elevation of this protein is suggestive of
   a. Fetal lung immaturity
   b. Immunologic deficiencies
   c. Neural tube defects
   d. Phenylketonuria

6. A woman is 34 weeks pregnant. Her amniocentesis revealed an increased bilirubin level as compared with levels performed a week ago. This rising bilirubin level is indicative of
   a. Possible fetal jeopardy caused by hemolytic disease
   b. Normal liver functioning
   c. Renal immaturity
   d. Fetal distress caused by hypoxia

7. The physician is concerned because a too early cesarean delivery may predispose an infant to respiratory distress syndrome (RDS). Which of these tests of amniotic fluid is used to assess lung maturity in the fetus?
   a. Surfactant-to-albumin ratio
   b. Creatinine levels
   c. Karyotyping of chromosomes
   d. Spectrophotometric analysis of bilirubin levels

8. A client who has diabetes is near term with her second pregnancy. Her other pregnancy was a stillbirth. She has been admitted to the obstetric unit for a possible early delivery. She is scheduled for amniocentesis this afternoon to assess fetal maturity. The client asks the nurse about the procedure. The nurse should explain to the client that
   a. Premedication will be used to relax her
   b. Local anesthesia must be used to eliminate pain
   c. Ultrasound will be performed to visualize the placenta and fetus
   d. Radiography of the abdomen is routine after the procedure is completed

9. A biophysical profile (BBP) for antepartum assessment combines a nonstress fetal monitoring with
   a. Amniocentesis
   b. Ultrasound measurements
   c. Chorionic villus sampling
   d. Tests for fetal maturity

References

Barron, M. L., & Fehring, R. (2005). Basal body temperature assessment: Is it useful to couples seeking pregnancy? *MCN: American Journal of Maternal/Child Nursing, 30*(5), 290–296.

Bornstein, J., Ohel, G., Sorokin, Y., Reape, K. Z., Shnaider, O., Kessary-Shoham, H., et al., (2009). Effectiveness of a novel home-based testing device for the detection of rupture of membranes. *American Journal of Perinatology, 26*(1), 45–50.

Capitulo, K. L. (2005). Evidence for healing interventions with perinatal bereavement. *MCN: American Journal of Maternal/ Child Nursing, 30*(6), 389–396.

DeCherney, A. H., Nathan, L., Goodwin, T. M., & Lauter, N. (Eds.) (2007). *Current diagnosis & treatment: Obstetrics & gynecology* (10th ed.). New York: McGraw-Hill.

Deglin, J. H., Vallerand, A. H., & Sanoski, C. A. (2011). *Davis's drug guide for nurses* (12th ed.). Philadelphia: F. A. Davis.

Hay, W. W., Levin, M. J., Sondheimer, J. M., & Deterding, R. (Eds.). (2011). *Current diagnosis and treatment: Pediatrics* (20th ed.). New York: McGraw-Hill.

Hutti, M., Armstrong, D. S., & Myers, J. (2011). Healthcare utilization in the pregnancy following a perinatal loss. *MCN:*

American Journal of Maternal Child Nursing, 36(2), 103–111.

Limbo, R., & Kobler, K. (2010). The tie that binds: Relationships in perinatal bereavement. *MCN: American Journal of Maternal Child Nursing, 35*(6), 316–321.

McGrath, J. M., Samra, H. A., Zukowsky, K., & Baker, B. (2010). Parenting after infertility: Issues for families and infants. *MCN: American Journal of Maternal Child Nursing, 35*(3), 156–163.

Oepkes, D., Seaward, P. G., Vandenbussche, F. P., Windrim. R., Kingdom, J., & Beyene, J. (2006). Doppler ultrasonography versus amniocentesis to predict fetal anemia. *New England Journal of England, 55*(2) 192–194.

Skirton, H. (2005). Huntington disease: A nursing perspective. *MEDSURG Nursing, 14*(3), 167–172.

Sun, H., Sinclair, M., Kernohan, W. G., Chang, T., & Paterson, H. (2011). Sailing against the tide: Taiwanese Women's journey from pregnancy loss to motherhood. *MCN: American Journal of Maternal Child Nursing, 36*(2), 127–133.

Whitaker, C., Kananaugh, K., & Klima, C. (2010). Perinatal grief in Latino parents. *MCN: American Journal of Maternal Child Nursing, 35*(6), 341–345.

Websites

www.americanpregnancy.org (Information on tests done during pregnancy including at home tests.)

www.fertell.com (Information on Fertell the first home test for sperm concentration in the male and FSH for egg quality in the female.)

www.resolve.org (National Infertility Association for information on infertility.)

Answers

1. d, 2. a., 3. c, 4. d, 5. c, 6. a, 7. a, 8. c, 9. b

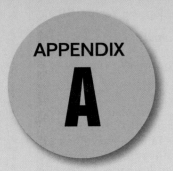

Reference Values for Newborns and Children Compared with Adult Values

Name of Test	Change in Value	Explanation for Change Found In
Acid phosphatase	Higher in newborns and children	Chap. 12
Aldolase	Higher in newborns and children	Chap. 12
Alkaline phosphatase	Higher until puberty	Chap. 12
ALT (SGPT)	Higher in newborns	Chap. 12
Ammonia	Higher in newborns, particularly premature infants Also higher in children	Chap. 10
Amylase	Low or absent in newborns	Chap. 12
AST (SGOT)	Higher in newborns and children	Chap. 12
Bicarbonate	Lower in newborns and slightly lower in children	Chaps. 5, 6
Bilirubin	Higher until 1 month of age	Chap. 11
BUN	Slightly lower in newborns and infants	Chap. 4
C3, C4	Lower at birth	Chap. 14
Calcium	Lower in newborns first few days; slightly higher in children	Chap. 7
Carbon dioxide content	Lower in infants and children	Chaps. 5, 6
Cholesterol	Lower in children	Chap. 9
Creatinine	Lower in children; increases with age; higher in males after puberty	Chap. 4
Creatine kinase	Higher in newborns	Chap. 12
Fibrinogen	Lower in newborns	Chap. 13
GGTP	Five times higher in newborns	Chap. 12
Gonadotropins (FSH and LH)	Lower in children	Chap. 15
Glucose	Lower in newborns and slightly lower in children	Chap. 8
Growth hormone (GH)	Higher in newborns and children	Chap. 15
Hgb, Hct, and RBC	High in newborns, lower by 1 year of age, and adult levels by 8–13 years; infants have some fetal Hgb	Chap. 2

Name of Test	Change in Value	Explanation for Change Found In
Immunoglobulins— IgG, IgA, etc.	Newborns contain some from mother, varies with age	Chap. 10
17-Ketogenic steroids	Low in newborns and increases with age	Chap. 15
LDH	Very high in newborns, child 1–2 times adult	Chap. 12
Magnesium	Slightly lower	Chap. 7
Metanephrines (urine)	Higher in infants	Chap. 15
pH	Lower in newborns	Chap. 6
Pao$_2$	Lower in newborns	Chap. 6
Phosphorus	Highest in newborns, levels decline by puberty	Chap. 7
Potassium	Slightly higher in newborns	Chap. 5
Pregnanediol	Lower in children	Chap. 15
Pregnanetriol	Lower in children	Chap. 15
PT (prothrombin time)	Higher in newborns	Chap. 13
PTT (partial thromboplastin time)	Higher in newborns	Chap. 13
Platelets	Slightly lower in newborns	Chap. 13
Reticulocytes	Higher in newborns	Chap. 2
Sedimentation rate	Slower in newborns and children	Chap. 2
Specific gravity	Lower until 2 years of age	Chap. 3
Testosterone	Much lower in children	Chap. 15
Total protein	Slightly lower in children	Chap. 10
Triglycerides	Lower in children	Chap. 9
T$_4$	Higher in children and especially newborns	Chap. 15
Uric acid	Lower values until puberty	Chap. 4
Urine osmolality	Lower in newborns	Chap. 4
WBC	Extremely high in newborns, differential also different in children	Chap. 2

Note: Also see other references for specific tests in each chapter. Note that the values for premature infants are not the same as for newborns at term. Consult a specialty text for high-risk neonate care.

References for Appendix A

DeCherney, A. H., Nathan, L., Goodwin, T. M., & Lauter, N. (Eds.). (2007). *Current diagnosis & treatment: Obstetrics & gynecology* (10th ed.). New York: McGraw-Hill.

Hay, W. W., Levin, M. J., Sondheimer, J. M., & Deterding, R. (Eds.). (2011). *Current diagnosis and treatment: Pediatrics* (20th ed.). New York: McGraw-Hill.

Wu, A. H. (Ed.). (2006). *Tietz clinical guide to laboratory tests* (4th ed.). St. Louis, MO: Saunders Elsevier.

Possible Alterations in Reference Values for the Aged

Name of Test	Change in Value	Explanation for Change Found In
Albumin	Slight decrease	Chap. 10
Alkaline phosphatase	Increase	Chap. 12
Amylase	Increase	Chap. 12
Antinuclear antibodies (ANA)	May be present	Chap. 14
AST	Increase	Chap. 12
Bilirubin	Slight increase	Chap. 11
Blood sugar, fasting and 2-hour p.c.	Increase	Chap. 8
BUN	Increase	Chap. 4
C3, C4	Increase	Chap. 14
Calcium	May decrease, but still in normal range	Chap. 7
Cholesterol	Increase until older than 70 years	Chap. 9
Cold agglutinins	Increase	Chap. 14
Creatinine clearance	Decrease	Chap. 4
Glucose tolerance test (GTT)	Change in curve	Chap. 8
Gonadotropins (LH, FSH)	Eventual decrease, but increase postmenopausal	Chap. 15
Immunoglobulins	Decrease and alterations	Chap. 10
Lymphocytes	May decrease	Chap. 2
17-Ketosteroids	Decrease	Chap. 15
Magnesium	Slight decrease	Chap. 7
Pao$_2$	Decrease	Chap. 6
Phosphorus	May decrease with age	Chap. 7
Pregnanediol	Decrease in women	Chap. 15
Rheumatic factor (RF)	May be present	Chap. 14
Sedimentation rate (ESR)	Increase	Chap. 2

Name of Test	Change in Value	Explanation for Change Found In
T$_3$ RIA	Decrease	Chap. 15
Triglycerides	Increase except in very elderly	Chap. 9
Transaminases (SGOT, SGPT)	Slight increase	Chap. 12
Uric acid	Slight increase	Chap. 4
VDRL	May become reactive?	Chap. 14
Vitamin B$_{12}$	Slight decrease	Chap. 2
WBC	Decrease	Chap. 2

Note: Also see the reference values for specific tests in each chapter. Note that the effect of age on many tests is not known. The figures used for normal may sometimes be more reflective of the common underlying chronic diseases of the elderly rather than of a normal healthy stage. For example, hypertension affects many elderly clients, and it can cause some renal changes that can change the values of various laboratory tests.

References for Appendix B

Edwards, N. & Baird, C. (2005). Interpreting laboratory values in older adults. *MEDSURG Nursing, 14*(4), 220–229.

McPhee, S. J., Papadakis, M. A., & Rabow, M. W. (Eds.). (2011). *Current medical diagnosis and treatment* (50th ed.). New York: McGraw-Hill.

Wu, A. H. (Ed.). (2006). *Tietz clinical guide to laboratory tests* (4th ed.). St. Louis, MO: Saunders Elsevier.

Altered Reference Values for Common Laboratory Tests in Normal Pregnancies

Name of Test	Change in Value	Explanation for Change Found In
ACTH	Decrease	Chap. 15
Aldosterone	Increase	Chap. 15
Alkaline phosphatase	Marked increase	Chap. 12
Albumin	Decrease	Chap. 10
Bilirubin	Occasional increase	Chap. 11
Bicarbonate	Decrease	Chap. 6
Blood glucose	Variations in trimesters	Chap. 8
BUN	Decrease	Chap. 4
C-Reactive protein	Increase	Chap. 14
Calcium	Decreases with albumin levels	Chap. 7
$Paco_2$	Decrease	Chap. 6
Cholesterol	Increase	Chap. 9
Cortisol	Increase	Chap. 15
Creatinine clearance	Increase	Chap. 4
Creatinine (serum)	Decrease	Chap. 4
Fibrinogen levels	Increase	Chap. 13
Folic acid levels	Decrease	Chap. 2
GGTP	Increase	Chap. 12
Hemoglobin, hematocrit	Decrease (dilutional)	Chap. 2
Iron	Decrease	Chap. 2
Magnesium	May decrease	Chap. 7
Phosphorus	May decrease	Chap. 7
Protein electrophoresis	Change in pattern	Chap. 10
PT	May decrease or same	Chap. 13
PTT	May decrease	Chap. 13

Name of Test	Change in Value	Explanation for Change Found In
Platelets	Increase after delivery	Chap. 13
Reticulocytes	Increase	Chap. 2
Sedimentation rate	Increase	Chap. 2
T_3-T_4 and thyroid-binding globulin	Altered values	Chap. 15
Triglycerides	Increase	Chap. 9
Uric acid	Decrease in early pregnancy	Chap. 4
Vitamin B_{12}	Decrease	Chap. 2
WBC	Increase in total and in neutrophils	Chap. 2

Note: Increases or decreases are in relation to the woman's prepregnancy values.

Also see references for specific tests discussed in each chapter.

References for Appendix C

DeCherney, A. H., Nathan, L., Goodwin, T. M., & Lauter, N. (Eds.). (2007). *Current diagnosis & treatment: Obstetrics & gynecology* (10th ed.). New York: McGraw-Hill.

Wu, A. H. (Ed.). (2006). *Tietz clinical guide to laboratory tests* (4th ed.). St. Louis, MO: Saunders Elsevier.

APPENDIX D

Units of Measure

cc	cubic centimeter (same as mL, 1/1,000 L, which is the preferred term)
cm	centimeter
dL	deciliter (1/10 of a liter)
g	gram (1/1,000 of a kilogram, 15 grains)
hpf	high-power field (microscope)
G%	grams in 100 milliliters
IU	international unit
kg	kilogram (1,000 g, or 2.2 pounds)
L	liter (1,000 mL or 1,000 cc)
lpf	low-power field (microscope)
μg	micrograms (1/1,000 mg)
mCi	millicurie
mEq	milliequivalent (*see* Chap. 5 for formula)
Mg	milligram (1/1,000 g)
mg%	milligrams in 100 milliliters (same as dL)
mIU	milliinternational unit (1/1,000 IU)
mL	milliliter (1/1,000 L, same as cc)
mm	millimeter (1/10 cm)
mm^3	cubic millimeter (*see* RBC, Chap. 2)
mm Hg	millimeters of mercury (*see* blood gases, Chap. 6)
mmol	millimoles (*see* Chap. 1 on SI units)
mOsm	milliosmoles (*see* Chap. 4)
ng	nanogram (1/1,000 μg, *see* Chap. 1)
pg	picogram (1/1,000 ng, *see* Chap. 1)
QNS	quantity not sufficient
SI	international system (*see* Chap. 1)
U	international enzyme unit
μ	micro

w/v	weight/volume
μCi	microcurie (1/1,000 of a mCi)
WNL	within normal limits
WNR	within normal range
<	less than
>	greater than

SI Conversion Factors

SI Conversion Factors for Values in Clinical Chemistry

Component	Present Reference Intervals (Examples)	Present Unit	Conversion Factor	SI Reference Intervals	SI Unit Symbol	Suggested Minimum Increment
Acetone (B,S)	0	mg/dL	172.2	0	μmol/L	10 μmol/L
Acid phosphatase (S)	0–5.5	U/L	16.67	0–90	nkat/L	2 nkat/L
Adrenocor-ticotropin (ACTH) (P)	20–100	pg/mL	0.2202	4–22	pmol/L	1 pmol/L
Alanine ami-notransferase (ALT) (S)	0–35	U/L	0.01667	0–0.58	μkat/L	0.02 μkat/L
Albumin (S)	4.0–6.0	g/dL	10.0	40–60	g/L	1 g/L
Aldolase (S)	0–6	U/L	16.67	0–100	nkat/L	20 nkat/L
Aldosterone (S) normal salt diet	8.1–15.5	ng/dL	27.74	220–430	pmol/L	10 pmol/L
Alkaline phosphatase (S)	30–20	U/L	0.01667	0.5–2.0	μkat/L	0.1 μkat/L
Alpha$_1$-anti-trypsin (S)	150–350	mg/dL	0.01	1.5–3.5	g/L	0.1 g/L
Alpha-fetopro-tein (S)	0–20	ng/mL	1.00	0–20	μg/L	1 μg/L
Ammonia (vP) as ammonia (NH$_3$)	10–80	μg/dL	0.5872	5–50	μmol/L	5 μmol/L
Amylase (S)	0–130	U/L	0.01667	0–2.17	μkat/L	0.01 μkat/L
Aspartate ami-notransferase (AST) (S)	0–35	U/L	0.01667	0–0.58	μkat/L	0.01 μkat/L
Bilirubin, total (S)	0.1–1.0	mg/dL	17.10	2–18	μmol/L	2 μmol/L

Component	Present Reference Intervals (Examples)	Present Unit	Conversion Factor	SI Reference Intervals	SI Unit Symbol	Suggested Minimum Increment
Bilirubin, conjugated (S)	0–0.2	mg/dL	17.10	0–4	µmol/L	2 µmol/L
Calcium (S)						
Male	8.8–10.3	mg/dL	0.2495	2.20–2.58	mmol/L	0.02 mmol/L
Female, 50 years	8.8–10.0	mg/dL	0.2495	2.20–2.50	mmol/L	0.02 mmol/L
Female >50 years	8.8–10.2	mg/dL	0.2495	2.20–2.56	mmol/L	0.02 mmol/L
	4.4–5.1	mEq/L	0.500	2.20–2.56	mmol/L	0.02 mmol/L
Calcium ion (S)	2.00–2.30	mEq/L	0.500	1.00–1.15	mmol/L	0.01 mmol/L
Calcium (U), normal diet	<250	mg/24 h	0.02495	<6.2	mmol/24 h	0.01 mmol/24 h
Carbon dioxide content (B,P,S) (bicarbonate + CO_2)	22–28	mEq/L	1.00	22–28	mmol/L	1 mmol/L
Chloride (S)	95–105	mEq/L	1.00	95–105	mmol/L	1 mmol/L
Cholesterol (P)						
<29 years	<200	mg/dL	0.02586	<5.20	mmol/L	0.05 mmol/L
Complement, C3 (S)	70–160	mg/dL	0.01	0.7–1.6	g/L	0.1 g/L
Complement, C4 (S)	20–40	mg/dL	0.01	0.2–0.4	g/L	0.1 g/L
Cortisol (S) 0800 h	4–19	µg/dL	27.59	110–520	nmol/L	10 nmol/L
Creatine kinase						
Isoenzymes (S)	0–130	U/L	0.01667	0–2.16	µkat/L	0.01 µkat/L
MB fraction	>5	%	0.01	>0.05	1	0.01
Creatinine (S)	0.6–1.2	mg/dL	88.40	50–110	µmol/L	10 µmol/L
Desipramine (P) therapeutic	50–200	ng/mL	3.754	170–700	nmol/L	10 nmol/L
Digoxin (P) therapeutic	0.5–2.2	ng/mL	1.281	0.6–2.8	nmol/L	0.1 nmol/L
	0.5–2.2	µg/L	1.281	0.6–2.8	nmol/L	0.1 nmol/L
Electrophoresis, protein (S)						
Albumin	60–65	%	0.01	0.60–0.65	1	0.01
Alpha$_1$-globulin	1.7–5.0	%	0.01	0.02–0.05	1	0.01
Alpha$_2$-globulin	6.7–12.5	%	0.01	0.07–0.13	1	0.01
Beta-globulin	8.3–16.3	%	0.01	0.08–0.16	1	0.01

Component	Present Reference Intervals (Examples)	Present Unit	Conversion Factor	SI Reference Intervals	SI Unit Symbol	Suggested Minimum Increment
Gamma-globulin	10.7–20.0	%	0.01	0.11–0.20	1	0
Estrogens (S) (as estradiol) Female	20–300	pg/mL	3.671	70–1100	pmol/L	10 pmol/L
Ethanol (P) legal limit (driving)	<80	mg/dL	0.2171	<17	mmol/L	1 mmol/L
Toxic	>100	mg/dL	0.2171	>22	mmol/L	1 mmol
Ferritin (S)	18–300	ng/mL	1.00	18–300	µg/L	10 µg/L
Fibrinogen (P)	200–400	mg/dL	0.01	2.0–4.0	g/L	0.1 g/L
Folate (Erc)	140–960	ng/mL	2.266	550–2200	nmol/L	10 nmol/L
Follicle-stimulating hormone (FSH) (P) female	2.0–15.0	mIU/mL	1.00	2–15	IU/L	1 IU/L
Peak production	20–50	mIU/mL	1.00	20–50	IU/L	1 IU/L
Male	1.0–10.0	mIU/mL	1.00	1–10	IU/L	1 IU/L
Galactose (P) (children)	<20	mg/dL	0.05551	<1.1	mmol/L	0.1 mmol/L
Gases (aB)						
Po_2	75–105	mm Hg (= Torr)	0.01333	10.0–14.0	kPa	0.1 kPa
Pco_2	33–44	mm Hg (= Torr)	0.01333	4.4–5.9	kPa	0.1 kPa
Gamma-glutamyltransferase (GGT) (S)	0–30	U/L	0.01667	0–0.50	µkat/L	0.01 µkat/L
Glucose (P)-fasting	70–110*	mg/dL	0.05551	3.9–6.1	mmol/L	0.1 mmol/L
Growth hormone (P,S)						
Male (fasting)	0.0–5.0	ng/mL	1.00	0.0–5.0	µg/L	0.5 µg/L
Female (fasting)	0.0–10.0	ng/mL	1.00	0.0–10.0	µg/L	0.5 µg/L
Haptoglobin (S)	50–220	mg/dL	0.01	0.50–2.20	g/L	0.01 g/L
Hemoglobin (B)						
Male	14.0–18.0	g/dL	10.0	140–180	g/L	1 g/L
Female	11.5–15.5	g/dL	10.0	115–155	g/L	1 g/L
Imipramine (P) therapeutic	50–200	ng/mL	3.566	180–710	nmol/L	10 nmol/L

Component	Present Reference Intervals (Examples)	Present Unit	Conversion Factor	SI Reference Intervals	SI Unit Symbol	Suggested Minimum Increment
Insulin (P,S)	5–20	µU/mL	7.175	35–145	pmol/L	5 pmol/L
Iron (S)						
Male	80–180	µg/dL	0.1791	14–32	µmol/L	1 µmol/L
Female	60–160	µg/dL	0.1791	11–29	µmol/L	1 µmol/L
Iron-binding capacity (S)	250–460	µg/dL	0.1791	45–82	µmol/L	1 µmol/L
Lactate (P) (as lactic acid)	0.5–2.0	mEq/L	1.00	0.5–2.0	mmol/L	0.1 mmol/L
	5–20	mg/dL	0.1110	0.5–2.0	mmol/L	0.1 mmol/L
Lactate dehy-drogenase (S)	50–150	U/L	0.01667	0.82–2.66	µkat/L	0.02 µkat/L
Lead (B)-toxic	>60	µg/dL	0.04826	>2.90	µmol/L	0.05 µmol/L
		mg/dL	48.26		µmol/L	0.05 µmol/L
Lipase (S)	0–160	U/L	0.01667	0–2.66	µkat/L	0.02 µkat/L
Lipoproteins (P) low density (LDL) as cholesterol	50–190	mg/dL	0.02586	1.30–4.90	mmol/L	0.05 mmol/L
Lithium ion (S) therapeutic	0.50–1.50	mEq/L	1.00	0.50–1.50	mmol/L	0.05 mmol/L
Luteinizing hormone (S)						
Male	3–25	mIU/L	1.00	3–25	IU/L	1 IU/L
Female	2–20	mIU/L	1.00	2–20	IU/L	1 IU/L
Metaneph-rines (U) (as normetaneph-rine)	0–2.0	mg/24 h	5.458	0–11.0	µmol/ 24 h	0.5 µmol/ 24 h
Osmolality (P)	280–300	mOsm/kg	1.00	280–300	mmol/kg	1 mmol/kg
Osmolality (U)	50–1200	mOsm/kg	1.00	50–1200	mmol/kg	1 mmol/kg
Phenobarbital (P) therapeutic	2–5	mg/dL	43.06	85–215	µmol/L	5 µmol/L
Phenytoin (P) therapeutic	10–20	mg/L	3.964	40–80	µmol/L	5 µmol/L
Phosphate (S) (as phospho-rus, inorganic)	2.5–5.0	mg/dL	0.3229	0.80–1.60	mmol/L	0.05 mmol/L
Potassium ion (S)	3.5–5.0	mEq/L	1.00	3.5–5.0	mmol/L	0.1 mmol/L
		mg/dL	0.2558		mmol/L	0.1 mmol/L
Potassium ion (U) (diet dependent)	25–100	mEq/ 24 h	1.00	25–100	mmol/ 24 h	1 mmol/24 h

Component	Present Reference Intervals (Examples)	Present Unit	Conversion Factor	SI Reference Intervals	SI Unit Symbol	Suggested Minimum Increment
Pregnanediol (U)						
Normal	1.0–6.0	mg/24 h	3.120	3.0–18.5	µmol/ 24 h	0.5 µmol/ 24 h
Pregnancy	depends on gestation					
Pregnanetriol (U)	0.5–2.0	mg/24 h	2.972	1.5–6.0	µmol/ 24 h	0.5 µmol/ 24 h
Procainamide (P)						
Therapeutic	4.0–8.0	mg/L	4.249	17–34	µmol/L	1 µmol/L
Toxic	>12.0	mg/L	4.249	>50	µmol/L	1 µmol/L
N-Acetylpro- cainamide (P)						
therapeutic	4.0–8.0	mg/L	3.606	14–29	µmol/L	1 µmol/L
Progesterone (P)						
Follicular phase	<2	ng/mL	3.180	<6	nmol/L	2 nmol/L
Luteal phase	2–20	ng/mL	3.180	6–64	nmol/L	2 nmol/L
Prolactin	<20	ng/mL	1.00	<20	µg/L	1 µg/L
Protein, total (S)	6.0–8.0	g/dL	10.0	60–80	g/L	1 g/L
Quinidine (P)						
Therapeutic	1.5–3.0	mg/L	3.082	4.6–9.2	µmol/L	0.1 µmol/L
Toxic	>6.0	mg/dL	3.082	>18.5	µmol/L	0.1 µmol/L
Salicylate (S) (salicylic acid) Toxic	>20	mg/dL	0.07240	>1.45	mmol/L	0.05 mmol/L
Sodium ion (S)	135–147	mEq/L	1.00	135–147	mmol/L	1 mmol/L
Sodium ion (U)	Diet dependent	mEq/24 h	1.00	diet dependent	mmol/ 24 h	1 mmol/24 h
Testosterone (P)						
Female	0.6	ng/mL	3.467	2.0	nmol/L	0.5 nmol/L
Male	4.6–8.0	ng/mL	3.467	14.0–28.0	nmol/L	0.5 nmol/L
Theophylline (P)						
Therapeutic	10.0–20.0	mg/L	5.550	55–110	µmol/L	1 µmol/L
Thyroid tests Thyroid-stirnu- lating hormone (TSH) (S)	2–11	µU/mL	1.00	2–11	mU/L	1 mU/L
Thyroxine (T_4) (S)	4.0–11.0	µg/dL	12.87	51–142	nmol/L	1 nmol/L
Thyroxine- binding globulin (TBG) (S) (as thyroxine)	12.0–28.0	µg/dL	12.87	150–360	nmol/L	1 nmol/L

Component	Present Reference Intervals (Examples)	Present Unit	Conversion Factor	SI Reference Intervals	SI Unit Symbol	Suggested Minimum Increment
Thyroxine, free (S)	0.8–2.8	ng/dL	12.87	10–36	pmol/L	1 pmol/L
Triiodothyro-nine (T_3) (S)	75–220	ng/dL	0.01536	1.2–3.4	mmol/L	0.1 nmol/L
T_3 uptake (S)	25–35	%	0.01	0.25–3.4	1	0.01
Transferrin (S)	170–370	mg/dL	0.01	1.70–3.70	g/L	0.01 g/L
Triglycer-ides (P) (as triolein)	<160	mg/dL	0.01129	<180	mmol/L	0.02 mmol/L
Urea nitrogen (S)	8–18	mg/dL	0.3570	3.0–6.5	mmol/L	0.5 mmol/L
Urea nitrogen (U)	2.0–20.0	g/24 h	35.700	450–700	mmol/24 h	10 msmol/24 h
Urobilinogen (U)	0.0–0.4	mg/24 h	1.693	0.0–6.8	µmol/24 h	0.1 µmol/24 h

*See Chapter 8 for newer reference values for fasting glucose.
Note: P=plasma, S=serum U=urine

Reference for Appendix E

Young, D. (1987). Implementation of SI units for clinical laboratory data. *Annals of Internal Medicine, 106*, 114–129.

Diagrams of Laboratory Results

A shorthand way to document laboratory results is to diagram them as follows:

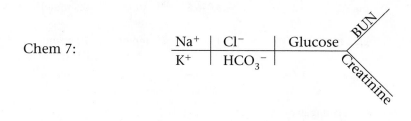

Chem 7:

$$\frac{Na^+ \mid Cl^-}{K^+ \mid HCO_3^-} \mid Glucose \underset{Creatinine}{\overset{BUN}{<}}$$

CBC:

$$WBC > \frac{Hgb}{Hct} < Platelets$$

Coagulation:

$$\frac{PT}{PTT} < INR$$

Liver tests:

AST $\times$ ALT, Total bilirubin, ALP

Other electrolytes:

Ionized or Total Calcium

$$Mg^+ \mid Phosp^-$$

Note: These diagrams are not standard and may vary in different institutions.

Index

A

Abdominal sonograms, 589–91
ABO grouping, 336–37
Acetaminophen, 463
Acetylcysteine, 463, 515, 656
Acetylsalicylic acid (ASA), 462–63
Acid-base balance, 128–31
  imbalances, steps to
    determine, 129
Acid-base balance imbalances,
    129–31
  reasons for, 131
  steps to determine, 129
Acidosis, 128, 134–35
Acid phosphatase, 275, 279. *See
    also* Prostatic acid
    phosphatase (PAP)
Aclonal, gamma globulins,
    239–40
ACTH–adrenal axis, 381, 382
Activated clotting time (ACT),
    300, 313
Addisonian crisis, 386–87
Adrenal cortex, 375, 481–82
Adrenal medulla, 375
Adrenocorticotropic hormone
    (ACTH), 376
  dexamethasone suppression
    test, 383
  preparation of client and collection
    of sample, 382
  reference value, 382
  stimulation test with
    metyrapone, 383
  use of Cosyntropin to stimulate
    cortisol production, 383
Advanced breast biopsy instrument
    (ABBI), 642
α-Fetoprotein (AFP), 477, 478, 690
  detect neural tube defects,
    690–92
  preparation of client and collection
    of sample, 478
Agranulocytosis, 50–51
Alanine aminotransferase (ALT),
    279–81
  decreased, 282
  increased, 280–81
  preparation of client and collection
    of specimen, 280

Albumin, serum
  decreased, 232–33
  functions of, 229, 230
  increased, 232
Alcohol
  legal limits, 465
  monitoring, transdermal, 465–66
Aldolase, serum, 289–90
Aldosterone plasma and urine, 390
  decreased, 393
  increased, 392
  preparation of client and
    collection of sample, 391
Alkaline phosphatase, 274–78
  decreased, 277–78
  increased, 276–77
  isoenzymes, 274
  preparation of client and
    collection of sample, 276
Alkalosis, 128–29, 133–34
Alpha-1-antitrypsin. *See* Alpha-1-
    protease inhibitor
Alpha-1-protease inhibitor, 237
Ambulatory electrocardiography,
    609–10
Amebiasis, 360
Aminoglycosides
  preparation of client and collection
    of sample, 452–53
Ammonia, serum, 243–45
  increased, 244
  preparation of client and collec-
    tion of sample, 243
Amniocentesis
  α-fetoprotein levels to detect neu-
    ral tube defects, 690–92
  in isoimmune disease (Rh factor),
    692–93
  karyotyping for chromosome
    study, 689–90
  for prenatal diagnosis of genetic
    defects, 689
  purposes, 689, 690, Table 28.2
Amniotic fluid, 692
  bilirubin in, 269
Amylase, serum, 290–93
Amylin, 181
Anaerobic cultures, 416–17
Anemia, 26–27
Angiography, 526–27

Anion gap, 106, 142, 143
Anions, 105, 168
Anisocytosis, 44
Ankle-brachial index (ABI), 585–86
Anterior pituitary gland, 374
  releasing factors stimulating,
    375–76
Antiarrhythmic drugs, 460–61
Antibiotics, 452–54
Antibody screening test, 341–42
Antibody to delta antigen (anti-
    delta), 343, 344
Anticonvulsants, 454–57
Antinuclear antibodies (ANAs),
    366, 367
Anti-streptodornase-B, 356, 357
Anti-streptolysin-O, 356, 357
Apolipoproteins A, B, and E, 223
Arterial blood gases, 131–33
  preparation of client and collec-
    tion of sample, 131–33
Arteriography, 526–28
Arthrograms, 532–33
Arthroscopy, 533, 678–79
Aschheim–Zondek (AZ) test, 475
Aspartate aminotranferase (AST),
    281–82
Aspirin resistance test, 320
Atypical lymphocytes, 44
Australian antigen, 343
Azotemia, 85

B

Bacteria, classification of (microscopic
    examination), 415
Bacterial vaginosis, 437
  rapid tests for, 436
Barbiturates, 466
Barium enema radiographs
  client preparation, 522
  instructions for, 522, Table 20.3
  posttest nursing implications, 523
  purpose, 521–22
Basal body temperature (BBT), 683–84
Base deficit, 140, 141–44. *See also*
    Bicarbonate, serum
  causes, 142
  nursing diagnoses, 143–44
Base excess, 140–41. *See also*
    Bicarbonate, serum

Basophilic stipplings, 44
Beta-2-microglobulin (B2M), 91, 247
Bicarbonate, serum, 123, 139–44
  decreased, 141–44
  direct and indirect methods to
      measure, 139–40
  increased, 140–41
Bilirubin, 524
  in amniotic fluid, 269
  combination of conjugated
      and unconjugated
      elevations, 263
  conjugated (direct), 257, 262–63
  excretion, pathway of, 258–59
  metabolism, tests to measure,
      257–70
  total, 259–60 (*See also* Total
      bilirubin)
  unconjugated (indirect), 257,
      261–62
  urine, 263–64
Biophysical profile (BPP), 696
Biopsy. *See* Bone marrow aspiration
β-lactamases, 418
Bladder sonograms, 595–96
Bladder tumor–associated antigen
      (BTA) test, 251
Blasts, 45
Blood alcohol, 464
  legal definitions of
      intoxication, 464
  preparation of client and collection
      of sample, 465
  relation of alcohol to other
      laboratory tests, 465
  transdermal monitoring, 465–66
Blood cells, formation and
      maturation of, 24
Blood cultures
  general indications, 425–26
  preparation of client and collection
      of sample, 426–27
Blood glucose monitoring devices
  alternative site testing, 187
  continuous glucose monitoring
      devices, 187
  guidelines, 186
  preparation of client and collec-
      tion of sample, 185–86
Blood lactate, 151–52
  POC test, 152
  preparation of client and collec-
      tion of sample, 152
Blood transfusions
  low hematocrit and, 31
  nursing diagnoses, 337–38
  purpose of, 335
  Rh factor in, 339
  screening, 335–36
  typing and crossmatching of
      blood, 336
  typing and screening, 336
  typing for packed cells, 336
Blood urea nitrogen (BUN)
  BUN-to-creatinine ratio, 84
  decreased, 87

increased, 83
  nephrotoxic drugs,
      monitoring, 84
  nursing diagnoses related to
      increased, 84–87
  nursing diagnosis related to
      decreased, 87
  preparation of client and collec-
      tion of sample, 83
Blood volume studies, 577
B-Natriuretic peptide (BNP), 288–89
  preparation of client and collection
      of samp, 288
Body scans, 540
Bone marrow aspiration, 633–34
Bone scans, 567–68
Bone/skeletal radiographs
  client preparation, 520
  nursing implications, 520
  purpose, 519–20
Bone sonograms, 595
Brachial arteriogram, 528
Brain electrical activity mapping
      (BEAM), 611
Brain mapping. *See* Quantitative
      electroencephalograms
      (qEEG)
Brain scans, 568
BRCA 1 and 2 (Breast Cancer
      genes), 252
Breast biopsy, 641–42
Breast cancer, estrogen and proges-
      terone receptors in, 408–9
Breast-feeding, and jaundice, 262
Breast scan with somatostatin recep-
      tor scintigraphy (SRS), 570
Breast sonograms, 595
Bronchodilators, 458–59
Bronchoscopy, 669–70
Buffy coat, 27
BUN-to-creatinine ratio, 84

C
CA 15–3, 249
CA 19–9, 250
CA 27.29, 249
CA 125, 248–49
Calcitonin, 397
Calcium, serum, 158–66
  decreased, 163–66
  food sources, 159
  increased, 160–63
  intake, recommended, 159
  NIH and, 159
  preparation of client and collec-
      tion of sample, 160
Canavan disease, 484
Cancer
  colorectal, screening tests, 326–27
  genetic screening for, 252–53
Capsule endoscopy (CE), 673
Captopril, 575
Carbamazepine, 456
Carbohydrate-deficient transferrin
      (CDT), 279

Carcinoembyronic antigen (CEA),
      245, 248
  reference values, 248
Carcinoid tumors, 76
Cardiac analyzers, as point-of-
      care, 287
Cardiac catheterization, 654–59
  posttest nursing diagnoses,
      658–59
  pretest nursing diagnoses, 657
  pretest nursing implications, 656
Cardiac markers, troponin as,
      286–87
Cardiac scans
  infarction scans, 572
  multiple gated acquisition scan,
      574–75
  myocardial imaging with Tc-99m
      sestamibi, 573
  perfusion scans, 572–73
  pharmacologic stress testing
      with dipyridamole/
      adenosine, 573
  pre/posttest nursing
      implications, 574
Cardiovascular diagnostic proce-
      dures, 649, Table 26.1
Carotid arteriogram, 528
Carotid artery scans for intimal
      medial thickness, 587
Case studies, 496–504
Catecholamines, 394
  deficiency, 395
  increased catecholamines in
      urine, 395
  nursing diagnoses related to
      increased, 395
  preparation of client and collec-
      tion of specimen, 394
Catheter-associated urinary tract
      infections (CAUTI), 423
Cations, 168
CD4 counts, 352
Cellular immunity, 230–31
Central line infection, 426–27
Cerebral circulation scans, 586
Cerebrospinal fluid (CSF)
  abnormal findings, 631–33
  pressure, measures, 630
Cerebrospinal fluid culture, 442–43
Cervical biopsy, 640–41
Cervical cytology, 638
Cervical epithelium, 641
Chemical electrical neutrality, 105
Chest radiographs, 517–18
  client preparation, 517–18
  nurse's role with portable chest
      radiography, 518
Chest x-rays, 517–18
Childbearing years, 681
Chlamydia, 436
  rapid tests for, 435–36
Chloride, serum
  decreased, 122–23
  increased, 121–22
Cholangiograms, 523–25

Cholesterol, serum, 210–17
  abnormal, recommendations for
    follow-up, 212–13
  home testing for, 211
  increased, 211–12
  preparation of client and collec-
    tion of sample, 210–11
  skin test for, 211
Chorionic villus sampling, 695
Christmas disease, 310, 315
Chromogranin A (CgA), 396
Chronic obstructive pulmonary
  disease (COPD), 237, 518
Cinchonism, 460
Cineography, 655
Circadian rhythms, 376–77
Classic hemophilia, 315
Claudication, 651
Client confidentiality, protecting, 7
Clinical Laboratory Improvement
  Act (CLIA), 10–11
Clopidogrel resistance test, 320
Clostridium difficile
  clinical significance in stool
    cultures, 441
Clot retraction test, 320
Cluster of differentiation (CD)
  lymphocyte immunophenotyping
    by, 54–55
Coagulation factors, deficiency in,
  316–17
Coagulation process, 298–300
Cobalamin deficiency, nursing diag-
  nosis related to, 38
Coccidioidomycosis, 363–64
Colonoscopy, 675–76
Colorectal cancer
  preparation of client and collection
    of sample for FOBT (guaiac),
    326–27
  preparation of client and collection
    of sample for FOBTi (immu-
    noassay), 326–27
  screening tests to detect, 326–27
Color flow imaging, 586
Colposcopy, 640–41
Complement fixation (CF), 363
Complete blood count (CBC), 23
Compression ultrasound of veins
  (CUS), 586
Computed tomography (CT), 508
  of abdomen, 538
  colonography, 542
  coronary artery calcium scores
    (CACS), 543
  description, 540–41
  EBCT for coronary artery screen-
    ing, 542–43
  MDCT for coronary artery screen-
    ing, 543
  MRI, comparison of, 539,
    Table 21.1
  multi-detector CT, 541
  newer types of CT scans, 541
  nursing diagnoses, 544–45
  posttest nursing implications, 545

purposes, 542
  to screen for lung cancer, 544
  virtual colonoscopy, 542
Condyloma, 640
Congenital adrenal hyperplasia
  (CAH), 388–89
Conjugated (direct) bilirubin (BC),
    257, 262–63
  increased level, 262–63
Continuous glucose monitoring
  (CGM) system, 187
Contrast-induced nephropathy, 515
Cooley's anemia (Thalassemia),
    35, 483
Coombs' test, 341
CO-oximetry, 150–51
Cord blood banking, 491
Coronary artery calcium scores
    (CACS), 543
Coronary artery disease, risk
    factors, 224
Corticosteroids, 181
Cortisol plasma levels, 383–84
C-peptide levels, 202–3
C-reactive protein (CRP) routine,
    365–66
Creatine kinase/phosphokinase
    (CK), 274, 275, 282–84
Creatinine, serum, 88–90
  decreased, 90
  increased, 89
  preparation of client and collec-
    tion of sample, 88
Creatinine clearance test, 90–91
Crigler–Najjar syndrome, 261
Critical test results, 13
Critical thinking
  in judging laboratory data value,
    6–7
Culture growths, 415–17
  anaerobic cultures, 416–17
  cultures for fungus, 417
  cultures for viruses, 417
Cultures
  anaerobic, 416–17
  blood, 425–27
  cerebrospinal fluid, 442–43
  eye, 434
  fungus, 417
  joint fluid, 443
  nasal swabs and nasopharyngeal,
    431–32
  peritoneal fluid, 443
  pleural fluid, 443
  and sensitivity tests, 417–18
  sputum, 427–28
  stool, 439–42
  throat, 430–31
  urine, 423–25
  vaginal, 434–35
  viruses, 417
  wound, 432–33
Culture–specimen collection
  amounts needed, 421
  nursing diagnosis, 422–23
  nursing implications, 420–21

Cushing's syndrome, 384, 385
Cyclosporine, 454
Cystatin C, 91
Cystic fibrosis (CF), tests for, 489–90
Cystoscopy, 676–77
Cytomegalovirus (CMV), 362

D

D-dimer screen, 322–23
Deep vein thrombosis (DVT), 586
  D-dimer test, 322
Delta agent, 343
Delta-aminolevulinic acid, 76
Delta bilirubin, 258
Deoxyribonuclease-B, 357
Dexamethasone suppression test
    (DST), 383
Diabetes mellitus
  gestational diabetes, 183
  type 2 diabetes in adults, 182
  type 2 diabetes in children, 183
  type 1.5 in adults, 183
Diagnostic testing (new technology),
    14–16
Digital radiographs, 511
Digital subtraction angiograms,
    526–28
Digitoxin, 459–60
Digoxin, 459–60
Dimercaptosuccinic
    acid (DMSA), 575
Dimeric inhibin A, 480
Dipstick method
  dipsticks for pH of gastric con-
    tents, 65
  urinalysis, 59
Direct antiglobulin test, 341
Disseminated intravascular coagula-
    tion (DIC), 319, 321
  D-dimer test, 322
  platelet count, low, 319
DNA banking, 15–16
DNA probes for gonorrhea and Chla-
    mydia, 435–36
DNA testing, 15
Döhle bodies, 45
Doppler techniques, 584–85
Down syndrome, screening tests,
    478–80, Table 18.3
Dual energy x-ray absorptiometry
    (DEXA)
  client preparation, 546
  description and purpose, 545
  nursing implications, 546
  osteoporosis, risk reduction
    method, 546, Table 21.2
  reporting of results, 546
Duodenoscopy, 666
Duplex scanning, 586

E

EBCT for coronary artery screening,
    542–43
Echocardiograms, 581
Echoencephalograms, 594

Electrocardiographic imaging
(ECGi), 605–8
Electrocardiography, 609–10
abnormal P wave, 603
arrhythmias, 603
basic components of, 602
cardiac arrest, ECG documentation
of, 604
description, 601–2
ectopic/premature beats, 603
Holter monitor, 609
nursing diagnosis, 609–10
PR interval, 603–4
P wave, 603
QRS complex, 604
QT interval, 604–5
sinus rhythm, characteristics of,
602–3
ST segment, 605
T wave, 604
Electroencephalography, 610–11
Electrolytes, 102–23, 168–76. *See also*
specific entries
reference values, 107
serum, reports interpretation,
103–4
Electromyelography, 612–13
Electrophoresis, 229
Electrophysiologic studies (EPS),
660–61
Endocrine tests
ectopic hormone production, 377
hypophyseal portal system, 376
methods to control hormone
production, 376
negative feedback system for
endocrine functioning, 376
screening and definitive tests, 377
Endometrial biopsy, 640–41
Endoscopes, 665, 666, 671
areas visualized, 666, Table 27.1
complications, 666–67
hollow organs/body cavities,
visualization of, 665
posttest nursing diagnoses, 668–69
pretest nursing diagnoses, 668
Endoscopic cholangiopancreatography, 524
Endoscopic retrograde cholangiopancreatography (ERCP), 672
Endoscopic ultrasound (EUS), 672
Enzyme immunoassay (EIA), 15, 334
Enzyme-linked immunosorbent
assay (ELISA), 15, 322, 334
Enzyme replacement therapy, 484
Eosinophilia, 51
Epilepsy, 610
Epinephrine, 181, 191
Erythema infectiosum, 358–59
Erythroblastosis fetalis, 261,
339–40, 692
Erythrocyte indices, 33–35
classification of anemias by, 36
mean corpuscular hemoglobin
concentration (MCHC), 35
mean corpuscular hemoglobin
(MCH), 34

mean corpuscular volume
(MCV), 33–34
preparation of client and collection
of sample, 33
Erythrocyte sedimentation rate
(ESR), 365
decreased, 46
increased, 46
nursing diagnosis related to
elevated, 46
preparation of client and collec-
tion of sample, 45
Erythrocytosis, 25–26
Erythropoietin (EPO) assay, 27
preparation of patient and
collection of sample, 43
urine test as drug screen, 44
Esophageal motility studies, 570
Esophagogastroduodenoscopy
(EGD), 671, 672
Estradiol and other forms of
estrogen, 407
Estriol levels, 485
Estrogen, 181
Estrogen receptors, 408–9
Ethnic neutropenia, 50
Evidence-based practice
and nursing process, 3–6 (*See also*
Laboratory reports and
nursing process)
striving for, 7
Evoked potential (EP) studies, 610
Exercise treadmill testing (Bruce
protocol), 651, Table 26.4
Exfoliative cytology, identifying
malignant cells, 638
Extractable nuclear antigens
(ENA), 367
Eye cultures
nursing diagnosis, 434
preparation of client and collection
of sample, 434
reference values, 434

F

Factor V Leiden, 324–25
False-positive tests and false-negative
tests, 14
sensitivity, 14
specificity, 14
Fasting blood sugar (FBS), 183–84
prediabetes, 184
preparation of client and collection
of sample, 184
reference values, 184
FDG-PET, 553
Fecal occult blood testing
(FOBT), 326
Fecal urobilinogen, 265
Femoral arteriogram, 527
Fern test, for ruptured membranes,
696–97
Ferritin, 39
Fertility testing, 682–83
antinuclear antibodies (ANA), 687
basal body temperature, 683–84
FSH/LH, levels of, 687

home, 685
hysterosalpingogram, 687
measurement of hormones, 687
nursing diagnoses, 682, 688
ovulation tests for LH, 684
pelvic inflammatory disease
(PID), 682
Rubin's test, 684, Table 28.1
saliva ferning tests to detect ovulation (home tests), 685
screening tests performed during
pregnancy, 689
screening tests performed preimplantation, 688
semen analysis, 685–86
Sims-Huhner test, 686
sterility, 682
treatment options, 687–89
tubal patency tests, 684,
Table 28.1
Fetal fibronectin (fFN) test, 486
Fetal maturity, tests for assessing
phosphatidylglycerol (PG), 693–94
surfactant-to-albumin ratio (S/A
ratio), 693
Fetal monitoring nonstress test,
695–96
Fibrinogen (factor I), 299, 321
decreased, 321–22
preparation of client and collection of sample, 321
Fibronectin, 486
"Fifth disease," 358–59
Fluoroscopy, 508
Folic acid and vitamin B12, serum
nursing diagnosis related to, 38
preparation of client and collection of sample, 37
Follicle-stimulating hormone (FSH),
475, 685
home test, 406
peptide regulator of, 480
preparation of client and collection
of sample, 406
Fosphenytoin, 454
Free light chains, 242
Free phenytoin, 455
Free PSA, 251
Friedman test, 475
Fructosamine assay
decreased blood glucose level,
197–201
elevated blood glucose level,
190–95
Fungal antibodies, 363–64
Fungal antigens, 364
Fungus, cultures for, 417

G

Galactosemia, 489
serum test for, 204
Gallbladder scans, 570
Gallium citrate (Ga-67), 568
Gallium scans, 568–69
Gamma globulins, 239–40
Gamma-glutamyl transferase (GGT),
275, 278–79

Gastric emptying studies, 571
Gastroesophageal reflux studies, 570
Gastrointestinal bleeding studies, 571
Gastrointestinal scans, 570–71
Gastroscopy, 670–71
Gaucher disease, 484
Genetic counseling, 689
Genetic defect, helping family of
 child with, 490–91
Genetic diseases
 probability of, 482, Table 18.4
 screening, 479, Table 18.2
Genetic disorder, management of, 694
Genetic Information Nondiscrimina-
 tion Act (GINA), 15
Genetic screening, 15–16
 for cancer, 252–53
 GINA, 15
 HNPCC, 253
Genetic testing and identification,
 use of DNA samples, 491–92
Genomics, 252
Gestational diabetes, 183
Gestational diabetes mellitus
 (GDM), 187
GI absorption of vitamin K, 524
Gilbert's syndrome, 261
Globulins
 functions of, 229, 230–31
 types, 229, 230
Glomerular filtration rate (GFR)
 estimation, 91
Glucagon, 181
Glucocorticoids, 191, 381, 382
Glucose
 metabolism, 181–82
 in urine, 70–71
Glucose-6-phosphate-dehydrogenase
 (G-6-PD), 41–42
 deficiencies, 42
 nursing diagnosis related to
 G-6-PD deficiency, 42
 preparation of client and collec-
 tion of sample, 41–42
Glucuronyl transferase, 258
Glutamic acid decarboxylase (GAD)
 65, 202
Glycated protein, 190–95
Glycosuria, 70–71
Gonadotropins and sex-related
 hormones, 405
Gonorrhea, 436
 rapid tests for, 435–36
Growth hormone (GH), 181,
 191, 378
 decreased, 380
 increased, 379
 preparation of client and collection
 of sample, 379
 reference values, 379
Guaiac tests, 326

H

Hantavirus, 363
HCG qualitative pregnancy tests,
 476, 477

HCG quantitative test, 476
Helicobacter pylori, serologic
 tests, 361
Hematocrit (Hct), 27–31, 667
 acute *vs.* chronically low, 29
 decreased, 28–31
 increased, 28
 nursing diagnoses related to
 decreased, 29–31
 nursing diagnosis related to
 elevated, 28
 preparation of client and collection of sample, 27
 reference values, 27
 relation to hemoglobin levels, 27
Hematology tests, 22–55
 EPO urine test as drug screen, 44
 erythrocyte indices, 33–35
 erythrocyte sedimentation rate,
 45–46
 erythropoietin assay, 43–44
 glucose-6-phosphate-dehydroge-
 nase, 41–42
 hematocrit, 27–31
 hemoglobin, 31–32
 home test hemoglobin, 33
 lymphocyte immunophenotyping
 by CD, 54–55
 methemoglobin, 33
 MMA and homocysteine levels, 37
 peripheral blood smear, 44–45
 red blood cell count, 25–27
 red blood cell distribution
 width, 35
 reticulocyte count, 42–43
 serum ferritin levels, 39
 serum folic acid and vitamin
 B$_{12}$, 37
 serum iron levels, 39
 total iron-binding capacity, 39
 total white blood cell count and
 differential, 46–54
 transferrin saturation, 39
Hemochromatosis (HFE gene), 40
Hemoglobin
 composition of, 31
 decreased, 32
 home test, 33
 increased, 32
 levels, hematocrit and, 27
 nursing diagnoses related to
 decreased, 32
 preparation of client and collection of sample, 31
 reference values, 31
Hemoglobin electrophoresis, 32
Hemoglobin (Hgb) A1C, 188–90
 nursing diagnoses, 189–90
 as point-of-care testing, 189
 preparation of client and collection of sample, 189
 reference values, 189
Hemoglobin S (HgbS), 481
Hemogram, 23
Hemolytic disease of newborn
 (HDN), 692
Hemophilia tests, 315

Heparin antifactor Xa assay
 (Anti-Xa), 314–15
Heparin monitoring
 low molecular weight heparins, 314
 unfractionated heparin, 314
Hepatitis, serologic testing for, 343
Hepatitis A
 nursing diagnoses, 346–47
 tests, 346–47
Hepatitis B, 343
 antigens, 343
 nursing diagnosis, 345
Hepatitis B surface antigen
 (HBsAg), 343
Hepatitis C, 343
 nursing diagnoses, 348–49
 tests, 347–49
Hepatitis D, 343
Hepatitis E, 343
Hepatobiliary scans, 570, 571
Hereditary Non-polyposis Colon
 Cancer (HNPCC), 253
HER-2/neu, 249
Herpes, 436–37
Herpes simplex virus (HSV), 361–62
High-density lipoprotein (HDL)
 cholesterol, 210, 220
 nursing diagnoses, 220
 preparation of client and collection of sample, 220
 ratio of total cholesterol to
 HDL, 220
 reference values, 220
Histoplasmosis, 363–64
HIV screening, 480–81
HIV testing, 349–50
 home tests for, 351
 major changes in guidelines
 for, 350
 nursing diagnoses, 351–52
 point-of-care testing, 351
 rapid test, 351
 viral load tests, 352–53
 Western blot HIV test, 350
Holter monitors, 600, 609, 611
Home drug test kits, 468
Home pregnancy test (HPT), 475–76
Home tests
 approved by FDA, 12
 for hemoglobin, 33
 serum cholesterol, 211
 for serum cholesterol, 211
Homocysteine levels, 37, 222
Hormones, measurement of, 687
Howell–Jolly bodies, 44
Human chorionic somatomammotropin (HCS), 191
Human papillomavirus (HPV)
 testing, 437
 infection, chronic, 639
 Papanicolaou smears of uterus,
 639–40
 posttest nursing implications, 640
 pretest nursing implications, 640
 vaccine for, 639
Human placental lactogen (HPL), 181
Hyperaldosteronism, 392

Hyperbilirubinemia, 265–69
Hypercalcemia, 160–63
  hyperparathyroidism, 160–61
Hypercapnia, 136–37
Hypercarbia. *See* Hypercapnia
Hyperchloremia, 121–22. *See also*
    Chloride
Hyperchromic erythrocytes, 35
Hypercoagulability, 325
Hyperglycemia, 190–95
  on serum osmolality, 192
Hyperkalemia, 115–17. *See also*
    Potassium
  drugs causing, 116
Hyperlipidemia, 209, 211–16
Hypermagnesemia, 173, 174–75
Hypernatremia, 108–11. *See also*
    Sodium
Hyperosmolar dehydration, 110
Hyperosmolar hyperglycemic non-
    ketotic coma (HHNK), 192
Hyperparathyroidism, 160–61
Hyperphosphatemia, 169–70
Hyperthyroidism, 401, 402
Hypertonic dehydration, 109
Hyperuricemia, 95–98
Hypoalbuminemia, 234–36
Hypocalcemia, 163–66
Hypocapnia, 138–39
Hypocarbia. *See* Hypocapnia
Hypochloremia, 122–23. *See also*
    Chloride
Hypochromic anemia, 32, 35, 36
Hypoglycemia, 193, 197–201
Hypokalemia, 118–20. *See also*
    Potassium
Hypolipidemia, 217
Hypomagnesemia, 173–74
Hyponatremia, 111–13. *See also*
    Sodium
Hypoparathyroidism, 163
Hypophosphatemia, 170–71
  reasons for, 169
Hypophyseal portal system, 376
Hypoprothrombinemia, 303–4
Hypothyroidism, 489
  in infants, 401, 403–4
  older children and adults, 404
Hysterosalpingograms, 528–29, 687

I
I-123, 561, 562, 564, 575
I-131, 559, 561, 562, 564, 576
Immune system, 230–31
  cellular immunity, 230–31
  humoral immunity, 231
Immunodiffusion (ID)
    techniques, 363
Immunoelectrophoresis (IEP), 229
  of urine, 243
Immunofluorescence antibody test
    (IFA), 334
Immunoglobulins, 241–42, 335
  defined, 241
  reference values, 241
Immunohematology
  serologic testing, 335–42

Immunologic tests, 364–65
Immunosuppressive agents, 454
Impaired fasting glucose, 184
Implantable cardioverter defibrilla-
    tor (ICD), 654
Implantable event recorder
    (ILR), 662
"Indirect" bilirubin, 258
Indirect Coombs' test, 341–42
Indium-labeled autologous
    leukocytes, 569
Indium scans, 569
Infarction scans, 572
Infectious hepatitis, 343
Infectious mononucleosis, 355–56
Infertility tests, 684, Table 28.1. *See
    also* Fertility testing
Influenza, rapid test for, 432
Infradian rhythms, 377
INR. *See* International Normalized
    Ratio (INR)
Insulin, 181
  administration, 194
Insulin autoantibodies (IAA), 202
International Normalized
    Ratio (INR)
  prothrombin time and,
    300–301, 302
  vitamin K for elevated, 304
Intestinal preparation, criteria sum-
    mary, 513, Table 20.1
Intoxication, legal definitions
    of, 464
Intravenous cholangiogram, 523
Intravenous pyelography (IVP),
    525–26, 575
Invasive diagnostic tests, 600, 622
  outpatient clinic, 623
  policy of, 623
Invasive tests (nurses role), 622
  adverse reactions to local anesthet-
    ics, 626
  arranging environment for
    test, 627
  equipment preparation, 626
  injectable local anesthetics, 626
  key points for nursing care, 625,
    Table 25.1
  local anesthetic cream, 626–27
  posttest nursing diagnoses, 628–29
  pretest nursing diagnoses, 623–25
  during procedure, 627–28
In vitro testing, 560
In vivo testing, 560–62
Ionized calcium, 160
Iron
  heme iron, 29
  lack of, clinical significance of, 40
  nonheme iron, 29–30
  nursing diagnosis related to iron
    deficiency, 29–30, 41
  nursing diagnosis related to iron
    overload, 41
  overload, clinical significance of,
    40–41
  preparation of patient and collec-
    tion of sample, 39–40

  reference values, 40
  serum ferritin levels, 39
  serum iron levels, 39
  total iron-binding capacity, 39
  transferrin saturation, 39
Islet cell autoantibodies (ICA), 201–2
Isoenzymes
  alkaline phosphatase, 274
  CK, 282
  LDH, 285
Isotonic dehydration, 109

J
Joint fluid culture, 443

K
Ketoacidosis
  diabetic coma, 193–94
Ketones, serum, 196–201
  positive tests for, 196–97
  preparation of client and collec-
    tion of sample, 196
  reference values, 196
Ketones in urine, 71–72
  nursing diagnoses, 72
  positive tests for, 196–97
  reference values, 71

L
Laboratory personnel
  cooperating with, 18–19
  medical technologist, 18
  pathologist, 18
Laboratory reports and nursing
    process, 3–6
  client/nurse goals, 5
  data collection, 4
  goal evaluation and expected
    outcomes, 6
  measurements, 16–17
  nursing diagnosis, 4–5
  nursing interventions, 5
Laboratory reports (measurements)
  conventional measurements, 16–17
  SI measurement system, 17
Laboratory values. *See* Reference
    values
Lactic dehydrogenase (LDH), 275,
    285–86
Lactose tolerance test, 203–4
Laminagram/planogram, 508
Laparoscopy
  Band-Aid operations, 678
  description and purposes, 678
  nursing implications, 678
Latent autoimmune diabetes in
    adults (LADA), 183
Law of partial pressure, 128
Lead, 468–69
Leg exercises, 654
Leg fatigue, 651
Leiden factor (factor V), 299, 324–25
Le Système Internationale d'Unités, 17
Leukocyte esterase
  reference values, 74
  urinalysis, 73–74

Lidocaine, 462
Lipase, serum, 294
Lipid metabolism, 210–24
Lipoprotein (a) levels, 222–23
Lipoprotein-associated phospholipase A_2(Lp–PLA$_2$), 223–24
Lipoprotein electrophoresis, 219–20
Lithium carbonate, 457
Liver and spleen scans, 571
Liver biopsy, 642–44
Low-density lipoprotein (LDL) cholesterol, 210, 221–22
    increased, nursing diagnoses related to, 221–22
    preparation of client and collection of sample, 221
    reference values, 221
    subclasses, 219–20
Low-molecular-weight (LMW) heparin, 314
Lp-PLA$_2$. *See* Lipoprotein-associated phospholipase A$_2$ (Lp-PLA$_2$)
L-Thyroxine serum concentration (Total T$_4$), 400
Lumbar puncture
    abnormal findings in CSF, 631–33
        (*See also* Cerebrospinal fluid (CSF))
    contraindications, 630–31
    description, 629–30
    manometer, 629
    positioning of client for, 629
    posttest nursing diagnoses, 630–31
    pretest nursing implications, 630
    purposes, 630
Lung scans, 571–72
Lupus anticoagulant, 311, 313
    anticardiolipin antibodies and, 313
    partial thromboplastin time and, 311
Luteinizing hormone (LH), 406, 684
    changes in FSH and LH serum levels, 407
    home test, 407
    ovulation tests for, 684
    preparation of client, 684
    preparation of client and collection of sample, 407
    reference values, 406
    urine samples, 684
Lyme disease, serologic testing, 360–61
Lymphadenopathy-associated virus (LAV), 349
Lymphocyte immunophenotyping by cluster of differentiation (CD)
    increased monocyte count, 55
    preparation of client and collection of sample, 54–55
    reference values, 55
Lymphocytosis, 52–53
Lymphopenia, 53–54

M

Macrocytic anemias, 36–37
Macroglobulinemia, 242

Magnesium, serum, 172–75
    decreased, 173–74
    increased, 173
    preparation of client and collection of sample, 172–73
    reference values, 173
Magnesium load test with 24 hour urine collection, 175–76
Magnetic resonance angiography (MRA), 549–50
Magnetic resonance imaging (MRI)
    acute tubular necrosis (ATN), 549
    claustrophobia problems, 548–49
    description, 547
    fetal imaging, 550
    gadolinium contrast, adverse effects of, 549
    hardware and software, 549
    magnetic resonance angiography (MRA), 549–50
    measurement of cardiac iron (T2*), 483
    MR spectroscopy (MRS) and functional MRI (fMRI), 550–51
    noise problems, 548
    nuclear magnetic resonance (NMR), 547
    nursing diagnoses, 551
    posttest nursing implications, 552
    in pregnancy, 550
    pretest nursing diagnoses, 551–52
    purposes, 549
    safety issues for magnet strength and radio frequency heating, 548
    safety issues for projectile items, 547–48
    use of, 549, 550
        detect breast cancer, 550
        pregnancy, 550
Mammograms
    barriers to mammograms, 530
    client preparation, 530–31
    description, 529
    posttest nursing implications, 531
    purposes, 530
Mammograms, digital, 529
Mean corpuscular hemoglobin concentration (MCHC), 23, 35
Mean corpuscular hemoglobin (MCH), 23, 34
    changes in, 35
    reference values, 34
Mean corpuscular volume (MCV), 23, 33–34
Mean platelet volume (MPV), 317
Medical technologist, 18
Metabolic panels, 17–18
Metamyelocytes, 44
Metanephrines, 394
Methemoglobin, 33
Methylmalonic acid (MMA) and homocysteine levels, 37
Metoclopramide, 520
Microalbuminuria, 68–69
Microbiologic serologic tests, 342–43, 342–64

Microcytic anemias, 36
Microvolt T-wave alternans (MTWA), 654
Milliequivalent (mEq), 16–17
    measurements by, 104–5
Mineralocorticoids, 381, 382
Minimal inhibitory concentration (MIC), 418–19
Minimum lethal concentration (MLC), 419–20
Modification of Diet in Renal Disease (MDRD), 90–91
Monoclonal, gamma globulins, 239
Mood stabilizers, 457
Multi-detector CT (MDCT), for coronary artery screening, 543
Multiple gated acquisition (MUGA) scan, 574–75
Multiwave oximeters, 150–51
Mutation, BRCA, 252–53
Myelocytes, 44
Myelograms
    client preparation, 532
    description, 531
    posttest nursing implications, 532
    purposes, 532
Myocardial imaging with Tc-99m sestamibi, 573
Myocardial ischemia, characteristic sign of, 651
Myxedema, 403

N

N-acetyl procainamide (NAPA), 461
Nasal swabs and nasopharyngeal cultures
    general indications, 431–32
    rapid test for influenza, 432
    rapid test for respiratory syncytial virus (RSV), 432
Needle aspiration, 641–42
Neonatal polycythemia, 26
Nephrotic syndrome, 69
Neuroblastomas, 395
Neutropenia, 49–51
Neutrophilia, 48–49
Newborn screening, 486–87
    characteristics, 486
    PKU, 487
Nitrazine test for ruptured membranes, 696
Nitric oxide breath test, 617–18
Nitrites
    reference values, 73
    urinalysis and, 72–73
Nitrogen balance, 88
NMP22, 252
Noninvasive diagnostic procedures, 600, Table 24.1
Noninvasive test, 600
    H. pylori, presence of, 618
    nursing diagnoses, 600–601
Nonketotic coma, 192
Nonstress test (NST), 695
    nursing implications, 695–96
Normal reference values, 12–13
Normetanephrine, 394

Normochromic anemias, 36
Normocytic anemias, 36
North American Nursing Diagnosis
    Association (NANDA), 4
NT-proBNP, 288
Nuclear medicine
    radiation hazards from radionu-
        clides, 563–64
    radionuclide diagnostic testing
        during pregnancy, 564
    radionuclides as low-level radioac-
        tive wastes, 564
    radionuclides as radioactive ele-
        ments, 559
    radionuclides used in diagnostic
        testing, 562–63
    radionuclide tests for elderly
        clients, 564
    radionuclide tests for infants and
        children, 564
    use of radionuclides as therapeutic
        agents, 559–60
    in vitro testing, 560, Table 22.1
    in vivo testing (scintigraphy),
        560–62, Table 22.2
    waste disposal for diagnostic test-
        ing materials, 564
Nurse-to-nurse orders, 5
Nursing diagnoses, 4–5
Nursing functions in laboratory
    testing
    blood and other specimen
        collection, 8
    client confidentiality, protecting, 7
    Clinical Laboratory Improvement
        Act, 10–11
    collection and transportation of
        specimens, 8–9
    critical thinking in judging labora-
        tory data value, 6–7
    laboratory data integration in
        nursing practice, 6
    order of collection tubes of blood,
        9–10
    point-of-care testing, 10–11
    preparation of client for laboratory
        test, 7–8
    reimbursement for laboratory
        tests, 7
    stat tests, 10, 11
    striving for evidence-based
        practice, 7
    use of home test kits, educating
        consumer about, 12
Nursing Interventions Classification
    (NIC) system, 5
Nursing process
    defined, 3
    use of laboratory data in, 3

O

Occult blood testing, 326
Octreotide scans, 563
Opioids, 521
Oral glucose tolerance test (OGTT),
    182, 187–88

Orthostatic proteinuria, 69
Osmolality
    hyperglycemia and, 192
    of serum, 92
    of urine, 92–93
Ovaries, 375
Ovulation tests for LH, 684
Oxygen saturation (Sao$_2$), 148–50
    decrease in, 148–49
    pulse oximeter to monitor, 149–50
Oxytocin challenge test (OCT), 585

P

Packed cell volume (PCV), 27
Pancreas, 375
Panic values, 13
Papanicolaou (Pap) smears, 639–40
Papanicolaou smears, 638
    identifying malignant cells, 638
    of uterus, 639–40
Paracentesis (abdominal tap),
    636–37
Parathormone, 396–97
    decreased, 397
    increased, 397
    preparation of client and collec-
        tion of sample, 396
Parathyroid, 375
    sonograms, 594–95
Partial pressure of carbon dioxide
    (Paco$_2$), 135–39
    hypercapnia, 136–37
    hypocapnia, 138–39
Partial pressure of oxygen (Pao$_2$,
    145–48
    decreased, 146–48
    increased, 145–46
Partial thromboplastin time (acti-
    vated) (APTT), 310–12
    decreased, 312
    increased, 310–12
    lupus anticoagulant, effect of, 311
    preparation of client and collec-
        tion of sample, 310
Partial thromboplastin time (PTT),
    450, 667
Parvovirus B19, 358–59
Pathologist, 18
Peak flow meters, 617
Pelvic examination, 686
Pelvic sonograms, 587–88
    Level II ultrasound scan, 587
    placenta position, 587
    pretest nursing diagnoses, 588
Perfusion scans, 572–73
Peripheral blood smear, 44–45
Peripheral inserted intravenous
    catheters, 596
Peripherally inserted central cath-
    eters (PICCs), 518
Peritoneal fluid culture, 443
pH
    arterial blood gases, 133–35
    of gastric contents, 65
    of urine, 63–65
    of vaginal secretions, 64

Pharmacogenetic testing for drug
    therapy, 448
Pharmacologic stress testing
    with dipyridamole/
        adenosine, 573
Phenobarbital, 456
Phenotyping for protease inhibitor
    genes, 237–38
Phenylalanine, reference values, 488
Phenylketonuria, 487–88
    client preparation and sample col-
        lection, 488
    nursing diagnoses, 488–89
    protein foods, found in, 487
Phenytoin, 454–55, 461
Pheochromocytoma, 395
Phosphatidylglycerol (PG), 693–94
    anticipatory grieving, 694
    fetal maturity, tests for assessing,
        693–94
    procedure, 694
Phosphorus/phosphates, 168–71
    decreased, 170–71
    increased, 169–70
    preparation of client and collec-
        tion of sample, 168–69
Physiologic anemia of pregnancy, 32
Physiologic shunting, 148
Picture archiving communication
    system (PACS), 511, 539–40
Pituitary tumors, 378
Plain radiographs, 519
Plasma drug levels
    caution in interpretation, 451
    nursing implications, 451–52
    reasons for monitoring, 448–50
    reasons for not monitoring,
        450–51
    use of laboratory tests to monitor
        for unwanted effects of
        drugs, 450–51
Plasminogen assay, 323–24
Platelet count
    increased, 317
    low, 318–19
    preparation of client and collec-
        tion of sample, 317
Pleural fluid culture, 443
Poikilocytosis, 44
Point-of-care (POC) testing, 10–11
    for arterial blood gases, 133
    for blood lactate, 152
    cardiac analyzers as, 287
    Hgb A1C as, 189
    for HIV, 351
Polyclonal, gamma globulins, 239
Polycystic ovary syndrome
    (PCOS), 409
Polycythemia vera, 25–26
    neonatal, 26
Polymerase chain reaction (PCR), 14
Porphyrins, urinary, 74–76
Positron emission tomography (PET)
    biochemical activity, 552
    description, 552
    fluorodeoxyglucose (FDG), 553
    posttest nursing implications, 554

pretest nursing implications, 553–54
purposes, 553
Postcoital examination, 686
preparation of client, 686
Sims–Huhner test, 686
Postprandial blood sugar (PPBS), 184–85
Postural orthostatic tachycardia syndrome (POTS), 661
Postural proteinuria, 69
Potassium
intake, recommended, 114
nursing diagnosis related to increased BUN, 85
reference values for serum, 115
reference values for urine, 121
serum, 114–20
urine, 120–21
Potassium chloride in oral preparations, 119
Pre-albumin, 233–34
Prediabetes, 184
Preeclampsia
platelet count, low, 319
Preeclampsia, tests for, 485
Pregnancy
reference value changes, 705–6
Rh factor in, 339–40
tests (See Pregnancy tests)
Pregnancy-associated plasma protein A (PAPPA), 480
Pregnancy tests, 475
human chorionic gonadotropin (HCG), 475
routine tests, 474, Table 18.1
serum HCG levels, 477
urine, 475–76
Pregnanediol (progesterone metabolite), 408
Prenatal screening for Down Syndrome, 478–80
Prenatal testing, nursing diagnoses, 682
Preterm labor, biochemical marker for, 486
Primigravidas, 689
Procainamide, 461
Proctoscopy, 673–75
Progesterone, 181, 408
Progesterone receptors, 408–9
Prolactin (PRL), 181, 380–81
Prostate-specific antigen (PSA), 250–51, 279
Prostatic acid phosphatase (PAP), 279
Protein
electrophoresis, 243
food sources, 236
nursing diagnosis related to increased BUN, 85
nursing diagnosis related to iron deficiency, 29–30
requirement across life span, 235
serum, tests of, 229
in urine, 68–70
Proteinuria, 68–70

nursing diagnosis, 70
qualitative method, 68
reference values, 68
Proteomics, test for cancer using, 252
Prothrombin time (PT), 300–309, 524
decreased, 309
increased, 303–4
international normalized ratio (INR), 300–301, 302
measurement in seconds, 301
nursing diagnoses related to increased, 305–9
preparation of client and collection of sample, 301
testing at home, 303
vitamin K, 524
Warfarin on, 301, 304
Pulmonary function tests (PFTs)
description, 613
findings from ventilation studies, 614–16
forced expiratory flow (FEF), 616
forced expiratory volume (FEV), 615
forced vital capacity (FVC), 614
maximal breathing capacity (MBC), 616
maximal voluntary ventilation (MVV), 616
nitric oxide breath test, 617–18
peak flow meters, 617
purposes, 613–14
spirometry, 613
urea breath test for *Helicobacter pylori*, 618
vital capacity (VC), 614
volume exhaled (VE), 616

Q

QuantiFERON-TB gold test (QFT-G), 429–30
Quantitative electroencephalograms (qEEG), 611–12
Quinidine, 460–61

R

Radiation detectors, deficient knowledge, 566
Radiation exposure, reducing the hazards, 508–11
benefit *vs.* risk, 510
14-day rule, 510
digital radiographs, 511
nursing diagnoses, 511–14
nursing implications for future care, 517
posttest nursing diagnoses, 515–16
teaching clients about x-rays, 509–10
Radiation protection, 509
Radiation therapy, 507
Radioactive iodine (RAI) test, 507
Radiographic procedures, nursing diagnoses, 511–16

Radiographs, 507–11
Radioimmunoassay (RIA), 14–15, 334
Radio-iodinated human serum albumin (RIHSA), 568
Radioisotope, 558, 559
Radiology information services (RIS)
digital images and computers, 539–40
Radionuclide(s), 558, 559, 560, 562, 563, 564
cold spots/cold nodules, 562
diagnostic testing during pregnancy, 564
diagnostic testing methods, 560–62
as low-level radioactive wastes, 564
nursing diagnoses, studies, 565–67
radiation hazards, 563–64
as radioactive elements, 559
tests for elderly clients, 564
tests for infants and children, 564
as therapeutic agents, 559–60
types used in diagnostic testing, 562–63
urine disposing, guidelines, 566–67
RAI uptake study, 576–77
nursing implications, 577
reference values, 576
Rapid tests, 11
Ratio of total cholesterol to HDL, 220
RBC antibody screen, 341
Reagent strips for urinalysis, 60
Reagin, 354
Recombinant immunoblot assay (RIBA), 347, 348
Red blood cell distribution width (RDW), 35–36
Red blood cells (RBCs) count. *See also* Erythrocyte indices
decreased RBC (*See* Anemia)
increased RBC (*See* Erythrocytosis; Polycythemia vera)
measurements of, 23
nursing diagnosis related to elevated, 26
preparation of client and collection of sample, 25
Red blood cell survival, 577
Refractometer, 65
Renal arteriogram, 528
Renal biopsy, 644–45
Renal function tests, 82–99
beta-2-microglobulin, 91
BUN test, 83
BUN-to-creatinine ratio, 84
creatinine clearance test, 90–91
creatinine levels in serum, 88–90
Cystatin C, 91
GFR, estimation, 91
osmolality, serum andurine, 92–95
uric acid, 96–99
urinary urea, 88
Renin, 393–94
Renograms, 525
Reptilase, 323
Respiratory syncytial virus (RSV), rapid test for, 432

Reticulocyte count, 23
  decreased, 43
  increased, 43
  preparation of client and collection
    of sample, 42
Rh antibody titer test, 340
Rheumatoid factor (RF), 367–68
Rh factor, 339–40
  in blood transfusions, 339
  nursing diagnoses, 340
  in pregnancy, 339–40
Rotavirus, clinical significance,
    441–42
Rouleaux formation, 44
Rubella, 357–58
Rubin's test, 684, Table 28.1

S

Salicylates, 462–63
Saliva-based drug tests, 468
Saliva ferning tests to detect ovulation
    (home tests), 685
Salivary cortisol
  decreased, 386–87
  increased, 384–85
  nursing diagnoses related to
    decreased, 387–88
  nursing diagnoses related to
    increased, 385–86
  preparation of patient and
    collection of sample, 384
Scans
  advantages and disadvantages,
    538–39
  full body scans for screening
    purposes, 540
  fusion/hybrid, 539
  picture archiving communication
    system (PACS), 539–40
  types of, 537
Secondary polycythemia, 25
Secure continuous remote alcohol
    monitor (SCRAM),
    465–66
Semen analysis, 685–86
Sentinel node scans, 569
Serologic testing, 332–68
  agglutinations and titer
    levels, 334
  enzyme immunoassay (EIA), 334
  enzyme-linked immunosorbent
    assay (ELISA), 334
  for *Helicobacter pylori*, 361
  for hepatitis, 343
  immunoglobulins G and M, 335
  immunohematology, 335–42
  immunologic tests, 364–68
  Lyme disease, 360–61
  microbiologic, 342–64
  radioimmunoassay (RIA), 334
  syphilis, 354–55
  techniques, 333–35
Serum glutamic-oxaloacetic trans-
    aminase (SGOT), 281–82.
    See also Aspartate amino-
    tranferase (AST)

Serum glutamic-pyruvic transami-
    nase (SGPT), 279–81. *See
    also* Alanine aminotrans-
    ferase (ALT)
Serum hepatitis, 343
Serum osmolality, 92–93
Serum protein electrophoresis
    (SPEP), 231–32
  preparation of client and collection
    of sample, 231
  reference values, 232
Sickle cell anemia, 481–82
Sigmoidoscopy, 673–75
Sims-Huhner test, 686
Single photon emission computed
    tomography (SPECT),
    554, 559
Sirolimus, 454
Skeletal radiographs. *See* Bone/
    skeletal radiographs
"Slapped cheek," 358–59
SLE. *See* Systemic lupus
    erythematosus (SLE)
Slow progressing type 1/1.5, 202
Small-bowel series, 520–21
SOB. *See* Shortness of breath (SOB)
Sodium
  content of food, 108
  nursing diagnosis related to
    increased BUN, 85
  reference values for serum, 108
  reference values for urine, 114
  serum, 107–13
  urine, 114
Sodium chromate (Cr-51), 562, 577
Somatostatin receptor scintigraphy
    (SRS), 563
  breast scan, 570
Somatotropin. *See* Growth hormone
Somnograms, 611
Specific gravity of urine, 65–68
  decrease in, 67
  increase in, 66
  nursing diagnosis related, 66–67
  reference values, 66
  testing, methods for, 65–66
  vs. urine osmolality test, 93
Spicules, 633
Sputum cultures and acid-fast bacillus
  general indications, 427–28
  nursing diagnoses, 429
  preparation of client and collection
    of sample, 428
  QuantiFERON-TB gold test
    (QFT-G), 429–30
  reference values, 429
  wet mounts of sputum specimens,
    428–29
Stat tests, 10, 11
Stem cell research, 491
Stem cells, 23–24
Stool cultures, 439–40
  nursing diagnoses, 442
  preparation of client and collection
    of sample, 440–42
  reference values, 440

Streptococcal infections, 356–57
Streptozyme test, 356, 357
Stress echocardiograms, 592
Stress tests, 648, 649–54
  assessing exercise tolerance, 652
  description, 649–50
  nuclear cardiology stress tests and
    echocardiography stress
    tests, 652
  posttest nursing implications,
    653–54
  pretest nursing implications,
    652–53
Surfactant to albumin (S/A
    ratio), 693
Syphilis, serologic testing, 354–55
  dark-field examination, 354
  nursing diagnoses, 355
  RPR, 354
  VDRL, 354
Systemic lupus erythematosus
    (SLE), 313
  tests for, 367

T

Tay-Sachs disease, 484
Technetium (Tc-99M), 562–63
Telemetry monitoring, 608–9
Testes, 375
Testosterone and other androgens,
    409–10
Tetany, 165
Thalassemia, 35, 483
Thallium scans, 572–73
Theophylline products, 458–59
Therapeutic life changes
    (TLCs), 210
Thoracentesis (pleural tap), 634–35
Thoracic sonograms, 594
Throat cultures, 430–31
  nursing diagnoses, 431
  preparation of client and collec-
    tion of sample, 430–31
  reference values, 431
Thrombin time, 323
Thrombocytopathy, 45
Thrombocytopenia, 318–20
Thrombocytosis, 317–18
Thrombophilia during pregnancy
    and postpartum,
    inherited, 485
Thyroglobulin test, 405
Thyroid gland, 397
  rapid test for TSH, 398
  screening for thyroid disease
    in asymptomatic
    clients, 398
  tests to diagnose thyroid
    disease, 398
Thyroid peroxidase (TPO), 368
Thyroid scans, 575–76
  I-131 whole-body imaging for
    thyroid tumor
    metastasis, 576
  nursing implications, 576
Thyroid sonograms, 594–95

Thyroid-stimulating hormone (TSH), 399, 475
  increased or decreased, 399
  preparation of client and collection of sample, 399
Thyroxin-binding pre-albumin. *See* Pre-albumin
Tilt table testing, 661
Tissue plasmin activating factor (TPA), 300
Tocainide, 462
Tomograms, 508
Tomography, 537
Total bilirubin, 259–60
  preparation of client and collection of sample, 259
Toxicology screens in blood and urine, 466–67
  chain-of-custody protocol, 467
  nursing diagnosis, 467
  preparation of client and collection of sample, 467
Toxoplasmosis (TPM), 359–60
Transcutaneous bilirubinometer, 269–70
Transesophageal echocardiogram (TEE), 592–93
  new window on heart, 592
  posttest nursing implications, 593
  pretest nursing implications, 593
Transferrin saturation, 39
Transhepatic cholangiography, 524
Transient aplastic crisis (TAC), 359
Transrectal ultrasound scanning, 591
Transthoracic echocardiogram (TTE), 591–92
  color flow Doppler, 593
  posttest nursing implications, 592
  pretest nursing implications, 592
  for valvular defects, 591
Transvaginal ultrasound scanning, 588–89
  digital rectal examination (DRE), 591
  posttest nursing implications, 589
  preparation of client, 589, Table 23.2
  pretest nursing implications, 589
  prostate-specific antigen (PSA) test, 591
  vaginal ultrasonography, 588
Treponema pallidum particle agglutination (TTPA), 355
  preparation of client and collection of sample, 353, 355
Trichomonas, 437
  rapid tests for, 436
Tricyclic antidepressants, 457–58
  nursing diagnosis, 458
  reference values, 458
Triglycerides, serum, 217–19
  decreased, 219
  increased, 218
  nursing diagnoses, 218–19

preparation of client and collection of sample, 217
  reference values, 217
Triiodothyronine serum concentration (T_3), 400
  decreased, 403
  increased, 401
  nursing diagnoses related to decreased, 403–5
  nursing diagnoses related to increased, 402–3
  preparation of client and collection of sample, 401
Troponin as cardiac markers, 286–87
T-tube cholangiography, 523–24
Tubal patency tests, 684, Table 28.1
Tuberculin skin test (TST), 429
Tuberculosis, rapid test for, 430
Tubes for venous sample collection
  color code, 8–9
  order of, 9
Tumor markers, 245–46, 252
Type 1 diabetes, 182
Type 2 diabetes, 182
  in adults, 182
  in children, 183
Type 1.5 in adults, 183

U

Ultrasound principles
  commercial mobile units for adult screening, 584
  cost *vs.* benefits of routine screening, 584
  description, 581–82
  fetal portraits with moving 3-D/4-D images, 584
  innovations, 582–83
  peripheral inserted intravenous catheters (PICC), 596
  pulse-echo method, 581, 582
  real-time imaging, 582
  risks, 583
  ultrasound as therapy, 581
  volumetric 3-D/4-D scans, 583
Unconjugated (indirect) bilirubin (BU), 257, 261–62
  increased levels, 261
Unfractionated heparin (UFH), 314
United Kingdom Prospective Diabetes Study (UKPDS), 195
Universal donor, 336–37
Universal recipient, 337
University of California, San Francisco (UCSF), 655
Upper GI endoscopy
  posttest nursing implications, 671
  pretest nursing implications, 671
Upper GI series, 520–21
  client preparation, 521
  posttest nursing implications, 521
Urea breath test for *Helicobacter pylori*, 618
Urechrome, 62
Uremic frost, 85
Ureteroscopy, 676–77

Uric acid, 96–99
  decreased, 99
  increased, 96–97
  nursing diagnoses related to increased, 97–98
  reference values, 96
Urinalysis and other urine tests
  collection of 24-hour urine specimens, 77–79
  collection of urine specimens, 61–62
  color of urine, 62
  culture and sensitivity, 61–62
  delta-aminolevulinic acid (Δ-ALA), 76
  as drug screen, EPO, 44
  examination of urine sediment, 74
  glucose in urine, 70–71
  ketones in urine, 71–72
  leukocyte esterase, 73–74
  nitrites, 72–73
  odor of urine, 62–63
  pH of urine, 63–65
  protein in urine, 68–70
  reagent strips for, 60
  reference values, 61
  specific gravity of urine, 65–68
  urinary 5-hydroxyindoleacetic acid for serotonin, 76–77
  urinary porphyrins, 74–76
Urinary amylase, 293
Urinary calcium, 166–67
  preparation of client and collection of sample, 166
  reference values, 166
Urinary cortisol levels, 390
Urinary 5-hydroxyindoleacetic acid for serotonin, 76–77
Urinary measurement of the adrenal cortex steroids, 390
Urinary phosphorus/phosphates, 171–72
Urinary urea nitrogen, 88
Urine collection, 10
Urine cultures
  general indications, 423
  nursing diagnosis, 425
  preparation of client and collection of sample, 423–24
  reference values, 424
Urine osmolality, 92–93
  decreased, 95
  increased, 93–94
  nursing diagnoses related to decreased, 95
  nursing diagnoses related to increased, 94
  reference values, 93
  vs. specific gravity test, advantages over, 93
Urine pregnancy tests
  biologic tests, 475
  home pregnancy tests (HPT), 475–76
  immunologic tests, 475
  preparation of client and collection of sample, 476

Urine test, 489
Urine urobilinogen, 264–65
Urinometer, 65
Urobilinogens, 258
  fecal, 265
  urine, 264–65

V
Vaginal and urethral smears
  cultures in children, 434–35
  preparation of client and collection of sample, 435
  reference values, 435
  use of NAA for gonorrhea and Chlamydia, 435–36
Vaginal infections, 640
Vaginal secretions, testing pH of, 64
Vaginal self-test for pH changes detection
  clinical significance of positive smears or cultures, 436–38
  nursing diagnoses, 438
  vaginal and rectal cultures to prevent transmission of neonatal group B streptococci disease, 439
Valproic acid, 455–56
Vancomycin, 453–54
Vancomycin-resistant enterococcus (VRE)
  clinical significance in stool cultures, 441
Van den Bergh reaction, 258

Vanillylmandelic acid (VMA), 394
Varicella-zoster antibody titer, 362–63
Venereal Disease Research Laboratory (VDRL), 354
  syphilis, 354
Venous samples, collection and transportation, 8–9
  color code for, 8–9
  precaution, 8–9
Very low density lipoproteins (VLDL), 219
Viral capsid antigen (VCA), 356
Viral load tests, 352–53
Viruses, cultures for, 417
Vital capacity (VC), 613
Vitamin B$_{12}$ deficiency, nursing diagnosis related to, 38
Vitamin D and calcium, 397
Vitamin D levels, 167–68
Vitamin K, for elevated INR, 304
Von Willebrand disease (vWD), screening for, 315–16

W
Warfarin
  genetic tests to determine dosage, 304–5
  on prothrombin time, 301, 304
Western blot HIV test, 350
West Nile virus (WNV) test, 353–54
White blood cell count and differential

changes in basophil count, 52
decreased eosinophil count, 51–52
decreased lymphocyte count, 53
decreased neutrophil count and agranulocytosis, 49–50
defined, 23
increased eosinophil count, 51
increased lymphocyte count, 52
increase in neutrophils and bands, 48–49
nursing diagnoses related to decreased neutrophils, 50–51
nursing diagnoses related to increased neutrophils, 49
Wound cultures, 432–33
  general indications, 432–33
  nursing diagnosis, 433
  preparation of client and collection of sample, 433
  reference values, 433

X
X-rays, 507
  nursing implications, 514, Table 20.2
  teaching clients, 509–10

Y
Yalow, Rosalyn, 14
Yeast infection, 437